HANDBOOK OF NEUROPSYCHOLOGY, 2nd Edition

Series Editors

FRANÇOIS BOLLER
INSERM, Unité 324, Centre Paul Broca, 75014 Paris, France

and

JORDAN GRAFMAN
National Institute of Neurological Disorders and Stroke, National Institutes of Health, Bethesda, MD 20892, USA

Volume 8, Part II

CHILD NEUROPSYCHOLOGY, PART II

Editors

SID J. SEGALOWITZ
Department of Psychology, Brock University, 500 Glenridge Avenue, St. Catharines, ON L2S 3A1, Canada

and

ISABELLE RAPIN
Department of Neurology, Albert Einstein College of Medicine, K 807, Bronx, NY 10461, USA

ELSEVIER

Amsterdam – Boston – London – New York – Oxford – Paris
San Diego – San Francisco – Singapore – Sydney – Tokyo

2003

ELSEVIER SCIENCE B.V.
Sara Burgerhartstraat 25
P.O. Box 211, 1000 AE Amsterdam, The Netherlands

First edition 1993
Second edition, first printing 2003

Library of Congress Cataloging in Publication Data
A catalog record from the Library of Congress has been applied for.

British Library Cataloguing in Publication Data
A catalogue record from the British Library has been applied for.

ISBN series 0 444 50376 5 (HB)
ISBN series 0 444 50377 3 (PB)
ISBN this edition (hardbound) 0 444 50955 0
ISBN this edition (paperback) 0 444 50956 9

∞ The paper used in this publication meets the requirements of ANSI/NISO Z39.48-1992 (Permanence of Paper).
Printed in The Netherlands

HANDBOOK OF NEUROPSYCHOLOGY, 2nd Edition

VOLUME 8, PART II

CHILD NEUROPSYCHOLOGY

Preface

We are pleased to present the eighth volume of the second edition of the Handbook of Neuropsychology. As already demonstrated by the first edition and by the first seven volumes of the second edition of the Handbook, neuropsychology is a field of science that has undergone extraordinary growth and changes in recent years. Planning for the first edition of the Handbook started over sixteen years ago and even though the more recent volumes of the first edition were designed to reflect some of the changes that have taken place in the field of neuropsychology, we have decided, with the encouragement of the Publisher, that it would be worthwhile to prepare a new edition. As the series co-editors, we intend to ensure that the new edition of the Handbook of Neuropsychology remains the principal reference source in the field, continuing to provide comprehensive and current coverage of both experimental and clinical aspects of neuropsychology. To this end, we have asked the authoritative chapter authors to produce new in-depth reviews that go beyond a summary of their results and point of view. Each chapter is up-to-date, covering the latest developments in methodology and theory. Discussion of 'bedside' evaluations, laboratory techniques, as well as extensive discussions of theoretical models are all to be found in the Handbook. The Handbook also presents the latest findings and methodologies of functional neuroimaging techniques such as PET, fMRI, and transcranial magnetic stimulation (TMS).

We are confident that the Handbook will continue to be an essential reference source for clinicians such as neuropsychologists, neurologists, psychiatrists, and psychologists, as well as for all scientists engaged in research in the cognitive neurosciences. This second all-new edition is designed to update chapters covering research domains where considerable developments have occurred. In addition, there has been an in-depth reorganization of content areas that have spawned new approaches since the first edition. All the chapters included in this new edition will provide the most recent data and references for further studies and research.

The first volume included an Introduction section that focused on practical and theoretical issues of general interest. Two chapters covered, in a novel and comprehensive fashion, clinical evaluation and neuropsychological assessment, with an emphasis not so much on the description of tests, but on their rationale. One of the features of Neuropsychology in recent years has been the spectacular comeback of single case studies and that is why the chapter on statistical approaches compared statistical procedures appropriate for groups to those of single cases. Hemispheric specialization remains an important topic, which was examined in the introduction under two different points of view. One chapter summarized the contribution to neuropsychology provided by the commissurotomy ('split brain') model, while another chapter reviewed experimental assessments of hemispheric specialization in normal individuals. An introduction to current neuroimaging techniques used language disorders as an illustration.

Neurophysiological techniques were reviewed with an emphasis on evoked potentials (ERPs). Several chapters dealt with the application of theoretical models to neuropsychology including a discussion of the lesion method and of computer modeling.

In the first volume, the Introduction was followed by the Section on Attention edited by Giacomo Rizzolatti. It included four chapters. Two of them concerned selective attention.

The first was essentially devoted to visuospatial attentional phenomena, while the focus of the second was on the temporal aspects of attention. The phenomenon of failure to orient, neglect and neglect related phenomena was dealt with in the third chapter. This chapter included a large section devoted to the anatomical localization of lesions producing neglect in humans. Finally, the last chapter reviewed the anatomy and the neurophysiological properties of the circuits whose lesion produces neglect deficits in primates. In that chapter, the various theories of neglect were reviewed and their validity discussed from a neurophysiological perspective.

The second volume of the Handbook was a special 'in memoriam' volume. It was dedicated to the memory of Laird Cermak who, despite his grave illness, vigorously and resolutely took on the task of preparing a new section on memory and its disorders. The volume included chapters on animal models and neuropsychological assessment. Memory was discussed from the anatomical and clinical viewpoints, and memory disorders resulting from specific diseases such as herpes simplex encephalitis and Alzheimer's disease were considered in detail. The section further provided a cognitive neuropsychological analysis of various forms of memory, including explicit memory, remote memory and semantic memory. Chapters on confabulation and on functional amnesia were also included. We were all deeply saddened by the news of Laird's untimely death. We are very much indebted to Mieke Verfaellie for supervising the final stages of the preparation of this volume for the revised handbook.

The third volume, edited by Rita Sloan Berndt, covered traditional approaches to, as well as new techniques for, investigating language disorders by leading researchers in the field of language and aphasia research. The volume is divided into four parts. The first part, entitled the study of aphasia, includes a chapter on historical developments, a discussion of the relationship between neuroanatomy and language, one on sign language, one on cross-lingual studies and a review of aphasia in bilinguals and polyglots. The second section ('understanding the symptoms of aphasia') discussed and analyzed the symptoms of aphasia and related disorders including reading and writing. The next section went further into related disorders with chapters that discuss the relationship between language and memory and attention as well as disorders of skilled movements, of body representation and of number processing. The volume concluded with a review of emerging methods for the study of language and aphasia including neuroimaging, ERP, TMS and studies of 'split brain' subjects.

Volume 4, edited by Marlene Behrmann, covered disorders of visual behavior. The volume began with a chapter reviewing the neurophysiology of spatial vision with special emphasis on single unit recordings in non-human primates. The next three chapters reviewed the recent work on recognition deficits for faces (prosopagnosia), objects (visual object agnosia) and words (peripheral dyslexias). Disorders of spatial representation, of color processing and of mental imagery, were presented next including a detailed discussion of the neuropsychological behavior as well as the underlying neural substrate of these disorders. Additional chapters dealt with Balint's syndrome, with blindsight and with visuospatial or constructional disorders. Finally, the relationship between eye movements and brain damage has been described in detail.

The fifth volume, edited by Guido Gainotti, covered emotional behavior and its disorders. It included introductory chapters dealing with basic theoretical and anatomical issues in the neuropsychological study of emotions. A central part of this volume addressed the problem of hemispheric asymmetries in emotional representation and a final group of chapters examined the neural mechanisms of the stress response and reviewed the main emotional disorders. In the introductory chapters, an effort was made to present both neurobiologically oriented and cognitively oriented theories of emotion. Both the detailed anatomo-clinical and theoretical aspects of the anatomical substrates of emotions were covered in depth. In the central part of the volume, the claims for right hemisphere dominance for emotions and emotional communication were contrasted with those assuming a different hemispheric specialization for positive versus negative emotions and with models assuming asymmetric cortico-limbic control of human emotion. Finally, in the last chapters of the volume, individual differences in the hemispheric control of the stress response were discussed and the neural mechanisms of affective/emotional disturbances were approached with neuropsychological methods and with functional neuroimaging techniques.

The sixth volume of the Handbook, edited by François Boller and Stefano Cappa, was devoted to topics related to Aging and Dementia. The volume began with two chapters dealing with age-related cognitive and neurobiological alterations in animals, including a detailed review of data obtained with transgenic and knockout mouse technology. The next chapter reviewed the cognitive changes associated with normal aging. The gamut of symptoms that occur in Alzheimer's disease (AD) were then described and analyzed. They include effects on attention, language, memory, non-verbal functions with emphasis on spatial abilities, olfaction and the motor system. The discussion of dementia syndromes was presented in two sections. The first concerned AD, discussed from the points of view of epidemiology, neuropathology and neurochemistry, concluding with a review of current and future treatments. The other section dealt with non-AD dementias including fronto-temporal and Lewy body dementias and specific conditions such as Parkinson's and Huntington's disease, as well as HIV infection. The volume included a review of brain imaging and cerebral metabolism findings in aging and dementia. The final chapters reviewed the relations between culture and dementia and the special syndrome of severe dementia.

Volume 7 comprises a completely revamped section on the Frontal Lobes edited by Jordan Grafman. A chapter on the neural architecture/anatomy of the prefrontal cortex leads off this volume. Animal research has contributed greatly to our understanding of the special capability of the frontal lobes to respond to a variety of input from 'lower order' sensory and posterior association cortex and this and other observations are reported in this volume. Functions dependent on the frontal lobes emerge late in ontogeny and appear to decline early in normal aging. These findings are reviewed and their implications for neuropsychology discussed. Over the last 15 years, the functioning of the frontal lobes has become associated with the term working memory. In this volume the concept of working memory is discussed in relationship to both functional neuroimaging and patient studies. Gross distinctions in the functioning of the prefrontal cortex have divided it topographically into dorsolateral and ventromedial sectors. This volume offers chapters highlighting the role of each sector from both neuroimaging and lesion perspectives. Many of the views of the prefrontal cortex characterize it as involved in 'processing'. A chapter in this volume takes a slightly different perspective and attempts to characterize the nature of knowledge representation within the frontal lobes. Many theories of the frontal lobes suggest that they are concerned with maintaining information across time. A chapter reviews the role of the frontal lobes in temporal processing. Since the frontal lobes are affected by many neuropsychiatric disorders, a chapter in this volume places their dysfunction in the context of the parallel fronto-subcortical networks and suggests that each network, when damaged, contributes specific symptoms to the patient's clinical presentation. Finally, computational modeling has taken center-stage in cognitive neuroscience and its usefulness in testing different theoretical stances about the role of the frontal lobes in information processing is presented in a concluding chapter.

The Child Neuropsychology Section consists of Volume 8, Parts I and II, edited by Sid Segalowitz and Isabelle Rapin. They rest on the fact that the impact of acquired and degenerative disorders in childhood is strongly colored by the immaturity of the brain, so that what is said in other volumes of the Handbook rarely applies directly to children. The first part considers theoretical perspectives in bridging developmental neuroscience with child psychology, with the role of neuroscience furthering our understanding of the child's mental development, and a separate chapter outlines the importance of plasticity in this growth. Chapters also cover methodological issues arising from epidemiological perspectives and from psychometric concepts and issues. Methods for measuring biological brain function and structure and their particular application to child neuropsychological disorders are covered next, including ERP, PET, SPECT, MRI and fMRI technologies. Included here is a chapter devoted to childhood seizure disorders. Next follow separate chapters on neuropsychological assessment in infancy, in the preschool child, and in school-aged children. Following this are presentations on the development of motor control, including handedness, and somatosensory perception. The second part begins with chapters on visual development and on development in visually impaired children, followed by chapters on cognitive development in deaf children and on central auditory functions and their evaluation. This is followed by chapters on early language development and its neural correlates, developmental language disorders, and on acquired aphasia in childhood. Two chapters on dyslexia and another on dyscalculia follow. Next are presented a chapter on disorders of memory with a special focus on temporal lobe disease and autism, one on attention disorders, and one on executive functions in normal and abnormal development. Following this are chapters on the development of emotional regulation and on mechanisms and influences on addiction in children and adolescents. Final chapters include one on eating disorders, and another focussing on autism spectrum disorders.

The final volume on Rehabilitation, edited by Jordan Grafman and Ian Robertson, contains topics not specifically covered in the previous edition of the Handbook. In particular, we were so impressed by the advances and current direction of studies on neuroplasticity and rehabilitation that we thought the time was right to include these topics in the new edition of the Handbook of Neuropsychology. Neuroplasticity is among the most exciting areas of research in cognitive neuroscience. In this volume, there are chapters on animal models of neuroplasticity, cortical map changes with practice and following brain damage, cross-modal reassignment of function, auditory system reassignment following learning and brain damage, the effects of amputation on phantom limb and pain perceptions, the effects of age on plasticity, the ability of the non-damaged hemisphere to take over functions of the damaged hemisphere, and the effects of cognitive skill learning on neural organization and function. A section describing how basic science findings can be translated into practical rehabilitation of patients follows. Rehabilitation programs for neglect, language, executive functions, and motor skills are described. The use of functional neuroimaging to provide a neural window on cognitive plasticity is discussed. The last section of the Handbook has traditionally been reserved for a discussion of the state-of-the-art of new technologies. Here we provide updates on MRI, fMRI, PET, transcranial magnetic stimulation, and other technologies that have burst upon the cognitive neuroscience scene in the last ten years.

As can be seen, there are important changes between the first edition and the present one in terms of organization and content. Other changes include timing, presentation and availability. The eleven volumes of the first edition appeared over a span of ten years because in most cases, volumes were written and edited consecutively.

In the second edition, several volumes have been concurrently planned and we estimate that the entire series will appear over a span of approximately two years. The first edition consisted of hardbound volumes that were followed by paperback volumes after an interval ranging from two to three years. In the current edition, the paperback edition appears at the same time as the hardbound one and its price will make it more easily available to students and fellows.

Besides the printed second edition of the Handbook of Neuropsychology that you have in your hands, there are already plans for a web-based version. This will make it easier to adapt the Handbook to changes that will undoubtedly occur in the near future. For example, neuroimaging techniques are rapidly developing, opening new in-roads into the mapping of brain and behavior relationships. The rising interest in the aging population is also very likely to increase even further, as new advances will occur concerning the early detection of cognitive impairment and the maintenance of cognitive functions into old age. The same advances will undoubtedly also occur for the developing brain.

Many people have contributed to the successful preparation of the Handbook. We again wish to emphasize our appreciation for the commitment of the Volume Editors who have spent long hours in the planning stage and in the actual compiling of the various sections. Throughout the development and production of the Series, the editorial staff of Neurology and Neuroscience of Elsevier Science B.V. in Amsterdam has provided invaluable assistance.

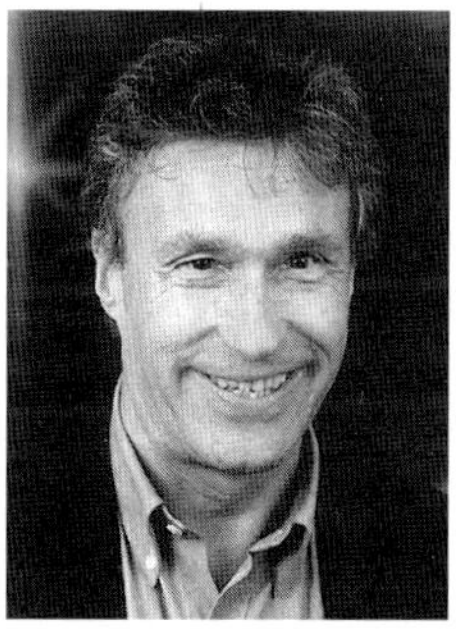

François Boller

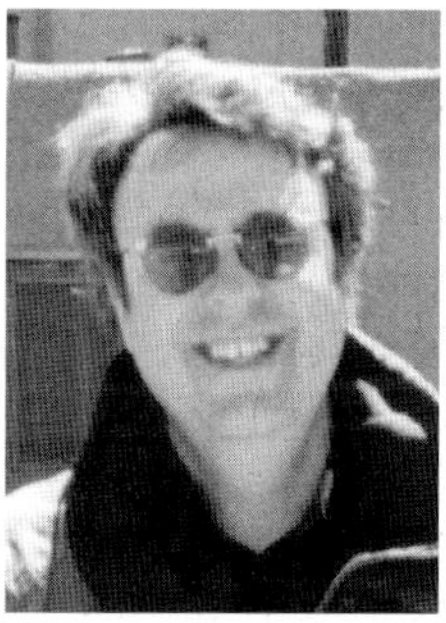

Jordan Grafman

List of Contributors

Allen, D.A. [†]	Division of Child Psychiatry, Albert Einstein College of Medicine, Bronx, NY 10461, USA
Barron, R.W.	Department of Psychology, University of Guelph, Guelph, ON N1G 2W1, Canada
Bates, E.	Center for Research in Language, University of California, San Diego, 9500 Gilman Drive, La Jolla, CA 92093-0526, USA
Bennetto, L.	Clinical and Social Sciences in Psychology, Meliora Hall, University of Rochester, Rochester, NY 14627, USA
Berlin, C.I.	Department of Otorhinolaryngology and Biocommunication, Kresge Hearing Research Laboratory of the South, Louisiana State University Health Sciences Center, 533 Bolivar Street, New Orleans, LA 70112, USA
Clancy, B.	Department of Psychology, 248 Uris Hall, Cornell University, Ithaca, NY 14853, USA
Constable, R.T.	Department of Diagnostic Radiology, Yale University School of Medicine, New Haven, CT 06510, USA
DeLong, G.R.	Department of Pediatrics (Neurology), Duke University Medical Center, Durham, NC 27710, USA
Dunn, M.	Saul R. Korey Department of Neurology, Rose F. Kennedy Center, Room 808, Albert Einstein College of Medicine, 1410 Pelham Parkway South, Bronx, NY 10461, USA
Erickson, K.	Mood and Anxiety Disorders Program, NIMH, Bethesda, MD 20892, USA
Finlay, B.	Department of Psychology, 248 Uris Hall, Cornell University, Ithaca, NY 14853, USA
Fletcher, J.M.	Department of Pediatrics, University of Texas Medical School, Houston, TX, USA
Fulbright, R.K.	Department of Diagnostic Radiology, Yale University School of Medicine, New Haven, CT 06510, USA
Gilmore, R.O.	Department of Psychology, Pennsylvania State University, University Park, PA 16802, USA

[†] Deceased

Gore, J.C. Departments of Diagnostic Radiology and Applied Physics, Yale University School of Medicine, New Haven, CT 06510, USA

Habib, K. Clinical Neuroendocrinology Branch, NIMH, Bethesda, MD 20892, USA

Hatton, D.D. Frank Porter Graham Child Development Center, University of North Carolina, Chapel Hill, NC, USA

Hood, L.J. Department of Otorhinolaryngology and Biocommunication, Kresge Hearing Research Laboratory of the South, Louisiana State University Health Sciences Center, 533 Bolivar Street, New Orleans, LA 70112, USA

Lovett, M.W. Brain and Behaviour Research Program, The Hospital for Sick Children, University of Toronto, 555 University Avenue, Toronto, ON M5G 1X8, USA

Lyon, G.R. Child Behavior and Learning Branch, National Institute of Child Health and Development, National Institutes of Health, Bethesda, MD 20892, USA

Mayberry, R.I. School of Communication Sciences and Disorders, McGill University, 1266 Pine Avenue West, Montreal, PQ H3G 1A8, Canada

Mencl, W.E. Department of Pediatrics, and Haskins Laboratories, Yale University School of Medicine, P.O. Box 3333, New Haven, CT 06510-8064, USA

Meyer, J.A. Department of Psychology, Lousiana State University, 2356 Drusilla Lane, Baton Rouge, LA 70809, USA

Minshew, N.J. Department of Psychiatry and Neurology, University of Pittsburgh School of Medicine, 3811 O'Hara Street, Suite 430, Bellefield Towers, Pittsburgh, PA 15213, USA

Pennington, B.F. Department of Psychology, Frontier Hall, University of Denver, Denver, CO 80208, USA

Pugh, K.R. Department of Pediatrics, and Haskins Laboratories, Yale University School of Medicine, P.O. Box 3333, New Haven, CT 06510-8064, USA

Rapin, I. Saul R. Korey Department of Neurology, and Department of Pediatrics, Rose F. Kennedy Center for Research in Mental Retardation and Human Development, Albert Einstein College of Medicine, 1410 Pelham Parkway South, Bronx, NY 10461, USA

Santesso, D.L. Department of Psychology, McMaster University, Hamilton, ON L8S 4K1, Canada

Schmidt, L.A. Department of Psychology, McMaster University, Hamilton, ON L8S 4K1, Canada

Schulkin, J.	Department of Physiology and Biophysics, Georgetown University, School of Medicine, Washington, DC 20007, USA
Shalev, R.S.	Neuropediatric Unit, Shaare Zedek Medical Center, P.O. Box 3235, Jerusalem 91031, Israel
Shaywitz, B.A.	Departments of Pediatrics and Neurology, Yale University School of Medicine, P.O. Box 3333, New Haven, CT 06510-8064, USA
Shaywitz, S.E.	Department of Pediatrics, Yale University School of Medicine, P.O. Box 3333, New Haven, CT 06510-8064, USA
Skudlarski, P.	Department of Diagnostic Radiology, Yale University School of Medicine, New Haven, CT 06510, USA
Tannock, R.	Brain and Behaviour Research Program, The Hospital for Sick Children, University of Toronto, 555 University Avenue, Toronto, ON M5G 1X8, USA
Thal, D.	Center for Research in Language, University of California, San Diego, 9500 Gilman Drive, La Jolla, CA 92093-0526, USA
Van Hout, A.	Service de Neurologie Pédiatrique, Université Catholique de Louvain, Cliniques Universitaires Saint Luc, 10 Avenue Hippocrate, 1200 Brussels, Belgium
Waldstein, S.R.	Department of Psychology, University of Maryland, Baltimore County, and Division of Gerontology, Department of Medicine, University of Maryland School of Medicine, and Geriatrics Research Education and Clinical Center, Baltimore, MD, USA
Walker, A.	Department of Psychiatry, Division of Child and Adolescent Psychiatry, Albert Einstein College of Medicine/Montefiore Medical Center, 3317 Rochambeau Avenue, Bronx, NY 10467, USA
Warren, D.H.	Department of Psychology, University of California, Riverside, CA 92521, USA

Contents

Handbook of Neuropsychology, 2nd Edition, Vol. 8, Part II
S.J. Segalowitz and I. Rapin (Eds)

CHAPTER 17

Toward a neuropsychology of visual development

Rick O. Gilmore *

Department of Psychology, Penn State University, University Park, PA 16802, USA

> One cannot guess how great the changes of growth would be; but it is conceivable, that if one knew where to look for the evidence, one would find marked differences of identity in the perceptions of child and adult.
>
> *Hebb, 1949*

Introduction

Many consider Donald Hebb the father of modern neuropsychology. He is perhaps best known today for proposing a simple, but powerful principle to describe the process of learning and synaptic change at the level of single neurons. However, as the quotation indicates, Hebb believed that these ideas have potentially profound implications for understanding not just learning in mature systems, but also the origins of adaptive behavior early in development. Of course, many have shared Hebb's view that perception might differ profoundly in infants from older children or adults. Indeed, it is safe to say that a driving factor in infant perceptual research has been an effort to determine just how infant perception differs from the mature state. Hebb's neuropsychology text is now more than fifty years old, and so in the context of this volume, it seems fitting to consider how well Hebb's conjecture fits with our current understanding of the developing human visual system.

Vision holds a commanding position among the primate senses, and visual information processing engages a dominant share of the primate brain (Van Essen, Anderson and Felleman, 1992). In the fifty years since the publication of Hebb's text, there has been enormous progress in understanding the behavioral, biological, and computational (Marr, 1982) bases of visual perception and cognition (Palmer, 1999). If the goal of a neuropsychology of vision is to understand the neural bases of visual perception and cognition, then the goals of a neuropsychology of visual development ought to be to describe what and how well young children see, how their vision changes, and how changes in vision are related to development in the nervous system. We are nowhere near achieving this ambitious goal, but in the past several decades we have made significant progress. Indeed, what was before mostly speculation about young children's capacities to see has moved into the realm of rough description, and in some domains, even to suggestions about mechanism. In the spirit of celebrating that progress, this chapter summarizes some of what we currently know about these questions in the first year of life. A number of other more detailed treatments of these topics can be found in the literature (Atkinson, 2000; Kellman and Arterberry, 1998; Simons, 1993; Vital-Durand, Atkinson and Braddick, 1996).

The first section discusses some of the biological milestones in nervous system development in general, and some of their implications for the study of vision in particular. The second section summarizes what is known about the functional development of visual systems from the retina to extrastriate cortical processing. The third section describes behavioral evidence regarding developments in visual

* Corresponding author. Tel.: +1-814-865-3664;
E-mail: rogilmore@psu.edu

processing in the first year. The general conclusion arising from this evidence is that Hebb was essentially correct in suggesting that visual perception is profoundly simpler in young infants than in older children or adults. Nevertheless, several lines of evidence support the argument that while early vision is simpler, it is adaptive for the specific niche that infants occupy. The chapter concludes with a discussion about what questions remain and what promise for answering them the future holds.

The functional development of visual circuitry

Describing the anatomical and physiological characteristics of the mature human visual system poses considerable challenges by itself. Notable progress has been made in the last 40 years in associating visual functions in adults with the processing of specific neural circuits, but many unanswered questions remain. Clearly, the challenge of understanding the neural bases of visual processing is magnified when one considers how the visual system's complexity emerges in development. In this section, we review what is known about the anatomical and physiological development of visual circuitry, and what factors influence the mature functional state.

Milestones of nervous system development

The basic phases of visual system development are identical to those that govern maturation in other parts of the nervous system. Table 1 depicts the principal events in neural development. These phases are described in a sequential fashion, but there is considerable overlap in the timing of the phases and considerable variability in their duration from region to region. The reader may wish to consult one of several excellent treatments on nervous system development for additional detail (Daw, 1995; Rakic, 1992). Here, the major milestones of nervous system development can be briefly summarized. The vast majority of neurons are generated during a limited period early in the embryonic period. Cells migrate to their proper position in the target structure with which they are associated. There, the cells differentiate into neurons of various types or die spontaneously. Surviving cells extend both axonal and dendritic processes. Their axons migrate to projection sites, and once they have reached their target locations, begin to form synapses. Some synapses are stabilized and strengthened, others diminish in strength and disappear. Finally, the axons and dendrites of neurons that have formed functional circuits are coated with an insulating myelin sheath.

For the scientist whose primary interest is in understanding the origins of visual function, the specific details of these processes may seem like distracting detail. However, knowledge about nervous system development can be quite important for understanding the sequence of visual development. To the extent that aspects of visual processing can be associated with specific visual circuits, understanding that different components of the visual system achieve these milestones at different times and at different rates can provide fundamental constraints about the pattern of visual development. Furthermore, knowledge about the onset and timing of nervous system development can help to answer questions about the relative influence of different causal factors. For example, neurogenesis, migration, and

TABLE 1

Major events in human brain development and their relative timing

Event	Relative timing	Comments
Neurogenesis	Prenatal	Limited postnatal neurogenesis may occur
Migration	Prenatal	Inside out pattern in cortex
Differentiation	Prenatal	Includes determination of neurotransmitter type
Axon sprouting and migration	Prenatal	Deeper layers before shallower ones
Dendritic arborization	Pre/postnatal	Deeper layers before shallower ones
Neuronal death	Prenatal	Considerable in cortex of non-human species; controversial in humans
Synapse formation	Pre/postnatal	Largely postnatal in human cerebral cortex
Synapse loss	Pre/postnatal	Largely postnatal in human cerebral cortex
Myelination	Pre/postnatal	Largely postnatal in human cerebral cortex

differentiation begin and end in most areas of the visual system well before the onset of physiological function in the participating neurons. These events, therefore are almost certainly regulated by intrinsic control factors, such as gene expression, since the neurons are not yet active. On the other hand, the most intensive period of synapse formation and loss in the cerebral cortex occurs postnatally and over an extended timecourse, suggesting that neural activity driven by visual information may play, at least in principle, an important role in shaping the set of synapses that are strengthened and stabilized.

Indeed, one of the insights that has come from detailed studies of visual development has been the recognition that some characteristics of the basic neural architecture may be dependent on physiological activity, but not necessarily on visual experience. Conventionally, many have tended to believe that all relevant neuronal activity stems, at least indirectly, from external sources in the environment. However, recent studies of development in the retina and thalamus (Shatz, 1996) have shown that the spontaneous activity of ganglion cells in the retina is crucial for normal development in the thalamus. These spontaneous patterns of activity occur prior to birth and to functional activity in the photoreceptors. Therefore these patterns are independent of light stimulation, but cause important activity-dependent effects. In addition to the determination of whether certain aspects of the structure of the visual system are dependent on activity-based processes, a consideration of the specifics of the development of visual circuitry forces one to ask other questions, such as: To what extent does the development of 'input' structures lag or lead the development of target systems? What is the timing of development in circuits that provide modulatory or feedback projections? Ultimately, a detailed understanding of the neural basis of visual processing will demand answers to these sorts of questions for every component of the visual system. At present, however, we know far more about functional development of the earliest stages of visual processing than we do about higher level processing systems. We now turn to that evidence. The interested reader is encouraged to consult more detailed accounts (Daw, 1995; Rakic, 1992) for additional information.

Development of the eye and retina

Based on studies of the macaque monkey whose visual system is quite similar to the human, cells that comprise the retina appear to be generated during an extended period in embryonic development that begins in the first half of gestation, before the onset of neurogenesis in the lateral geniculate nucleus (LGN) or in cortex. Neurogenesis in the retina also extends beyond the end of neurogenesis in these other structures (Rakic, 1992). There is a gradient in the onset of neurogenesis such that neurons are generated centrally, near the fovea, early on and peripheral cells are generated later. Neurogenesis in the retina continues up to the time of birth (LaVail, Rapaport and Rakic, 1991) even though cell formation has long ended in the LGN and visual cortex. Roughly 60% of the initially produced ganglion cells are lost by the time of birth due to programmed cell death (Rakic and Riley, 1983). Many features of the retinal architecture appear to develop early, and are largely independent of functional activity. For example, the distribution of rods and cones in the fetal retina appears roughly adult-like prior to the onset of functional synaptic contacts with horizontal or bipolar cells (Nishimura and Rakic, 1987; Wikler and Rakic, 1991). Nevertheless, there is considerable evidence that the retina of the newborn is quite immature (Abramov et al., 1982) along a number of dimensions. The newborn retina does not have the dense packing of photoreceptors in the central foveal region characteristic of adults, nor have the outer, light sensitive segments of the photoreceptors reached their mature length. Large scale photoreceptor migration toward the fovea and increases in outer segment length occur during the first year of life (Hendrickson, 1993), but other subtle morphological changes occur up to the age of 4 years (Yuodelis and Hendrickson, 1986).

In addition to changes in the microcircuitry of the retina, there are other large scale changes that may influence visual processing in important ways, such as growth in the eye. The distance from the cornea to the retina increases by about 25% by 1 year of age and increases another 25% by adolescence (Hirano, Yamamoto, Takayama et al., 1979; Larsen, 1971). Simply based on the reduction in retinal image size associated with the smaller size of the neonatal eye, theoretical calculations predict a one-third reduction in visual acuity (Banks and Bennett, 1988; Kellman and Banks, 1998).

Development of subcortical visual structures

While retinal ganglion cells project to several subcortical target structures, including the superior colliculus, the pretectum, and the hypothalamus, we will restrict our discussion to the LGN to which roughly 90% of retinal ganglion axons project. Neurogenesis in the LGN begins later and ends sooner than in the retina, and the proportion of initially produced cells that die appears smaller (Rakic, 1992). The period of cell death in the LGN ends before cell elimination in the retina begins, suggesting that intrinsic factors control the process. Moreover, LGN cell death occurs before the emergence of LGN layers or the establishment of feedback projections from visual cortex. Initial projections from ganglion cells in the retinae from both eyes connect broadly throughout the LGN. Cells appear to project in an orderly fashion which maintains the retinal topography. This process appears to be under genetic control. For example, in addition to other phenotypic features, albino humans and other animals have more extensive visual projections from the contralateral eye to the LGN than do normals. Moreover, the process of topographic projection occurs prior to the onset of physiological activity in the ganglion cells (Daw, 1995; Rakic, 1992).

Not all of the anatomical features of the LGN emerge as a result of intrinsic, activity independent factors, however. As mentioned previously, Shatz and colleagues have recently shown that the formation of eye-specific layers in the LGN depends upon activity in retinal ganglion cells (Shatz, 1996). Blocking the propagation of action potentials to the LGN abolishes the development of eye-specific layers. It now appears that the ganglion cells of the retina generate waves of action potentials spontaneously in the absence of input from the light-sensitive photoreceptors. Indeed, the waves of activity occur before the photoreceptors have matured sufficiently to respond to light stimulation. How do the spontaneous waves of activity in the retina induce the formation of eye-specific layers in the LGN? Shatz argues that ganglion cell inputs compete for functional synapses at the LGN, by means of an activity-dependent learning mechanism in which correlated or synchronous inputs cause synapses with target LGN cells to increase in strength.

More than 50 years ago, Hebb (1949) proposed the existence of synapses which would increase in strength whenever activity in the presynaptic and postsynaptic cells occurred simultaneously. There is now ample evidence for Hebbian-type synapses that undergo long-term potentiation (LTP), or synaptic strengthening, in many areas of the nervous system, including the hippocampus and cerebral cortex. Moreover, this type of learning mechanism is widely used to simulate processes of learning and plasticity. In the LGN, Shatz demonstrates that synapses between ganglion cells and LGN neurons undergo LTP, and that the synaptic strengthening can be prevented by chemicals which block LTP in other areas of the brain. Thus, Shatz and colleagues appear to have identified a plausible mechanism for activity-related plasticity in the LGN.

Many questions remain, however. One is how an activity-dependent mechanism could cause the eye-specific layers in the LGN to form in such a regular and precise way. Shatz argues that the random waves of spontaneous activity cause ganglion cells within one eye to fire in a more correlated fashion than those in the other eye. The relative difference in correlations causes recipient cells in the LGN to strengthen synapses with inputs from one or the other eye. A similar idea underlies computational models of the formation of ocular dominance columns in primary visual cortex (Miller, Keller and Stryker, 1989). However widespread sensitivity to relative strengths of correlations might be in the visual system, it is likely that other intrinsic and extrinsic factors contribute to the formation of eye-specific layers in the LGN. Shatz speculates that intrinsic activity may play an important role in shaping connectivity in other areas of the brain, including the cerebral cortex. If so, then spontaneous patterns of activity may provide another mechanism, beyond regularities in the external environment, for achieving a high precision of connectivity in the brain without the need for detailed genetic specification.

There are, of course, other potential influences on the ultimate functional properties of LGN neurons. One of them is feedback from activity in deep cortical neurons in primary visual cortex (V1). Axons from LGN cells project to V1 in a retinotopic fashion that appears driven largely by intrinsic factors such as gradients of nerve growth factors (Payne, Pearson and Cornwell, 1988). LGN axons initially make synaptic contacts with cells located below the cortical plate, so-called subplate neurons. At first, these subplate neurons drive Layer IV and VI cells. Eventually, LGN axons will migrate upward and drive Layer IV cells directly, as they do in the mature system. But, they do not reach these targets if the subplate neurons are eliminated. Moreover, at the same time that LGN axons are migrating toward the cortex, feedback projections from deep layer VI neurons are projecting toward the LGN (Rakic, 1992). In other words, during the time period in which LGN axons are modifying their pattern of connectivity with cortical neurons, LGN neurons are receiving feedback signals from cortex. Furthermore, in the human and presumably other species, there are large changes in the volume of the LGN in the first 6 postnatal months (Huttenlocher, De Courten, Garey and Van der Loos, 1982), in addition to more subtle morphological changes at the level of individual cells (Leuba and Garey, 1982). How multiple intrinsic and activity-related factors are integrated to yield the highly and regularly structured thalamic nucleus is not yet known. However, it is clear that the mechanisms exist for visual system integrity to be affected by visual input and processing within the first several months after birth.

Development of primary visual cortex

The primary visual cortex has been the focus of an intensive investigation of how the anatomical and functional dimensions of visual development relate to one another. Neurogenesis in monkey primary visual cortex begins several days later than in the retina or LGN, but unlike the retina, appears to end well before birth (Rakic, 1992). As is the case for other areas of the cerebral cortex, there is an orderly sequence in the timing of neurogenesis among neurons in V1. Neurons destined for deep layers are generated in the deep ventricular zone first, with neurons slated to occupy superficial layers generated later (Rakic, 1974). Neurons migrate up radially projecting glial cells that span the distance from the subplate zone below layer VI to the outermost portion of Layer I. This results in an 'inside-out' pattern of neuronal migration. For the most part, the laminar structure of visual cortex appears to be largely immune to activity-dependent control, but is instead regulated by nerve growth factors and selective gene expression. This is supported by the finding that gene mutations, such as that found in the 'reeler' mouse, cause selective errors in the final laminar targets reached by cortical cells. Further, cell migration occurs over a prolonged time course. In the cat, some cells do not reach their target layers until some 2 weeks after birth (Shatz and Luskin, 1986). In the macaque, there appears to be a relatively large degree of cell death (Rakic, 1992), but whether this occurs at all in the human is controversial (Huttenlocher, 1990).

One of the most important facets of anatomical development in primary visual cortex from the point of view of activity-dependent mechanisms is the onset and pattern of synaptogenesis. In several mammalian species, synaptogenesis in visual cortex begins prenatally, but increases rapidly reaching a peak during the early postnatal period, then is followed by a period of synaptic loss. This progressive and regressive pattern has been measured in humans as well (Huttenlocher, 1990; Huttenlocher and De Courten, 1987; Huttenlocher et al., 1982), with the notable observation that synaptic density in newborns is low, but increases rapidly after birth reaching a peak between 4 and 5 months before beginning a gradual period of decline. Levels of cerebral metabolic activity show similarly low initial levels and subsequent increases (Chugani, Müller and Chugani, 1996; Chugani and Phelps, 1986), suggesting that these measures may be related to one another. The important point is that unlike the formation of the topographic projections or the establishment of basic processing circuitry, the period of most rapid synapse formation occurs when externally driven activity dependent mechanisms can hold influence. On the other hand, it is unlikely that visual stimulation per se regulates the rate of synapse production, but instead modifies and eliminates preexisting synapses (Rakic, 1992).

With respect to other functional features of neurons in primary visual cortex, such as orientation selectivity, direction of motion selectivity, and ocular dominance, these dimensions appear also to be influenced by both intrinsic and activity-dependent mechanisms. In the cat, crude sensitivity to orientation develops prenatally (Wiesel and Hubel, 1974), and therefore forms without visual experience. The selectivity in orientation selective cells continues to increase postnatally, and appears to be disrupted by blocking neural activity (Daw, 1995) or if visual experience is impaired (Bonds, 1979). Similarly, there is some degree of direction of motion selectivity found in V1 neurons from shortly after birth (Hubel and Wiesel, 1963), but substantial enhancement direction selectivity occurs postnatally (Bonds, 1979). The story is similar with regard to ocular dominance, or the extent to which neurons respond most strongly to input from one eye or the other. As with initial projections from the retina to the LGN, LGN afferents to cortex from each eye specific lamina overlap initially (Rakic, 1976). Within the first 6 weeks of life, cells have segregated into bands which respond largely or exclusively to input from one eye or the other. Blocking neural activity eliminates the process of segregation. The prevailing view is that the ultimate formation of ocular dominance columns is driven by a process of competitive interaction at the synaptic level among inputs from both eyes (e.g. Miller, 1990). Unlike the process described for the segregation of eye specific layers in the LGN, however, the formation of ocular dominance columns seems to be influenced by visual information, not spontaneous patterns of activity alone.

Development beyond V1

Unfortunately, there is remarkably little detailed evidence about how cortical structures outside of V1 develop. We know that while V1 does not receive projections via the corpus callosum from the opposite hemisphere, V2 and subsequent areas do. Those projections are initially widespread, but many axons eventually retract (Dehay, Kennedy, Bullier and Berland, 1988). It is generally known that output from mature V1 to higher order cortical areas originates in layers 2 and 3 while projections to the LGN originate in layer 6. Projections to subcortical areas such as the superior colliculus and to the cortical motion processing area V5 originate from layers 4B and 5. Accordingly, based on the generally consistent observation that deeper layers of the cortex mature earlier than do more superficial layers (Conel, 1939–1967; Purpura, 1975; Rabinowicz, 1979), it has been suggested that output from V1 to higher order cortical areas may be delayed relative to connections with subcortical structures (Johnson, 1990). Some of the behavioral evidence related to this hypothesis will be discussed in the next section. Similarly, there is limited information about the timing of synaptogenesis and morphological change in human extrastriate visual regions (Conel, 1939–1967), but the existing evidence suggests that the timing of synaptogenesis and its associated peak varies considerably from one region of the cortex to another (Huttenlocher, 1990; Huttenlocher and Dabholkar, 1997). These data are in rough accord with those showing gradual increases in resting metabolic activity that vary in onset from region to region (Chugani et al., 1996; Chugani, Phelps and Mazziotta, 1987). For example, in the inferior temporal (IT) cortex, which is a central component in the ventral, form processing visual stream, metabolic activity is barely detectable in infant monkeys and does not reach adult levels until 6 months (Hagger, Brickson and Bachevalier, 1988).

Despite the relative lack of data, several investigators have taken these patterns of anatomical development as the launching point for accounts of how visual function in young infants might be directly linked to the emergence of function in specific circuits in visual cortex and its associated structures (Atkinson, 1984; Bronson, 1982; Johnson, 1990). In general, these accounts point to the relatively low synaptic density in the visual cortex of newborns and the subsequently rapid increase as evidence that subcortical visual circuits control the majority of visual processing in neonates, and in particular, that as the primary input to higher order visual processing areas, immaturities in connectivity within V1 may render newborns' vision largely dependent on subcortical mechanisms. This view is controversial in part because newborns have been shown to have several visual capacities such as size constancy and slant perception that presumably depend on cortical processing (Slater, 1993; Slater, Mattock and Brown, 1990; Slater and Morison, 1985). Nevertheless, there is considerable evidence that vision in young infants is diminished in ways that are consistent with initially immature processing both in V1 and in other areas of cortex. The next section summarizes some of that evidence.

The development of visual processing

It is widely known that infants see poorly relative to adults, and that vision improves rapidly and dramatically in the first year of life. What may not be so widely appreciated is the fact that vision early in life differs from the adult form along a number of basic sensory dimensions. Moreover, with few exceptions, there is relatively little research which attempts to create a comprehensive characterization of infant vision based on the combined influence of multiple sensory and perceptual factors (Banks and Bennett, 1988; Banks and Shannon, 1993). The existing work suggests that developments in visual perception early in life stem from changes at multiple levels of the visual system, from changes in the optics of the eye to the maturation of cortical visual processing circuitry. Several excellent and more comprehensive treatments of this material can be found elsewhere (Atkinson, 2000; Kellman and Arterberry, 1998; Kellman and Banks, 1998; Simons, 1993). We discuss low-level and high-level vision in turn.

Low-level vision

Optical factors

The formation of a focused, undistorted visual image on the retinal surface is the first step in the process of visual perception. It appears that full term neonates are on average hyperopic, or far-sighted, under normal viewing conditions, and approximately twenty to fifty percent of neonates are astigmatic (Atkinson, Braddick and French, 1980; Mohindra, Held, Gwiazda and Brill, 1978). While the evidence is somewhat mixed, both types of refractive errors appear to decline over the first several years of life (Atkinson et al., 1980; Banks, 1980; Howland, 1993; Mohindra and Held, 1981). Whether moderate levels of refractive error have important consequences for visual development are not precisely known, but Banks and colleagues (Banks and Bennett, 1988) have argued that young infants' poor visual acuity and greater depth of field probably diminish the impact of optical imperfections.

Visual field size

Similarly, there are considerable changes visual field size in the first year. While different behavioral methods show measurement variability, newborns have measurable binocular visual fields that are only 15–25% of the 160–170° values typical of the average human adult (Mayer and Fulton, 1993; Sireteanu, 1996). Binocular visual field sizes begin to increase at about 1–2 months of age, but do not reach adult values until 12–24 months. Monocular field size has a somewhat more rapid developmental time course. For large, statically presented targets, field size rapidly improves from birth, approaching adult levels by approximately 4 months (Lewis and Maurer, 1992; Maurer and Lewis, 1991). Moreover, field size for static targets develops more rapidly in the temporal visual field than in the nasal field. Field sizes to moving targets grow more slowly; adult levels are not reached until approximately the end of the first year of age (Mohn and Van Hof-van Duin, 1986). Further, there are no notable differences between temporal and nasal visual fields. What causes differences in the rate of development in the nasal and temporal fields is not known. A variety of explanations have been offered which attribute the differences to peripheral factors — differential timing in the maturation of cone photoreceptors or retinal ganglion cells — or central factors — crossed (temporal hemifield) versus uncrossed (nasal hemifield) projections to cortex, or projections from cortex to subcortical oculomotor nuclei. The answers to this and other questions, such as the extent to which visual sensitivity varies with visual field size early in life, will have to wait further research (Mayer and Fulton, 1993; Sireteanu, 1996).

Grating acuity

Within the effective visual field, the ability to resolve detailed features of the visual image is critical for the recognition of form. There are several measures of visual acuity used in testing vision in young children. Grating acuity is the most widely assessed, due in part to the laudable work of Teller and colleagues (Teller, McDonald, Preston et al., 1986) in developing and extensively testing a system for assessing grating visual acuity in young infants. Since these techniques and terms may be unfamiliar to the nonspecialist, Fig. 1 illustrates some of the dis-

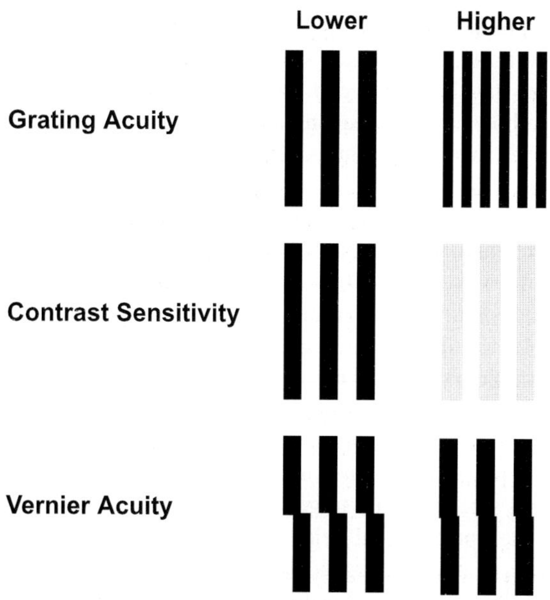

Fig. 1. Grating acuity, contrast sensitivity, and vernier acuity are three dimensions of visual function that are commonly assessed in children. Normally developing children move from lower levels of acuity or sensitivity toward higher levels as they mature. The figure illustrates the visual consequences of development along each dimension.

plays commonly used to assess visual function in children. In the Teller Acuity Card procedure, acuity is measured using a Forced Choice Preferential Looking technique (Teller, 1979). Infants are shown a series of high contrast cards with black and white stripes of varying widths appearing on the left or right side of the card. The stripes are measured in terms of spatial frequency, or the number of black and white cycles per degree of visual angle. An observer who does not know which side the stripes appear on, gazes through a peep hole to determine whether the infant looks toward the stripes or toward a gray region that reflects the same amount of light as the striped region. Studies using this technique have suggested that binocular grating acuity in neonates is roughly 0.5–1.5 cycles/deg — roughly the width of an adult's finger held at arm's length. Acuity improves rapidly over the next few months, reaching 3–6 cycles/deg by 6 months. Over the next 6 months acuity changes more slowly. At 1 year, the rate of change increases, resulting in adult-like acuity values of roughly 30 cycles/deg by age 3 (summarized in Teller et al., 1986). Monocular acuity lags binocular acuity, unlike adults who show minimal differences between monocular and binocular thresholds (Sireteanu, 1996). Moreover, in a finding similar to the pattern observed for field size changes, the nasal field acuity apparently lags temporal field acuity. The specific causes of grating acuity development are not known, but theoretical analyses suggest that optical and retinal factors do not account for all of the measured deficits in young infants' vision (Banks and Bennett, 1988); this would appear to implicate a narrowing in the receptive fields of thalamic or cortical neurons perhaps via synaptic remapping or lateral inhibition.

Vernier acuity

Vernier acuity involves the detection of small offsets between the segments of similarly oriented line segments. It is thought to be a form of hyperacuity because adult levels of sensitivity exceed estimates of photoreceptor density on the retina (Westheimer, 1981). As a result, the emergence of vernier acuity is thought to reflect processing in later stages of the visual processing stream, particularly in visual cortex. In adults, Vernier acuity exceeds grating acuity; however, in infants and young children vernier acuity sharply lags grating acuity. Vernier thresholds are approximately ten times lower than adult levels in 1-year-olds (Skoczenski and Norcia, 1999) compared with grating acuities which are roughly half the adult value. Moreover, Vernier acuity has a slower developmental course. Adult values are not reached until approximately age 4 years (Carkeet, Levi and Manny, 1998), and developmental visual disorders such as amblyopia impair Vernier acuity more severely than grating acuity (Levi and Carkeet, 1993). While the specific neural systems which give rise to Vernier acuity are not yet known, the bulk of the evidence suggests that striate and extrastriate visual circuits jointly contribute.

Chromatic sensitivity

Extensive reviews of the development of infants' sensitivity to chromatic information have been published elsewhere (Teller, 1997; Teller and Bornstein, 1987). Chromatic vision originates in specialized photoreceptive cells in the retina, called cone, that are sensitive to three specific wavelengths of light.

These cones are informally known by the color that corresponds to their peak sensitivity: blue for short wavelength cones, green for medium wavelength cones, and red for long wavelength cones. In general, young infants do not discriminate colors well, and there is evidence that sensitivity to shorter (i.e., blue) wavelengths may be especially impaired. There is a general consensus that sensitivity to red–green differences appears to emerge in the second month after birth and discrimination of blue–yellow differences some time later. A number of factors have been associated with the development of color vision in human infants. Most investigators have emphasized the impact of maturation in the photoreceptors. However, Banks and Bennett (1988) have argued that much of young infants' insensitivity to color discriminations may be due to reduced sensitivity to changes in luminance alone, not wavelength per se. Nevertheless, there is general agreement that the roughly sequential emergence of sensitivity to red/green and tritan or blue/yellow contrasts suggest that the short wavelength (blue) channel matures at a slower rate. What role development in primary visual cortex or downstream areas such as V2 and V4 that contribute to adult color processing might play in the process of color perception remains relatively unexplored.

Motion

Two broad classes of motion sensitivity are critical for visual perception (Banton and Bertenthal, 1997). One is the perception of relative motion, such as that generated by an object moving relative to a static background. The other is the perception of uniform motion, such as those generated by eye or head movements. Adult observers depend on relative motion to perceive the form, position, and direction of moving objects while uniform patterns of motion may be used in perceiving the observer's motion within a static environment. Primitive capacities to detect and respond to relative visual motion have been observed in newborns, and several lines of evidence suggest that sensitivity to global patterns of motion develops somewhat more slowly (Banton and Bertenthal, 1997). Both types of perceptual processes depend upon the accurate detection of both the direction and speed of moving elements.

Some behavioral measures, such as the image-stabilizing optokinetic nystagmus (OKN) reflex, suggest that newborns have crude selectivity to the direction of motion (Atkinson, 1979). However, in young infants OKN is asymmetric. When moving patterns are viewed monocularly, OKN can only be driven by motion in the nasal-ward direction. Some, but not all, of the asymmetry in early monocular OKN has been attributed to the influence of a simpler, subcortical motion processing pathway from the retina to the nucleus of the optic tract in the pretectum. By 3–5 months, monocular OKN and cortical evoked responses (Norcia et al., 1991) are directionally symmetric, suggesting that cortical motion processing circuits gradually begin to modulate the largely subcortical OKN response. Studies examining other visual behavior related to motion sensitivity paint a similar picture. There is minimal evidence for direction-selective VEPs in infants younger than 7–8 weeks (Wattam-Bell, 1996). But, there is gradual development in direction selectivity; direction thresholds reach 17° by 18 weeks (Banton, Bertenthal and Dobkins, 2000). Adults detect direction differences of less than 1° (De Bruyn and Orban, 1988), so direction discrimination clearly undergoes significant development in older infants. Behavioral and physiological methods that both the maximum and minimum speeds infants detect under relative motion conditions increase rapidly in the first several months after birth (Wattam-Bell, 1996). Moreover, sensitivity to changes in visual direction under relative motion conditions emerges at 6–8 weeks and subsequently improves. On the other hand, minimum velocity thresholds do not appear to change between 6 and 18 weeks in response to uniform motion patterns (Banton and Bertenthal, 1995). Why sensitivity to relative motion develops slowly and sensitivity to uniform motion emerges early and develops minimally in this time period is not known. However, Banton and Bertenthal (1995) suggest that relative motion sensitivity may be more dependent on the development of complex motion detectors in higher order visual areas, such as MST, which receive convergent input from directionally selective cells in MT. Recent evidence from my own laboratory regarding the discrimination of another form of uniform motion — heading direction from optic flow — suggests that this account may not be fully adequate.

In addition to changes in direction discrimination, the velocity ranges over which relative changes in direction can be detected also grows postnatally. The minimum and maximum speeds detectable by 8–10 week-olds are an order of magnitude worse than in adults (see review by Wattam-Bell, 1996). By 15–20 weeks, infants are sensitive to speeds up to 30°/s, but sensitivity remains substantially below adult levels which reach 100°/s in some cases. Furthermore, there is minimal evidence about the development of velocity sensitivity in infants older than 15–20 weeks, so how and when speed sensitivity approaches adult levels is not known.

Orientation perception

One of the hallmarks of visual processing in primary visual cortex is orientation selectivity. Initially it was thought that the detection of dynamic 45° changes in grating orientation were not detected until 6–8 weeks of age in the human (Braddick, Wattam-Bell and Atkinson, 1986). However, subsequent studies using static patterns showed that newborns could discriminate large changes in orientation (Atkinson, Hood, Wattam-Bell et al., 1988; Slater, Morison and Somers, 1988). Based on evoked responses from visual cortex, sensitivity to smaller changes in orientation appears to develop gradually over the first several months after birth (Atkinson, 2000). By 12 weeks, more than half of all infants show discernible evoked responses to orientation changes of 10°. Taken together the evidence suggests that, like the monkey and cat, systems in visual cortex which underlie orientation selectivity in human neonates undergo substantial postnatal development.

Binocularity

Ocular dominance, or the tendency of a neuron to respond more strongly to inputs from one eye, is also a common feature of many cells in V1. The segregation of inputs by their eye of origin is thought to be an essential first step prior to the determination of retinal disparity, and ultimately distance in depth. Of course, it is difficult to measure ocular dominance or its absence using behavioral means. Nevertheless, several ingenious paradigms have been devised for measuring binocular interaction and stereopsis in infants. One, for example, presents infants with displays in which information is presented to each eye separately and in a way that is either consistent or inconsistent. Using this sort of technique, infants show visual evoked potentials (VEPs) activated by binocular correlation between 8 and 20 weeks (Braddick, Wattam-Bell and Atkinson, 1983) and a rather abrupt onset of disparity sensitivity between 12 and 20 weeks (Birch, Gwiazda and Held, 1982; Held, Birch and Gwiazda, 1980). Thereafter, the minimum retinal disparity that can be detected appears to increase rapidly (Birch et al., 1982). The sudden onset and rapid development of stereoacuity led some to speculate that a specific neurological milestone was the root cause, namely, the formation of ocular dominance columns (Held, 1985).

We now know that cells from each eye specific layer of the LGN project widely throughout V1 (Hubel and Wiesel, 1963) and that some of these projections are selectively withdrawn as a result of competitive interactions among neurons projecting from each LGN in a process that appears analogous to that described previously regarding the formation of eye specific layers (Wiesel and Hubel, 1965). Furthermore, in both the cat (Pettigrew, 1974) and monkey (LeVay, Wiesel and Hubel, 1980), the process of ocular dominance column segregation continues for several weeks postnatally, and the completion of segregation occurs at about the time of the onset of stereopsis (O'Dell, Quick and Boothe, 1991; Timney, 1981). As a result, it does appear that the onset of stereopsis may be quite closely associated with the completion of ocular dominance formation in V1 although questions about why binocular function appears so abruptly in the face of gradual ocular dominance formation, among others, remain.

Higher-level vision

The preceding discussion of changes in low-level vision suggest that in the first months after birth there are changes occurring at multiple levels of the visual system which may interact with one another in complex, and in as yet poorly understood ways. While some low-level visual changes can be linked to specific anatomical or physiological changes, the multiple, interacting influences make detailed accounts of the anatomical and physiological basis of change in higher-level vision especially difficult. Nevertheless, there are a number of domains in which investigators have examined development in selected aspects of higher level vision that have reasonably well defined

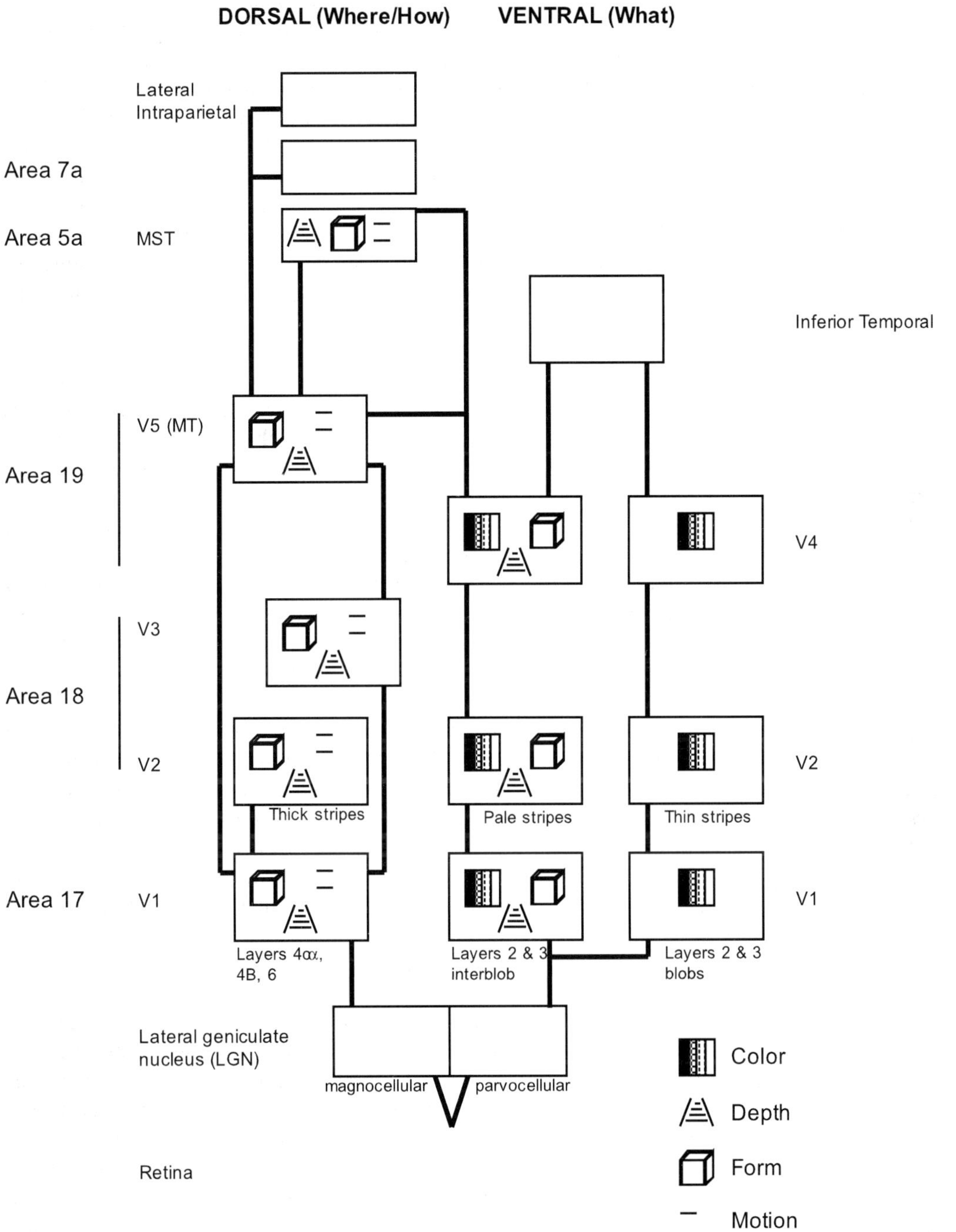

Fig. 2. The primate visual system is thought to consist of two interconnected, but functionally parallel processing streams which may begin segregating at early stages of visual processing. The dorsal stream, so named because it projects dorsally from primary visual cortex toward the parietal lobe, largely specializes in processing information related to space and action planning. The ventral stream, named for its terminations in the ventrally located temporal lobe, specializes in processing shape, color, and form. The figure presents a simplified version of our current knowledge of the way these pathways originate and interconnect. Adapted from DeYoe and Van Essen, 1988.

biological substrates. In general, these lines of work have been motivated by the search for behavioral changes which might reveal or index the functional properties of specific functional neural systems. This is a broad and growing area of research, so our discussion will be limited to a small set of representative examples. In accord with the conventional view that visual processing may be divided both on logical, and to a certain extent, neuroanatomical grounds into relatively separate systems for spatial and object-related processing (Goodale and Milner, 1992; Ungerleider and Mishkin, 1982), Fig. 2 illustrates how the dorsal (spatial processing) and ventral (object processing) streams, while densely interconnected, might begin to separate at very early stages in the mature visual system. We will discuss some recent evidence for development in each type of processing system in turn.

Vision for spatial perception and action planning

The central challenge for the visual system in extracting spatial information is to determine the direction, distance, and orientation of objects and surfaces in the environment. Most accounts of mature spatial processing and action planning accord a central role to areas in the occipital, parietal, and temporal lobes that comprise the dorsal visual processing stream (Ungerleider and Mishkin, 1982; Goodale and Milner, 1992). These areas appear to represent spatial relationships in multiple, interacting coordinate systems in which visual and non-visual sources of information are systematically integrated (Andersen, 1997; Stein, 1992).

Previous research regarding the determination of visual direction had indicated that young infants initially perceive spatial locations using body-centered or egocentric coordinates then gradually shift to using environment-centered representations (Acredolo, 1990; Piaget and Inhelder, 1948). However, it was not known whether body-centered representations for action were prespecified and present from birth, or whether they emerged gradually over the first year from an even more primitive coordinate system. Mark Johnson and I (Gilmore and Johnson, 1997a,b) addressed this question by adapting for use with infants a simple eye movement task. The double-step saccade task (e.g. Hallett and Lightstone, 1976a,b) distinguishes between different forms of spatial information that might guide eye movement planning — visually-centered information based on the position of a visual target on the retina, and head or body-centered information that incorporated eye or head position. In a series of experiments, we (1997a,b) observed a change in type of information that governed young infants' saccade planning. Infants 3 to 5 months of age were more likely to make saccade sequences based on visually centered information alone, but 6- to 7-month-olds were more likely to base their responses on body-centered information. The systematic integration of visual and eye position or movement information is associated with single cell responses in areas 7a and LIP of the dorsal visual processing stream (Andersen, 1997) of the monkey and with normal parietal function in humans (Duhamel, Colby and Goldberg, 1993). Consequently, we interpreted these results as suggesting that retinocentric representation of space, based largely on the activity in a primitive subcortical orienting system, dominates spatial perception and saccade planning in young infants. In turn, gradual development of cortical circuitry permits functional body-centered representations to emerge between 3 and 7 months of age. The findings suggested that other mechanisms associated with perceiving body-centered direction might undergo considerable development in infancy.

Accordingly, my students and I have recently sought evidence about the precision with which infants can discriminate their direction of self-motion, or heading, from optic flow. Adults determine their direction of heading from optic flow to within 1° of visual angle (Royden, Crowell and Banks, 1994; Warren, Morris and Kalish, 1988). Furthermore, neurophysiological studies have shown that in monkeys optic flow selectively activates the dorsal portion of the medial superior temporal cortex (MSTd), a region of visual association cortex (Duffy and Wurtz, 1991; Duffy and Wurtz, 1997). A homologous area has been found in human adults by means of brain imaging (De Jong, Shipp, Skidmore et al., 1994). We examined the extent to which young infants discriminate changes in heading in an effort to assess the relative state of development of this system.

In one series of experiments (Gilmore and Rettke, in press), we habituated 4-month-old infants to an optic flow display depicting motion in one direction.

Then, once looking times reached an habituation criterion, we measured changes in looking time to the familiar direction and novel ones. Infants' average looking times increased when the changes in direction were large (180°), but not when the differences were of an intermediate size (4°, 8°, or 16°). A subsequent study used a more sensitive Forced Choice Preferential Looking technique in which we estimated that the threshold for detecting changes in heading direction at 4 months of age was about 40° or 8 times larger than adults'. Accordingly, it appears that 4-month-old infants do not accurately discriminate their direction of translational self motion from optic flow, at least relative to adults. We do not yet know when heading discrimination approaches adult levels; however these data and the previous data regarding the emergence of body-centered representations are broadly consistent with the possibility that there is a prolonged period of development in dorsal stream cortical areas. The possibility that dorsal stream processing has a delayed or prolonged developmental timecourse has been suggested by others, as well (Atkinson, 2000).

The perception of distance information has been more widely studied, but has in general been less directly linked to specific neural substrates. More extensive reviews of the evidence can be found elsewhere (Kellman and Arterberry, 1998; Kellman and Banks, 1998). In general, behavioral evidence points to the possibility that like the perception of direction, there is a sequence in the emergence of sensitivity to different visual cues that provide information about distance.

The earliest emerging cues to distance appear to based on motion. Among the many dynamic cues to depth, infants show earliest sensitivity to the pattern of optical expansion that is generated by an object approaching the viewer. Newborn animals of a variety of species produce eye, head, and other avoidance behaviors in response to approaching or looming patterns (Schiff, 1965). In humans, however, collision avoidance behavior develops more slowly. While avoidance behaviors can be observed in infants as young as 6 weeks, blinking and head movements do not occur reliably until about 3 months (Yonas, Pettersen and Lockman, 1979), and these behaviors become increasingly selective to the form of the approaching object or surface over the next several months (Carroll and Gibson, 1981; Nañez and Yonas, 1994; Schmuckler and Li, 1998). Sensitivity to the relative ordering of surfaces in depth that is specified by the accretion and deletion of texture shows a similar trend. By 5 to 7 months, infants appear to be able to reach toward the 'nearer' of two surfaces when the depth order is specified by the accretion or deletion of texture (Craton and Yonas, 1990). Finally, sensitivity to the depth relations specified by motion parallax or motion perspective information generated by lateral movement of the head may also emerge early. 4-month-old infants under some conditions may be able to discriminate the visual consequences of their own passive lateral movement from motion of an object alone (Von Hofsten, Kellman and Putaansuu, 1992). Because these studies suggested that infants have sensitivity to optical velocities an order of magnitude below velocity sensitivity measured via other techniques (Kellman and Banks, 1998), they should be interpreted cautiously. Little is known about the specific visual circuits that give rise to extracting depth information from motion, but these abilities are likely to engage the motion processing systems mentioned earlier.

The emergence of sensitivity stereoscopic depth between 3 and 5 months of age was discussed earlier, so we will move to a discussion of pictorial cues to depth. There are a variety of such cues, but all of them depend upon a relatively high degree of visual acuity and relatively sophisticated processing of the retinal image. Accordingly, it is not surprising that not until around 7 months of age do infants show systematic sensitivity to pictorial cues to depth (Yonas, Arterberry and Granrud, 1987; Yonas and Granrud, 1985). There is some evidence that younger infants can discriminate the rudimentary features of certain depth relations (Bhatt and Waters, 1998), but these demonstrations do not indicate that younger infants perceive these elements as indicating specific spatial relationships. Like the determination of depth relations from motion, little is known about the neural mechanisms which give rise to this process. However, most existing theories suggest that these aspects of processing are likely to depend on extrastriate visual areas, and may require an interaction between information extracted from the dorsal and ventral processing streams (Palmer, 1999).

Overall, these data about the development of spatial vision imply that there is a fundamental transformation in the way that young infants perceive direction and distance information between birth and 7 months of age, with notable changes occurring in the last half of this time period. While some of these behavioral changes have been associated with the functional operation of relatively prescribed neural systems, others have not, and on the whole, the evidence for these associations remains indirect, at least for the time being.

Vision for object recognition

The process of perceiving the three dimensional form of objects is enormously complex and remains poorly understood. We have already discussed several aspects of low-level vision that contribute to the perception of form, such as development in sensitivity to high spatial frequencies, to the orientation of line segments, to motion direction, and to color. A detailed treatment of the developmental data on this topic is unfortunately beyond the scope of this chapter, but there are several excellent sources in literature (Kellman, 1996; Kellman and Arterberry, 1998; Kellman and Banks, 1998). Here, I will describe several examples which seem to indicate that relatively sophisticated object recognition abilities seem to emerge rather early in life.

Perhaps the most striking of these lines of evidence is the finding that newborn infants appear to discriminate face-like patterns from other stimuli, including inverted face-like patterns equated on a number of low-level visual characteristics (for a detailed treatment see Johnson and Morton, 1991). Indeed, 3-day-olds appear to discriminate their mother's face from visual information alone (Bushnell, Sai and Mullin, 1989) although recent evidence suggests that visual information from the outer contour of the head and the hairline, not internal facial features, influences infants' behavior (Pascalis, De Schonen, Morton et al., 1995) at least for the first 2 months. At about one month, the initial orienting preference disappears, but by 2 months, it reappears, but in a more sophisticated form that suggests a reorganization has occurred in infants' face processing. In particular, it appears from a Linear Systems Analysis based on models of low-level visual acuity that whereas newborns' visual preferences for faces are driven largely by the degree of stimulus energy or visibility of the pattern (i.e., the amplitude spectrum), at 2 months, infants show sensitivity to the specific characteristics (i.e. phase information) of faces as images (Kleiner and Banks, 1987; Mondloch et al., 1999). Based on this and other evidence Johnson and Morton (1991) have proposed that early face-preferences are due to a simple, early developing neural mechanism that gives rise to a general preference to orient toward simple face-like patterns. The subsequent disappearance and reorganization of face recognition is due to the maturation of a more sophisticated, later developing system that controls, among other things, learning about the specific characteristics of faces. The neural substrates of these proposed systems have not been specified, but Johnson and Morton (1991) have suggested that the first system is based in subcortical systems and the second system within the cerebral cortex. Neuroimaging data have suggested that faces activate regions of the fusiform gyrus in infants, much as they have been shown to do in adults (Tzourio, De Schonen, Mazoyer et al., 1992); moreover, there appears to be a right hemisphere advantage for face processing (De Schonen and Mathivet, 1990). In short, while there is considerable change in face processing, along a number of dimensions it appears that face processing assumes many functional characteristics similar to adults relatively early in life.

Other examples of the relatively early emergence of form perception pertain to the discrimination of object form from motion. Arterberry and Yonas (1988, 2002) have shown that 8-week-old infants can discriminate three dimensional shape when form is specified by differential patterns of optic flow alone. Other investigators have shown that 4-month-old infants appear to perceive that line segments or object parts that translate or rotate behind an occluding screen are part of the same object (Kellman and Short, 1987; Kellman and Spelke, 1983). Similarly, 3- to 5-month-olds discriminate inversions in the orientation of a display depicting biological motion (Bertenthal, Proffitt and Kramer, 1987), and by 5 months show evidence of sensitivity to the local phase relationships among the moving elements that suggest the perception of actual human movement (Bertenthal, 1993). Again, the specific neural mechanisms that support the perception of object form from motion are not well understood, but it has been suggested that these abilities engage ventral stream systems and higher order motion processing such that observed in areas MT and MST (Atkinson, 2000).

This brief survey of evidence regarding visual object recognition early in life suggests that at relatively early ages, infants begin to demonstrate the capacity to perceive and discriminate object form using a variety of sources of visual information. There are notable developments in these capacities in the first several months and many of the changes have been linked to the functional maturation of specific visual processing systems in the extrastriate cortex. Nevertheless, we are a long way from being able to offer a comprehensive account of the neuropsychology of early object processing.

Toward a neuropsychology of visual development

The previous discussion has illustrated some of the remarkable progress that has been made over the past several decades in describing how the visual system develops at the structural and functional level. In this concluding section, I will briefly summarize the state of our progress toward the goal of a comprehensive understanding of the neurological bases of visual development.

The data concerning the anatomical and physiological development of visual system structures suggest several broad generalizations. The process of establishing the basic functional architecture in the retina, LGN, and primary visual cortex occurs during the embryonic and fetal period. The generation of neurons, their migration, differentiation, pattern of initial axonal projection, and death are largely regulated by genetic factors although there are important effects of spontaneous neural activity in some instances. In contrast, the fine-tuning of the visual architecture by means of synapse formation, strengthening, and loss and the differentiation of dendritic arbors begins in the late fetal period and continues for an extended period after birth. These processes appear to be quite dependent on neuronal activity, and specifically, visually driven activity derived from visual input that is 'typical' for young primates. Many functional characteristics of neurons in the retina, in LGN, and in cortex emerge in a crude or imprecise form prior to birth and the onset of patterned visual experience, but the further development of these characteristics appears highly dependent on visual experience. In the human infant, there is a small, but consistent body of evidence suggesting that there is considerable development at all levels of the visual system in the months following birth. The eye grows; photoreceptors mature, lengthen, and migrate toward the fovea; the LGN grows in size; synaptic density in visual cortex accelerates rapidly, reaches a peak, then begins a slow period of decline; resting metabolic rates slowly grow toward adult levels. The evidence regarding development in structures further down the processing stream is sparse, but it appears that different cortical areas undergo rapid synaptogenesis and metabolic rate increases at different point in time during postnatal development.

Regarding the behavioral correlates of visual development, the emergence of new sophisticated techniques for measuring visual capacities in young children has brought with it a wealth of new data. These suggest that some of the most dramatic changes in visual capacities occur in the first 6 months after birth, but that visual development continues at a somewhat slower rate well into the preschool years. Among the low-level capacities that improve rapidly in the first 6 months are grating and vernier acuity, visual field size, sensitivity to chromatic (color) contrasts, sensitivity to orientation, and the direction and speed of motion. Moreover, during the same time period, we observe changes in higher-order visual processing of spatial and object-based information. For example, it appears that the perception of direction and distance is far simpler in young infants and is based on a more limited set of information than is available to and used by older children. On the other hand, capacities to use multiple sources of information in the discrimination of object form seems to emerge somewhat earlier. A number of investigators have sought to associate changes in low-level (Banks and Bennett, 1988; Held, 1985) and high-level vision with the development or functional maturation of specific neural systems (Atkinson, 2000; Bronson, 1982; Johnson, 1990; Johnson and Morton, 1991). These efforts have had some degree of success, but they have a number of limitations, not the least of which is the fact that our knowledge of the detailed anatomy and physiology of visual processing remains incomplete.

The current state of knowledge leaves many important questions unanswered. Regarding the neurobiology of vision, while studies of the retina, LGN, and V1 should continue, clearly, additional information about the patterns of anatomical and physiological development in extrastriate visual areas should be a research priority. These data are essential for making progress in determining how the visual architecture gets built. Indeed, it may well be that understanding how this enormously complex system is constructed will yield important insights about the functioning of the mature system.

In the realm of visual behavior, it is striking how differently scientists who study lower level perceptual processes view infants' capacities in comparison with those who study higher-level visual perception or cognition. With regard to infant visual cognition, there is a dominant theme in the literature that relatively sophisticated aspects of core knowledge about physical principles emerge early in life (e.g. Spelke, Breinlinger, Macomber and Jacobsen, 1992). But, how are we to reconcile these sorts of views with findings from perceptual development that suggest young infants have rather poor, but rapidly changing visual capacities? In other words, it seems vital for a developmental neuropsychology of vision to reconcile eventually these somewhat disparate views of perceptual and cognitive development early in life. One possibility is that visual development is highly action specific in the way that recent observations suggest is true for motor development (Adolph, 1997; Adolph, Eppler and Gibson, 1993). An account along these lines may help to explain why there might be different rates of development or differences in timing among visual capacities related to spatial versus object processing. It may be that young infants are more advanced in perceiving object form, in part, because they are relatively immobile (Kellman, 1993) and that, as others have observed, locomotion and other sorts of spatial action, which emerge later in infancy put different demands on visual processing.

This line of argument raises a final set of unanswered questions about the role of visually-driven experience in shaping functional development. There is extensive evidence that self-produced locomotion affects the development of many visual and visuomotor capacities (Bertenthal, Campos and Kermoian, 1994), including the now legendary demonstration that self-produced motion is superior to its passively experienced equivalent (Held and Hein, 1963) in shaping normal perceptual and motor development. Yet, the possible role of passive visual experience has been of relatively little interest. This seems surprising given that human infants accrue a substantial amount of passive visual experience in the first several months after birth and that this coincides with rapid increases in functional brain activity and in visual capacities. Moreover, passive experience is deemed vital in the domain of speech perception and language development (e.g. Kuhl, 1994), but we do not actually know to what extent passive visual experience contributes to the normal emergence of visual function in humans. Furthermore, questions about the timing and duration of critical periods in the normal development of the visual system are central to understanding how abnormal visual experience such as strabismus, amblyopia, and cataract affect vision and to what extent their effects might be remediated.

For example, recent evidence from children born with cataracts provide provocative data about the extent to which early visual experience shapes subsequent development. A cataract is an opacity in the lens of the eye that blurs vision and scatters light. For children whose cataracts are in the middle of their lens and of sufficient density, visual function and tracking are prevented. Increasingly infants with cataracts are identified and treated early, within the first several months after birth, usually by the removal of the cataract, and the subsequent fitting for contact lenses to compensate for the removed lens. Nevertheless, prior to surgery, these children have suffered a particular form of visual deprivation in which they were exposed to variations in overall light intensity, but not to focused light or visual patterns. In an elegant series of studies, Maurer, Lewis and colleagues have examined the visual acuity of children with cataracts from the first moments after patterned vision was restored to several months or years after corrective surgery. Their results suggest that the normal postnatal development in visual acuity depends on patterned visual input. Immediately after the restoration of focused, patterned vision in children with cataracts in both eyes, visual acuity was indistinguishable from that of newborns. This finding is all the more remarkable given that the children were treated and tested over a wide age range, from 1 week to 9 months. After an hour of visual input, eight of ten children showed measurable increases in visual acuity, followed by somewhat slower changes over the subsequent month. Thus, these results suggest that the human visual system retains considerable plasticity over an extended time period that can be rapidly expressed when normal patterned visual input is restored (Maurer, Lewis, Brent and Levin, 1999). On the other hand, children who have had surgical correction for congenital cataract show deficits relative to normally developing children in acuity, contrast sensitivity, and eye movement control that appear to persist indefinitely (Maurer and Lewis, 1993). And, somewhat paradoxically, it appears that children with a single monocular cataract fare somewhat worse than children with opacities in both eyes. Take together, these studies indicate that despite an extended period of developmental plasticity and the capacity for rapid recovery, even short periods of visual deprivation can have long lasting, perhaps even permanent effects. Indeed, Maurer and Lewis argue that normal visual input is required for some aspects of visual development for up to 10 years after birth (Maurer and Lewis, 2001) and that the neurological changes that underlie ongoing developmental plasticity probably occur at multiple levels of the visual system.

These data and others provide a number of reasons to be optimistic about the future of developmental visual neuropsychology. Not only is continued progress being made in studying the development of visual behavior in human children and in the emergence of mature circuitry in non-human primates, but visual scientists are placing increasing evidence on quantitative or computational models of visual processing (Banks and Bennett, 1988; Miller, 1990; Wilson, 1993). These techniques allow more specific hypotheses about the nature of visual processing and its neural underpinnings to be more rigorously assessed. Coupled with new and refined techniques for physiological recording and brain imaging that are becoming increasingly available for research in young children, the field is poised to make significant progress in the coming decade.

In conclusion, regarding Hebb's original conjecture that vision early in life is profoundly different from that of the adult, the bulk of the evidence seems to agree. To Hebb we can also give credit for the simple, but profound insight about how some aspects of visual development that are driven by correlated neural activity might be captured within a scheme for strengthening individual synapses. However, despite the notable progress made since Hebb's book in characterizing how early vision operates and how it changes, we do not yet have a fully satisfying account either of the development of visual behavior or its neural underpinnings. How the dynamic interplay of forces gives rise to the mature visual system and whether the understanding of development will have consequences for other areas of neuropsychology remain questions for future investigators.

Acknowledgements

I thank Robin Smail for her assistance and Sid Segalowitz and Isabelle Rapin for comments on the text.

References

Abramov I, Gordon J, Hendrickson A, Hainline L, Dobson V, Laboussier E: The retina of the newborn human infant. Science: 217; 265–267, 1982.

Acredolo L: Behavioral approaches to spatial orientation in infancy. Annals of the New York Academy of Sciences: 608; 596–612, 1990.

Adolph KE: Learning in the development of infant locomotion. Monographs of the Society for Research in Child Development: 62(3, Serial No. 251); 1997.

Adolph KE, Eppler MA, Gibson EJ: Crawling versus walking infants' perceptions of affordances for locomotion over sloping surfaces. Child Development: 64(4); 1158–1174, 1993.

Andersen RA: Multimodal integration for the representation of space in the posterior parietal cortex. Philosophical Transactions of the Royal Society of London: 352; 1441–1428, 1997.

Arterberry ME, Yonas A: Infants' sensitivity to kinetic information for three-dimensional object shape. Perception and Psychophysics: 44; 1–6, 1988.

Arterberry ME, Yonas A: Perception of three-dimensional shape specified by optic flow by 8-week-old infants. Perception and Psychophysics: 62(3); 550–556, 2000.

Atkinson J: Development of optokinetic nystagmus in the human infant and monkey infant: An analogue to development in kittens. In Freeman RD (Ed), Developmental Neurobiology of Vision. New York: Plenum Press, pp. 277–287, 1979.

Atkinson J: Human visual development over the first six months of life: A review and a hypothesis. Human Neurobiology: 3; 61–74, 1984.

Atkinson J: The Developing Visual Brain. Oxford: Oxford University Press, 2000.

Atkinson J, Braddick O, French J: Infant astigmatism: Its disappearance with age. Vision Research: 20; 891–893, 1980.

Atkinson J, Hood B, Wattam-Bell J, Anker S, Tricklebank J: Development of orientation discrimination in infancy. Perception: 17; 587–595, 1988.

Banks MS: Infant refraction and accommodation. Internationl Ophthalmology Clinics: 20; 205–232, 1980.

Banks MS, Bennett PJ: Optical and photoreceptor immaturities limit the spatial and chromatic vision of human neonates. Journal of the Optical Society of America A: 5(12); 2059–2079, 1988.

Banks MS, Shannon E: Spatial and chromatic visual efficiency in human neonates. In Granrud CE (Ed), Visual Perception and Cognition in Infancy. Hillsdale, NJ: Lawrence Erlbaum Associates, pp. 1–46, 1993.

Banton T, Bertenthal BI: Infants' sensitivity to uniform motion. Vision Research: 36(11); 1633–1640, 1995.

Banton T, Bertenthal BI: Multiple developmental pathways for motion processing. Optometry and Vision Science: 74(9); 751–760, 1997.

Banton T, Bertenthal BI, Dobkins K: Infant direction discrimination thresholds. Vision Research: 41(8); 1049–1056, 2001.

Bertenthal BI: Infants' perception of biomechanical motion: Intrinsic image and knowledge-based constraints. In C.E. Granrud CE (Ed), Visual Perception and Cognition in Infancy. Hillsdale, NJ: Lawrence Erlbaum, pp. 175–214, 1993.

Bertenthal BI, Campos JJ, Kermoian R: An epigenetic perspective on the development of self-produced locomotion and its consequences. Current Directions in Psychological Science: 3(5); 140–145, 1994.

Bertenthal BI, Proffitt DR, Kramer SJ: Perception of biomechanical motions by infants: Implementation of various processing constraints. Journal of Experimental Psychology: Human Perception and Performance: 13; 577–585, 1987.

Bhatt RS, Waters SE: Perception of three-dimensional cues in early infancy. Journal of Experimental Child Psychology: 70(3); 207–224, 1998.

Birch EE, Gwiazda J, Held R: Stereoacuity development for crossed and uncrossed disparities in human infants. Vision Research: 22; 507–513, 1982.

Bonds AB: Development of orientation tuning in the visual cortex of kittens. In Freeman RD (Ed), Developmental Neurobiology of Vision. New York: Plenum Press, 1979.

Braddick OJ, Wattam-Bell J, Atkinson J: The onset of binocular function in human infants. Human Neurobiology: 2; 65–69, 1983.

Braddick OJ, Wattam-Bell J, Atkinson J: Orientation-specific cortical responses develop in early infancy. Nature: 320; 617–619, 1986.

Bronson GW: Structure, status and characteristics of the nervous system at birth. In Stratton P (Ed), Psychobiology of the Human Newborn. Chichester: Wiley and Sons, pp. 99–118, 1982.

Bushnell IWR, Sai F, Mullin JT: Neonatal recognition of the mother's face. British Journal of Developmental Psychology: 7; 3–15, 1989.

Carkeet A, Levi DM, Manny RE: Development of Vernier acuity in childhood. Optometry and Visual Science: 74; 741–750, 1998.

Carroll JJ, Gibson EJ: Infants differentiation of an aperture and an obstacle. Paper presented at the Society of Research in Child Development, Boston, 1981.

Chugani HJ, Phelps ME: Maturational changes in cerebral function in infants determined by [18]FDG positron emission tomography. Science: 231; 840–843, 1986.

Chugani HT, Müller RA, Chugani DC: Functional brain reorganization in children. Brain Development: 18; 347–356, 1996.

Chugani HT, Phelps ME, Mazziotta JC: Positron emission tomography study of human brain functional development. Annals of Neurology: 22; 487–497, 1987.

Conel JL: The Postnatal Development of the Human Cerebral Cortex, Vols. I–VIII. Cambridge, MA: Harvard University Press, 1939–1967.

Craton LG, Yonas A: The role of motion in infants' perception of occlusion. In James TE (Ed), Advances in Psychology: 69. The Development of Attention: Research and Theory. Amsterdam, The Netherlands: North-Holland, 1990.

Daw NW: Visual Development. New York: Plenum Press, 1995.

De Bruyn B, Orban GA: Human velocity and direction discrimination measured with random dot patterns. Vision Research: 28; 1323–1335, 1988.

De Jong BM, Shipp S, Skidmore B, Frackowiak RSJ, Zeki S: The cerebral activity related to the visual perception of forward motion in depth. Brain: 117; 1039–1054, 1994.

De Schonen S, Mathivet E: Hemispheric asymmetry in a face discrimination task in infants. Child Development: 61; 1192–1205, 1990.

Dehay C, Kennedy H, Bullier J, Berland M: Absence of interhemispheric connections of area 17 during development in the monkey. Nature: 331; 348–350, 1988.

DeYoe EA, Van Essen DC: Concurrent processing streams in the monkey visual cortex. Trends in Neuroscience: 11; 219–226, 1988.

Duffy CJ, Wurtz RH: The sensitivity of MST neurons to optic flow stimuli. I. A continuum of response selectivity to large field stimuli. Journal of Neurophysiology: 65; 1329–1345, 1991.

Duffy CJ, Wurtz RH: Medial superior temporal area neurons respond to speed patterns in optic flow. Journal of Neuroscience: 17(8); 2839–2851, 1997.

Duhamel JR, Colby CL, Goldberg ME: The updating of the representation of visual space in parietal cortex by intended eye movements. Science: 255; 90–92, 1993.

Gilmore RO, Johnson MH: Body-centered representations for visually-guided action emerge during early infancy. Cognition: 65; B1–B9, 1997a.

Gilmore RO, Johnson MH: Egocentric action in early infancy: Spatial frames of reference for saccades. Psychological Science: 8(3); 224–230, 1997b.

Gilmore RO, Rettke HR: Four-month-olds' discrimination of optic flow patterns depicting different directions of observer motion. Infancy, 4(2), in press.

Goodale MA, Milner AD: Separate pathways for perception and action. Trends in Neuroscience: 15(1); 20–25, 1992.

Hagger C, Brickson M, Bachevalier J: Functional maturation of inferior temporal cortex in infant monkeys. Neuroscience Abstracts: 14(2); 1988.

Hallett PE, Lightstone AD: Saccadic eye movements to flashed targets. Vision Research: 114; 107–114, 1976a.

Hallett PE, Lightstone AD: Saccadic eye movements towards stimuli triggered by prior saccades. Vision Research: 16; 99–106, 1976b.

Hebb DO: The organization of behavior: A Neuropsychological Theory. New York: John Wiley and Sons, 1949.

Held R: Binocular vision: Behavioral and neuronal development. In Mehler J, Fox R (Eds), Neonate Cognition: Beyond the Blooming, Buzzing Confusion. Hillsdale, NJ: Lawrence Erlbaum, 1985.

Held R, Birch E, Gwiazda J: Stereoacuity in human infants. Proceedings of the National Academy of Sciences: 77; 5572–5574, 1980.

Held R, Hein A: Movement produced stimulation in the development of visually guided behavior. Journal of Comparative Physiological Psychology: 56(5); 872–876, 1963.

Hendrickson AE: Morphological development of the primate retina. In Simons K (Ed), Early Visual Development, Normal and Abnormal. Oxford: Oxford University Press, pp. 287–295, 1993.

Hirano S, Yamamoto Y, Takayama H, Sugata Y, Matsuo K: Ultrasonic observation of eyes in premature babies: Part 6. Growth curves of ocular axial length and its components. Acta Societatis Ophthalmologicae Japonicae: 83; 1679–1693, 1979.

Howland HC: Early refractive development. In Simons K (Ed), Early Visual Development: Normal and Abnormal. Oxford: Oxford University Press, pp. 3–13, 1993.

Hubel DH, Wiesel TN: Receptive fields of cells in striate cortex of young visually inexperienced kittens. Journal of Neurophysiology: 26; 994–1002, 1963.

Huttenlocher PR: Morphometric study of human cerebral cortex development. Neuropsychologia: 28; 517–527, 1990.

Huttenlocher PR, Dabholkar AS: Regional differences in synaptogenesis in human cerebral cortex. Journal of Comparative Neurology: 387; 167–178, 1997.

Huttenlocher PR, De Courten C: The development of synapses in the striate cortex of man. Human Neurobiology: 6; 1–9, 1987.

Huttenlocher PR, De Courten C, Garey LG, Van der Loos H: Synaptogenesis in human visual cortex — evidence for synapse elimination during normal development. Neuroscience Letter: 33; 247–252, 1982.

Johnson MH: Cortical maturation and the development of visual attention in early infancy. Journal of Cognitive Neuroscience: 2(2); 81–95, 1990.

Johnson MH, Morton J: Biology and Cognitive Development: The Case of Face Recognition. Oxford, UK: Blackwell, 1991.

Kellman PJ: Kinematic foundations of infant visual perception. In Granrud C (Ed), Visual Perception and Cognition in Infancy. Hillsdale, NJ: Lawrence Erlbaum Associates, 1993.

Kellman PJ: The origins of object perception. In Epstein W, Rogers S (Eds), Handbook of Perception and Cognition. New York: Academic Press, pp. 3–48, 1996.

Kellman PJ, Arterberry M: The Cradle of Knowledge: Development of Perception in Infancy. Cambridge, MA: MIT Press, 1998.

Kellman PJ, Banks MS: Infant visual perception. In Kuhn D, Siegler RS (Eds), Handbook of Child Psychology: Cognition, Perception, and Language, (5th ed., Vol. 2). New York: John Wiley and Sons, pp. 103–146, 1998.

Kellman PJ, Short KR: Development of three-dimensional form perception. Journal of Experimental Psychology: Human Perception and Performance: 13(4); 545–557, 1987.

Kellman PJ, Spelke ES: Perception of partly occluded objects in infancy. Cognitive Psychology: 15; 483–524, 1983.

Kleiner KA, Banks MS: Stimulus energy does not account for 2-month old preferences. Journal of Experimental Psychology: Human Perception and Performance: 13; 594–600, 1987.

Kuhl PK: Learning and representation in speech and language. Current Opinion in Neurobiology: 4; 812–822, 1994.

Larsen JS: The sagittal growth of the eye: IV. Ultrasonic measurement of the axial length of the eye from birth to puberty. Acta Ophthalmologica: 49; 873–886, 1971.

LaVail MM, Rapaport DH, Rakic P: Cytogenesis in the monkey retina. Journal of Comparative Neurology: 309; 86–114, 1991.

Leuba G, Garey LJ: A morphometric developmental study of dendrites in the lateral geniculate of the monkey. Neuroscience: 7 (Suppl) 131; 1982.

LeVay S, Wiesel TN, Hubel DH: The development of ocular dominance columns in normal and deprived monkeys. Journal of Comparative Neurology: 191; 1–51, 1980.

Levi DM, Carkeet A: Amblyopia: A consequence of abnormal visual development. In Simons K (Ed), Early Visual Development, Normal and Abnormal. Oxford: Oxford University Press, pp. 391–408, 1993.

Lewis TL, Maurer D: The development of the temporal and nasal visual fields during infancy. Vision Research: 32; 903–911, 1992.

Marr D: Vision. Cambridge, MA: MIT Press, 1982.

Maurer D, Lewis TL: The development of peripheral vision and its physiological underpinnings. In Weiss MJ, Zelazo PR (Eds), Newborn Attention: Biological Constraints and the Influence of Experience. Norwood, New Jersey: Ablex, pp. 218–255, 1991.

Maurer D, Lewis TL: Visual outcomes after infantile cataract. In Simons K (Ed), Early Visual Development, Normal and Abnormal. New York: Oxford University Press, 1993.

Maurer D, Lewis TL: Visual acuity: The role of visual input in inducing postnatal change. Clinical Neuroscience Research: 2001.

Maurer D, Lewis TL, Brent HP, Levin AV: Rapid improvement in the acuity of infants after visual input. Science: 286(5437); 108–110, 1999.

Mayer DL, Fulton AB: Development of the human visual field. In Simons K (Ed), Early Visual Development, Normal and Abnormal. New York: Oxford University Press, 1993.

Miller KD: Correlation-based models of neural development. In Gluck MA, Rumelhart DE (Eds), Neuroscience and Connectionist Theory. Hillsdale, NJ: Erlbaum, pp. 267–353, 1990.

Miller KD, Keller JB, Stryker MP: Ocular dominance column

development: Analysis and simulation. Science: 245; 605–615, 1989.

Mohindra I, Held R: Refraction in humans from birth to five years. Documenta Ophthalmologica: 28; 19–27, 1981.

Mohindra I, Held R, Gwiazda J, Brill S: Astigmatism in infants. Science: 202; 329–330, 1978.

Mohn G, Van Hof-van Duin J: Development of the binocular and monocular visual fields during the first year of life. Clinical Vision Sciences: 1; 51–64, 1986.

Mondloch CJ, Lewis TL, Budreau DR, Maurer D, Dannemiller JL, Stephens BR, Kleiner-Gathercoal KA: Face perception during early infancy. Psychological Science: 10(5); 419–422, 1999.

Nañez JE, Yonas A: Effects of luminance and texture motion on infant defensive reactions to optical collision. Infant Behavior and Development: 17(2); 165–174, 1994.

Nishimura Y, Rakic P: Development of the rhesus monkey retina: II. A three-dimensional analysis of the sequences of synaptic combinations of the inner plexiform layer. Journal of Comparative Neurology: 262; 290–313, 1987.

Norcia AM, Garcia H, Humphry R, Holmes A, Hamer RD, Orel-Bixler D: Anomalous motion VEPs in infants and in infantile esotropia. Investigative Ophthalmology and Visual Science: 32; 346–439, 1991.

O'Dell CD, Quick MW, Boothe RG: The development of stereoacuity in infant Rhesus monkeys. Investigative Ophthalmology and Visual Science (Supplement): 32; 1044, 1991.

Palmer SE: Vision Science. Cambridge, MA: MIT Press, 1999.

Pascalis O, De Schonen S, Morton J, Deruelle C, Fabre-Grenet M: Mother's face recognition by neonates: A replication and an extension. Infant Behavior and Development: 18; 79–85, 1995.

Payne BR, Pearson HE, Cornwell P: Development of connections in cat visual and auditory cortex. In Peters A, Jones EG (Eds), Cerebral Cortex: Development and Maturation of Cerebral Cortex. New York: Plenum Press, pp. 309–389, 1988.

Pettigrew JD: The effect of visual experience on the development of visual specificity by kitten cortical neurons. Journal of Physiology: 237; 49, 1974.

Piaget J, Inhelder B: The Child's Conception of Space (Langdon, FJ, Lunzer JL, Trans.). London: Routledge and Kegan Paul, 1948.

Purpura DP: Normal and aberrant neuronal development in the cerebral cortex of human fetus and young infant. In Buchwald NA, Brazier MAB (Eds), Brain Mechanisms of Mental Retardation. New York: Academic Press, 1975.

Rabinowicz T: The differential maturation of the human cerebral cortex. In Falkner F, Tanner JM (Eds), Human Growth vol. 3. Neurobiology and Nutrition. Plenum, New York: Plenum Press, 1979.

Rakic P: Neurons in rhesus monkey visual cortex: Systematic relation between time of origin and eventual disposition. Science: 183; 425–427, 1974.

Rakic P: Prenatal genesis of connections subserving ocular dominance in the rhesus monkey. Nature: 467–471, 1976.

Rakic P: An Overview — Development of the Primate Visual System: From Photoreceptors to Cortical Modules. In Lent R (Ed), The Visual System: From Genesis to Maturity. Boston: Birkhauser, pp. 1–17, 1992.

Rakic P, Riley KP: Overproduction and elimination of retinal axons in the fetal rhesus monkey. Science: 209; 1411–1444, 1983.

Royden CS, Crowell JA, Banks MS: Estimating heading during eye movements. Vision Research: 34(23); 3197–3214, 1994.

Schiff W: The perception of impending collision: A study of visually directed avoidant behavior. Psychological Monographs: 79(11, Whole No. 604); 1965.

Schmuckler MA, Li NS: Looming responses to obstacles and apertures: The role of accretion and deletion of background texture. Psychological Science: 9(1); 49–52, 1998.

Shatz CJ: Emergence of order in visual system development. Proceedings of the National Academy of Sciences: 93(2); 602–608, 1996.

Shatz CJ, Luskin MB: The relationship between the geniculocortical afferents and their cortical target cells during the development of the cat's primary visual cortex. Journal of Neuroscience: 6; 3655–3668, 1986.

Simons K (Ed): Early Visual Development, Normal and Abnormal. Oxford: Oxford University Press, 1993.

Sireteanu R: Development of the visual field: Results from human and animal studies. In Vital-Durand F, Atkinson J, Braddick OJ (Eds), Infant Vision. Oxford: Oxford University Press, pp. 17–31, 1996.

Skoczenski AM, Norcia AM: Development of VEP vernier acuity and grating acuity in human infants. Investigative Ophthamology and Visual Science: 40(10); 2411–2417, 1999.

Slater A, Mattock A, Brown E: Size constancy at birth: Newborn infants' responses to retinal and real size. Journal of Experimental Child Psychology: 49(2); 314–322, 1990.

Slater A, Morison V: Shape constancy and slant perception at birth. Perception: 14(3); 337–344, 1985.

Slater AM: Visual perceptual abilities at birth: Implications for face perception. In De Boysson-Bardies B, De Schonen S, Jusczyk P, MacNeilage P, Morton J (Eds), Developmental Neurocognition: Speech and Face Processing in the First Year of Life. Dordrecht: Kluwer Academic Press, pp. 125–134, 1993.

Slater AM, Morison V, Somers M: Orientation discrimination and cortical function in the human newborn. Perception: 17; 597–602, 1988.

Spelke ES, Breinlinger K, Macomber J, Jacobsen K: Origins of knowledge. Psychological Review: 99(4); 605–632, 1992.

Stein JF: The representation of egocentric space in the posterior parietal cortex. Behavioral and Brain Sciences: 15; 691–700, 1992.

Teller DY: The forced preferential looking procedure: A psychophysical technique for use with human infants. Infant Behavior and Development: 2; 77–86, 1979.

Teller DY: First glances: The vision of infants. Investigative Ophthalmology and Visual Science: 38; 2183–2203, 1997.

Teller DY, Bornstein M: Infant color vision and color perception. In Salapatek P, Cohen L (Eds), Handbook of Infant Perception, Vol I: From Sensation to Perception. Orlando, FL: Academic Press, 1987.

Teller DY, McDonald MA, Preston K, Sebris SL, Dobson V: Assessment of visual acuity in infants and children: The Acuity Card procedure. Developmental Medicine and Child Neurology: 28; 779–789, 1986.

Timney B: Development of binocular depth perception in kittens. Investigative Ophthalmology and Visual Science: 21; 493–496, 1981.

Tzourio N, De Schonen S, Mazoyer B et al.: Regional cerebral blood flow in two-month-old alert infants. Society for Neuroscience Abstracts: 18(2); 1121, 1992.

Ungerleider LG, Mishkin M: Two cortical visual systems: Separation of appearance and location of objects. In Ingle DL, Goodale MA, Mansfield RJW (Eds), Analysis of Visual Behavior. Cambridge, MA: MIT Press, pp. 549–586, 1982.

Van Essen DC, Anderson CH, Felleman DJ: Information processing in the primate visual system: An integrated system perspective. Science: 255; 419–422, 1992.

Vital-Durand F, Atkinson J, Braddick OJ: Infant Vision. Oxford: Oxford University Press, 1996.

Von Hofsten C, Kellman P, Putaansuu J: Young infants' sensitivity to motion parallax. Infant Behavior and Development: 15(2); 245–264, 1992.

Warren WH, Morris MW, Kalish M: Perception of translational heading from optic flow. Journal of Experimental Psychology: Human Perception and Performance: 14; 646–660, 1988.

Wattam-Bell JRB: Development of visual motion processing. In Vital-Durand F, Atkinson J (Eds), Infant Vision. Oxford: Oxford University Press, 1996.

Westheimer G: Visual hyperacuity. Progress in Sensory Physiology: 1; 1–30, 1981.

Wiesel TN, Hubel DH: Comparison of the effects of unilateral and bilateral eye closure on cortical unit responses in kittens. Journal of Neurophysiology: 28; 1029–1040, 1965.

Wiesel TN, Hubel DH: Ordered arrangement of orientation columns in monkeys lacking visual experience. Journal of Comparative Neurology: 158; 307–318, 1974.

Wikler KC, Rakic P: Emergence of the photoreceptor mosaic from a protomap of early-differentiating cones in the primate retina. Nature: 352; 397–400, 1991.

Wilson HR: Theories of Infant Visual Development. In Simons K (Ed), Early Visual Development, Normal and Abnormal. Oxford: Oxford University Press, pp. 560–572, 1993.

Yonas A, Arterberry ME, Granrud CE: Space perception in infancy. In Vasta R (Ed), Annals of Child Development, Vol. 4. London: JAI, pp. 1–34, 1987.

Yonas A, Granrud CE: Development of visual space perception in young infants. In Mehler J, Fox R (Eds), Neonate Cognition: Beyond the Blooming Buzzing Confusion. Hillsdale, NJ: Lawrence Erlbaum, 1985.

Yonas A, Pettersen L, Lockman J: Young infants' sensitivity to optical information for collision. Canadian Journal of Psychology: 33; 268–276, 1979.

Yuodelis C, Hendrickson A: A qualitative and quantitative analysis of the human fovea during development. Vision Research: 26; 847–855, 1986.

© 2003 Published by Elsevier Science B.V.
Handbook of Neuropsychology, 2nd Edition, Vol. 8, Part II
S.J. Segalowitz and I. Rapin (Eds)

CHAPTER 18

Cognitive development in children with visual impairments

David H. Warren [a,*] and Deborah D. Hatton [b]

[a] *Department of Psychology, University of California, Riverside, CA 92521, USA*
[b] *Frank Porter Graham Child Development Center, University of North Carolina, Chapel Hill, NC, USA*

Introduction

In a word, cognition is thought. Cognition allows the human being to go beyond perception, to deal with aspects of the world without actually being in perceptual contact with them. Freedom from perceptual contact allows a person to deal with things that are remembered (no longer within perceptual contact), abstract (not available for perceptual contact), or even imaginary (what if people had three legs?). In all of these cases, cognition depends on representation: the person deals with mental concepts in various ways, rather than with direct and immediate experience.

Human neonates do not think in the same way 5-year-olds do, and even 10-year-olds do not enjoy the same flexibility of thought processes that adults do. In short, cognition develops.

When cognition develops under conditions of visual impairment, there is potential for the developmental process to differ from sighted development. One major purpose of this chapter is to outline what is known about the similarities and differences in cognitive development when vision is and is not impaired. The second major purpose is to present what is known about the variables that affect cognitive development under conditions of visual impairment. Our orientation will be to both population characteristics and individual differences. In particular, we attempt to identify those factors that produce variability around population norms. These factors include both status variables (such as functional vision, prematurity, or additional disabilities) and environmental variables.

The traditional use of the term 'cognitive', as applied to representation and thought process, is gradually being expanded to apply to many areas of human function which either feed into thought or depend in some sense on thought. In this chapter, we adopt this larger usage: thus we will treat thought not only in the traditional usage, but also in relation to areas such as spatial orientation, language, attention, and memory.

Our treatment of this area will be selective of the literature and, for that matter, of the specific topics. Not all possible topics are considered, and not all available sources are mentioned. Our goal is to provide a representative, not an exhaustive, treatment.

The larger plan of the chapter is to deal first with the traditional issues of the development of concepts and representation. We will then turn to specialized areas within cognition such as language development, attention, and spatial concepts. A short section on electrophysiological and neuroimaging correlates will be followed by a discussion of assessment and research methodology

Infancy

Research in developmental psychology and neuroscience has affirmed the important contribution of vision to early development. Infants have an innate

* Corresponding author. E-mail: david.warren@ucr.edu

ability to recognize faces visually even a few hours after birth (Johnson, 1999; Johnson, Dziurawiec, Ellis and Morton, 1991), and innate reflexes prime both the caregiver and infant for intersubjective interactions (Aitken and Trevarthen, 1997; Bigelow, 1995; Preisler, 1995, 1997) and attachment. The primacy of vision in facilitating attachment, affective development, and prelinguistic communication has been documented by researchers of both sighted and blind children (Fraiberg, 1977; Mundy and Willoughby, 1996; Preisler, 1991, 1995; Rogers and Puchalski, 1984; Rowland, 1984). Additionally, visual imitation, a predictor of language development and therefore inextricably tied to cognition, is not possible for infants who are blind (Bigelow, 1995; Preisler, 1995, 1997). Without the lure of vision, blind infants have little interest in objects and the external world during their first 12–18 months (Bigelow, 1995; Preisler, 1995, 1997), further placing cognitive development at risk. Schore (1996) theorizes that the reciprocal gaze of caregiver and infant stimulates neural growth in the prefrontal cortex, suggesting that blindness may fundamentally alter the structure or processes of the brain.

The fundamental importance of vision is such that visual impairment can have a variety of impacts on the course of development. During infancy cognitive, motor, affective, communicative, and perceptual development are completely interwoven. Perhaps the most fundamental is the social–emotional phenomenon of attachment.

Attachment and social–emotional development in infancy

Early in the first year of life the infant begins to make various responses, such as smiling and vocalizing, to the initiation of social interactions by other people. Midway during the first year these responses begin to narrow in their target, such that they occur not indiscriminately but in response to a small number of people, typically the mother and/or father. Accompanying this narrowing of positive responses is a developing wariness of strangers. The development of attachment depends not only on the infant's exhibiting the appropriate behaviors (e.g., smiling, vocalizing) but on the parent's perceiving and responding appropriately to them. In turn, the parent's presence and responsiveness must be perceived by the infant.

The 'security' of the attachment relationship is thought to be related to the infant's willingness to venture outward into the environment to explore and experience it, and therefore develop understanding of the physical world. The infant's earliest social–emotional responses serve not only to maintain the proximity of other people for protection and sustenance, but also to set the stage for the development of more mature social relationships.

Because of the importance of vision as a communicative vehicle, the infant with visual impairment is at risk in these developments. Indeed, Rogers and Puchalski (1988) found indices of attachment at around 13 months in visually impaired infants, in contrast to the normative age of 6–9 months for sighted infants. The dynamics of this are evident. A parent who may already be distressed by the fact of a visual impairment may be inclined to mute the quality and quantity of his/her emotional responses to the infant's initiations, and an adverse cycle may occur. Evidence bears out this scenario. From two months on, the infant without vision does not respond to caregivers or to the external world in the same manner as sighted infants (Bigelow, 1995; Fraiberg, 1977; Preisler, 1991, 1997). Adaptive strategies such as stilling or freezing to better attend to sound may be interpreted as rejection by parents (Fraiberg, 1977; Preisler, 1991). Being picked up unexpectedly without sound cues might startle the child in a way not found in sighted infants who can see and anticipate such actions. Rogers and Puchalski (1984) and Rowland (1984) found that normatively, blind infants were less productive of behaviors that tend to elicit positive maternal affective response, and that in turn, mothers were less likely to visually engage the infant and were therefore likely to miss the signals that the infants *did* produce. Preisler (1991, 1995) described similar interactions in her study of blind infants in Sweden.

However, Als, Tronick and Brazelton (1980) and Preisler (1991, 1995) documented positive adaptations in some mother–infant dyads that compensated for the lack of vision. Als et al. (1980) described interactions in which the mother was highly responsive to the blind infant and created a situation of 'affective reciprocity' with the infant by engaging in a set of highly interactive behaviors that effectively engaged the infant and resulted in what would currently be described as affect attunement. Preisler (1991) used videotapes of parent–child interactions with parents that facilitated the ability of parents to read and respond to their children's cues. Specialized early intervention is now more accessible to families and children and should facilitate this process. Indeed, recent research reveals that early interventionists recognize the importance of helping parents learn to read their infants' cues and respond in ways that may not be instinctual. As affirmation, parents report that specialized early intervention has helped them and their children by providing guidance and access to resources (Hatton and Waring, 1999).

Thus while visual impairment does create a condition of risk, the development of attachment is not necessarily impeded. More uncertain, however, is how lack of vision impacts relationships outside the family. Insight into the challenges facing infants and toddlers in the development of social relationships with others can be gained by examining the development of communication.

The basis for communication

In recent years infancy researchers have turned their attention to the dynamic communicative processes developing in the first year that form the basis for the infant's acquisition of concepts of, and an orientation to, the external world. The fundamental basis for these communicative processes appears to be the affective relationship between infant and primary caretaker; thus early communication is closely intertwined with attachment. Increasingly, we are coming to understand the critical communicative link with the caregiver as the functional basis for these developments.

Vision is an important element in this process. Consider the nature of the infant–caregiver interaction in the first year. In the first few months the interaction is characterized by a face-to-face dyadic relationship with eye-to-eye contact and vocalization accompanied by touching. Indeed, the infant's early reaching is often to features of the parent's face, and this is accompanied by mutual vocalization. As the infant's interest becomes captured by other events in mid-year, the dyadic relationship begins to include external events that become the focus for shared attention, imitation, vocalization, and eventually shared referential labeling. These events also become a vehicle for the infant's expression of intentionality, as the infant learns that the caregiver can become the instrument of operation on events. Consequently, the infant learns effective ways of communicating intentionality, whether by directing the caregiver's gaze to a desired object by shared eye-contact or by vocal or gestural means. At the same time, the infant begins to understand that the caregiver is a distinct person with his/her own needs and actions that are separate from those of the infant (and not always immediately accessible to address the infant's desires).

Numerous researchers have documented the impact of blindness on early communication (Bigelow, 1987, 1990; Fraiberg, 1977; McConachie and Moore, 1994; Preisler, 1991, 1995, 1997; Rowland, 1984; Urwin, 1984). Preisler's longitudinal qualitative study of five blind infants in Sweden probably best describes the potentially adverse impact of blindness on prelinguistic communication. Rogers and Puchalski (1984) also demonstrated difficulties inherent in the earliest communication between blind infants and their caregivers.

However, positive outcomes are possible as well. Preisler (1991, 1995, 1997) and Als et al. (1980) showed that responsive interactions with parents can facilitate prelinguistic communication. Responsive caregivers used body-touching games to help infants anticipate actions. Initially, infants produced subtle signs, gestures, or actions that show that they anticipated the next action. These types of activities, and responsiveness to and imitation of new sounds made by the infant, facilitate the acquisition of communication abilities.

These interactions illustrate how aspects of early development are inextricably woven together and that impediments in any one area may transact to impact the other areas. For example, infants who are securely attached are motivated to communicate with their caregivers. These communicative interactions help the infant learn about others and eventually the external world. Interactions with the outside world expand communicative abilities and serve as the basis for cognitive development. Cognitively, the emerging interpersonal understandings of imitation, shared attention, and turn-taking are part of the infant's emerging 'theory of mind' or development of intersubjectivity (Bigelow, 1995). We will address this issue in the section on perspective-taking.

Early motor development

In considering the relationship between cognitive and motor development in infancy, we return briefly to attachment and affective development. Secure attachment is associated with a child's willingness to move out into the world and explore. Using social referencing, sighted infants typically move out from their mothers to explore new territory with frequent looks back to assess the mother's emotional expression and location.

Initially, then, the blind infant is at a disadvantage because s/he lacks the innate visual lure that facilitates attachment to parents as well as motivating movement into and acquiring knowledge of the world. Fraiberg (1977) and Preisler (1991, 1995, 1997) documented that caregivers' reactions to the disability can affect the affordances available for children. Indeed, infants who are blind are uniquely dependent on their caregivers as mediators of the environment since they are less able to acquire incidental information about the world (Bigelow, 1995; Nesker-Simmons and Davidson, 1992; Preisler, 1991, 1995, 1997).

Sighted infants acquire concepts of space, distance, and location/orientation as they begin to sit, crawl, pull to stand, and walk. Along the way, they see many interesting objects that elicit exploration through vision, mouthing, and touch. Thus, as sighted children acquire motor milestones, their world is enlarged, and cognitive development is facilitated. Parents of blind infants must be extraordinarily persistent in motivating their children to move out into the world. In doing so, they often must overcome their own fearfulness and tendency to be overly protective.

One notable characteristic of infants who are blind is the lack of visual regard of the hands. Visual regard of the hands facilitates midline orientation and hand–eye and hand–mouth coordination and typically begins around three months of age. An infant without vision may be observed with hands and shoulders rotated outward, often with hands held at shoulder height. This posture does not facilitate haptic exploration of objects, and consequently does not facilitate cognitive development. Additionally, it tends to impede midline exploration, transfer of objects, and reaching. Combined with an early lack of interest in toys/objects (Preisler, 1991, 1995, 1997), these factors may contribute to and transact with a deficiency in understanding objects and their relationship to the infant and to each other that impedes optimal cognitive development in children without vision.

Although sighted infants typically begin to crawl in the third quarter of the first year, clinical and research reports indicate that on the average, blind infants do not begin to crawl until the beginning of the second year (Adelson and Fraiberg, 1974; Norris, Spaulding and Brodie, 1957; Tröster, Hecker and Brambring, 1994). And whereas sighted infants typically take their first steps by the end of the first year, this is correspondingly delayed for blind infants. Subsequent locomotor activities involving the gross musculature are delayed in infants with visual impairments (e.g., Adelson and Fraiberg, 1974; Norris et al., 1957; Preisler, 1995; Sonksen, Levitt and Kitzinger, 1984; Tröster et al., 1994). Additionally, delays in postural skills and righting reactions have also been reported (Jan, Sykander and Groenveld, 1990; Sonksen et al., 1984).

There are multiple reasons for these apparent delays. One possibility is that the large musculature develops more slowly, thereby delaying those behaviors that depend on it. The evidence does not favor this explanation: for example the developmental item 'stands alone' does not typically show as much normative delay as the item 'walks alone'. Furthermore, blind infants are observed to be poised on hands and knees, apparently ready to crawl from a muscular point of view, well before they actually do crawl. Indeed, Tröster et al. (1994) found several infants who walked before they crawled. On the other hand, hypotonia is often noted in blind infants as well as in many children with developmental delays (Jan et al., 1990; Sonksen et al., 1984). Passivity and lack of opportunity to move are associated with hypotonia, and this is undoubtedly a factor in the delayed acquisition of motor skills in some blind infants (Jan, Robinson, Scott and Kinnis, 1975; Sonksen et al., 1984).

Nor does the simple lack of vision hold a ready explanation. Studies that have examined the variance in the onset of locomotor indicators typically find a wide variance, with some infants beginning to crawl and walk well within normative ranges for sighted infants (Norris et al., 1957).

While lack of vision may not have a direct causal effect, the evidence is good that it has an indirect effect (Ferrell, 1998; Ferrell, Trief, Deitz et al., 1990; Tröster et al., 1994). Infants do not crawl or walk just for the sake of accomplishing those activities, but rather to accomplish some end. Vision may well serve as an external stimulus to engage in crawling or walking, such as obtaining a toy which is not within reach. Indeed, there is some evidence that young children with limited vision have better motor skills than those who have no visual function (Hatton, Bailey, Burchinal and Ferrell, 1997; Reynell, 1978). Of course, other sensory modalities (hearing, smell) might signal the existence of an object to be attained but not with the simultaneous and detailed quality of vision. Fraiberg (1968) did not find earlier crawling despite continued attempts to induce reaching and crawling in response to an external sounding object.

The inability to see and imitate the actions of others directly impacts motor development in blind children. Such simple activities as waving bye-bye and patty cake become more difficult in the absence of vision. Sighted children typically acquire many motor skills through incidental learning and visual imitation of others. These skills must be modeled through other senses in the absence of vision, or language must be used to guide the child through the steps. In that case, the child is required to cognitively construct a representation of a motor activity, rather than simply basing it on perception. In the case of modeling through other senses, the representation that results from touch and movement is likely different from that acquired perceptually through vision.

An important factor is the provision of opportunity and encouragement to crawl and walk. Norris et al. (1957) noted impressive individual differences in their sample of infants and found that those who were delayed in locomotion were 'typically those who were not given appropriate opportunities' (p. 39). Similarly, Brambring (1996) found considerable variability in outcomes to be related to positive parental interactions and encouragement of activity. It is clear that the provision of appropriate opportunities to the infant is an important factor in the onset of locomotion. Tröster et al. (1994) suggested that vision may also serve to reduce the anxiety associated with locomotion such as by being able to see the parent's face indicating that 'it's OK'.

Perhaps most important of all factors to the onset of locomotion is the acquisition of the object concept. Bigelow (1986, 1990, 1992), Fraiberg (1977), Rogers and Puchalski (1988), and Tröster and Brambring (1993) have documented critical relationships between motor and cognitive development. The general finding is that reaching for objects, crawling/walking, or other movements outward to the environment do not occur until blind infants have acquired the object concept. Interestingly, young blind children may use words before they acquire the object concept, but they do not move out into the environment prior to the acquisition of this important milestone.

The object concept

When a child's behavior indicates that he or she regards an object as continuing to exist, despite not receiving immediate perceptual information about it, the child is said to have achieved the object concept (or the concept of object permanence). This acquisition is viewed as an index of cognitive growth because the child's knowledge is no longer dependent on specific sensory stimulation. Acquisition of the object concept represents the beginnings of conceptual memory.

Piaget (1970) emphasized the role of vision in the acquisition of the object concept. The distal senses, audition and vision, both may convey information about the continued existence of an object when it is out of tactual contact, but auditory information is typically discontinuous. Thus without vision, according to Piaget's argument, it is more difficult for the child to understand that the object does not cease to exist when it is not in tactual contact, and thus the blind child should develop the object concept more slowly, though presumably in the same order. Corroborating Piaget's expectation, Bigelow (1986) provided solid evidence that blind infants progress through the stages of object concept attainment in the same order that sighted infants do. In addition numerous studies have found evidence for the expected delays: normatively, visually impaired infants' progress in achieving the object concept is slower than that of sighted infants (Bigelow, 1986, 1990; Ferrell et al., 1990; Fraiberg, 1968; Reynell, 1978; Rogers and Puchalski, 1988).

Although on the average the course of attainment of the object concept is slower, there are sufficient counter-examples to suggest that visual impairment does not necessarily interfere with that attainment. Fraiberg, Siegel and Gibson (1966) and Als et al. (1980) have provided examples of behaviors that show children with visual impairments to have attained components of the object concept at normative or near-normative ages, and other studies show substantial individual variation (Bigelow, 1986; Schwartz, 1984). Rogers and Puchalski (1988) tested 20 infants over time with a variety of suitably adapted tasks. On the average, the acquisition of substage behaviors was substantially delayed. However, the standard deviations were large, and Rogers and Puchalski also reported the range of ages at acquisition in addition to the means. For virtually every test item, there were blind infants in the sample who passed the item well within the normative age range for sighted children. This is a critical finding, since it suggests that visual impairment does not necessarily impede the acquisition of the object concept.

We thus turn to the variables that might affect the rate of acquisition. One such variable is functional vision, and indeed the evidence (e.g., Bigelow, 1990; Fraiberg, 1968; Reynell, 1978) suggests that residual vision is beneficial in this development. A second general factor is experience, and this can take several forms. One is the quality of motor and locomotor engagement with the spatial environment: it is likely that restricted motor experience restricts the acquisition of spatial concepts. Another experiential factor has to do with the quality of perceptual experience. Fraiberg's 'educational' program provided the infants with a variety of toys designed to unite tactual and auditory experience, and these may have facilitated object concept acquisition by drawing the infants' attention to their spatial surroundings. Finally, Als et al. (1980) argued that the quality of the emotional bond between parent and infant is critical in providing the infant with a sense of security sufficient to allow effective engagement of the physical environment.

Infants who have a fully mature object concept not only search for a disappeared object in the several locations in which they have previously experienced it, but also search in other possible locations even if they have not experienced the object there. For example, Fraiberg et al. (1966) reported that none of their children exhibited this level of activity even by three years of age, whereas the normative age for this acquisition is one and a half to two years. It may be that the very clear difficulties that severely visually impaired infants and young children have with the acquisition of spatial concepts makes attainment of the mature object concept particularly difficult, and this is undoubtedly tied to the typically delayed emergence of locomotor activity at just this period of development. Again, separating cognition from other areas of development proves to be a very difficult and ultimately unrewarding pursuit.

In sum, while acquisition of the object concept proceeds more slowly in the absence of vision, the dramatic individual differences illustrated in the literature suggest that typical development may be facilitated by the provision of an appropriate experiential basis.

Classification

Much of human conceptual behavior involves the creation and manipulation of classes of events and information. As development proceeds, children acquire the ability to form conceptual classes, to add new experiences appropriately to them, and to modify them as they prove inadequate to accommodate new experiences and information. They come to recognize that while the members of a given conceptual class share some attributes in common, they also differ on other attributes; therefore, alternative classifications are possible and important. They understand that various concepts are subordinate and/or superordinate to one another. In short, the development of mature thought requires adequate ability to deal with classification.

Higgins (1973) evaluated classification skills of blind and visually impaired children aged 5–11 years, of average IQ, and with at most light perception. Higgins reached two key conclusions. First, the development of aspects of classification emerged with age in much the same way that Piaget and others had found for sighted children: the general principle of cognitive growth, that the emergence of operational skills depends on the prior acquisition of preoperational thought, applies to blind and visually impaired as well as to sighted children. Second, there was a pattern of divergence between abstract and concrete concepts, with the former lagging behind the latter as expected. Higgins concluded that experience, not visual status, is the primary factor influencing the course of cognitive development.

Other factors influence the emergence of classification. Hatwell (1966, 1985) compared congenitally blind (defined as visual loss within the first year) with adventitiously blind (vision for at least 4 years) children on several tasks, and found a significant advantage of the latter group on several classification tasks. The role of partial vision was examined by Friedman and Pasnak (1973) using verbal and tactual tests of seriation and classification. For the younger (8- and 11-year-old) groups, children with some functional vision made generally fewer errors than the totally blind children on the tactual tasks, but not on the verbal tasks. The oldest group (14 years) did not show this difference.

Several studies (Higgins, 1973; Tillman, 1967a,b; Zweibelson and Barg, 1967) have examined the performance of visually impaired children on tests involving abstract and concrete items, particularly intelligence test items, and have typically reported relatively weaker performance on the abstract material than on the concrete. Unfortunately, none of these studies has examined the relationship between the abstract–concrete dimension and the child's experiential history or general intellectual level. Hammill and Powell (1967) found no differences between blind and partially sighted children, but both chronological age and IQ were significantly correlated with scores on the abstraction test.

In the work discussed up to this point, the youngest subjects have been 5 years of age. Gerhardt (1982) reported a classification study of a single blind infant at the ages of 14, 16, and 18 months. Over the 4-month span, the infant showed the predicted progress from grouping dissimilar items to making similarity-based classifications. Although research with infants is difficult, full understanding of the development of classification skills in older children will depend on complete study of blind infants and preschool children, particularly in relation to the child's accumulating experiences.

Several studies (Adkins, 1965; Friedman and Pasnak, 1973; Lebron-Rodriguez and Pasnak, 1977) show success in training of classification skills. The relationships among the skills to be trained, the training materials, and the child's general level of accomplishment and specific experiential history need careful study, as does the training outcome in relation to its practical function in the child's educational and everyday experience.

Conservation

Conservation refers in general to conceptual understanding of properties of the physical world. Many aspects of conservation have been studied: those that have been most thoroughly studied with blind and visually impaired children are substance (mass), weight, and displacement volume.

With sighted children, these tasks are typically performed based on visual presentation of the materials. The usual adaptation for visually impaired children is to give the child haptic exposure to the stimulus materials; in the case of partially sighted subjects, the available vision is usually occluded.

A spectrum of studies (Gottesman, 1973; Hatwell, 1985; Miller, 1969; Stephens and Simpkins, 1974; Swanson, Minifie and Minifie, 1979; Wan-Lin and Tait, 1987) have addressed conservation abilities with blind and partially sighted children. In general, the acquisition of conservation abilities appears delayed in relation to chronological age, but the order of acquisition of the various concepts is similar to that of sighted children. However, there is a great deal of variation in results. Likely sources of variation include current visual status, age of onset of impairment, and school–home characteristics.

Several studies (e.g., Wan-Lin and Tait, 1987) compared groups of partially sighted and totally blind children and found each conservation ability in the partially sighted group to precede that of the totally blind group by a year to several years. Other studies (e.g., Hatwell, 1985) found that adventitiously blind subjects are developmentally earlier to show conservation of weight and substance than children who were blind at birth or became blind within their first year. This advantage of children with a period of early vision is a pervasive one in the literature.

Another factor that is complex but of potential interest is school and home environments. Samples vary in their selection of children from residential schools and regular schools, and consequently from institutional and home environments. In complex ways, this combination of characteristics may affect the acquisition of cognitive skills. In general, studies which have used mainly visually impaired children who were educated within the public school setting (e.g., Gottesman, 1973) tend to show earlier acquisition of conservation than those whose subjects were primarily from residential schools for the blind (e.g., Stephens and Simpkins, 1974).

Other studies have evaluated the home–school setting variable directly. For example, Brekke, Williams and Tait (1974) found a significantly better conservation of weight by children living at home than by those in the institutional setting. Finally, Wan-Lin and Tait (1987) and Tait (1990) found that naturally occurring cultural differences in specific experiences had systematic relationships to acquisition of conservation concepts.

Language development

As described earlier in this chapter, the impact of vision loss on prelinguistic communication between infant and caregiver is considerable and impacts other areas of development. Studies of language development in young children with visual impairment have primarily focused on comparative studies, sometimes with conflicting results. An exception is the longitudinal study of development across domains described by Hatton et al. (1997).

In this longitudinal study of 186 children with visual impairments aged 12–73 months, the Battelle Developmental Inventory was used as a standardized index of development in order to plot individual and group growth curves for both overall development and development across cognitive, communication, motor, personal–social, and adaptive domains (Hatton et al., 1997). The presence of additional disabilities and the amount of vision significantly affected the mean level of communication development. This finding was consistent for overall development and development in all other domains. Additional disabilities also had a significant impact on the rate of development; communication developed at about half the rate of children without additional disabilities. Interestingly, however, amount of vision seemed to impact language development to a lesser extent than that observed in any other domain for children with and without additional disabilities. When compared to the other domains, children with visual function of 20/800 or worse scored higher on communication than on any other domain including cognition. These findings are consistent with those reported by Reynell (1978) who also found that language seemed to be less affected by amount of vision than sensori-motor understanding or exploration of the environment.

In contrast to Hatton et al.'s (1997) study that provided a relatively gross measure of communication development across a wide age-span, researchers from a variety of disciplines have looked at various aspects of language using microanalytic methods. Researchers examining the acquisition of words, or the lexicon, of children with visual impairment have reported contradictory findings. Delays in the emergence of first words have been reported by some researchers (Fraiberg, 1977; McConachie and Moore, 1994; Norris et al., 1957; Reynell, 1978) while others have noted that language emerges within the normal range for sighted children (Bigelow, 1990; Mulford, 1988). It must be noted, however, that Bigelow's study included only 3 subjects and that Mulford's study was based on a re-analysis of 16 case studies previously described in the literature. Mulford acknowledged that although acquisition might be within the typical ranges for children with vision, there were major qualitative differences in language and how it was used by children without vision. In fact, qualitative differences in the language of young children with visual impairment form a pervasive theme in this literature (Andersen, Dunlea and Kekelis, 1984; Dunlea, 1989; McConachie and Moore, 1994; Mills, 1988; Mulford, 1988). Differences have been documented in acquired word types and their use (Andersen et al., 1984; McConachie and Moore, 1994). Additionally, difficulties in reciprocity, pragmatics (Andersen et al., 1984; Bigelow, 1987; Dunlea, 1989; McConachie and Moore, 1994; Mills, 1988; Mulford, 1988), illocutionary force or strength of intentionality (Dunlea, 1989), referential communication (Dunlea, 1989; Preisler, 1991), and morphological development (Dunlea and Andersen, 1992) have been identified as qualitative differences between the language of children with and without vision.

Specifically, young children with visual impairment acquire words that are directly related to themselves and their own experiences. They seldom extend words as sighted children do (e.g., calling a cow a dog); and they do not drop words from their vocabularies. As could be expected and as discussed in the infancy section, lack of access to the visual world and to the nonverbal communication of others impedes development of reciprocity, referential communication, and pragmatics. The inability to visually detect the interest of others based on eye gaze and to catch a person's eye makes initiation and maintenance of conversations challenging, particularly at the preschool level, where nonverbal communication facilitates engagement with play groups and individuals. The Kekelis (1996) study of discourse skills in young children without vision demonstrated differences in discourse between two children without vision and their mothers and two children with vision and their mothers. Children without vision were less likely to respond contingently to questions or directives, and they produced fewer utterances per turn than children with vision. Kekelis noted the importance of these skills in pragmatics and suggested that these differences may account for the lack of fluent discourse between young children with visual impairments and communicative partners reported in other studies (Kekelis, 1992; Kekelis and Sacks, 1992; MacCuspie, 1992).

The impact of parents on the development of communication in children with visual impairment has been described in three studies. Kekelis and Andersen (1984) examined the influence of parents' communication and found that parents of children with visual impairment tend to label objects rather than providing rich descriptions of form and function that might compensate for a lack of vision. In addition, parents of children with visual impairment used more imperatives.

Moore and McConachie (1994) conducted a study with ten subjects, rather than four, and their findings were similar. However, they found a difference in language input from parents depending on whether the child was totally blind or severely visually impaired. (Severely visually impaired subjects had object perception or better while subjects considered blind had light perception at best.) Request for actions was the most frequent type of utterance by parents of both groups. Parents of children with severe visual impairment used more imperatives, and they were more likely to talk about topics within the current context and to describe the attributes of objects. Parents of children who were blind tended to talk about topics in a future context, rather than the here and now, an omission that deprives children of information related to the nonverbal context. Additionally, parents of children who were blind made significantly more initiations than did the parents of children with severe visual impairment. Finally, in a correlational study of 18 toddlers (20–36 months) who were legally blind, Dote-Kwan (1995) found that maternal responsiveness, as compared to mother initiation, was positively related to developmental outcome. Specifically, the children of mothers who responded to the initiations of their children (i.e., paraphrased or repeated the child's communicative acts and then expanded the acts by adding new information) and facilitated turntaking, or reciprocity, in vocal interactions (i.e., pacing their speech and pauses in speech) had better developmental scores on the Maxfield–Buchholz and Reynell–Zinkin Scales (Dote-Kwan, 1995).

In examining the relationship between cognition and communication, Bigelow (1990), McConachie and Moore (1994), and Rogers and Puchalski (1988) found that the acquisition of language is not tied to the object concept, a marker for symbolic representation. However, Rogers and Puchalski did find that symbolic play was related to language development in that children who were able to use 'no' and 'you' appropriately also engaged in symbolic play. Although Piaget suggested that experiences form the basis for language development, evidence from studies of language in young children with visual impairment call this theory into question. Repeatedly, authors discuss how blind children seem to acquire more advanced language without having the concrete experiential base that might be thought to be a prerequisite. Both Bigelow (1990) and Dunlea (1989) suggest that a shared base underlies language and cognitive development in these children, particularly since the object concept does not seem to be a prerequisite for language acquisition. The finding that expressive language was higher than receptive by McConachie and Moore (1994) and that communication scores of children with visual function of 20/800 or worse were markedly higher than cognitive scores by Hatton et al. (1997) provide further evidence. These results must be tempered by acknowledging that it is difficult to assess cognitive status in very young children with visual impairment. However, the microanalyses reported by Bigelow (1990) and Rogers and Puchalski (1988) are consistent with the results of both Hatton et al. (1997) and McConachie and Moore (1994).

Dunlea and Andersen (1992) demonstrated the importance of studying language acquisition as a process in their study of morphological development. In addition, they found evidence that cognition and language acquisition vary from child to child and that one may facilitate development of the other, depending on particular words and concepts. Their discussion of the relationship between cognition and language in children without vision was as informative as their finding that the morphological development of children with no vision or with reduced vision varies from each other and from that of sighted children.

Several authors suggest that the inability to decenter or share the perspective of others interferes with language and cognitive development in young children with visual impairment (Andersen et al., 1984; Bigelow, 1990; Dunlea, 1989). Others suggest that anomalies in cognitive structures themselves may account for language differences. Hatwell's (1985) description of the disruption of accommodation and assimilation provides the most eloquent treatment of this subject. She argues convincingly that the cognitive development of children without vision must be different because of their inability to abstract the criterial features of objects and the environment. The lack of over-extensions reported in studies of the language of young children without vision provides support for this theory.

Studies of language development have provided the richest descriptions of the development of children with visual impairment to date. Although it is apparent that the acquisition and use of language is quite different in young children with visual impairment, it is also apparent that its emergence heralds a dynamic new stage of development. Language appears to be used in a compensatory fashion to facilitate the acquisition of abstract thought (Hatwell, 1985; Reynell, 1978), as well as a tool for initiating interactions. The inability to use eye gaze to initiate interactions at younger ages likely impedes both communication and social development. Thus language acquisition, though delayed and qualitatively different, offers a powerful tool to facilitate growth in those areas as well as a means to assess and facilitate cognitive development, and to enhance motor and adaptive skill acquisition (e.g., through verbal descriptions of skills that cannot be seen).

Perceptual and cognitive perspective-taking

Several specific and general phenomena are related to the child's understanding of another person's perception and thought. These phenomena have been studied under various rubrics for many years but have in the past decade been increasingly, and usefully, referred to as *Theory of Mind.* Flavell (1988) has provided important conceptual frameworks for the more recent work, which generally shows an emerging capability to understand perspective-taking over the preschool and elementary school years.

Cratty (1969) observed that a pair of blind twins discovered around the age of 4 or 5 years that they could 'hide' from one another simply by remaining silent, whereas they could not do this with their (sighted) mother. This instance illustrates an emerging awareness of the role of perception and specifically the limitations on visual perception by the blind child, and it is of interest as a cognitive phenomenon.

Bigelow (1988, 1992) evaluated the emergence of this kind of perceptual understanding in two blind brothers over the age range 4–8 years. The essential task involved asking the child to 'show' an item to a sighted or a blind (i.e., the child's brother) observer. Responses suggested that even at the youngest age, there was a fundamental understanding that an object did not need to be within the sighted observer's tactual grasp, but that this was requisite for 'showing' an object to the blind sibling. On the other hand, there was incomplete understanding of the importance of sight lines even at the upper age studied.

Bigelow (1991) reported similar findings in the context of sightlines and the requirements for an object to be hidden. Interestingly, some children equated self-exposure with the mouth rather than with the eyes as tends to be the case with sighted children.

Farrenkopf and Davidson (1992) evaluated the emergence of perspective-taking using larger samples of early-blind children with at most light perception over the 3–8-year age range. They did not find strong evidence of age-related improvement in perspective-taking, although the data trends were in the expected direction. The authors discussed the importance of framing the experimental situation and the questions in a way that is clearly understandable to children; indeed, this may have been the primary difficulty with the study, or it may be that reliable age trends would have emerged with the inclusion of older children.

An interesting point of semantics is suggested by Bigelow's work and reflects a point made by Landau and Gleitman (1985), who noted that young blind children whom they studied consistently used the word 'look' to mean 'search' (i.e., look for), and the word 'see' to mean 'perceive'. The point is a cautionary one that blind children may not invest particular words with the same semantic value that sighted children (or researchers!) do.

Minter, Hobson and Bishop (1998) carried the corresponding issue into the realm of cognition by evaluating blind children's ideas of what other children believe. The paradigm involved inducing the subject child to have a false (i.e., counter-intuitive) belief about an event (the contents of a teapot), then correcting that belief, then ascertaining whether the child would attribute the same false belief to another (visually impaired) peer. Sighted children were tested as well. The age range was 5–9 years. More of the blind children than the sighted children supposed that the peer would hold the corrected (counter-intuitive) belief rather than the false belief. Children who performed correctly tended to have higher mental age and IQ. It should be noted that though there were significant differences between blind and sighted groups, considerable numbers of the blind children gave correct responses on the various tasks, and it can be concluded that there is more similarity than difference between the groups.

The emerging literature on theory of mind should prove to be a valuable tool in our quest to understand the nature of the visually impaired child's understanding of perception and cognition.

Attention and memory

The development of concepts and of conceptual abilities depends heavily on perceptual information. Selective attention is the ability to pick important information out of the vast quantity of information that is usually present in the surrounding environment. Attention has not been investigated extensively in the blind and visually impaired literature, but there are several examples of excellent and important work.

Berlá (1974) and Berlá and Murr (1974) found improvement in tasks involving spatial reorientation and tactile maps over the second to eighth grade range, as well as differences within grade levels. With advances in grade level, children tended increasingly to attend to and use distinctive features of the figures, and at a given grade level, the quality of performance was positively related to the tendency to use distinctive features. Similarly, Davidson, Dunn, Wiles-Kettenmann and Appelle (1981) found typical improvements over the 10–17-year age range on conservation of mass tasks. Again, cross-age and within-age variation in performance was related to the maturity of the children's tactile strategies in examining the stimulus. Clearly strategies of attention are involved in this kind of spatial conceptual task.

The causality of the attention–performance relationship is unclear, however. It is certain that performance is facilitated by appropriate attentional strategies, but it is also possible that children who have more organized strategies of information acquisition develop cognitive skills better as a result of their better attentional habits. This relationship deserves careful exploration, particularly in view of the possibility that attentional strategies can be taught (e.g., Berlá and Butterfield, 1977).

Witkin, Oltman, Chase and Friedman (1971) used a test of auditory embedded figures in addition to other tests of perception. Congenitally blind adolescents were better at this task than comparable sighted subjects. Witkin et al. explained this finding as a more highly developed auditory selective attention; this superiority is not a general attentional superiority, however, since the same blind subjects were not as good as the sighted on a test of tactile embedded figures.

Another line of evidence with respect to auditory attention is seen in studies of the obstacle sense. It has long been known (e.g., Supa, Cotzin and Dallenbach, 1944) that the ability that many blind people show to detect surfaces in the environment is in fact dependent on their ability to attend effectively to auditory echo information; furthermore, sighted subjects can learn relatively quickly to attend to the relevant stimulus qualities. Little developmental work has been done on the phenomenon, but Worchel, Mauney and Andrew (1950) found clear evidence that blind adolescents are quite good at obstacle detection.

Related to these findings are various reports that blind children have a very good verbal memory span, as measured by tests such as the Digit Span subscale of the Wechsler Intelligence Scale for Children (WISC). For example, Tillman and Osborne (1969) examined the profiles of WISC subscale performance for blind and sighted children, aged 7–11, where the overall WISC score was equated. The blind group showed significantly better performance on the Digit Span scale but not on other subscales.

Spatial concepts

There is a great deal of research literature as well as common experience that forces rejection of the simple supposition that without vision, effective spatial behavior is not possible. The question arises, though, whether the process of acquisition of spatial concepts, or the end result of that process, is different under conditions of visual impairment. The answer, briefly, is that both process and product are different, but that many situational variables come into play.

We noted earlier that in the later stages of acquisition of the object concept, there is difficulty moving from a primarily egocentric organization of space to an allocentric understanding that spatial relationships retain their quality regardless of the child's position in the space. Contributing to this difficulty are the generally lower level of locomotor activity associated with visual impairment in infancy and the typical difficulty in integrating tactual and auditory information with respect to spatial structure (Schwartz, 1972).

Research on these issues with preschool and school-aged children has generally been oriented to the question of the process of constructing an understanding of spatial arrays. Siegal and White (1975) argued that the essence of this process is that landmarks are identified and gradually organized in relation to one another, both with regard to sequences of actions within the environment and the overall understanding of the structure of the environment. As the relationships among landmarks are understood, parts of the overall environment are organized in relation to one another, and the details are gradually incorporated. Infants demonstrate the rudiments of this development in relatively simple environments; it is in childhood that the full abilities develop. The question of the importance of vision arises in relation to these developments, and there is a long history of research on this issue.

A robust finding of this literature is that children who had a period of sight before the onset of visual impairment exhibit spatial understanding and perform spatial tasks better than those blind from birth. An excellent example is Dodds, Howarth and Carter (1982), who found that 11-year-old children with a history of early vision performed much better than congenitally blind children on learning routes within an array of several city blocks, and on identifying alternative routes to those specifically learned. Similarly, Fletcher (1980, 1981a,b) found substantial differences as a function of early vision. Children learned a room-sized spatial array either by free exploration or guided exploration, and they then answered questions designed to tap knowledge about routes within the array or overall spatial relations independent of routes. There was considerable variation in results of individual children, and early vision was a significant predictor of performance particularly for the questions about routes.

Of equal interest are studies of children's spatial understanding of environments with which they have some familiarity. Kephart, Kephart and Shwartz (1974) asked 5–7-year-olds questions about the layout of their own home, as well as their more extended neighborhood and region. The quality of knowledge increased with increasing age, and there was a progressive degradation of knowledge about the extended environment. Bigelow (1991) compared blind with partially sighted 5–8-year-olds in their ability to indicate directions from a familiar place in their house to other locations in the house, outside the house, and in the neighborhood. There was a dramatic advantage of the children with partial vision. Performance was initially best for locations on the same floor, then those in the yard, then those within the house but on a different floor. In a follow-up study with somewhat older (10–12 years) children, Bigelow (1996) differentiated between routes and Euclidean directions. Asked to indicate the direction of the route to take to target points, the totally blind children were generally better than if asked to indicate the point-to-point direction in three-dimensional space, and they showed the same sequence of acquisition that Bigelow (1991) reported. The partially sighted children performed well on both kinds of tasks from the onset of testing.

Thus there is considerable improvement in the understanding of spatial environments during the middle childhood years. It is clear that having some visual function facilitates this development. Given that, it is critical to offer children without visual function an effective array of experiences that will allow mature spatial understanding to develop. The study by Casey (1978) of totally blind children's understanding of the spatial layout of their residential school environment demonstrates that such a mature understanding is possible: the key is to offer the child an appropriate set of experiences to allow that understanding to be developed.

Electrophysiological and neuroimaging indicators

During the past 20 years, improved technology has greatly facilitated the study of the structure and function of the brain. Previous research on brain and behavior in individuals with blindness focused on electrophysiological activity as measured by electroencephalograms (EEGs). The work of Novikova (1973) suggested that electrical activity was related to amount of vision and age of onset of vision loss. Jan and Wong (1988) affirmed the relationship between visual acuity and electrical activity; however, they did not find differences related to age at vision loss. Methodological constraints may have prevented such relationships from emerging.

In any case, gross EEG activity has not proved to be a rewarding tool for the study of specific brain correlates of visual impairment. More recently, researchers interested in the plasticity of the brain and in cross-modal transfer have studied subjects with blindness using a variety of electrophysiological and neuroimaging techniques. Findings from this body of research seem to converge and suggest that the structure of the brain in sighted and blind subjects does not differ; however, there is increased blood flow and metabolic activity in the occipital areas of blind individuals during tactile and auditory discrimination tasks compared to sighted controls.

Presumably because the visual cortex of subjects totally blind from birth does not receive input, changes in this area of the brain might be expected. Using magnetic resonance imaging (MRI), Buchel, Price, Frackowiak and Friston (1998) and Kujala, Houtilainen, Sinkkonen et al. (1995a) found no structural differences in the macroanatomy of the brains in their blind subjects and sighted controls.

Studies of function have revealed differences in the activation of the visual cortex during tactile discrimination, Braille reading, and auditory discrimination. Specifically, using positron emission tomography (PET), Sadato, Pascual-Leone, Grafman et al. (1996) and Sadato, Pascual-Leone, Grafman et al. (1998) found that Braille reading and tactile discrimination tasks activated the primary visual cortex in subjects with early onset blindness. According to the authors, this finding suggests plasticity in the brain in that areas normally receiving visual input are used for somatosensory processing instead. They hypothesize that areas intended for visual shape discrimination might be used for tactile processing in subjects without vision. In the 1998 study, Sadato et al. extended their initial findings by using transcranial magnetic stimulation directed at the primary visual cortex to disrupt the identification of Braille letters in their subjects, leaving little doubt that the identification of Braille occurs in the visual cortex of subjects with early onset blindness.

Sadato et al.'s 1998 study followed one reported by Cohen, Celnik, Pascual-Leone et al. (1997) in which transcranial magnetic stimulation (TMS) was used with similar results with a smaller sample of subjects. Most recently, Cohen, Weeks, Sadato et al. (1999) reported that there appears to be a period of susceptibility for cross-modal transfer in individuals who are blind. In this study, TMS disrupted the reading of Braille in the primary visual cortex in individuals whose loss of vision occurred prior to 14 years of age. In addition, PET indicated differences in areas of activation in the primary visual cortex for individuals with early versus late onset blindness. The authors noted that this cut-off age for plasticity is similar to that seen in the acquisition of second languages and the upper limit for rehabilitation of individuals with amblyopia.

Using PET, Buchel et al. (1998) found similar activation patterns in Braille readers with early and late-onset blindness. These authors conceded that their findings suggest task-specific cross-modal transfer in the subjects with early-onset blindness, but suggested that visual imagery might be responsible for the activation observed in late-onset blindness.

Kujala, Alho, Kekoni et al. (1995b) used magnetoencephalography to confirm reports of activation of the occipital cortex during auditory discrimination in subjects with blindness using evoked response potentials (ERP; Alho, Kujala, Paavilainen et al., 1993; Kujala et al., 1995a). Similar ERP results have been reported for somatosensory discrimination in individuals with blindness (Kujala et al., 1995a; Roder, Rosler and Hennighausen, 1997). In the only reported use of single photon emission computed tomography (SPECT) for this purpose, Uhl, Franzen, Podreka et al. (1993) found evidence for increased cerebral blood flow in the occipital cortex of individuals who were blind from an early age, adding to the accumulating evidence that the occipital cortex is indeed active in individuals who have been blind from an early age. Finally, Sadato and Hallett (1999) reported similar results using functional MRI.

More recently, two groups of researchers have found that ERP responses are different in individuals blind from birth when compared to sighted controls. Specifically, Roder, Rosler and Neville (1999) examined the effects of interstimulus intervals on auditory event-related potentials and found that amplitude recovery was much more pronounced, and N2 responses were more posteriorly distributed in the blind subjects. Target detection times were shorter in the subjects without vision than in the sighted controls. The authors concluded that the differences observed in the congenitally blind subjects and sighted controls were probably due to compensatory adaptations that result from intermodal plasticity. Although the same brain systems appear to be involved in processing elementary auditory stimuli, they appeared to work more efficiently in the blind subjects. Leclerc, Saint-Amour, Lavoie et al. (2000) came to a similar conclusion in their study of sound localization using ERP. These authors noted that the visual areas of the brain appeared to be recruited for auditory functions in the blind subjects in their study, representing cross-modal brain reorganization that resulted in normal to superior performance on auditory stimulus feature analysis.

In summary, the results of electrophysiological and neuroimaging studies strongly suggest that with early onset blindness, the primary visual cortex is plastic and that neuronal pathways may be altered so that somatosensory and auditory information are rerouted to this area. Additionally, activation of the occipital cortex is task dependent. To date, activation has been proven during discrimination tasks involving tactile and auditory input. Although one group of researchers (Cohen et al., 1997) suggests that this plasticity may extend only to 14 years of age, more evidence is needed to support that specific finding.

Assessment and research methodology

Much of the existing research literature on blind and visually impaired children is less than satisfying, for a variety of reasons. Often research design is inappropriate to the task: much of the literature simply borrows research methodology from the tradition of research with sighted samples, typically using a normative rather than a differential approach to evaluation. That is, the concern is primarily with the mean value of a sample, rather than with the variability of values and the factors that produce that variability. This approach tends to hide, rather than reveal, differences among subjects, and it is particularly inappropriate for research on heterogeneous and low-incidence populations such as the blind and visually impaired (Warren, 1984, 1994).

Furthermore, the tendency in the literature has been to use the comparative approach, evaluating the characteristics of blind and visually impaired children in relation to those of sighted children.

This goal, too, tends to undervalue the analysis of variation within the blind and visually impaired population.

The issue of appropriate assessment is even more serious, however. Whether the goal of research is to compare blind with sighted samples or to analyze variation within blind samples, it is unfortunately the case that much evaluation of the blind is done with assessment techniques that have been designed for the sighted population and therefore are not ideal for, or worse yet misrepresent, the characteristics of the blind.

For example, the traditional conservation tasks for sighted children rely heavily on vision; their adaptation for the blind typically involves simple substitution of tactual for visual exposure to the stimulus materials. It is not at all clear that this adaptation produces a task which assesses the same cognitive characteristics in the blind child which the visual version taps in the sighted, and therefore comparison of blind and sighted children is suspect. Similarly, evaluation of object constancy in sighted infants usually depends heavily on vision, and it is not clear that a tactual adaptation of the task assesses the blind infant in comparable manner.

The assessment of intelligence is just as difficult. Most researchers have recognized that children's IQ tests, such as the WISC, cannot be used with blind and visually impaired children without modification. Furthermore, it is obviously inappropriate simply to omit the heavily vision-based performance scales and retain the verbal scales. In recognition of this, several tests of intelligence have been developed specifically for blind and visually impaired children. For example, the Perkins–Binet (Davis, 1980) is a thorough adaptation of the Stanford–Binet test; the Blind Learning Aptitude Test was developed by Newland (1979) specifically for blind and visually impaired children. However, the psychometric properties of many assessments designed for children who are visually impaired leaves much to be desired. The development of tests of intelligence for blind children and their norming on blind samples is clearly a more appropriate route to assessment than using portions of tests designed for the sighted. However, the use of such tests for blind children effectively precludes making any comparisons of their intelligence with that of sighted children, since these tests are equally inappropriate for the sighted.

Development of indicator tests suitable for blind and visually impaired children is a useful and important first step in conducting better research. However, there is another point on which the existing literature is very weak. A score derived from performance on an intelligence test is simply an indicator. Such a score is valuable only to the extent that the ability or characteristic which it represents is clearly conceptualized and to the extent that it is a valid indicator of that ability or characteristic. It is not enough simply to evaluate intelligence, for example, without inquiring what the functional significance of the resulting score is for the child's adaptive potential.

The IQ score is not inherently meaningful; to be meaningful, its relationship to adaptive behavior must be clear. The vast majority of research with blind and visually impaired children, and for that matter a good deal of research with sighted children, does not take this additional step. Validity must be a serious and ongoing concern among researchers with the blind. And although the immediate example concerns intelligence tests, the same point must be considered in relation to any task, such as those used to evaluate conservation abilities, which is used as an index of some aspect of cognitive or other functioning.

All of this is not to conclude that the existing literature on cognitive development of blind and visually impaired children is not useful, but that caution must be used in interpreting this literature. Future research must be more concerned with the use of appropriate research design and assessment techniques.

Conclusion

Instead of attempting the difficult and perhaps inappropriate task of summarizing the diverse material presented here, we will identify several important themes of the literature and propose suggestions about directions that our future research should explore.

Although a close comparison of the development of blind and visually impaired children with that of sighted children is inadvisable for both conceptual and methodological reasons, it is clear that in many aspects of cognitive development, visually impaired children may be developmentally delayed. More important, however, is the question of what, if anything, to do about this. We have argued elsewhere (e.g., Warren, 1994) that developmental equivalence is not an appropriate goal. Instead, we should recognize that children find different routes to adaptation to the demands of their existence. A more appropriate goal, then, is to ensure that the blind or visually impaired child is provided with every possible opportunity to find a path of successful adaptation.

The literature is helpful in this respect, in allowing delineation of those factors which have been found to be associated with more developmentally advanced cognition. It is convenient to divide these into two categories, 'status' variables such as IQ and functional vision, which are not readily amenable to manipulation, and 'environmental' variables, which may be readily varied.

It should not be surprising that children who have had a period of vision early in life show generally better indices of cognitive development. Furthermore, the literature is very clear in showing that children with some functional vision are at an advantage in cognitive development. Although the existence or amount of vision is not under our control, the encouragement of the child with low vision to use that visual capability is. Barraga (1976) has been persuasive in encouraging the effective use of any residual visual capability, and the present pattern of results bears out her argument forcefully. On the negative side, there is an emerging literature that clearly links adverse developmental outcomes to the presence of additional disabilities in addition to visual loss.

Other variables, which have an equally great impact on the course of development of cognitive abilities, are under our potential influence. We refer here to variables such as the provision of varied perceptual, motor, cognitive, and linguistic experience, the encouragement of the blind or visually impaired infant or child to seek and engage learning experiences, the provision of a supportive social–emotional environment, and the provision of effective educational opportunities. Although there is a great deal to be learned about these variables and how to arrange a suitable environment, there is sufficient evidence of their importance to support the conclusion that optimizing these factors should lead to optimal conceptual development.

The 'traditional' aspects of cognitive development, such as conservation and classification, have been thoroughly examined. Other areas that are related to the traditional topics, such as spatial cognition, language, and attention, have not been so completely studied. The interconnectedness of various aspects of development must be fully recognized, so that a more integrated overall picture may be realized.

As we look to future research on these issues, we will need to respond to four specific challenges. The first challenge is to escape existing research models, which are heavily oriented to evaluation of cognitive development in the visually impaired child by reference to norms of the sighted child. It is relatively easy to do research using the comparative model, but this research is not of real benefit. It is implicitly oriented to the assessment of the role of vision, and the effects of the severe impairment of vision, in cognitive development. Not only does the comparative model not yield useful information about these issues, but more importantly, these issues are not those to which we should be directing our attention. Instead, we should be examining the effects on cognitive development of variables related to visual impairment itself, such as etiology, visual history, severity of loss, and yet more importantly, the effects of such environmental characteristics as the nature of the learning environment. The development and use of such models will be more difficult, but vastly more rewarding, both to our understanding of cognitive development under conditions of visual impairment and to our ability to optimize that development in individual cases.

The second challenge stems from the first. Given that the comparative model is not an appropriate one for research with the visually impaired child, it is imperative that assessment instruments are developed that are appropriate for use with the visually impaired population. It is not sufficient simply to adapt a previously existing instrument for nonvisual use. Functional instruments must be developed for evaluation of the visually impaired child, and they must be adequately normed on that population. Furthermore, no assessment instrument is an end in itself. An assessment instrument is an indicator of fundamental capabilities which are in some sense adaptive for the individual's functioning. Therefore, in the development of appropriate assessment techniques and in their use in research, careful regard must be maintained for the adaptive capabilities and behaviors which the instrument is designed to assess.

Thirdly, the gap between our understanding of cognitive functioning in the visually impaired child and the neurological substrates for that functioning is vast. As developing psychobiological techniques allow ever more detailed relationships to be identified between cognitive behavior and the underlying physiology that enables that behavior, those techniques must be effectively and creatively applied to the case of the visually impaired child. There is a great need to learn, by the use of quantitative neuroimaging techniques, of advanced electrophysiologic tests of the functioning brain, as well as postmortem analyses, where possible, about the nature of the reorganization of brain structure and function that is associated with various degrees of visual loss.

Fourth, it will be imperative to adapt our research models to suit the ever-increasing proportion of individuals with multiple disabilities. Research on children with only vision loss, while important, is decreasingly relevant to the emerging population. In order for future research to be optimally useful, it must include and effectively address issues related to multiple disabilities.

Attention to these areas and methodologies of research in the future will, we believe, lead to a substantial improvement in our understanding of the nature of cognitive development under conditions of visual impairment, and consequently in our ability to facilitate the development of optimal cognitive functioning in visually impaired children.

References

Adelson E, Fraiberg S: Gross motor development in infants blind from birth. Child Development: 45; 114–126, 1974.

Adkins S: Effects of visual deficit on acquisition of classification concepts. Dissertation Abstracts: 26; 1769A, 1965.

Aitken K, Trevarthen C: Self/other organization in human psychological development. Development and Psychopathology: 9(4); 653–677, 1997.

Alho K, Kujala T, Paavilainen P, Summala H, Naatanen R: Auditory processing in visual brain areas of the early blind: Evidence from event-related potentials. Electroencephalography and Clinical Neurophysiology: 86; 418–427, 1993.

Als H, Tronick E, Brazelton T: Stages of early behavioral organization: The study of a sighted infant and a blind infant interaction with their mothers. In Field T (Ed), High-Risk Infants and Children: Adult and Peer Interactions. New York: Academic Press, 1980.

Andersen E, Dunlea A, Kekelis L: Blind children's language: Resolving some differences. Journal of Child Language: 11(3); 645–664, 1984.

Anderson D, Olson M: Word meaning among congenitally blind children. Journal of Visual Impairment and Blindness: 75; 165–168, 1981.

Barraga N: Visual Handicaps and Learning: A Developmental Approach. Belmont, CA: Wadsworth Publishing Company, 1976.

Berlá E: Tactual orientation performance of blind children in different grade levels. American Foundation for the Blind, Research Bulletin: 27; 1–10, 1974.

Berlá E, Butterfield LJ: Tactual distinctive features analysis: Training blind students in shape recognition and in locating shapes on a map. Journal of Special Education: 11; 335–346, 1977.

Berlá E, Murr M: Searching tactual space. Education of the Visually Handicapped: 6; 49–58, 1974.

Bigelow A: The development of reaching in blind children. British Journal of Developmental Psychology: 4; 355–366, 1986.

Bigelow A: Early words of blind children. Journal of Child Language: 14; 47–56, 1987.

Bigelow A: Blind children's concepts of how people see. Journal of Visual Impairment and Blindness: 82(2); 65–68, 1988.

Bigelow A: Relationship between the development of language and thought in young blind children. Journal of Visual Impairment and Blindness: 84(8); 414–419, 1990.

Bigelow A: The effects of distance and intervening obstacles on visual inference in blind and sighted children. International Journal of Behavioral Development: 14(3); 273–283, 1991.

Bigelow A: Locomotion and search behavior in blind infants. Infant Behavior and Development: 15; 179–189, 1992.

Bigelow A: The effect of blindness on the early development of the self. In Rochat P et al. (Eds), The Self in Infancy: Theory and Research, Vol. 112. Amsterdam: North-Holland/Elsevier Science Publishers, pp. 327–347, 1995.

Bigelow A: Blind and sighted children's spatial knowledge of their home environments. International Journal of Behavioral Development: 19(4); 797–816, 1996.

Brambring M: Early intervention with blind children: Main findings of the Beilefeld Longitudinal Study. In Brambring M, Rauh H, Beelmann A (Eds), Early Childhood Intervention: Theory, Evaluation, and Practice. New York: Walter de Gruyter, 1996.

Brekke B, Williams J, Tait P: The acquisition of conservation of weight by visually impaired children. Journal of Genetic Psychology: 125; 89–97, 1974.

Buchel C, Price C, Frackowiak S, Friston K: Different activation patterns in the visual cortex of late and congenitally blind subjects. Brain: 121; 409–419, 1998.

Casey S: Cognitive mapping by the blind. Journal of Visual Impairment and Blindness: 72; 297–301, 1978.

Cohen L, Celnik P, Pascual-Leone A, Corwell B, Faiz L, Dambrosia J, Honda M, Sadato N, Gerloff C, Catala M, Hallett M: Functional relevance of cross-modal plasticity in blind humans. Nature: 389; 180–183, 1997.

Cohen L, Weeks R, Sadato N, Celnik P, Ishii K, Mallett M: Period of susceptibility for cross-modal plasticity in the blind. Annals of Neurology: 45; 451–460, 1999.

Cratty B: Perceptual–Motor Behavior and Educational Processes. Springfield, IL: Charles C Thomas, 1969.

Davidson P, Dunn G, Wiles-Kettenmann M, Appelle S: Haptic conservation of amount in blind and sighted children. Journal of Pediatric Psychology: 6; 191–200, 1981.

Davis CJ: Perkins–Binet Tests of Intelligence for the Blind. Watertown, MA: Perkins School for the Blind, 1980.

Dodds A, Howarth C, Carter D: The mental maps of the blind: The role of previous experience. Journal of Visual Impairment and Blindness: 76; 5–12, 1982.

Dote-Kwan J: Impact of mothers' interactions on the development of their young visually impaired children. Journal of Visual Impairment and Blindness: 89; 47–58, 1995.

Dunlea A: Vision and the Emergence of Meaning. Cambridge: Cambridge University Press, 1989.

Dunlea A, Andersen E: The emergence process: Conceptual and linguistic influences on morphological development. First Language: 12; 95–115, 1992.

Farrenkopf C, Davidson I: The development of perspective-taking abilities in young blind children. RE:view: XXIV (Number 1); 7–22, 1992.

Ferrell K: Project PRISM: A longitudinal study of developmental patterns of children who are visually impaired (Final Report). Greeley, CO: Division of Special Education, University of Northern Colorado, 1998.

Ferrell K, Trief E, Deitz S, Bonner M, Cruz D, Ford E, Stratton J: The visually impaired infants research consortium: First year results. Journal of Visual Impairment and Blindness: 84(8); 404–410, 1990.

Flavell J: The development of children's knowledge about the mind: From cognitive connections to mental representations. In Asington J, Harris P, Olson O (Eds), Developing Theories of Mind. New York: Cambridge University Press, 1988.

Fletcher J: Spatial representation in blind children. 1: Development compared to sighted children. Journal of Visual Impairment and Blindness: 74; 381–385, 1980.

Fletcher J: Spatial representation in blind children. 2: Effects of task variations. Journal of Visual Impairment and Blindness: 75; 1–3, 1981a.

Fletcher J: Spatial representation in blind children. 3: Effects of individual differences. Journal of Visual Impairment and Blindness: 75; 46–49, 1981b.

Fraiberg S: Parallel and divergent patterns in blind and sighted infants. The Psychoanalytic Study of the Child: 23; 264–300, 1968.

Fraiberg S: Insights from the Blind: Comparative Studies of Blind and Sighted Infants. New York: Basic Books, 1977.

Fraiberg S, Siegel B, Gibson R: The role of sound in the search behavior of a blind infant. The Psychoanalytic Study of the Child: 21; 327–357, 1966.

Friedman J, Pasnak R: Accelerated acquisition of classification skills by blind children. Developmental Psychopathology: 9; 333–337, 1973.

Gerhardt J: The development of object play and classificatory skills in a blind child. Journal of Visual Impairment and Blindness: 76; 219–223, 1982.

Gottesman M: Conservation development in blind children. Child Development: 44; 824–827, 1973.

Hammill D, Powell L: An abstraction test for visually handicapped children. Exceptional Children: 33; 646–47, 1967.

Hatton D, Bailey D, Burchinal M, Ferrell K: Developmental growth curves of preschool children with vision impairments. Child Development: 68(5); 788–806, 1997.

Hatton D, Waring E: Parent perceptions of young children with visual impairments. Paper presented at the 20th International Seminar on Preschool Blindness, Pacific Grove, CA, 1999.

Hatwell Y: Privation Sensorielle et Intelligence. Paris: Presses Universitaires de France, 1966.

Hatwell Y: Piagetian Reasoning in the Blind. New York: American Foundation for the Blind, 1985.

Higgins L: Classification in Congenitally Blind Children, Vol. 25. New York: American Foundation for the Blind, 1973.

Jan J, Robinson G, Scott E, Kinnis C: Hypotonia in the blind child. Developmental Medicine and Child Neurology: 17; 35–40, 1975.

Jan J, Sykander A, Groenveld M: Habilitation and rehabilitation of visually impaired and blind children. Pediatrician: 17; 202–207, 1990.

Jan J, Wong P: Behavior of the alpha rhythm in electroencephalograms of visually impaired children. Developmental Medicine and Child Neurology: 30; 444–450, 1988.

Johnson M: Cortical plasticity in normal and abnormal cognitive development: Evidence and working hypotheses. Development and Psychopathology: 11(3): 419–437, 1999.

Johnson M, Dziurawiec S, Ellis H, Morton J: Newborns' preferential tracking of face-like stimuli and its subsequent decline. Cognition: 40; 1–19, 1991.

Kekelis L: A field study of a blind preschooler. In Sacks S, Kekelis L, Gaylord-Ross R (Eds), The Development of Social Skills by Blind and Visually Impaired Students. New York: American Foundation for the Blind, 1992.

Kekelis L: Blind and sighted children with their mothers: The development of discourse skills. Journal of Visual Impairment and Blindness: 90(5); 423–436, 1996.

Kekelis L, Andersen E: Family communication styles and language development. Journal of Visual Impairment and Blindness: 78(2); 54–65, 1984.

Kekelis L, Sacks S: The effects of visual impairment on children's social interactions in regular education programs. In Sacks S, Kekelis L, Gaylord-Ross R (Eds), The Development of Social Skills by Blind and Visually Impaired Students. New York: American Foundation for the Blind, 1992.

Kephart J, Kephart CP, Shwartz G: A journey into the world of the blind child. Exceptional Children: 40; 421–427, 1974.

Kujala T, Alho K, Kekoni J, Hamalainen H, Reinikainen K, Salonen O, Standerskjold-Nordenstam C, Naatanen R: Auditory and somatosensory event-related brain potentials in early blind humans. Experimental Brain Research: 104; 519–526, 1995b.

Kujala T, Houtilainen M, Sinkkonen J, Ahonen A, Alho K, Hamalainen M, Ilmoniemi R, Kajola M, Knuutila J, Lavinkainen J, Salonen O, Simola J, Standertskjold-Nordenstam C-G, Tiitinen H, Tissari S, Naatanen R: Visual cortex activation in blind humans during sound discrimination. Neuroscience Letters: 183; 143–146, 1995a.

Landau B, Gleitman L: Language and Experience: Evidence from the Blind Child. Cambridge, MA: Harvard University Press, 1985.

Lebron-Rodriguez D, Pasnak R: Introduction of intellectual gains in blind children. Journal of Experimental Child Psychology: 24; 505–515, 1977.

Leclerc C, Saint-Amour D, Lavoie ME, Lassond M, Lepore F: Brain functional reorganization in early blind humans revealed by auditory event-related potentials. NeuroReport: 11; 545–550, 2000.

MacCuspie P: The social acceptance and interaction of visually impaired children in integrated settings. In Sacks S, Kekelis L, Gaylord-Ross R (Eds), The Development of Social Skills by Blind and Visually Impaired Students. New York: American Foundation for the Blind, 1992.

McConachie H, Moore V: Early expressive language of severely visually impaired children. Developmental Medicine and Child Neurology: 36; 230–240, 1994.

Miller C: Conservation in blind children. Education of the Visually Handicapped: 1; 101–105, 1969.

Mills A: Visual handicap. In Bishop D, Mogford K (Eds), Language Development in Exceptional Circumstances. New York: Churchill Livingstone, 1988.

Minter M, Hobson R, Bishop M: Congenital visual impairment and 'theory of mind'. British Journal of Developmental Psychology: 16(2); 183–196, 1998.

Moore V, McConachie H: Communication between blind and severely visually impaired children and their parents. British Journal of Developmental Psychology: 12; 491–502, 1994.

Mulford R: First words of the blind. In Smith M, Locke JL (Eds), The Emergent Lexicon: The Child's Development of a Linguistic Vocabulary. New York: Academic Press, pp. 293–338, 1988.

Mundy P, Willoughby J: Nonverbal communication, joint attention, and early socioemotional development. In Lewis M, Sullivan M (Eds), Emotional Development in Atypical Children. Mahwah, NJ: Erlbaum Associates, 1996.

Nesker-Simmons J, Davidson I: Determinants of Development: Conceptualizing Young Blind Children. Ottawa, ON: Heron Press, 1992.

Newland TE: The Blind Learning Aptitude Test. Journal of Visual Impairment and Blindness: 73; 134–139, 1979.

Norris M, Spaulding P, Brodie F: Blindness in Children. Chicago, IL: University of Chicago Press, 1957.

Novikova L: Blindness and the Electrical Activity of the Brain. New York: American Foundation for the Blind, 1973.

Piaget J: Genetic Epistemology. New York: Columbia University Press, 1970.

Preisler G: Early patterns of interaction between blind infants and their sighted mothers. Child: Care, Health, and Development: 17; 65–90, 1991.

Preisler G: The development of communication in blind and deaf infants — similarities and differences. Child: Care, Health and Development: 21(2); 79–110, 1995.

Preisler G: Social and emotional development of blind children: a longitudinal study. In Lewis V, Collis G (Eds), Blindness and Psychological Development in Young Children. Leicester: British Psychological Society/New York: Raven Press, 1997.

Reynell J: Developmental patterns of visually handicapped children. Child: Care, Health, and Development: 4; 291–303, 1978.

Roder B, Rosler F, Hennighausen E: Different cortical activation patterns in blind and sighted humans during encoding and transformation of haptic images. Psychphysiology: 34; 292–307, 1997.

Roder B, Rosler F, Neville HJ: Effects of interstimulus interval on auditory event-related potentials in congenitally blind and normally sighted humans. Neuroscience Letters: 264; 53–56, 1999.

Rogers S, Puchalski C: Social characteristics of visually impaired infants play. Topics in Early Childhood Special Education: 3(4); 52–56, 1984.

Rogers S, Puchalski C: Development of object permanence in visually impaired infants. Journal of Visual Impairment and Blindness: 82; 137–142, 1988.

Rowland C: Preverbal communication of blind infants and their mothers. Journal of Visual Impairment and Blindness: 78(7); 297–302, 1984.

Sadato N, Pascual-Leone A, Grafman J, Deiber M, Ibanez V: Neural networks for Braille reading by the blind. Brain: 121; 1213–1229, 1998.

Sadato N, Pascual-Leone A, Grafman J, Ibanez V, Deiber M, Dold G, Hallett M: Activation of the primary visual cortex by Braille reading in blind subjects. Nature: 380(11); 526–528, 1996.

Sadato N, Hallett M: FMRI occipital activation by tactile stimulation in a blind man. Neurology: 52; 423, 1999.

Schore A: The experience-dependent maturation of a regulatory system in the orbital prefrontal cortex and the origin of developmental psychopathology. Development and Psychopathology: 8; 59–87, 1996.

Schwartz A: A comparison of congenitally blind and sighted elementary school children on intelligence, tactile discrimination, abstract reasoning, perceived physical health, perceived personality adjustment and parent–teacher perceptions of intellectual performance. Dissertation Abstracts International: 33; 5588A, 1972.

Schwartz M: The role of sound for space and object perception in the congenitally blind infant. In Lisett L, Rovee-Collier C (Eds), Advances in Infancy Research. Norwood, NJ: Ablex, pp. 23–56, 1984.

Siegal A, White S: The development of spatial representation of large-scale environments. In Reese H (Ed), Advances in Child Development and Behavior, Vol. 10. New York: Academic Press, pp. 9–25, 1975.

Sonksen P, Levitt S, Kitzinger M: Identification of constraints acting on motor development in young visually disabled children and principles of remediation. Child: Care, Health and Development: 10; 273–286, 1984.

Stephens B, Simpkins K: The Reasoning, Moral Judgment, and Moral Conduct of the Congenitally Blind, Report No. H233197: Office of Education, Bureau of Education for the Handicapped, 1974.

Supa M, Cotzin M, Dallenbach K: 'Facial vision': the perception of obstacles by the blind. American Journal of Psychology: 57; 133–183, 1944.

Swanson L, Minifie D, Minifie E: Conservation development in the partially sighted child. Psychology in the Schools: 16; 309–313, 1979.

Tait P: The attainment of conservation by Chinese and Indian children. Journal of Visual Impairment and Blindness: 84(7); 380–382, 1990.

Tillman M: The performance of blind and sighted children on the Wechsler Intelligence Scale for Children: Study I. International Journal for the Education of the Blind: 16(3); 65–74, 1967a.

Tillman M: The performance of blind and sighted children on the Wechsler Intelligence Scale for Children: Study II. International Journal for the Education of the Blind: 16(4); 106–112, 1967b.

Tillman M, Osborne R: The performance of blind and sighted children on the Wechsler Intelligence Scale for Children: interaction effects. Education of the Visually Handicapped: 1; 1–4, 1969.

Tröster H, Brambring M: Early motor development in blind infants. Journal of Applied Developmental Psychology: 14; 83–106, 1993.

Tröster H, Hecker W, Brambring M: Longitudinal study of gross-motor development in blind infants and preschoolers. Early Child Development and Care: 104; 61–78, 1994.

Uhl F, Franzen P, Podreka I, Steiner M, Deecke L: Increased regional cerebral blood flow in inferior occipital cortex and cerebellum of early blind humans. Neuroscience Letters: 150; 162–164, 1993.

Urwin C: Communication in infancy and the emergence of language in blind children. In Schiefelbusch R, Pickar J (Eds), The Acquisition of Communicative Competence. Baltimore, MD: University Park Press, pp. 479–524, 1984.

Wan-Lin M, Tait P: The attainment of conservation by visually impaired children in Taiwan. Journal of Visual Impairment and Blindness: 81; 423–428, 1987.

Warren D: Blindness and Early Childhood Development. 2nd ed., New York: American Foundation for the Blind, 1984.

Warren D: Blindness and Children: An Individual Differences Approach. New York: Cambridge University Press, 1994.

Witkin H, Oltman P, Chase J, Friedman F: Cognitive patterning in the blind. In Hellmuth J (Ed), Cognitive Studies, Vol. 2. New York: Brunner/Mazel, 1971.

Worchel P, Mauney J, Andrew J: The perception of obstacles by the blind. Journal of Experimental Psychology: 40; 747–751, 1950.

Zweibelson I, Barg C: Concept development in blind children. New Outlook Blind: 61; 218–222, 1967.

Handbook of Neuropsychology, 2nd Edition, Vol. 8, Part II
S.J. Segalowitz and I. Rapin (Eds)

CHAPTER 19

Central auditory function and evaluation of auditory processing disorders

Linda J. Hood * and Charles I. Berlin

Department of Otorhinolaryngology and Biocommunication, Kresge Hearing Research Laboratory of the South, Louisiana State University Health Sciences Center, 533 Bolivar Street, New Orleans, LA 70112, USA

Introduction

The broad definition of auditory perception or auditory processing encompasses function at all levels of the auditory system from the external ear to the cortex. Most hearing disorders in children and adults are due to problems in the middle ear or inner ear (cochlea). Middle-ear problems result in conductive hearing losses where sound is attenuated as it travels through the external and/or middle ears. Sensory impairments the cochlea and, along with attenuation of signals, also may result in distortion and increased difficulty when listening in noise (Plomp, 1978, 1986). Hearing problems may coexist at multiple sites; thus a patient may have a conductive or cochlear hearing loss as well as an auditory processing disorder.

While the incidence of auditory processing disorders of the peripheral and central nervous systems is lower than the more peripheral (middle-ear and cochlear) hearing disorders in children, it is significant both in occurrence and in the effects on speech perception and language learning. Children with auditory processing disorders often display normal peripheral auditory function but are unable to successfully utilize auditory stimuli, particularly in adverse listening conditions.

* Corresponding author. Tel.: +1-504-568-4785; Fax: +1-504-568-4460; E-mail: lhood@lsuhsc.edu

Controversy exists in the literature and in discussions among professionals regarding the sources, causes and characteristics of 'auditory processing' disorders. Often labeled auditory perception or central auditory processing disorders (CAPD), these terms refer to a broad range of functions and encompass a variety of processes. Little consensus is available on either the appropriate terminology to describe the problems, methods of measurement or what functions or dysfunctions appropriately encompass this area. For example, some suggest that auditory perception cannot be measured directly and therefore prefer the term 'auditory processing' as a term that more closely denotes directly measurable performance on specific tasks or series of stimuli. Auditory perception also has been differentially compared to speech perception. While some view speech and language perception as a unique 'top-down' or cognitive process, others report that children with severe language disabilities demonstrate auditory difficulties with both speech and non-speech stimuli (Tallal and Piercy, 1973, 1974).

In this chapter, we examine function of the normal auditory system related to perception of simple and complex auditory stimuli along with advantages and limitations of behavioral and electrophysiological measures in evaluating auditory processing and its disorders. We will present illustrative cases of disorders that adversely affect the normal development of auditory/verbal skills or cause interruption to this cycle, and we will briefly discuss management issues.

Development of auditory function

The normal development of speech and language is critically related to the ability of the auditory system to receive input through normal auditory channels. Human cochlear function has been recorded physiologically after 20 weeks gestational age (Elliot and Elliot, 1964; Johansson, Wedenberg and Westin, 1964) and brainstem responses can be recorded at 28–29 weeks conceptional age (Starr, Amlie, Martin and Sanders, 1977). Brainstem length is adult-like by 1 year of age (Ponton, Moore, Eggermont et al., 1994) while the brainstem auditory pathway continues to lengthen until about 3 years of age (Moore, Ponton, Eggermont et al., 1996). Functionally, brainstem conduction time is adult-like by the time of term birth and postnatal increases in conduction time appear to offset path length changes (Moore et al., 1996).

Auditory sensitivity progressively improves over approximately the first 6 months of life. Improved threshold sensitivity may relate to external and middle ear developmental changes as well as to cochlear and neural changes. Infants demonstrate varying degrees of frequency, intensity, and temporal discrimination ability (Bartoshuk, 1964; Eisenberg, 1976; Kearsley, Schneider, Richie et al., 1962; Steinschneider, Lipton and Richmond, 1966). Frequency resolution, as shown by auditory filter width and physiological studies, appears mature early in neonatal life. Ability to discriminate changes in intensity appears to mature through infancy and early childhood, though the amount of improvement and timing is less certain (Werner and Gray, 1998). Temporal resolving ability, studied using several measures of temporal resolution, appears to follow a relatively long developmental time course (e.g., Hall and Grose, 1994; Werner et al., 1992).

An infant is able to discriminate his/her mother's voice at birth and prefers that voice to others (DeCasper and Fifer, 1980). Such findings support the existence of auditory experience before birth that involves the ability to make distinctions in rhythm and intonation. Neonates and infants also demonstrate a preference for a certain type of speech, referred to as infant-directed speech, that is characterized by expanded frequency and intensity changes, slower speaking rate, and longer syllable durations (Cooper and Aslin, 1990; Fernald and Kuhl, 1987).

By 1 to 2 months of age, an infant can distinguish phonemic contrasts (Moffitt, 1969), linguistic stress (Spring and Dale, 1977), and perceive rhythm (Demany, McKenzie and Vurpillot, 1977). Discrimination of phonetic contrasts focuses on structures within a specific language during the first year of life (Eimas, 1978; Werker and Tees, 1984). Additional evidence of auditory processing documented in infants indicates that localization of sound begins by 4 months with localization along the horizontial plane maturing before vertical localization. By 6 months, an infant can localize very soft speech (Northern and Downs, 1991). In-depth discussions of the development of auditory function in infants can be found in Northern and Downs (1991), Werner and Gray (1998) and Eggermont and Stein (1996).

Maturation of auditory function is accompanied by the development of speech and language abilities. Beginning use of the auditory feedback loop is evidenced by an infant's first speech where the speech patterns reflect the signals received through the auditory system. Some lag occurs in the production of speech relative to the perception of speech in normal infants (Berko and Brown, 1960), and the specific relationship between development of speech production and auditory function is unclear (Menyuk, 1977).

The presence of a period of vocalization in deaf infants who obviously do not hear their parents' voices suggests the involvement of some reflexive, preadaptive behavior (Northern and Downs, 1991). There are clear differences in speech development in normally hearing versus deaf infants as demonstrated by Eilers and Oller (1994). Their studies show that the onset of well-formed production of syllables such as "da", "na", "bee" (canonical babbling) occurred in normal infants before 11 months of age, while infants who were deaf did not demonstrate canonical babbling until 11 months or older.

By the time speech emerges at about 12–18 months of age, an infant has received considerable auditory input. Deprivation of input due to an abnormal peripheral or central auditory system can seriously compromise development of speech and language. Early identification of peripheral hearing loss and early intervention are critical for normal speech and language development. It has been demonstrated that identification of peripheral hearing loss and initiation of management of that hearing loss before 6 months of age significantly influences language development (Yoshinaga-Itano et al., 1998). Those infants who are managed prior to 6 months are able to stay on track with their normal hearing peers in language.

Data from studies of children with severe or profound hearing loss since birth who subsequently received a cochlear implant suggest a critical age range associated with greater benefit and ability to succeed in normal educational environments. Children who are implanted before the age of 5 years tend to be more likely to perform better on speech production and perception tasks than those implanted later (e.g., Robinson, 1998). These observations are further supported by cortical evoked potential studies showing that auditory evoked potentials in cochlear implant users implanted in their teens are different from those of their normal hearing peers (e.g., Ponton and Eggermont, 2001).

Deprivation effects and critical periods of development as they relate to central auditory dysfunction are less well established. Auditory deprivation at critical ages affects brainstem development in certain rodents whose auditory systems are quite immature at birth (Webster and Webster, 1977), but similar findings are not observed in rodents who have more developed auditory systems at birth (Hood, Webster and Barlow, 1990; Webster and O'Connell, 1989) or in primates (Doyle and Webster, 1991). In addition, the critical period for such input to occur is very early in the developmental cycle.

Neural plasticity has been studied in relation to native and second language acquisition. Functional magnetic resonance imaging (fMRI) study of representation of native and second languages has shown that second languages acquired in adulthood are spatially separated in different regions of the cortex (Kim, Relkin, Lee and Hirsch, 1997). When a second language is learned at an early age (during an 'early' language acquisition stage), fMRIs show both languages represented in common frontal cortical areas (Kim et al., 1997).

Principles which can be applied to functional evaluation of the auditory nervous system

Several important characteristics of the auditory nervous system should be considered in selecting evaluation techniques, interpreting results, and planning management programs.

Neuromaturation of the auditory nervous system

Neural responses recorded even from peripheral portions of the auditory neural pathways continue to develop after birth, and some responses recorded from the cortex continue to mature to age 10 years and beyond. For example, the auditory brainstem response shows decreases in latency over the first 12–18 months of age (Starr et al., 1977) while cortical auditory evoked potentials become adult-like in the late teens (e.g., Albrecht, Suchodoletz and Uwer, 2000; Ponton, Don, Eggermont et al., 1996).

Cortical asymmetries correlated with speech-language function

Histological and radiological methods demonstrate anatomical asymmetries in the temporal lobes of human brains. The superior surface of the temporal lobe, presumed important for auditory function, is anatomically larger on the left in more brains than the right, and the planum temporale is longer on the left than right in the majority of human subjects (Geschwind, 1978; Geschwind and Levitsky, 1968), more so in males than females (Kulynych, Vlader, Jones and Weinberger, 1994). Such asymmetries are present in infants and children (Seidenwurm, Bird, Enzmann and Marshall, 1985; Wada, Clark and Hamm, 1975; Witelson, 1977). These anatomical asymmetries relate to functional differences between the right and left hemispheres and, in particular, to specialization for speech and language in the left hemisphere (Kimura, 1961; Studdert-Kennedy and Shankweiler, 1970). Newer techniques, such as positron emission tomography (PET), functional MRI (fMRI), and magnetic source imaging enhance ability to study hemispheric asymmetries and relationships between structural and functional differences (e.g., Belin, Zilbovicious, Crozier et al., 1998; Penhune, Zattore, MacDonald and Evans, 1996; Syzmanski, Perry, Gage et al., 2001).

Primary representation of stimuli via contralateral pathways

The primary neuroanatomical pathway from the ear to the cortex takes a contralateral route with the first decussation occurring at the level of the cochlear nucleus to the contralateral pathways via the trapezoid body. While this pattern is well known, knowledge of specific generators of certain responses and the relation between performance and sites of dysfunction remain unclear. Consideration of contralateral pathways and crossover of neural pathways at cortical and subcortical levels is important in relating peripheral deficits and performance on auditory processing tests.

Tonotopic organization

Frequency specificity and tuning in the auditory system begin at the level of the cochlea and are accurately preserved as signals travel to the cortex.

Speech intelligibility

Natural speech signals contain multiple sources of information and perception of all components is generally not necessary for understanding. Effective speech tests of auditory processing use stimuli where difficulty is increased by methods such as filtering, temporal changes, or competing messages (Bocca and Calearo, 1963; Jerger, 1973).

Processing at the peripheral level

The auditory sensory organ, the cochlea, is composed of inner and outer hair cells that serve very different functions. The main sensory receptors within the cochlea are the inner hair cells that have the majority of the afferent connections to the cochlear branch of the VIIIth cranial nerve. The cochlear outer hair cell system is related to an active process (cochlear amplifier) that is thought to enhance auditory sensitivity. The presence of this active process supports observations that frequency tuning and much processing of signals occur in the periphery. The outer hair cells are primarily connected to efferent neural fibers comprising the olivocochlear pathways. Modulation of outer hair cell function via the efferent olivocochlear system may contribute to the ability to process speech in background noise (e.g., Liberman and Guinan, 1998). Measurement of cochlear or otoacoustic emissions, discussed later in this chapter, provides information about outer hair cell system function and may help to distinguish peripheral from central disorders.

Neural plasticity

Though conventional wisdom might suggest that the nervous system in humans, once fully developed, could not undergo either self-repair or further arborization, clinical observations show that normal humans continue to learn new skills well into their seventies. Reports of patients who had undergone total hemispherectomy and continued to learn new tasks support the re-organization of brain function around remaining strengths. The remarkable recovery of hemispherectomized children was ascribed to the plasticity of their 'young brains' and the still incomplete nature of their development, which could then be recruited to compensate for the hemispherectomy. Thus, evidence supports reorganization of the nervous system, or neural plasticity, throughout life as demonstrated through successes in post-injury recovery and specific skill training programs.

Evaluating auditory processing

Individuals with deficits of the auditory neural pathways most often show normal results on measures of the auditory system that involve tonal or speech stimuli presented only to one ear and without competition. Routine measures of pure tone thresholds and speech recognition in quiet are generally insensitive to auditory processing deficits. Tests that are sensitive to auditory processing disorders introduce a temporally competing signal in either the same ear (monotic) or opposite ear (dichotic), use binaural presentation to test interaction of signals, or involve some type of distortion which alters the frequency, intensity or temporal characteristics of signals.

Behavioral and physiological measures are sensitive to auditory processing disorders. The following sections contain a discussion of the advantages and limitations of these measures in children. This discussion is not exhaustive of all measures used in auditory processing evaluation, and more detailed information is available from sources such as Willeford (1985a), Katz and Wilde (1985) and Baran and Musiek (1999), and texts by Keith (1977), Pinhiero and Musiek (1985), and Bellis (1996).

Several factors should be considered when developing a clinical strategy for evaluation of auditory processing disorders. First, most auditory processing tests are indicative of central pathology only after a loss of peripheral sensitivity has been ruled out. Because the results of many auditory processing tests are influenced by peripheral hearing loss, proper interpretation of test results is not possible without knowledge of peripheral hearing sensitivity. Second, many behavioral tests exhibit considerable inherent variability, particularly when used with younger age groups. Therefore it is advisable to use a battery, or group, of tests in all evaluations and to perform these tests in a suitable acoustic environment. And finally, we always include at least one and generally several physiological measures in an auditory processing test battery.

Behavioral measures of auditory processing using monaural stimuli

Behavioral monaural (monotic) measures of auditory processing include *filtered speech*, *time altered speech*, signals with *ipsilateral competing messages*, and *pattern recognition* of non-speech stimuli. Limiting the frequency content of speech by removing high-frequency components (through low-pass filtering) reduces the redundancy of natural speech signals and challenges the auditory nervous system. Abnormal performance on *filtered speech* tests occurs most often in the ear contralateral to a cortical lesion or may show reduced performance bilaterally (Bocca and Calearo, 1963; Lynn and Gilroy, 1975).

Monaural presentation of speech in the presence of a *competing noise* or a *competing signal* may reflect potential difficulty that children experience in noisy classroom environments. The use of linguistic competition, such as single or multiple competing messages, may serve to better reflect real-life listening situations. While most of these tests were developed for adults, the Pediatric Speech Intelligibility (PSI) Test (Jerger, 1980; Jerger, Lewis, Hawkins and Jerger, 1980) is a competing message task that was constructed specifically for children. This test utilizes a series of target sentences along with competing stimuli presented either ipsilateral to the target (monaural test) or contralateral to the target (dichotic test). Performance on the PSI has been shown to be consistently abnormal in children with confirmed CNS lesions affecting auditory areas while performance is normal for children with non-auditory confirmed lesions (Jerger, Jerger and Loiselle, 1988). Children with suspected central auditory processing disorders and those with confirmed temporal lobe lesions showed decreased performance on dichotic, but not monotic, measures (Jerger et al., 1988).

Several auditory processing measures use stimuli other than speech. For example, Pinhiero (1977) developed a test of auditory processing in adults and children involving recognition of pitch patterns that permits evaluation of *pattern perception* and *temporal sequencing* ability. In Pinhiero's Pitch Pattern Test, subjects are presented three tones, two of one frequency and one of a different frequency, arranged in various orders. Patients with brain lesions and children with learning disabilities generally are able to correctly hum these patterns but cannot reproduce the patterns verbally or manually (Musiek and Guerkink, 1980; Pinhiero, 1977; Pinhiero, 1978; Pinhiero, Jacobsen and Boller, 1982). This type of test paradigm allows adaptation of response modes to the ability of the patient which adds to its application in various age ranges and ability groups.

Behavioral measures of auditory processing using dichotic stimuli

Several dichotic measures are used in evaluating auditory processing in children including *dichotic consonant–vowel syllables* (Berlin and McNeil, 1976), *spondees* (two syllable words with equal stress on both syllables) that partially overlap in time (Staggered Spondaic Words; Katz, 1962), *dichotic digits* (Kimura, 1961), and *competing sentences* (Willeford, 1985b). As with many monaural speech tests, dichotic measures generally were developed on adults and subsequently applied to the evaluation of children.

Dichotic *consonant–vowel nonsense syllables* (CVs) are particularly sensitive to lesions of the temporal lobe (Berlin, Lowe-Bell, Jannetta and Kline, 1972). Simultaneous and time-staggered presentation of two different CVs to normal children indicated that they have an adult-like right-ear advantage from 5 years of age (Berlin, Hughes, Lowe-Bell and Berlin, 1973; Mirabelle, Porter, Hughes and Berlin, 1978) and show improvement in performance for double-correct responses with increasing age (Berlin, 1976). Double-correct responses seem to be especially vulnerable in patients with confirmed brain lesions and in children with auditory processing deficits. Performance of such children lags their normal peers by 3 to 5 years. Much information is available regarding performance of adults on the *Staggered Spondaic Word* (SSW) Test (Katz, 1962), which uses partially overlapping spondaic words as stimuli. Information is also available on use of this test with children (see text by Arnst and Katz, 1982).

Behavioral measures of auditory processing using binaural stimuli

In binaural tests utilizing speech, portions of stimuli are presented to each ear and normal function at some point in the central auditory nervous system is presumed necessary to integrate stimuli into a single message. Examples of such binaural measures are *binaural fusion*, *alternating speech* and *masking level differences (MLD)*. In *binaural fusion* tasks, a low-frequency portion of a message may be presented to one ear and a high-frequency portion to the other ear. While neither stimulus is intelligible alone, integration of the two results in an intelligible message.

Tests using *alternating speech*, where the stimulus material is switched back and forth between the two ears, are sensitive to some lesions in the lower pons (Lynn and Gilroy, 1977). Alternating speech tests are relatively easy to administer to children. However, positive results have been shown on only a small percentage of children with learning disabilities (Willeford and Billger, 1978), and it is not considered a particularly useful test of central function (Willeford, 1985b).

The *masking level difference* (MLD) is quite sensitive to caudal brainstem disorders and is particularly useful when peripheral hearing is normal (Olsen, Noffsinger and Carhart, 1976). The MLD assesses binaural function with regard to phase sensitivity where antiphasic presentation of masking signals results in a "release from masking of a primary signal." The MLD can be administered quickly and easily to children using tones or spondees, but abnormal results are limited to cases where function of the caudal brainstem is compromised. Because of its ease of administration and well-documented sensitivity to these lesions, the MLD test is useful to include in a test battery, but the test will not reveal dysfunction at sites central to the caudal brainstem.

Physiological measures of the central auditory nervous system

Physiologic measures take on particular importance when evaluating the integrity of the auditory system in infants and children. Physiological tests offer an advantage over behavioral measures due to their objectivity and the absence of a need for cooperative participation by the subject. While these tests cannot measure the 'moment' of hearing, they are useful in determining the mechanical and neural integrity of the auditory system, which are critical factors in normal hearing. Physiological analysis is critical in identifying patients with neural synchrony disorders (auditory neuropathy) as discussed later (Case 2). Of particular clinical value are *middle ear muscle reflexes (MEMR), otoacoustic emissions (OAEs), and auditory evoked potentials.*

The *middle ear muscle reflex* is one of two auditory efferent reflexes that can be evaluated in patients. This reflex involves measurement of the contraction of the stapedius muscle of the middle ear in response to high intensity sounds and is used to evaluate the function of the reflex arc which passes through the caudal brainstem (Jerger, 1975). Stimulation of one ear with high intensity stimuli normally results in bilateral contraction of the stapedius muscles, provided that the middle ear, as well as pathways of the seventh and eighth cranial nerves and lower brainstem tracts through the superior olivary complex, are intact. While a very sensitive measure, the middle ear muscle reflexes are compromised by conductive (middle-ear) disorders, cochlear hearing losses greater than moderate in degree, and neural abnormalities affecting the VIIth or VIIIth nerves and/or brainstem pathways. Both the presence of middle-ear disease and cochlear hearing loss must be taken into account prior to interpreting MEMRs relative to any neural disorder. The prevalence of middle-ear problems in young children can limit the utility of this measure in evaluating auditory processing in children with middle-ear disorders. Middle-ear muscle reflexes are generally measured with both ipsilateral and contralateral stimulation, and comparison of responses provides insight into the nature and possible area of a problem. For example, the presence of ipsilateral reflexes and absence of contralateral reflexes is pathognomic for caudal brainstem dysfunction. Because of the effectiveness of MEMR measurement and the brief amount of time necessary to obtain information, its routine use in clinical practice is highly recommended.

In 1978, Kemp published his now landmark paper outlining the existence of *otoacoustic emissions* (OAEs), also referred to as cochlear echoes or cochlear emissions (Kemp, 1978). OAEs are low-amplitude acoustic signals which are emitted from the ear and are associated with normally functioning outer hair cells of the cochlea. OAEs do not provide information about function of the cochlear inner hair cells. Transient-evoked OAEs and distortion product OAEs are the most common OAE measures used clinically and responses are expected in individuals whose hearing threshold sensitivity is better than 30–40 dB HL and middle ear function is normal. OAEs are widely used as a hearing screening test for newborns and infants and as a component of the overall clinical battery of hearing tests used to assess peripheral versus central function in patients of all ages. Otoacoustic emissions, when used in conjunction with auditory evoked potentials, are particularly helpful in distinguishing disorders (such as in patients with auditory neuropathy/dys-synchrony described below and in Case 2) that selectively affect the sensorineural pathway while leaving outer hair cell function intact.

A second efferent reflex in the auditory system, the *olivocochlear reflex* (OCR), reflects activity at the level of the caudal brainstem that affects outer hair cell function. The OCR can be measured by *efferent suppression of OAEs*. This response occurs as a result of activation of the medial efferent pathways descending via the olivocochlear bundle to the outer hair cells. Efferent suppression can be measured using continuous noise in the ear contralateral to the OAE stimulus (e.g., Collet, Kemp, Veuillet et al., 1990; Berlin, Hood, Wen et al., 1993) or by presenting a suppressor stimulus contralaterally, ipsilaterally, or binaurally using a forward masking paradigm (Berlin, Hood, Hurley et al., 1995). (In a forward masking paradigm, the suppressor stimulus, which may be thought of as the 'masker' in forward masking terminology, precedes the OAE evoking stimulus in time in order to avoid interactions between two stimuli presented simultaneously through the same earphone.) Efferent suppression is characterized by amplitude decreases and phase shifts in the OAEs (e.g., Berlin et al., 1993; Ryan, Kemp and Hinchcliffe, 1991). The ability to measure efferent suppression of otoacoustic emissions depends on the presence of OAEs and normal middle-ear function. Efferent suppression of OAEs is abnormal in patients with vestibular nerve section (Williams, Brookes and Prasher, 1993), patients with auditory neuropathy (Berlin, Hood, Hurley and Wen, 1994; Starr, Picton, Sininger et al., 1996), and in many patients with tumors affecting the VIIIth (auditory) nerve (Maurer, Beck, Mann and Mintert, 1992).

Auditory evoked potentials assess neural activity in the auditory pathways from the VIIIth nerve and brainstem through cortical levels. Auditory evoked potentials are useful in the evaluation of neural integrity in children who present with suspected auditory processing problems. Determining the presence or absence of functional abnormalities in the neural pathways can be used to support observed behavioral difficulties on auditory tasks. The most commonly used auditory evoked potentials are the auditory brainstem response (ABR), middle latency response (MLR) and late responses (N1–P2, P300, and mismatch negativity or MMN). The literature on these topics is vast, and the reader is referred to Davis (1976), Hall (1992), Hood (1998), and Jacobson (1994) for detailed information.

The ABR is present at 26–28 weeks gestational age and reaches maturity by 12–18 months of age in normal term infants. The ABR has an elevated threshold in patients with cochlear hearing losses exceeding the moderate hearing loss range and is absent with severe or profound peripheral hearing

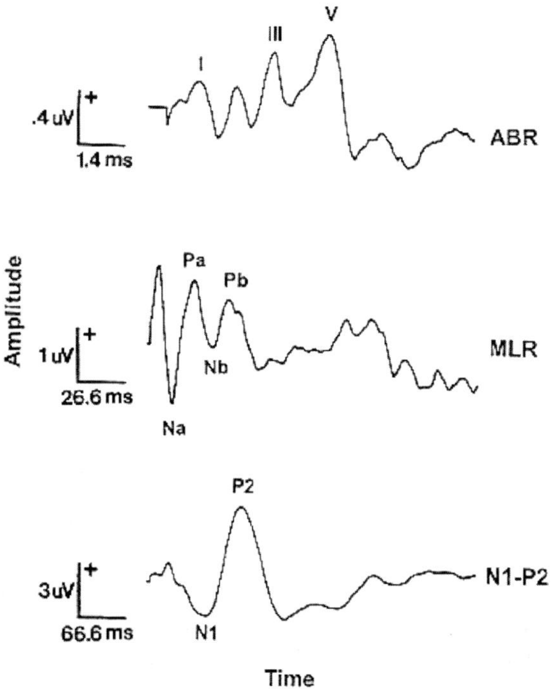

Fig. 1. Normal auditory brainstem response (top tracing), middle latency response (middle tracing) and N1–P2 cortical response (bottom tracing).

losses. ABR abnormalities are observed in neurologically compromised patients (Kraus, Ozdamar, Stein and Reed, 1984) and the ABR is sensitive to space-occupying lesions affecting the VIIIth nerve and/or brainstem (Starr and Achor, 1975). The ABR is generally absent in patients with auditory nerve dys-synchrony (Starr et al., 1996) but is generally normal in children with auditory processing disorders at thalamic and higher levels in the auditory system (Hood, Berlin and Allen, 1994). Thus, a normal ABR does not rule out deficits that may interfere with normal development of speech and language. A normal ABR is shown in Fig. 1 (top tracing).

The middle latency response (MLR) is an auditory evoked potential characterized by two primary vertex-positive components noted as Wave Pa at approximately 30 ms post stimulation and Wave Pb at 50–55 ms (Fig. 1, middle tracing). While the MLR generators have not been conclusively isolated, centers in the thalamus (medial geniculate) and primary cortical projections in auditory areas are likely candidates (Erwin and Buchwald, 1986; Kraus, McGee and Comperatore, 1990; Ozdamar and Kraus, 1983). There are distinct primary and non-primary pathways with components that are differentially affected by arousal state and have different maturational time courses (McGee and Kraus, 1996). MLRs may be recorded in young children but may not reach normal values until 8–10 years of age. The MLR is sensitive to handedness with left-handed listeners generally showing longer Wave Pb latencies than right-handed listeners (Hood, Martin and Berlin, 1990).

Cortical auditory evoked potentials appear promising in evaluating and understanding various aspects of auditory perception in children (e.g., Cheour, Leppanen and Kraus, 2000; Kraus, McGee, Carrell et al., 1995; Tonnquist-Uhlen, 1996). Cortical responses include both those obtained to like stimuli either in quiet or in competing message situations (e.g., N1–P2 response; Fig. 1, bottom tracing) as well as those involving discrimination between different stimuli where a response is required (e.g., P300, Fig. 2) or where no response is necessary (e.g., mismatch negativity).

Cortical potentials such as the P300 response and mismatch negativity (MMN) are ‘event-related potentials’ that occur when the brain makes a decision about whether one stimulus differs from another. For these responses, two different stimuli are presented randomly with one of the stimuli occurring only rarely. The patient’s task in recording the P300 response is to count the number of ‘different’ or rarely occurring stimuli. Changes in vertex N1–P2 and P300 cortical responses have been demonstrated in children and adults in pre- and post therapy or training conditions as well as in relation to cochlear implant success in comparisons of responses obtained to auditory stimuli before and after auditory training therapy (Jirsa, 1992; Kileny, Boerst and Zwolan, 1997).

Mismatch negativity, described as a change-detection response, is recorded without participation of the patient, other than remaining quiet, making the MMN particularly useful in evaluating infants and young children. Unlike other cortical auditory potentials, the MMN is quite stable developmentally and can be obtained from even preterm infants (Cheour-Lutanen, Ahlo, Sainio et al., 1996). Amplitude shows little change across age and latency reaches adult-like values by school-age years.

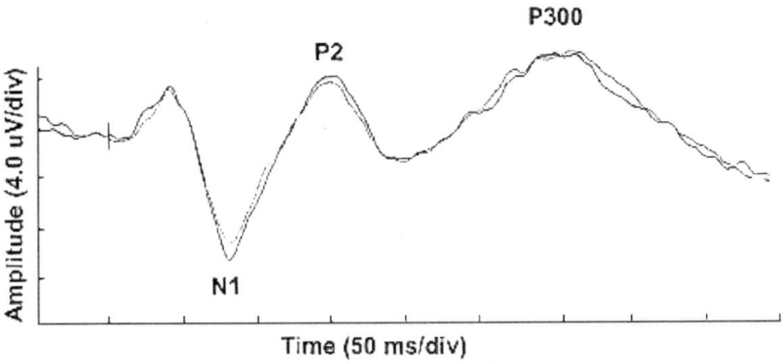

Fig. 2. Normal P300 response to tones.

MMNs appear to be a promising technique in understanding various auditory perception abilities in infants and children as well as adults, assessing the effectiveness of cochlear implants, and monitoring the effectiveness of intervention programs (e.g., Kraus et al., 1995; Kraus, McGee and Koch, 1998). Phoneme discrimination has been demonstrated with the MMN technique in children and adults and in relation to foreign language learning and foreign versus native language processing (Kraus et al., 1995; Naatanen, Lehtokoski, Lennes et al., 1997; Winkler, Lehtokoski, Alku et al., 1999. The MMN also has been used to demonstrate phoneme discrimination ability in infants as young as 30–34 weeks conceptional age (Cheour-Lutanen et al., 1996) and to study development of language specific discrimination abilities (Cheour, Ceponiene, Lehtokoski et al., 1998).

Middle latency and cortical responses display abnormalities in patients with disorders at suprathalamic/supra-collicular levels of the auditory system. Abnormal MLRs are reported in individuals with unilateral and bilateral lesions of the temporal lobes (Kileny, Paccioretti and Wilson, 1987; Kraus, Ozdamar, Hier and Stein, 1982; Ozdamar, Kraus and Curry, 1982). Abnormal cortical responses are associated with a number of neurological disorders including Huntington disease, Parkinson disease, HIV, Alzheimer disease, schizophrenia, autism, and dementia. Middle latency responses and cortical potentials are affected by sleep and sedation, are susceptible to muscle activity, and have longer neuromaturational time courses than the ABR. While these responses may be more difficult to record reliably in young children, they hold significant value in learning about central auditory processing in normal and abnormal systems. In order to successfully record responses in young children, researchers and clinicians have developed techniques to distract or involve children according to the requirements of the protocol. In-depth discussions of the middle latency and cortical responses can be found in Kraus and McGee (1992) and McPherson (1996).

Imaging studies and central auditory nervous system function

Penfield and Roberts (1959) mapped the living human cortex by applying mild electrical pulses to various portions of the open brains of living patients who were undergoing surgery for epileptic foci and temporarily leaving behind numbered (sterile) tickets as a map, noting and recording the resultant behaviors. The criticisms leveled at the work noted that none of the patients were 'normal' in the sense that all had epileptic disease for which they were undergoing craniotomy. However, their general findings, which have been since verified non-invasively in healthy humans, showed a four-part tree in the brain for mediating speech and language perception and production (medial geniculate to pulvinar to primary auditory cortices on each side and then across the anterior commissure and corpus callosum to the left hemisphere for speech–language related information directed to the right hemisphere). Their still viable concepts show that the pulvinar (part of the thalamus that is not part of the primary auditory pathway), and its projections to temporal occipital and frontal areas form the primary and association pathways to the structures in the human brain that are most active in comprehension, processing and expression of language in both speech and writing.

Confirmation of Penfield and Roberts observations came from many sources. Lassen, Ingvar and Skinhoj (1978) asked volunteers to inhale Xe-133, a radioactive gas that binds to hemoglobin. The volunteers then underwent various perceptual and production tasks while the scientists studied metabolic rates and regional cerebral flow inferred by the density of the Xe-133 molecules. The scientific findings confirmed the dominance of the temporal areas for auditory processing, the frontal areas for motor speech production, and the implied importance of the arcuate fasciculus in facilitating functional connections between posterior and anterior portions of the brain (Webster, 1999).

Current techniques for studying brain function include Positron Emission Tomography (PET) to study cerebral blood flow and Magnetic Resonance Imaging (MRI) that offers detailed pictures of brain structures that allow for the location and study of lesions of the brain. Functional MRI (fMRI) permits the analysis of molecular and chemical events that accompany hearing and speech functions.

During speech perception and production there is a feedback loop running to and from Broca's and Wernicke's areas, via the arcuate fasciculus. This feedback loop is clinically testable by a delayed auditory feedback technique. In patients with disconnection aphasia there is no interference with speech production because there is no monitoring (Geschwind, 1965). There also is no monitoring in the truly deaf patient. Delayed auditory feedback has been used to study the integrity of the connection in hearing impaired, normal hearing, and cochlear implant patients (Berlin and Svirsky, 1989).

Limitations of auditory processing measures

Subject factors

Subject factors can influence results obtained on measures of auditory processing. Degree and configuration of peripheral hearing loss, symmetry of hearing between the two ears, and speech recognition for undistorted stimuli can affect test results, and significant peripheral hearing loss can seriously compromise the validity of auditory processing testing. Other subject factors such as age, drugs, medication, attention, motivation, reading ability, educational background, linguistic function and fatigability can also affect results and must be considered in interpretation.

Adaptations of tests constructed for adults

Many of the measures used to evaluate auditory processing in children are adaptations of tests originally developed and validated in adults. Vocabulary and level of difficulty of stimuli are sometimes inappropriate, especially for young children. For example, filtered speech tests generally have been validated on adults (Bocca and Calearo, 1963; Lynn and Gilroy, 1975) and then applied to evaluation of children (Willeford and Billger, 1978). An exception is the Pediatric Speech Intelligibility (PSI) Test where stimuli were generated based upon descriptions of pictures by children and careful evaluation of vocabulary level (Jerger et al., 1980).

Variability of responses in children

Children from 5–10 years of age show considerable variability in performance on auditory processing tests. For example, Willeford's (1985a) norms for the filtered speech test show that differences in performance between ears are greater in children (about 5%) than in adults (less than 1%), and the range of normal performance varies by as much as 40% in younger children compared to 20% in adults. Language is a critical factor in auditory processing testing and the appropriateness of stimuli to the language level of a child can affect results (Wilson and Thompson, 1984). Based on the wide variability in performance, it may be advisable to consider scores abnormal only when the score for one or both ears falls below the lower range boundary for the child's age group, or when a marked difference in performance exists between the two ears (Willeford, 1985a).

Maturation appears to be a factor in performance variability on many, but not all, auditory processing measures. For example, Rupp (1983) noted an 11% improvement in speech-in-noise scores for monosyllables in children from kindergarten through grade 5, suggesting that some age-related changes may affect speech-in-noise abilities. Willeford (1977) reports maturation of binaural fusion ability from ages 5 through 9 based on changes in norms across this age range. In contrast, data from Diefendorf (1981) showed that 6-month-old infants demonstrated success on a binaural fusion task, suggesting that changes in binaural fusion scores may not be related to maturation.

Broader variation in responses in younger children than in older children and adults also occurs in evaluation of some psychoacoustic abilities. For example, while children aged 3–5 years could attend well to a temporal resolution task, threshold variability from run to run was substantial, which may have been related to attentional factors (Wightman, Allen, Dolan et al., 1989).

Inability to isolate site of lesion

Auditory processing disorders may reflect specific localizable damage to the central nervous system or diffuse, non-localizable disorders evidenced by below average performance on a series of skills. Both types of problems are difficult to isolate based upon symptomatology and a series of test results. Specific localizable lesions may be supported by radiological abnormalities, making quantification easier, while below normal or low average function unaccompanied by physical evidence of a lesion usually presents the greatest diagnostic challenge. Regardless of the type of disorder, it is difficult to isolate lesion sites precisely due to multiple overlapping pathways and the limits of current knowledge of generators within the central auditory nervous system.

Importance of the test battery

No single measure of auditory processing ability is perfect for identifying disorders. This, combined with the complexity of the auditory system, the variability in performance and many subject factors which can influence test results, points to the necessity of using a series of tests in the evaluation of patients suspected to have an auditory processing disorder. Various studies noted throughout this chapter have compared performance of different auditory processing tests and reported those in which performance separated normal from abnormal groups. When examining these studies, it is important to carefully compare one's own clinical population with those sampled prior to drawing any conclusions or adapting a test for use in one's own clinical practice.

Association of test results with specific disorders

The relationship among *delayed language*, *learning disabilities* and other disorders such as *attention deficit/hyperactivity disorders* occupies many chapters and entire texts. Test performance varies considerably and appears to be closely tied to the test material, mode of presentation, task difficulty and subject definition. For example, a large percentage of learning disabled children demonstrated difficulty with certain auditory processing tasks (Katz and Burge, 1971; Willeford and Billger, 1978), but the range of performance varied widely (Willeford, 1977). Interpretation of results can also be affected by scoring techniques and which ear is tested first (White, 1977). Even some of the 'more objective' measures show considerable variability among studies. For example, Sweetow and Reddell (1978) and Stecker (1983) differentiated learning disabled and normal children with the MLD while Roush and Tait (1984) found no differences in MLDs between controls and language learning-disabled children.

Careful consideration of what a test is measuring is necessary for appropriate application and interpretation. For example, Roush and Tait (1984) measured binaural fusion, masking level differences and the ABR in normal and language/learning-disabled children aged 6–12 years. The language/learning-disabled group performed poorly for all conditions, while the MLD and ABR did not differentiate groups. This finding suggests that the lower overall performance may have been due to the distortion produced by filtering rather than dysfunction of binaural synthesis. This is further supported by the observation that the two groups differed on filtered speech tasks but not on tests with non-linguistic stimuli (MLD and ABR). While evidence supports the usefulness of auditory processing tests in identifying children with language and/or learning disorders, specific cause–effect relationships are still speculative.

Distinguishing auditory processing disorders from other categories of disorders is also problematic.

For example, Gascon, Johnson and Burd (1986) described a series of children defined as having *attention deficit disorders* who exhibited short attention spans, distractibility, hyperactivity and impulsivity. When such children were given CNS stimulants for their attention deficit disorder, performance on tests of auditory processing improved in 79% of the children. Gascon suggests, based on these results, that the clinical picture of an auditory processing disorder is indistinguishable from an attention deficit disorder. It is clear that, while performance on auditory tests may be more likely to be abnormal in children with attention disorders, they would not be an appropriate way to actually test for attention deficits.

Case studies of children with auditory processing disorders

Children with auditory processing disorders often demonstrate such characteristics as poor auditory attention, difficulty listening in situations with background noise, difficulty with auditory integration or sequencing, and/or problems following rapid changes in speech. Depending on the underlying etiology, auditory processing problems may be accompanied by other sensory deficits. Reading and spelling often are the most deficient academic areas. Auditory processing deficits may range from a mild difficulty isolated to particular tasks or areas of function to a severe central problem that renders the child unable to utilize auditory stimuli in a meaningful manner. While characteristics consistent with auditory dysfunction may be similar among patients, the underlying abnormalities may be very different, as distinguished in Patients 1 and 2 below.

Localizable central hearing defects

Patients with cortical deafness, also referred to as central auditory deafness, auditory aphasia, or verbal auditory agnosia present unique evaluation and habilitation challenges (e.g., Goldstein, 1974; Graham, Greenwood and Lecky, 1980; Jerger, Weikers, Sharbrough and Jerger, 1969; Kaga, Shindo and Tanaka, 1997; Landau, Goldstein and Kleffner, 1957; Landau and Kleffner, 1957; Michel, Peronnet and Schott, 1980). Of particular interest is the case reported by Landau et al. (1957) of a child who by 6 years of age had not developed speech, despite apparent adequate intelligence. Reactions were observed to low-frequency sounds but no comprehension of spoken language was apparent. At 8 years a functional vocabulary of about 175 words was present via reading, speaking and writing. Following death at age 10 due to cardiac complications, the brain was obtained for examination. The brainstem was grossly normal; however, cortical degeneration of the parietal, temporal and occipital lobes was observed and the medial geniculate nuclei were severely degenerated. This case demonstrated severe anatomical damage to the primary auditory projection pathways bilaterally and the near complete effect upon speech and language development. This patient, and the patient described in the next section, fit the characteristics of Landau–Kleffner syndrome, or acquired aphasia with convulsive disorder (Landau and Kleffner, 1957), with approximately 200 cases reported in the literature (Klein, Tuchman and Rapin, 2000).

Patient One: bilateral temporal lobe lesions resulting in cortical deafness

We have followed Patient One, identified as a child with true cortical deafness, for more than 20 years. Following a high fever at about one year of age, several misdiagnoses were made over the years that followed including peripheral deafness, learning disability, emotional disturbance, retardation, and autism. When we first saw her she was 5 years old, unable to follow verbal instructions, and demonstrated speech quality that is characteristic of individuals with profound hearing loss. Peripheral auditory sensitivity was difficult to quantify due to inconsistent responses; thresholds for speech stimuli were in the normal to mild hearing loss range. Middle-ear muscle reflexes were normal. Good peripheral hearing sensitivity was confirmed by auditory brainstem responses to low- and high-frequency stimuli where latency–intensity functions showed responses to very faint stimuli for each ear. Thus peripheral sensitivity was considered normal bilaterally. Middle latency responses were absent bilaterally which was consistent with bilateral absence of large portions of the temporal lobes shown by computed tomography (CT) and later by magnetic resonance imaging (MRI). Late cortical responses showed presence of some synchronous activity, but with delays in latency and asymmetries in amplitude. The patient's inability to recognize speech stimuli precluded all speech-based behavioral central hearing tests. Localization testing showed inability to reliably localize any stimuli.

As would be expected, this child received little to no benefit from speech therapy or hearing aids. In fact, she rejected hearing aids and communicated primarily by reading and writing until learning sign language. Her language ability remains significantly delayed, and she relies upon manual communication which she used in her education at a state school for the Deaf.

Several conclusions can be reached from this case (Fig. 3). First, the importance of objective measures of auditory function cannot be over-emphasized. Secondly, objective tests such as the ABR and middle-ear muscle reflexes do not eliminate the possibility of a central hearing loss, and it is critical to use measures presumed to be sensitive to function at more central areas. Third, it is important to look beyond peripheral hearing regions when communication problems cannot be explained. And finally, early identification of problems at any level of the hearing system is important followed *immediately* by introduction of training toward some viable mode of communication.

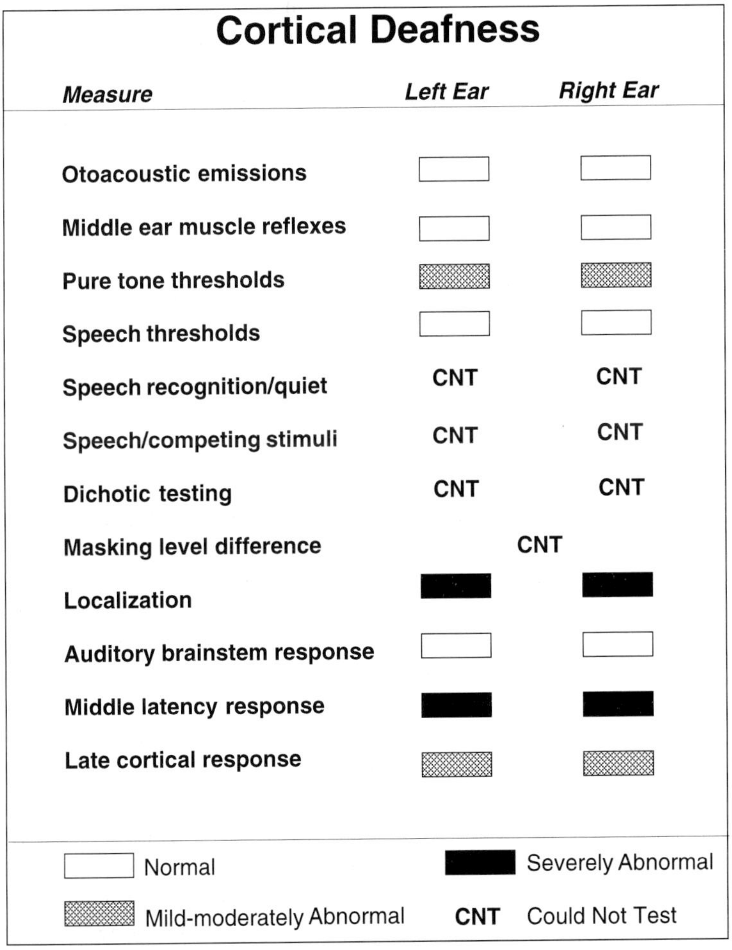

Fig. 3. Summary of behavioral and electrophysiological test results for Patient One who is an example of cortical deafness. Greatest abnormalities were observed for localization and middle latency responses. CT scans and MRI show bilateral absence of large portions of the temporal lobes. With an inability to utilize any auditory information, this patient communicates using American Sign Language.

An auditory processing problem due to poor neural synchrony and a peripheral neuropathy

Recently, patients ranging in age from infants to adults have been described with an auditory disorder termed auditory neuropathy or auditory dys-synchrony (Berlin et al., 1993; Berlin, Hood, Morlet and Keats, 2001; Starr et al., 1996). These patients have normal otoacoustic emissions, suggesting normal outer hair cell function, and abnormal ABRs, demonstrating a neural dys-synchrony. While the term neuropathy suggests pathology of the auditory nerve, abnormal inner hair cell function and input to the nerve or a problem at the synaptic juncture could also result in neural dys-synchrony necessary to disrupt the ABR.

Auditory neuropathy/dys-synchrony should be clearly distinguished from more 'central' auditory processing disorders. They are very different types of disorders and are contrasted by site of the disorder, pattern of test results, and viable management options. For example, cochlear implants have been successful in the majority of auditory neuropathy/dys-synchrony patients implanted, while implants are not a management option for more central auditory processing types of disorders.

Patients with auditory neuropathy/dys-synchrony show normal CT and MRI results which distinguishes them from patients with space-occupying lesions or disorders such as multiple sclerosis. Some patients with auditory neuropathy/dys-synchrony demonstrate timing problems (Starr, McPherson, Patterson et al., 1991; Zeng, Oba, Garde et al., 1999) which are suggestive of a disturbance in neural synchrony. Most patients with auditory neuropathy/dys-synchrony show bilateral symptoms, though function is often asymmetric between ears and a few cases of unilateral auditory neuropathy/dys-synchrony have been documented.

Patients with an auditory neuropathy/dys-synchrony show variable pure-tone thresholds ranging from normal sensitivity to the severe or profound hearing loss range (e.g., Berlin et al., 1993, 1994; Gorga, Stelmachowicz, Barlow and Brookhouser, 1995; Kaga, Nakamura, Shinogami et al., 1996; Starr et al., 1991). Normal outer hair cell function is evidenced by the presence of otoacoustic emissions and cochlear microphonics. Abnormal synchrony is reflected by abnormal ABRs and absent MEMRs. While there may initially appear to be an ABR response, close examination shows that there is no increase in latency with decreasing stimulus intensity, as should occur with neural responses. Furthermore, when the polarity of the stimulus is reversed (rarefaction versus condensation clicks), the peaks of the recorded response reverse (Berlin, Bordelon, St John et al., 1998). Both of these characteristics are consistent with a cochlear microphonic rather than neural response. Fig. 4 shows an ABR with condensation clicks only and with condensation and rarefaction clicks obtained in an infant with auditory neuropathy/dys-synchrony. Patients generally show no masking level difference, consistent with abnormalities in processing of timing and phase information. Speech recognition is quite variable though generally much poorer than expected.

The classification of auditory neuropathy/dys-synchrony most likely describes several different specific sites of abnormality, all of which result in the clinical observation of normal outer hair cell responses accompanied by poor neural synchrony. Some patients, both children and adults, have no known etiology and no other identified neurological abnormalities. In other patients, the auditory findings may be associated with other peripheral neuropathies such as hereditary motor sensory neuropathy (HMSN; Charcot–Marie–Tooth disease). Of particular interest is the number of infants and young children who have been identified with auditory dys-synchrony. Infants with neonatal abnormalities, including prematurity, exchange transfusion, low birth weight, hyperbilirubinemia, etc. have been reported (Deltenre, Mansbach, Bozet et al., 1997; Stein, Tremblay, Pasternak et al., 1996), and there are cases where a genetic basis is suspected due to multiple affected family members (Berlin et al., 2001).

The mechanisms of auditory neuropathy/dys-synchrony presently are unclear, and several mechanisms and etiologies most likely exist. Most writers agree with Starr et al. (1991) that this is a timing disorder that may be axonic, dendritic, or even primarily sensory in nature. The mechanical transduction or other functional characteristics of the inner hair cells could be abnormal, the synaptic juncture between the inner hair cells and the cochlear branch of the vestibulocochlear (eighth) nerve could be affected,

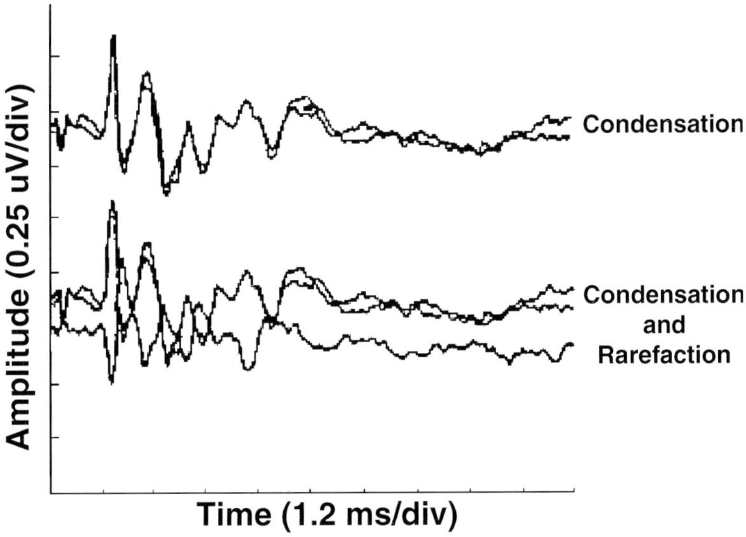

Fig. 4. Auditory brainstem response to condensation clicks (top tracing) and to condensation and rarefaction clicks (bottom tracing) obtained from an infant with auditory neuropathy/dys-synchrony. The inversion of all waves with the stimulus polarity change is consistent with a cochlear microphonic rather than neural response.

or the axons or cell bodies of the eighth nerve itself could be the site. Uneven conduction velocities, especially in cases where there is demyelinization, could underlie the poor synchrony observed.

Management of patients with auditory neuropathy/dys-synchrony with standard amplification (hearing aids) generally has not been beneficial though some patients benefit from FM (frequency modulation) devices, most likely due to improved signal-to-noise ratios that provide a clearer signal to a system that cannot cope with interference. Management for all children with auditory neuropathy/dys-synchrony should include use of some visual system (such as cued speech or sign language) to facilitate development of language and communication skills. While patients do well with Auditory/Verbal therapy post cochlear implant, auditory cues alone are insufficient for language development in these patients. The majority of patients with auditory neuropathy/dys-synchrony who have been managed with cochlear implants demonstrate good benefit. Further confounding management issues related to infants and children with auditory neuropathy/dys-synchrony are reports that auditory function may change over time. The majority of patients show either no change in auditory function or a worsening of responses over time, but there are a few who have appeared to develop some auditory abilities though their ABR remains dys-synchronous (Berlin et al., 1998; Stein et al., 1996).

Patient two: abnormal peripheral neural synchrony ('auditory neuropathy'/'auditory dys-synchrony')

This patient was first evaluated at age thirteen years, upon failure of a hearing test at school. He was reported to be an average student who worked hard in school to maintain a 'C' average. Math was his best subject and he enjoyed math problems. His history indicated that he began to walk late (at 21 months), had a history of middle ear problems, and had poor balance. Audiological test results indicated decreased hearing in the high frequencies for pure tones bilaterally and a mild loss in the mid-frequency range for the left ear as well (Fig. 5). At the time of the initial testing, speech recognition in the left ear was very poor in quiet and in noise, while speech presented to the right ear was intelligible in quiet but compromised in noise. The very poor speech recognition in the left ear precluded dichotic testing. The masking level difference showed no release of masking at all when the phase of the noise was shifted.

This patient has been followed for the past 8 years, during which time he subsequently was di-

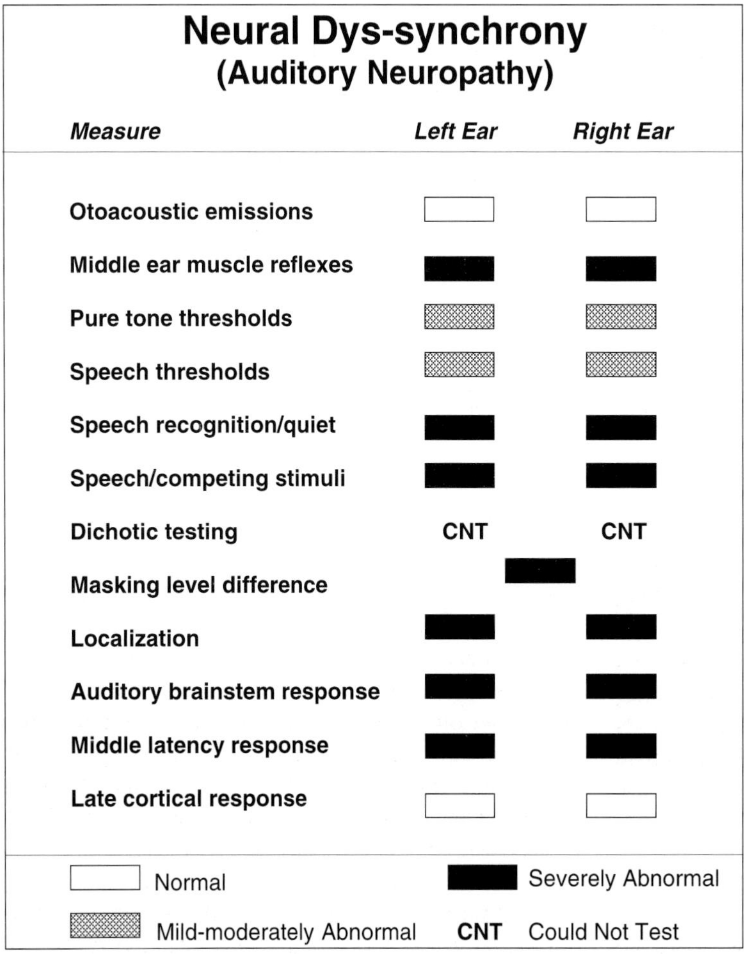

Fig. 5. Summary of behavioral and electrophysiological test results for Patient Two who is an example of neural dys-synchrony or auditory neuropathy. Poor performance, to a greater extent for the left ear, was observed on most behavioral measures. Despite poor understanding of speech and absence of some electrophysiological responses, this individual has normal speech and attends normal classes. He uses visual information via lipreading, notetaking services, and closed captioning.

agnosed with Charcot–Marie–Tooth disease, based upon the finding of reduced nerve conduction velocities, consistent with a demyelinating neuropathy. Over the course of several years, pure-tone thresholds gradually decreased to a moderate to severe hearing loss. Word recognition progressively decreased to an inability to understand single words or connected speech, even in quiet, without visual cues. The patient continues to show robust transient evoked and distortion product otoacoustic emissions, but no efferent suppression of transient evoked otoacoustic emissions. Middle-ear function (tympanometry) has been normal on all tests though no MEMRs have been recorded. Absence of both efferent reflexes (OAE suppression and MEMR) is most likely related to poor afferent input (Hood, Berlin, Bordelon et al., 2000). Auditory brainstem and middle latency responses are absent though late responses (N1–P2 cortical potentials) are present.

An absent ABR in the presence of normal otoacoustic emissions is the classic indicator of an auditory dys-synchrony or auditory neuropathy. Absent middle-ear muscle reflexes and auditory brainstem and middle latency responses in the presence of normal late (cortical) responses suggest difficulty with synchronous information from the lower brainstem, thalamus and primary auditory areas, but some successful cortical integration. An FM (frequency modulation) system was tried with little benefit. The patient depends primarily on lipreading, notetaking service for classes, closed captioning, and other visual cues for communication. Additional information regarding test findings for this patient can be found in articles by Berlin et al. (1993, 1994).

Pseudo central hearing loss

There are a number of conditions under which peripheral damage to the cochlea can simulate the characteristics of an auditory processing disorder. When any sharp slope or sharp discontinuity in auditory sensitivity occurs, due to cochlear abnormalities, a peculiar set of circumstances can co-exist. Patients can hear environmental noises and identify them with considerable success, but they cannot understand speech. This pairing of circumstances is often erroneously taken as a sign of an auditory processing disorder. In this section, we will review conditions under which these peripheral losses can simulate central loss, how to identify such conditions and how to manage them.

Downward sloping high-frequency loss

In young children, a sharply sloping high-frequency loss with normal hearing up to about 500 Hz (Fig. 6) can give a child the ability to respond to simple stimuli (his name, the dog's name, repetition of syllables "ba–ba–ba") often used in sound field testing to see if a child alerts to speech. Since this alerting can and often does occur at very faint levels (15–25 dB Hearing Level), diagnosticians often use this as an 'index of normal hearing.' The rest of the audiogram is then 'constructed' based on a preconceived notion that the child has normal hearing since he has normal sensitivity for speech sounds. What has actually happened is that the low-frequency vocalic carrier of the speech or the low frequency side band of any abrupt sound falls into the normal hearing zone of the child, and he/she, in fact, hears but does not understand. This particular effect is commonly seen in children for whom no other objective tests are run. To prevent such a misdiagnosis, astute audiologists use tympanometry, ipsilateral and contralateral middle-ear muscle reflexes showing symmetry of all the reflexes at normal levels, auditory brainstem responses, otoacoustic emissions tests, and in some instances a special middle-ear muscle reflex test comparing broadband, low-pass and high-pass noise (SPAR: Sensitivity Prediction using the Acoustic Reflex; Jerger, Burney, Mauldin and Crump, 1974). Children with this type of peripheral loss will show language delay and characteristic speech patterns, should they develop language, which show omission or distortion of high-frequency consonants. If the high frequency loss extends down to 250 Hz, leaving 125 Hz as the nearly normal frequency, for all practical purposes the child will behave deaf to all but broadband environmental sounds including the male voice. Screening with the Ling Five-Sound Test will show that patients like this respond to the vowels "ah" and "oo" but give no response to the consonants "s" and "sh" with a borderline response possible to the vowel "ee" at normal levels.

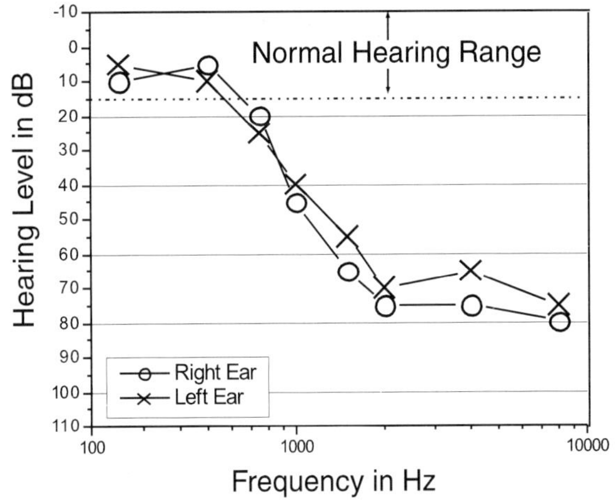

Fig. 6. Audiometric configuration of a downward sloping sensorineural hearing loss.

Upward sloping low-frequency hearing loss

Some years ago we uncovered a type of hearing loss that had been hitherto undocumented in the literature (Berlin, Wexler, Jerger et al., 1978). In this loss, hearing is quite poor throughout the standard audiometric range, but there is an upward slope to the audiogram such that by 10–12 kHz (ranges

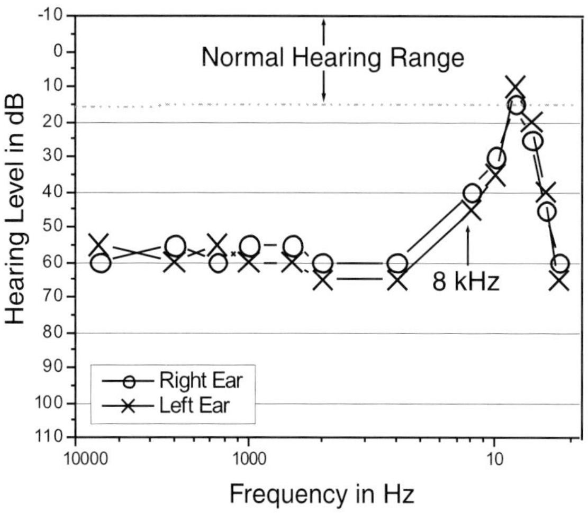

Fig. 7. Audiometric configuration of an upward sloping sensorineural hearing loss.

usually outside the standard audiogram) the patient has normal or nearly normal hearing (Fig. 7). Such patients respond to environmental noises of very high frequencies, very faint /s/ or /sh/ phonemes but not to vocalic sounds. They too are often labeled centrally deaf, autistic or receive some other arcane diagnosis because their peripheral hearing loss has not been objectively assessed.

Patient three: mild peripheral sensory loss mistaken for an auditory processing impairment

This child was brought to us at age 4 with a diagnosis of an auditory processing disorder. He was at that time 1.5 years delayed in language, had many speech and articulation errors and seemed to be unresponsive to everyday conversation. He had a longstanding 25–35 dB HL sensory loss in both ears that had been confirmed both behaviorally and electrophysiologically on a number of occasions. However, the professional told the family that this much hearing loss was fundamentally inconsequential to speech and language development and that the child's failure to develop adequate speech and language was secondary to some more central problem.

We did not concur with this diagnosis and fitted the child with mild gain hearing aids. He has made a major improvement in speech, language, behavior and orientation. Basically, what this child was forced to do was learn a new language with a decrement in his hearing abilities that could have been considered inconsequential only if he already knew English, all of its rules of grammar, and all its nuances of phonology. Since he had this hearing loss all his life, he was unable to acquire these cues easily and was ignoring them. Armed with hearing aids, he made sufficient recovery to be in regular school and to catch up on his language skills with the aid of Fast ForWord, a very valuable tool in our experience for compensating for auditory deprivation. Test results for Patient Three are shown in Fig. 8.

General rules to separate pseudocentral hearing loss from an auditory processing disorder

In general, the application of immittance (impedance) audiometry, otoacoustic emissions, and electrophysiology in clinical evaluation will pick up most, if not all, peripheral losses masquerading as central hearing losses. In acquiring auditory brainstem responses, frequency specific stimuli such as well-defined tonebursts or other spectrally limited stimuli should be used to rule out sharply sloping audiometric configurations that would be 'masked' by use of only broad band stimuli such as clicks. ABR via bone conduction, along with immittance measures can be used to identify conductive components to the hearing loss.

Peripheral contributions to auditory processing disorders

Mild conductive hearing loss

Infants and young children have a high incidence of conductive hearing loss (Northern and Downs, 1991). A history of fluctuating hearing loss in early life may place a child at risk for difficulties in auditory processing later in life (Jerger, Jerger, Alford and Abrams, 1983; Weber, Folsom and Thompson, 1983). Even a slight conductive hearing loss with thresholds on the order of 15–25 dB Hearing Level can inhibit accurate perception of speech sounds, especially in background noise, and be a handicapping loss (Dobie and Berlin, 1979; Downs and Blager, 1982; Northern and Downs, 1991).

Some children with mild conductive hearing loss demonstrate the same results on language tests that

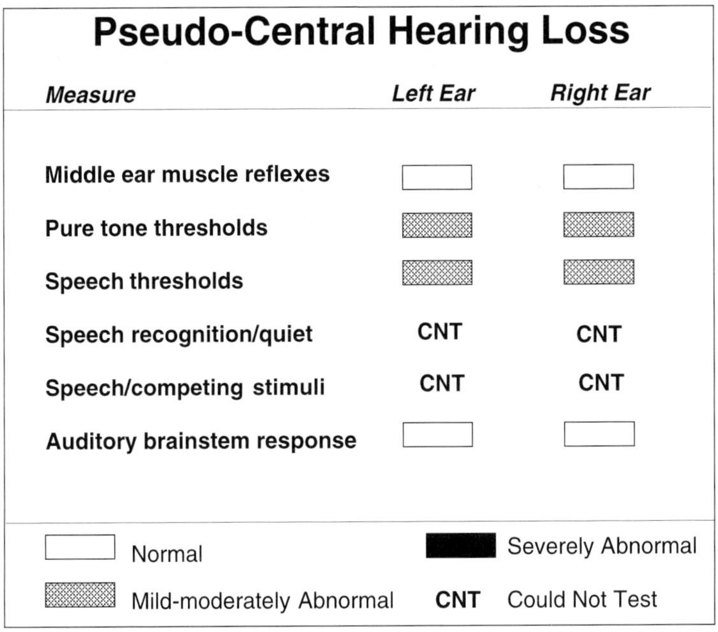

Fig. 8. Summary of behavioral and electrophysiological test results for Patient Three who is an example of a pseudo-central hearing disorder. Though reports of evaluations suggested a central hearing disorder as the basis for his delayed speech and language development, this child was found to have a mild peripheral hearing loss and benefits well from mild gain hearing aids.

have been reported as classic “central processing disorders” (Downs, 1985). Performance demonstrates (1) lower verbal scores than performance on IQ tests, (2) lower scores on test items considered sensitive to auditory perceptual problems, (3) lower scores on items describing receptive and auditory learning skills, and (4) lower scores on auditory than visual items.

The long term effects of otitis media with effusion (OME) indicate no residual peripheral hearing loss in the standard audiometric range after the condition has resolved (e.g., Gravel and Wallace, 2000). However, data also show that a history of chronic OME may result in cochlear hearing loss in frequency regions above those normal tested clinically (i.e., above 8000 Hz) (Hunter, Margolis, Ryyken et al., 1996). Poorer performance on binaural processing tasks has been reported in children with history of middle-ear problems (Hall, Grose and Pillsbury, 1995). Electrophysiological evidence of longstanding effects of conductive hearing loss has been observed in the auditory brainstem responses, particularly the binaural interaction component, where responses differ from those in normal individuals (Dobie and Berlin, 1979; Gunnarson and Finitzo, 1991).

The long-term effects of OME, after it has resolved, on language and learning suggest long-term effects in some areas of speech and language development though much variability exists among studies with regard to documentation of OME, the types of measures used, populations studied, and issues addressed. Prospective studies of children with a history of OME, which provide ability to carefully document OME histories, suggest an association of hearing loss during the first year of life with speech delays and difficulties in language processing during the early years (e.g., Gravel and Wallace, 1995; Shriberg, Friel-Patti, Flipsen and Brown, 2000). Preliminary comparisons of children with positive and negative histories of OME also have shown poorer phonological perception in those with positive histories of OME (Petinou, Schwartz, Gravel and Raphael, 2001). Still other studies have failed to show significant relationships between early OME history and language skills in the preschool or school years (Augustsson and Engstand, 2001; Klausen, Moller, Holmfjord et al., 2000; Roberts, Burchinal, Jackson et al., 2000).

Unilateral sensory hearing loss

Patients with unilateral hearing loss, where one ear is normal and the other ear exhibits a severe to total hearing loss, are often considered to have no handicapping hearing condition (Bess and Tharpe, 1986). However, problems exhibited by persons with unilateral sensory hearing loss are often quite similar to those observed in central hearing disorders. Elimination of 'two-eared' listening compromises ability to localize and the ability to use the binaural system to squelch background noise and obtain a release from masking (Bess, Tharpe and Gibler, 1986). This increases difficulty when listening in noisy environments which reduces understanding and can cause problems in classroom situations.

Management of pseudocentral, conductive and unilateral hearing losses

With respect to downward sloping high-frequency hearing losses, specialized hearing aids are now available to address this problem either directly or indirectly. The most effective direct method is a combined use of specialized ear molds (Libby horns, CFA adapters) and programmable hearing aids. Hearing aids of this sort have expanded frequency responses and very flat insertion gains which should be monitored by real ear probe microphone measurements. The importance of a real ear probe microphone measurement cannot be overstressed since resonant peaks and valleys in the ear canal can generate enormous unintentional degradation of the signal-to-noise ratio.

Upward sloping low-frequency hearing losses were best managed years ago by upward shifting translator hearing aids (Cullen, Berlin and Halperin, 1982). This was necessary because of the limitations in frequency response of speakers and the insertion loss caused by solid ear molds. Now, although we have translators available, we first try to have patients use broad band input automatic gain control hearing aids. Also, hearing aids with 2 : 1 compression or similar output control and a broad frequency response can be used with some success. Again, real ear measurement and monitoring of the sound pressure at the ear drum is essential.

Conductive hearing losses can respond to virtually any kind of hearing aid since amplification of sound across a broad frequency range is the general goal. In patients with unilateral sensory hearing loss, CROS type hearing aids (where the signal is picked up on the side with poor hearing with one hearing aid and routed into the good ear by another hearing aid) have been used successfully in the past. In another method, used with individuals with unilateral hearing losses, a powerful behind the ear hearing aid is placed on the side of the impaired ear and signals are routed via bone conduction to the good ear, bypassing the need for a second hearing aid (Sullivan, 1988). Some patients report considerable success with such a system, while others feel it is simply adding noise to an already difficult listening situation. Wearable FM systems and related assistive listening devices are also used with unilateral hearing loss patients and evidence suggests that such systems with limited maximum output and very little amplification can be quite helpful in patients with unilateral hearing losses (Bess, Klee and Culbertson, 1986).

Management of auditory processing disorders

When an auditory processing problem is suspected or identified, measures should be taken to improve the child's listening environment, such as the classroom (Katz and Wilde, 1985). Such improvements may include reduction of background noise, increasing the quality of the primary signal, and enhancing non-auditory cues to the child.

In general, improvement of the signal-to-noise ratio with assistive listening systems is often helpful to children with central hearing problems. Children, especially those who show poor MLDs, disturbed ability to follow signals in noise, etc., will benefit from either infrared assistive listening devices or the more commonly available FM systems. These systems basically enhance the signal-to-noise ratio in all listening situations. The usual listening signal-to-noise ratio for common, everyday experiences is 6–8 dB; that is, the human voice reaches the listener about 6 feet away at approximately 50–55 dB hearing level. The background noise corrected for audibility is usually between 45 and 50 dB A scale in most rooms. That means that the common listening situations rarely give enormous advantages of the signal over the noise. By measuring the physical output of the voice at the mouth, one sees that the human voice can generate approximately 105–115 dB SPL right at the point of origin for vocalic utterances. These speech sounds can then be delivered by FM radio or infrared systems to the ear of the listener so that, for practical purposes, the ear of the listener is always at the mouth of the speaker no matter what the actual physical distance might be. This improves the signal-to-noise ratio from about 6 dB to close to 50 dB and markedly enhances information transfer.

Our experience with children with mild or moderate auditory processing problems suggests that assistive listening devices can sometimes be of value. In the severe cases of auditory agnosia and bilateral absence of the temporal lobes (Patient One), we have found no successful assitive listening systems to engender speech/language production and have found that the patients are comfortable using sign language and being raised in a Deaf culture.

In addition to assistive listening devices, Matkin (1982) suggests several management techniques which include simultaneous visual input as a supplement to auditory stimuli, limitation of the length and complexity of the message, gaining the child's attention, and monitoring the child's comprehension of the message.

Neural plasticity and auditory processing

There are many lessons to be learned from the natural reorganization of the brain after injury or surgery. Among them is that brains and nervous systems organize themselves based on experiences and learning; thus, strictly speaking, any learning experience changes the brain. It was also clear to visionary scientists like Hebb, Skinner, Mountcastle, and their professional descendants that, if training could be carefully controlled, the nature of the brain's organization could be manipulated. The principle was clear: if we knew what had to be taught, and we could put it in a form that the nervous system could use, changes through learning would likely take place.

Michael Merzenich, one of Mountcastle's professional descendants, reasoned, against the conventional wisdom of the 1950s, that one nervous system was just like another. If one wanted to understand, for example, how the central auditory nervous system organized itself, Merzenich suggested studying the more accessible somatosensory cortex and input pathways and make discoveries relevant to all systems. Merzenich and his colleagues found that when monkeys had to re-learn a complex manipulation task after availability of some of their fingers changed, the somatosensory cortex reorganized itself to allow the task to be performed (Merzenich, Recanzone and Jenkins, 1990). However, the reorganization was haphazard unless the task was re-taught in a very specific manner reinforcing only correct performance, fractionating the task into accessible bits, and manipulating accurate performance by carefully controlled increments. These experiments showed plasticity of the somatosensory nervous system and that successful reorganization was based on systematic hours-long retraining methods.

Along a separate line of research, many scientists had found that people with language and auditory comprehension problems, some categorized as 'Auditory Processing Disorders,' showed deficits in processing rapidly successive or concatenated stimuli. Some of the original work by Efron (1970) showed that patients with temporal lobe disorders required over 600 ms to establish a proper temporal order judgment either auditorily *or* visually. Children with language delays traceable to auditory temporal processing problems or phonological problems were much slower to recognize temporal intervals and orders than were phonologically normal individuals (e.g., Tallal, Stark and Mellits, 1985). Such children could not perceive the critical microstructure of spoken syllables with sufficient accuracy to allow the development of phonologic awareness which is critical to speech perception and suitable translation into reading success. Work in our laboratory in the 1970s demonstrated that normal children were very slow to perceive a 'crossover' in a voiced–voiceless continuum compared to normal adults and suggested that children with language or reading disorders might be even slower. Later research showed that this indeed was the case, that children with phonological disorders were quite slow to perceive the rapid transitions that give consonants their unique percepts.

Adults with Broca's aphasia which usually leads to non-fluency and problems in speech motor control as well as word finding etc., may develop different temporal recall strategies than do other types of patients (Szelag, Von Steinbuchel and Poppel, 1997). Not all language problems are traceable to auditory temporal processing impairment (e.g., Bishop, Carlyon, Deeks and Bishop, 1999), but auditory temporal processing problems are clearly able to cause specific forms of auditory-based language impairment (Sussman, 1988; Tallal and Piercy, 1973; Wright, Lombardino, King et al., 1997).

We have found a commercially available system called Fast ForWord a clinically productive method of managing, and often ameliorating, problems of auditory temporal sequencing (Merzenich, Jenkins, Johnston et al., 1996; Tallal, Miller, Bedi et al., 1996). Preliminary evidence suggests that, after successful completion of the repetitive and long-lasting exercises that are part of Fast ForWord (100 minutes a day, 5 days a week for 6 weeks), changes are recordable not only in behavior but in middle latency evoked potentials (Berlin, unpublished data).

Some years ago, we noted that right handed normals show a Wave Pb in the middle latency responses (see Fig. 1) at around 50 ms, while left-handed normals show a response closer to 55 ms (Hood et al., 1990). When we study the middle latencies of children referred for auditory processing disorders and/or delayed language development, many of them show either no Wave Pb when the data are collected at extremely slow rates, or diffused waves with poorly defined peaks at or near 65–70 ms. Their ABRs and MLR Wave Pa are usually normal. When the data are collected with binaural stimulation, the responses are more robust and measurable than when one ear at a time is stimulated. In some children we observe well formed midline Wave Pb responses with little or no discernible response from electrodes over the temporal lobes. These observations, coupled with normal audiometry, reflexes, and emissions, suggest a physiological deficit in information processing and/or delay in the development at the hemispheric level.

Homologous changes are documented in functional MRI (fMRI) results on a small number of patients who were successful with the Fast ForWord program, with one unsuccessful patient showing NO changes (Temple, Poldrack, Protopapas et al., 2000) and two successful patients showing marked normalization of fMRI studies. In addition we have found that many of these children show very small or sometimes absent masking level differences.

We now have an effective therapy for some children who present with auditory processing disorders that involve a failure to process rapid concatenated syllables and involve poor hearing in noise. The Fast ForWord system works surprisingly well for children with temporally based language, speech, and reading disorders (Habib, Expresser, Rey et al., 1999; Talcott, Witton, McLean et al., 2000; Temple et al., 2000). It is also used in some children with hearing loss and in cochlear implant users who have suffered auditory deprivation and need to re-organize their nervous systems to make up for the lack of stimulation.

Summary

Auditory processing disorders can occur in various areas along the auditory pathways, alone or in conjunction with peripheral hearing problems, and some peripheral hearing problems can mimic more central deficits. While routine auditory tests are generally insensitive to central hearing problems, a number of physiologic and behavioral methods are available that use either monaural, dichotic or binaural presentation of stimuli. Each of these measures has advantages and limitations, and factors such as maturation and the wide range of normal performance in younger patients on behavioral tasks are additional important considerations when evaluating children.

The importance of identifying abnormal function at any level in the auditory system at an early age is critical. In addition, managing reversible disorders and seeking methods of instilling speech and language information into the young system (either via amplification or by using alternative communication modes), and providing appropriate training to overcome specific processing problems are all paramount to the successful development of verbal communication skills.

Acknowledgements

Preparation of this chapter was supported by the National Institute on Deafness and Other Communication Disorders, Deafness Research Foundation, Oberkotter Foundation, National Organization for

Hearing Research, and KAM's Fund for Hearing Research.

References

Albrecht R, Suchodoletz Wv, Uwer R: The development of auditory evoked dipole source activity from childhood to adulthood. Clinical Neurophysiology: 111; 2268–2276, 2000.

Arnst D, Katz J (Eds): The SSW Test: Development and Clinical Use. San Diego CA: College-Hill Press, 1982.

Augustsson I, Engstand I: Otitis media and academic achievements. International Journal of Pediatric Otolaryngology: 57; 31–40, 2001.

Baran JA, Musiek FE: Behavioral assessment of the central auditory nervous system. Chapter 13 In Musiek FE, Rintelmann WF (Eds), Contemporary Perspectives in Hearing Assessment. Boston: Allyn and Bacon, pp. 375–413, 1999.

Bartoshuk AK: Human neonatal cardiac responses to sound: A power function. Psychonomic Science: 1; 151–152, 1964.

Belin P, Zilbovicious M, Crozier S, Thivard L, Fontaine A, Masure MC, Samson Y: Lateralization of speech and auditory temporal processing. Journal of Cognitive Neuroscience: 10; 536–540, 1998.

Bellis TJ: Assessment and Management of CAPD in the Educational Setting. San Diego CA: Singular Publishing Group, 1996.

Berko J, Brown R: Psycholinguistic research methods. In Mussen PH (Ed), Handbook of Research Methods in Child Development. New York: John Wiley and Sons, 1960.

Berlin CI: New developments in evaluating central auditory mechanisms. Annals of Otology, Rhinology and Laryngology: 85; 833–841, 1976.

Berlin CI, Hood LJ, Wen H, Szabo P, Cecola RP, Rigby P, Jackson DF: Contralateral suppression of non-linear click-evoked otoacoustic emissions in humans. Hearing Research: 71; 1–11, 1993.

Berlin CI, Bordelon J, St John P, Wilensky D, Hurley A, Kluka E, Hood LJ: Reversing click polarity may uncover auditory neuropathy in infants. Ear and Hearing: 19; 37–47, 1998.

Berlin CI, Hood LJ, Hurley A, Wen H: Contralateral suppression of otoacoustic emissions: An index of the function of the medial olivocochlear system. Otolaryngology-Head Neck Surgery: 100; 3–21, 1994.

Berlin CI, Hood LJ, Hurley A, Wen H, Kemp DT: Bilateral noise suppresses click-evoked otoacoustic emissions more than ipsilateral or contralateral noise. Hearing Research: 87; 96–103, 1995.

Berlin CI, Hood LJ, Morlet T, Keats BJ: Managing and renaming auditory neuropathy (AN) as part of a continuum of auditory dys-synchrony (AD). ARO Abstracts: 24; 137, 2001.

Berlin CI, Hughes LF, Lowe-Bell SS, Berlin HL: Dichotic right ear advantage in children 5 to 13. Cortex: 9; 393–401, 1973.

Berlin CI, Lowe-Bell SS, Jannetta PJ, Kline DG: Central auditory deficits after temporal lobectomy. Archives of Otolaryngology: 96; 4–10, 1972.

Berlin C, McNeil M: Dichotic listening. In Lass N (Ed), Contemporary Issues in Experimental Phonetics. New York: Academic Press, 1976.

Berlin CI, Svirsky M: Delayed auditory feedback in multichannel cochlear implant patients. ARO Abstracts: 12; 275–276, 1989.

Berlin CI, Wexler KF, Jerger JF, Halperin HR, Smith S: Superior ultra-audiometric hearing: A new type of hearing loss which correlates highly with unusually good speech in the 'profoundly deaf'. Otolaryngology: 86; 111–116, 1978.

Bess FH, Klee T, Culbertson JL: Identification, assessment, and management of children with unilateral sensorineural hearing loss. Ear and Hearing: 7; 43–51, 1986.

Bess FH, Tharpe AM: An introduction to unilateral sensorineural hearing loss. Ear and Hearing: 7; 3–13, 1986.

Bess FH, Tharpe AM, Gibler AM: Auditory performance of children with unilateral sensorineural hearing loss. Ear and Hearing: 7; 20–26, 1986.

Bishop DV, Carlyon RP, Deeks JM, Bishop SJ: Auditory temporal processing impairment: neither necessary nor sufficient for causing language impairment in children. Journal of Speech, Language, Hearing Research: 42; 1295–1310, 1999.

Bocca E, Calearo C: Central hearing processes. In Jerger J (Ed), Modern Developments in Audiology. New York: Academic Press, 1963.

Bocca E, Calearo C, Cassinari V: A new method for testing hearing in temporal lobe tumors. Acta Otolaryngologica: 44; 219–221, 1954.

Cheour M, Ceponiene R, Lehtokoski A, Luuk A, Allik J, Ahlo K, Naatanen R: Devleopment of language-specific phoneme representations in the infant brain. Nature Neuroscience: 1; 351–353, 1998.

Cheour M, Leppanen PHT, Kraus N: Mismatch negativity (MMN) as a tool for investigating auditory discrimination and sensory memory in infants and children. Clinical Neurophysiology: 111; 4–16, 2000.

Cheour-Lutanen M, Ahlo K, Sainio K et al.: The ontogenetically earliest discriminative response of the human brain. Psychophysiology: 33; 478–481, 1996.

Collet L, Kemp DT, Veuillet E, Duclaux R, Moulin A, Morgon A: Effect of contralateral auditory stimuli on active cochlear micro-mechanical properties in human subjects. Hearing Research: 43; 251–262, 1990.

Cooper RP, Aslin RN: Preference for infant-directed speech in the first month after birth. Child Development: 61; 1584–95, 1990.

Cullen JK, Berlin CI, Halperin H: Auditory signal translation for persons with residual high frequency hearing. Proceedings of the International Congress of Rehabilitative Medicine, 1982.

Davis H: Principles of electric response audiometry. Annals of Otology, Rhinology and Laryngology: Supplement 28; 4–96, 1976.

DeCasper AJ, Fifer WP: Of human bonding: Newborns prefer their mother's voices. Science: 208; 1174–1176, 1980.

Deltenre P, Mansbach AL, Bozet C, Clercx A, Hecox KE: Auditory neuropathy: a report on three cases with early onsets and major neonatal illnesses. Electroencephalography and Clinical Neurophysiology: 104; 17–22, 1997.

Demany I, McKenzie B, Vurpillot E: Rhythm perception in early infancy. Nature: 266; 718–719, 1977.

Diefendorf AO: An investigation of one aspect of central auditory function in an infant population utilizing a binaural resynthesis (fusion) task. Unpublished doctoral dissertation, University of Washington, 1981.

Dobie RA, Berlin CI: Influence of otitis media on hearing development. Annals of Otology, Rhinology and Laryngology: 88(Supplement 60); 48–53, 1979.

Downs MP: Effects of mild hearing loss on auditory processing. Otolaryngologic Clinics of North America: 18; 337–344, 1985.

Downs MP, Blager FB: The otitis prone child. Developmental and Behavioral Pediatrics: 3; 106–113, 1982.

Doyle WJ, Webster DB: Neonatal conductive hearing loss does not compromise brainstem auditory function and structure in rhesus monkeys. Hearing Research: 54; 45–51, 1991.

Efron R: The relationship between the duration of a stimulus and the duration of a perception. Neuropsychologia: 8; 37–55, 1970.

Eggermont JJ, Stein L (Eds): Maturation of the Auditory System. Ear and Hearing: 17; 359–446, 1996.

Eilers RE, Oller DK: Infant vocalizations and the early diagnosis of severe hearing impairment. Journal of Pediatrics: 124; 199–203, 1994.

Eimas PD: Developmental aspects of speech perception. In Held R, Leibowitz HW, Teuber HL (Eds): Handbook of Sensory Physiology, Volume 8. Berlin: Springer-Verlag, 1978.

Eisenberg RB: Auditory competence in early life. Baltimore: University Park Press, 1976.

Elliot GB, Elliot KA: Some pathological, radiological and clinical implications of the precocious development of the human ear. Laryngoscope: 74; 1160–1171, 1964.

Erwin RJ, Buchwald JS: Midlatency auditory evoked responses: Differential recovery cycle characteristics. Electroencephalography and Clinical Neurophysiology: 64; 417–423, 1986.

Fernald A, Kuhl P: Acoustic determinants of infant perception for motherese speech. Infant Behavior Development: 10; 279, 1987.

Gascon GG, Johnson R, Burd L: Central auditory processing and attention deficit disorders. Journal of Child Neurology: 1; 27–33, 1986.

Geschwind N: Disconnexion syndromes in animals and man. I. Brain: 88; 237–294, 1965.

Geschwind N: Anatomical asymmetry as the basis for cerebral dominance. Federal Proceedings: 37; 2263–2266, 1978.

Geschwind N, Levitsky W: Human brain: Left-right asymmetries in temporal speech region. Science: 161; 186–187, 1968.

Goldstein MN: Auditory agnosia for speech ('pure word deafness'). Brain and Language: 1; 195–204, 1974.

Gorga MP, Stelmachowicz PG, Barlow SM, Brookhouser PE: Case of recurrent, reversible, sudden sensorineural hearing loss in a child. Journal of the American Academy of Audiology: 6; 163–172, 1995.

Graham J, Greenwood R, Lecky B: Cortical deafness: A case report and review of the literature. Journal of Neurological Sciences: 48; 35–49, 1980.

Gravel JS, Wallace IF: Early otitis media, auditory abilities, and educational risk. American Journal of Speech-Language Pathology: 4; 89–94, 1995.

Gravel JS, Wallace IF: Effects of otitis media with effusion on hearing in the first 3 years of life. Journal of Speech, Language, and Hearing Research: 43; 631–644, 2000.

Gunnarson AD, Finitzo T: Conductive hearing loss during infancy: effects on later auditory brain stem electrophysiology. Journal of Speech and Hearing Research: 34; 1207–1215, 1991.

Habib M, Expresser R, Rey V, Giraud K, Braus P, Gres C: Training dyslexics with acoustically modified speech: Evidence of improved phonological performance. Brain and Cognition: 40:143–146, 1999.

Hall JW III: Handbook of Auditory Evoked Responses. Boston: Allyn and Bacon, 1992.

Hall JW III, Grose JH: Development of temporal resolution in children as measured by the temporal modulation transfer function. Journal of the Acoustical Society of America: 96; 150–154, 1994.

Hall JW III, Grose JH, Pillsbury HC: Long-term effects of chronic otitis media on binaural hearing in children. Archives of Otolaryngology-Head and Neck Surgery: 121; 847–852, 1995.

Hood LJ: Clinical Applications of the Auditory Brainstem Response. San Diego CA: Singular Publishing Group, 1998.

Hood LJ, Berlin CI, Allen P: Cortical deafness: A longitudinal study. Journal of the American Academy of Audiology: 5; 330–342, 1994.

Hood LJ, Berlin CI, Bordelon J, Goforth-Barter L, Hurley A, Tedesco S: Patients with auditory neuropathy lack efferent suppression of evoked otoacoustic emissions. ARO Abstracts: 23; 159, 2000.

Hood LJ, Martin DA, Berlin CI: Auditory evoked potentials differ at 50 milliseconds in right- and left-handed listeners. Hearing Research: 45; 115–122, 1990.

Hood LJ, Webster DB, Barlow EK: Conductive hearing loss affects brainstem structures in altricial but not precocial rodents. Audiology Today: 2; 30, 1990.

Hunter LL, Margolis RH, Ryyken JR, Le CT, Daly A, Giebink GS: High frequency hearing loss associated with otitis media. Ear and Hearing: 17; 1–11, 1996.

Jacobson JT (Ed): Principles and Applications in Auditory Evoked Potentials. Boston: Allyn and Bacon, 1994.

Jerger J: Diagnostic audiometry. In Jerger J (Ed), Modern Developments in Audiology, Second Edition. New York: Academic Press, 1973.

Jerger J: Diagnostic use of impedance measures. In Jerger J (Ed), Handbook of Clinical Impedance Audiometry. Dobbs Ferry, NY: American Electromedics Corporation, 1975.

Jerger J, Burney P, Mauldin L, Crump B: Predicting hearing loss from the acoustic reflex. Journal of Speech and Hearing Disorders: 39; 11–22, 1974.

Jerger J, Weikers NJ, Sharbrough FW, Jerger S: Bilateral lesions of the temporal lobe: A case study. Acta Otolaryngologica: Supplement 258; 1–57, 1969.

Jerger S: Evaluation of central auditory function in young children. In Keith R (Ed), Central Auditory and Language Disorders in Children. Houston: College-Hill Press, pp. 30–60, 1980.

Jerger S, Jerger J, Alford BR, Abrams S: Development of speech intelligibility in children with recurrent otitis media. Ear and Hearing: 4; 138–145, 1983.

Jerger S, Jerger J, Loiselle L: Pediatric central auditory dysfunction. Comparison of children with confirmed lesions versus suspected processing disorders. American Journal of Otology: Suppl. 9; 63–71, 1988.

Jerger S, Lewis S, Hawkins J, Jerger J: Pediatric Speech Intelligibility Test I. Generation of test materials. International Journal of Pediatric Otorhinolaryngology: 2; 217–230, 1980.

Jirsa RE: The clinical utility of the P3 AERP in children with auditory processing disorders. Journal of Speech and Hearing Research: 35; 903–912, 1992.

Johansson B, Wedenberg E, Westin B: Measurement of tone response by the human fetus. Acta Otolaryngologica: 57; 188–192, 1964.

Kaga K, Nakamura M, Shinogami M, Tsuzuku T, Yamada K, Shindo M: Auditory nerve disease of both ears revealed by auditory brainstem responses, electrocochleography and otoacoustic emissions. Scandinavian Audiology: 25; 233–238, 1996.

Kaga K, Shindo M, Tanaka Y: Central auditory information processing in patients with bilateral auditory cortex lesions. Acta Oto-Laryngologica: (Supplement) 532; 77–82, 1997.

Katz J: The use of the staggered spondaic words for assessing the integrity of the central auditory nervous system. Journal of Auditory Research: 2; 327–337, 1962.

Katz J, Burge C: Auditory perception training for children with learning disabilities. Menorah Medical Journal: 2; 18–29, 1971.

Katz J, Wilde L: Auditory perceptual disorders in children. In Katz J (Ed), Handbook of Clinical Audiology. Baltimore: Williams and Wilkins, Chapter 33, pp. 664–688, 1985.

Kearsley R, Snider M, Richie R et al.: Study of relations between psychologic environment and child behavior. American Journal of Disorders in Children: 104; 12–20, 1962.

Keith RW (Ed): Central Auditory Dysfunction. New York: Grune and Stratton, 1977.

Kemp DT: Stimulated acoustic emissions from within the human auditory system. Journal of the Acoustical Society of America: 64; 1386–1391, 1978.

Kileny PR, Boerst A, Zwolan T: Cognitive evoked potentials to speech and tonal stimuli in children with implants. Otolaryngology-Head and Neck Surgery: 117; 161–169, 1997.

Kileny P, Paccioretti D, Wilson AF: Effects of cortical lesions on middle-latency auditory evoked responses. Electroencephalography and Clinical Neurophysiology: 66; 108–120, 1987.

Kim KH, Relkin NR, Lee KM, Hirsch J: Distinct cortical areas associated with native and second languages. Nature: 388; 171–174, 1997.

Kimura D: Cerebral dominance and the perception of verbal stimuli. Canadian Journal of Psychology: 15; 166–171, 1961.

Klausen O, Moller P, Holmfjord A, Reisaeter S, Asbjornsen A: Lasting effects of otitis media with effusion on language skills and listening performance. Acta Otolaryngologica: Suppl 543; 73–76, 2000.

Klein SK, Tuchman RF, Rapin I: The influence of premorbid language skills nd behavior on language recovery in children with verbal auditory agnosia. Journal of Child Neurology: 15; 36–43, 2000.

Kraus N, McGee T: Electrophysiology of the human auditory system. Chapter 6 In Popper AN, Fay RR (Eds), The Mammalian Auditory Pathway: Neurophysiology. New York: Springer-Verlag, pp. 335–403, 1992.

Kraus N, McGee T, Carrell TD, Sharma A, Koch D, King C, Tremblay K, Nicol T: Neurophysiologic bases of speech discrimination. Ear and Hearing: 16; 19–37, 1995.

Kraus N, McGee T, Comperatore C: Middle latency response in sleeping children: Evidence for subcortical contributions to Wave Pa of the human MLR. ARO Abstracts: 13; 158, 1990.

Kraus N, McGee TJ, Koch DB: Speech sound representation, perception, and plasticity: A neurophysiologic perspective. Audiology and Neuro-Otology: 3; 168–182, 1998.

Kraus N, Ozdamar O, Hier D, Stein L: Auditory middle latency responses (MLRs) in patients with cortical lesions. Electroencephalography and Clinical Neurophysiology: 54; 275–287, 1982.

Kraus N, Ozdamar O, Stein L, Reed N: Absent auditory brain stem response: Peripheral hearing loss or brain stem dysfunction? Laryngoscope: 94; 400–406, 1984.

Kulynych JJ, Vlader K, Jones DW, Weinberger DR: Gender differences in the normal lateralization of the supratemporal cortex: MRI surface-rendering morphometry of Heschl's gyrus and the planum temporale. Cerebral Cortex: 4; 107–118, 1994.

Landau WM, Goldstein R, Kleffner FR: Congenital aphasia: A clinicopathologic study. Neurology: 7; 915–921, 1957.

Landau WM, Kleffner FR: Syndrome of acquired aphasia with convulsive disorder in children. Neurology: 7; 523–530, 1957.

Lassen NA, Ingvar DH, Skinhoj E: Brain function and blood flow. Scientific American: 239; 62–71, 1978.

Liberman MC, Guinan JJ: Feedback control of the auditory periphery: Anti-masking effects of middle ear muscles vs. olivocochlear efferents. Journal of Communication Disorders: 31; 471–483, 1998.

Lynn G, Gilroy J: Effects of brain lesions on the perception of monotic and dichotic speech stimuli. Proceedings of a Symposium on Central Auditory Processing Disorders. Omaha: University of Nebraska Medical Center, 1975.

Lynn G, Gilroy J: Evaluation of central auditory dysfunction in patients with neurological disorders. In Keith R (Ed), Central Auditory Dysfunction. New York: Grune and Stratton, 1977.

Matkin N: Central auditory testing. Asha: 24; 759, 1982.

Maurer J, Beck W, Mann W, Mintert R: Veränderungen otoakustisher Emissionen unto gleichzeitiger Beschallung des Gegenohres bei Normalpersonen und bei Patientien mit einseitigem Akustikusneurinom. [Changes of amplitude of otoacoustic emissions under contralateral noise in normal hearing persons and in patients with unilateral acoustic neuroma.] Laryngology-Rhinology-Otology: 71; 69–73, 1992.

McGee T, Kraus N: auditory development reflected by middle latency response. Ear and Hearing: 17; 419–429, 1996.

McPherson DL: Late Potentials of the Auditory System. San Diego CA: Singular Publishing Group, 1996.

Menyuk P: Effects of hearing loss on babbling in the language-acquisition stage. In Jaffe B, Hearing loss in children. Baltimore: University Park Press, 1977.

Merzenich MM, Jenkins WM, Johnston P, Schreiner C, Miller SL, Tallal P: Temporal processing deficits of language-learning impaired children ameliorated by training. Science: 271; 27–28, 1996.

Merzenich MM, Recanzone GM, Jenkins WM: How the brain functionally rewires itself. In Arbib M, Robinson JA (Eds), Natural and Artificial Parallel Computations. New York: MIT Press, 1990.

Michel F, Peronnet F, Schott B: A case of cortical deafness: Clinical and electrophysiological data. Brain and Language: 10; 367–377, 1980.

Mirabelle PJ, Porter RJ, Hughes LF, Berlin CI: Dichotic lag effect in children 7 to 15. Developmental Psychology: 14; 277–285, 1978.

Moffitt AB: Speech perception by 20 to 24 weeks old infants. Paper presented at March Meeting of Society for Research in Child Development, Santa Monica, California, 1969.

Moore JK, Ponton CW, Eggermont JJ, Wu BJ-C, Huang JQ: Perinatal maturation of the auditory brain stem response: Changes in path length and conduction velocity. Ear and Hearing: 17; 411–418, 1996.

Musiek FE, Guerkink NA: Auditory perceptual problems in children: Considerations for the otolaryngologist and audiologist. Laryngoscope: 90; 962–971, 1980.

Naatanen R, Lehtokoski A, Lennes M et al.: Language-specific phoneme representations revealed by electric and magnetic brain responses. Nature: 358; 432–434, 1997.

Northern JL, Downs MP: Hearing in Children, Fourth Edition. Baltimore: Williams and Wilkins, 1991.

Olsen W, Noffsinger D, Carhart R: Masking level differences encountered in clinical populations. Audiology: 15; 287–301, 1976.

Ozdamar O, Kraus N: Auditory middle-latency responses in humans. Audiology: 22:34–49, 1983.

Ozdamar O, Kraus N, Curry F: Auditory brain stem and middle latency responses in a patient with cortical deafness. Electroencephalography and Clinical Neurophysiology: 53; 224–230, 1982.

Penfield W, Roberts L: Speech and Brain Mechanisms. Princeton NJ: Princeton University Press, 1959.

Penhune VB, Zattore RJ, MacDonald JD, Evans AC: Interhemispheric anatomical differences in human primary auditory cortex: Probabilistic mapping and volume measurement from magnetic resonance scans. Cerebral Cortex: 6; 661–672, 1996.

Petinou KC, Schwartz RG, Gravel JS, Raphael LJ: A preliminary account of phonological and morphophonological perception in young children with and without otitis media. International Journal of Language and Communication Disorders : 36; 21–42, 2001.

Pinhiero M: Tests of central auditory function in children with learning disabilities. In Keith R (Ed), Central Auditory Dysfunction. New York: Grune and Stratton, 1977.

Pinhiero M: Central auditory test profile in children with learning disabilities. In Bradford L (Ed), Communication Disorders: An Audio Journal for Continuing Education. New York: Grune and Stratton, 1978.

Pinhiero M, Jacobsen G, Boller F: Auditory dysfunction following a gunshot wound of the pons. Journal of Speech and Hearing Disorders: 47; 296–300, 1982.

Pinhiero ML, Musiek FE: Assessment of Central Auditory Dysfunction: Foundations and Clinical Correlates. Baltimore: Williams and Wilkins, 1985.

Plomp R: Auditory handicap of hearing impairment and the limited benefit of hearing aids. Journal of the Acoustical Society of America: 63; 533–549, 1978.

Plomp R: A signal-to-noise ratio model for the speech-reception threshold of the hearing impaired. Journal of Speech and Hearing Research: 29; 146–154, 1986.

Ponton CW, Don M, Eggermont JJ, Waring MD, Masuda A: Maturation of human cortical auditory function: Differences between normal-hearing children and children with cochlear implants. Ear and Hearing: 17; 430–437, 1996.

Ponton CW, Eggermont JJ: Of kittens and kids: Altered cortical maturation following profound deafness and cochlear implant use. Audiology and Neuro-Otology: 6; 363–380, 2001.

Ponton CW, Moore JK, Eggermont JJ, Wu BJ-C, Huang J: Relationship between auditory brainstem size and auditory brainstem response (ABR) response latency in human development. ARO Abstracts: 57, 1994.

Roberts JE, Burchinal MR, Jackson SC, Hooper SR, Roush J, Mundy M, Neebe EC, Zeisel SA: Otitis media in childhood in relation to preschool language and school readiness skills among black children. Pediatrics: 106; 725–735, 2000.

Robinson K: Implications of developmental plasticity for the language acquisition of deaf children with cochlear implants. International Journal of Pediatric Otorhinolaryngology: 46; 71–80, 1998.

Roush J, Tait CA: Binaural fusion, masking level differences, and auditory brain stem responses in children with language-learning disabilities. Ear and Hearing: 5; 37–41, 1984.

Rupp RR: Establishing norms for speech-in-noise skills in children. The Hearing Journal: 36; 16–19, 1983.

Ryan S, Kemp DT, Hinchcliffe R: The influence of contralateral acoustic stimulation on click-evoked otoacoustic emissions in humans. British Journal of Audiology: 25; 391–397, 1991.

Seidenwurm D, Bird CR, Enzmann DR, Marshall WH: Left-right temporal asymmetry in infants and children. American Journal of Neurology and Radiology: 6; 777–779, 1985.

Shriberg LD, Friel-Patti S, Flipsen P Jr., Brown RL: Otitis media, fluctuant hearing loss, and speech-language outcomes: a preliminary structural equation model. Journal of Speech, Language, Hearing Research: 43; 100–120, 2000.

Spring DR, Dale PA: Discrimination of linguistic stress in early infancy. Journal of Speech and Hearing Research: 20; 224–232, 1977.

Starr A, Achor LJ: Auditory brain stem responses in neurological disease. Archives of Otolaryngology: 32; 761–768, 1975.

Starr A, Amlie RN, Martin WH, Sanders S: Development of

auditory function in newborn infants revealed by auditory brainstem potentials. Pediatrics: 60; 831–839, 1977.

Starr A, McPherson D, Patterson J, Don M, Luxford W, Shannon R, Sininger Y, Tonokawa L, Waring M: Absence of both auditory evoked potentials and auditory percepts dependent on timing cues. Ear and Hearing: 16; 361–371, 1991.

Starr A, Picton TW, Sininger Y, Hood LJ, Berlin CI: Auditory neuropathy. Brain: 119; 741–753, 1996.

Stecker NA: A comparison of efferent auditory system functioning in three groups of children. Unpublished doctoral dissertation, State University of New York at Buffalo, 1983.

Stein L, Tremblay K, Pasternak J, Banerjee S, Lindemann K, Kraus N: Brainstem abnormalities in neonates with normal otoacoustic emissions. Seminars in Hearing: 17; 197–213, 1996.

Steinschneider A, Lipton EI, Richmond JB: Auditory sensitivity in the infant: Effect of intensity on cardiac responsivity. Child Development: 37:233–252, 1966.

Studdert-Kennedy M, Shankweiler D: Hemispheric specialization for speech perception. Journal of the Acoustical Society of America: 48; 579–594, 1970.

Sullivan RF: Transcranial ITE CROS. Hearing Instruments: 39; 11–12, 1988.

Sussman HM: The neurogenesis of phonology. In Whitaker H (Ed), Phonological Processes and Brain Mechanisms. New York: Springer-Verlag, pp. 1–23, 1988.

Sweetow R, Reddell R: The use of masking level differences in the identification of children with perceptual problems. Journal of the American Auditory Society: 4; 52–56, 1978.

Syzmanski MD, Perry DW, Gage NM, Rowley HA, Walker J, Berger MS, Roberts TP: Magnetic source imaging of late evoked field responses to vowels: Toward an assessment of hemispheric dominance for language. Journal of Neurosurgery: 94; 445–453, 2001.

Szelag E, Von Steinbuchel N, Poppel E: Temporal processing disorders in patients with Broca's aphasia. Neuroscience Letters: 235; 33–36, 1997.

Talcott JB, Witton C, McLean MF, Hansen PC, Rees A, Green GGR, Stein JF: Dynamic sensory sensitivity and children's word decoding skills. Proceedings of the National Academy of Sciences: 97; 2952–2957, 2000.

Tallal P, Miller SL, Bedi G, Byma G, Wang X, Nagarajan SS, Schreiner C, Jenkins WM, Merzenich MM: Language comprehension in language-learning impaired children improved with acoustically modified speech. Science 271:81–84, 1996.

Tallal P, Piercy M: Developmental aphasia: Impaired rate of non-verbal processing as a function of sensory modality. Neuropsychologia: 11; 389–398, 1973.

Tallal P, Piercy M: Developmental aphasia: Rate of auditory processing and selective impairment of consonant perception. Neuropsychologia: 12; 83–93, 1974.

Tallal P, Stark RE, Mellits ED: Identification of language-impaired children on the basis of rapid perception and production skills. Brain Language: 25; 314–322, 1985.

Temple E, Poldrack RA, Protopapas A, Nagarajan S, Salz T, Tallal P, Merzenich MM, Gabrieli JDE: Disruption of the neural response to rapid acoustic stimuli in dyslexia: Evidence from functional MRI. Proceedings of the National Academy of Sciences: 97; 13907–13912, 2000.

Tonnquist-Uhlen I: Topography of auditory evoked cortical potentials in children with severe language impairment. Scandinavian Audiology: (Supplement) 44; 1–40, 1996.

Wada JA, Clark R, Hamm A: Cerebral hemispheric asymmetry in humans. Cortical speech zones in 100 adults and 100 infant brains. Archives of Neurology: 32; 239–246, 1975.

Weber BA, Folsom RC, Thompson G: Auditory brainstem response in children with early recurrent middle ear disease. Annals of Otology, Rhinology and Laryngology: 92; 249–253, 1983.

Webster DB: Neuroscience of Communication, Second Edition. San Diego CA, Singular Publishing Group, 1999.

Webster DB, O'Connell NA: Neonatal conductive hearing loss affects cochlear nuclei in altricial rodents but not in precocial rodents. Society for Neuroscience Abstracts, 1989.

Webster DB, Webster M: Neonatal sound deprivation affects brainstem auditory nuclei. Archives of Otolaryngology: 103; 392–396, 1977.

Werker JF, Tees RC: Cross-language speech perception: Evidence for perceptual reorganization during the first year of life. Infant Behavior and Development: 7; 49–63, 1984.

Werner LA, Gray L: Behavioral studies of hearing development. In Rubel EW, Popper AN, Fay RR: Development of the Auditory System. New York: Springer, pp. 12–79, 1998.

Werner LA, Marean OC, Halpin CF, Spetner NB, Gillenwater JM: Infant auditory temporal acuity: gap detection. Child Development: 63; 260–272, 1992.

White EJ: Children's performance on the SSW Test and Willeford battery: Interim clinical data. In Keith R (Ed), Central Auditory Dysfunction. New York: Grune and Stratton, pp. 319–340, 1977.

Wightman F, Allen P, Dolan T, Kistler D, Jamieson D: Temporal resolution in children. Child Development: 60; 611–624, 1989.

Willeford JA: Assessing central auditory behavior in children: A test battery approach. In Keith R (Ed), Central Auditory Dysfunction. New York: Grune and Stratton, pp. 43–72, 1977.

Willeford J: Assessment of central auditory disorders in children. In Pinhiero ML, Musiek FE (Eds), Assessment of Central Auditory Dysfunction: Foundations and Clinical Correlates. Baltimore: Williams and Wilkins, Chapter 14, pp. 239–255, 1985a.

Willeford J: Sentence tests of central auditory dysfunction. In Katz J (Ed), Handbook of Clinical Audiology. Baltimore: Williams and Wilkins, Chapter 21, pp. 404–420, 1985b.

Willeford J, Billger J: Auditory perception in children with learning disabilities. In Katz J (Ed), Handbook of Clinical Audiology. Baltimore: Williams and Wilkins, pp. 410–425, 1978.

Williams EA, Brookes GB, Prasher DK: Effects of contralateral acoustic stimulation on otoacoustic emissions following vestibular neurectomy. Scandinavian Audiology: 22; 197–203, 1993.

Wilson WR, Thompson G: Behavioral audiometry. In Jerger J (Ed), Pediatric Audiology: Current Trends. San Diego: College-Hill Press, Ch. 1, pp. 1–44, 1984.

Winkler I, Lehtokoski A, Alku P et al.: Pre-attentive detection of vowel contrasts utilizes both phonetic and auditory memory representations. Brain Res Cogn Brain Res: 7; 357–369, 1999.

Witelson SF: Anatomic asymmetry in the temporal lobes: Its documentation, phylogenesis, and relationship to functional asymmetry. Annals of the New York Academy of Sciences: 299; 328–354, 1977.

Wright BA, Lombardino LJ, King WM, Puranik CS, Leonard CM, Merzenich MM: Deficits in auditory temporal and spectral resolution in language-impaired children. Nature: 387; 176–178, 1997.

Yoshinaga-Itano C, Sedley AL, Coulter DK, Mehl AL: Language of early- and later-identified children with hearing loss. Pediatrics: 102; 1161–1171, 1998.

Zeng FG, Oba S, Garde S, Sininger Y, Starr A: Temporal processing deficits in auditory neuropathy. Neuroreport: 10; 29–35, 1999.

Handbook of Neuropsychology, 2nd Edition, Vol. 8, Part II
S.J. Segalowitz and I. Rapin (Eds)

CHAPTER 20

Cognitive development in deaf children: the interface of language and perception in neuropsychology

Rachel I. Mayberry *

School of Communication Sciences and Disorders, McGill University, 1266 Pine Avenue West, Montreal, PQ H3G 1A8, Canada

Introduction

What does the sense of hearing contribute to human development? To answer the question, we must ask what the sense of hearing gives the child. Hearing gives the child the acoustic correlates of the physical world: approaching footsteps, dog barks, car horns, and the pitter-patter of rain. Hearing also allows the child to revel in the patterned complexity of a Beethoven symphony or a mother's lullaby. Children who are born deaf clearly miss a great deal. However, hearing conveys much more to the growing child than the acoustics of the physical world. Hearing is the sensory modality through which children perceive speech — the universe of talk that ties individuals, families and societies together. Children born with bilateral hearing losses that are severe (70–89 dB loss) or profound (>90 dB loss) are referred to as deaf. They cannot hear conversational speech (approximately 60 dB) and consequently do not spontaneously learn to talk. Indeed, not talking at the right age is one of the first signs that a child cannot hear.

The primary consequence of childhood deafness is that it blocks the development of spoken language — both the acts of speaking and comprehending. This fact leads us to ask what spoken language contributes to the child's cognitive development. Because deafness impedes the development of spoken language, we must ask whether complex and logical thought can develop in the absence of spoken language. Can the child develop 'inner thought' or working memory without the ability to hear? Consider sign language. Can sign language foster the same kinds of abstract mental development and complex thought as speech? Now consider an even more complex situation, namely, the cognitive development of children who grow up with little or no exposure to any language in any form, be it signed or spoken, as a simple consequence of being born deaf. What are the effects of such linguistic and social isolation on the child's development of a mental life?

Each of these questions has been asked about deaf children in one form or another since the beginning of philosophical inquiry (Lane, 1984). At first glance, the answers would seem to be straightforward and, historically, have been treated as such. However, as we shall see, the answers to these questions quickly become complex for several reasons. First, cognitive development entails more than maturation of the child's brain. Cognitive development is the product of the child's attempts to understand the family, neighborhood, school and the world at large during this period of rapid brain growth and learning. The effects of deafness on cognitive development are, therefore, quite diverse and complex due to the multitudinous ways in which families, societies, and cultures, react to and interact with children who are born deaf and hence do not spontaneously learn to talk and comprehend speech. Against this enor-

* Corresponding author. Tel.: +1-514-398-4141;
E-mail: rachel.mayberry@mcgill.ca

mously varied backdrop, we explore here research on the cognitive development of deaf children.

We begin with the premise that cognition, or intelligence, is multi-faceted and reflected in the coordinated performance of numerous language and non-language tasks, including perception, memory, mental imagery, concept formation, problem solving, language learning, academic achievement, and navigating everyday life (Sternberg, 1989). Our focus here is on whether and how deafness affects the child's cognitive development across several domains that have been studied in some, but not equal, detail. The cognitive aspects we consider are the following: (1) Academic achievement; (2) reading development, (3) language development and the factors known to affect it; (4) performance on standardized intelligence tests; (5) visual–spatial and memory skills; (6) conceptual development, and (7) neuropsychological function. For each domain, we discuss the development of deaf children who use either signed or spoken language. However, because so little is known about them, we will only briefly discuss the cognitive development of deaf children who grow up with little or no exposure to conventional language (in any form, spoken or signed). We begin with academic achievement because it illustrates the unique developmental challenge congenital deafness poses for the young child.

Academic achievement

Population profiles

The Gallaudet Research Institute regularly collects and analyzes demographic data on the academic achievement of deaf children in the United States based on the Stanford Achievement Test (Allen, 1994). The median math computation skills of 15-year-old deaf children in the USA are at the 7th grade level. Age-matched hearing children perform at the 10th grade level (Allen, 1989). These statistics show that deafness, by itself, does not impede the child's ability to learn and manipulate abstract symbols and symbolic relations. By contrast, the median reading achievement of 17–21-year-old deaf students leaving American secondary schools is at the 4th grade level (Allen, 1994). This wide performance gap between language tasks as compared to non-language tasks is a common profile among deaf children worldwide (Conrad, 1979). These academic performance patterns illustrate the great difficulty experienced by deaf children perceiving and learning spoken language and visual representations of speech, namely written and read language. Indeed, the effects of deafness on spoken language development increase as degree of hearing loss increases. For example, students with mild to moderate hearing losses read at lower levels than do students with normal hearing. Furthermore, students with severe to profound hearing losses read more poorly than do students with moderate losses but on math computation they show equivalent achievement (Allen and Schoem, 1997).

The primary effect of degree of hearing loss on language development, in turn, interacts with factors extraneous to deafness, such as socioeconomic and ethnic status and additional handicaps. Deaf children from lower socioeconomic status homes perform less well than middle-class deaf children. For example, only 5% of Black and 6% of Hispanic deaf students (17–21 years old, severely to profoundly deaf) read at or above the 6th grade level whereas 15% of White deaf students read above this level (Allen, 1994). Deaf children who have motor or sensory impairments in addition to deafness, such as poor vision or cerebral palsy, perform less well as a group than deaf children without additional impairments (Allen, 1989). Together these data indicate that the academic achievement of deaf students is predicted to a large extent by the same factors that predict the academic achievement of normally hearing students in North America, that is, social class, ethnic and racial background, and other handicapping conditions. This means that deafness, by itself, does not determine academic success or failure but rather interacts with many other factors in complex ways.

Reading development

The median reading level of the deaf, high school population does not reach the level required for a person to be considered literate (i.e., the 6th to 8th grade level and beyond). Indeed, the median reading levels of the deaf student population have not changed much over the past century (Chamberlain and Mayberry, 2000). This discouraging, but often replicated, finding suggests that something about deafness creates a barrier to reading development. However, if the barrier were insurmountable, no deaf students would read proficiently. It is important to remember that these reading statistics are median reading levels. Half of deaf high school students read below the fourth grade level but half also read above this level.

Factors in reading development

Spoken language

Many deaf students read well. For example, in a study of 100 profoundly deaf 16–17-year-olds, Geers and Moog (1989) found 57% to read at or above the grade 7 level and 30% to read at the grade 10 level. The students shared several traits: above average performance on nonverbal IQ tests, parents who were college educated and professionally employed, and special education begun at or before preschool age. These facts mean that the students in this study all had access at an early age to high quality intervention services. In addition to high reading achievement, the students performed at high levels on a battery of spoken language tests.

Indeed, the spoken language development of deaf children, as measured by syntactic and vocabulary skills (independent of word decoding skills), has often been postulated to be a causal factor in reading development in the deaf population. Spoken language skills have been found to predict reading levels in deaf students, both those who use sign language ($r = +0.70$, Lichtenstein, 1983; Moores and Sweet, 1990) and those who use speech ($r = +0.83$, Geers and Moog, 1989). Sign language has historically been conceptualized as being unimportant or even detrimental to the reading development of deaf students, either because it has no sound patterning or because its grammatical structure is different from that of spoken language (Mayer and Wells, 1996; Moores and Sweet, 1990). In fact, whether sign language can provide the cognitive foundation that spoken language provides for reading development has been a matter of considerable debate for decades. Only recently has the question been investigated in a systematic fashion (Chamberlain and Mayberry, 2000). If sign language development interferes with reading development, then there should be a negative relation between deaf children's sign language skills and reading ability but recent research has found the opposite relation. Recent research shows a positive correlation between sign language skills and reading development.

Sign language

Mayberry and her colleagues (Mayberry, Chamberlain, Waters and Doehring, 2002) investigated the reading and sign skills of 48 severely and profoundly deaf students aged 7–15 years. They found 42% to read at the expected grade level and 67% to read above the fourth grade level. All the children were educated with sign language and spoken language (specifically 'Total Communication'). All the children additionally had average or above average performance on selected nonverbal IQ sub-tests and had begun to learn sign language through early intervention by age three. Unlike the orally trained children studied by Geers and Moog (1989), the reading levels of the children educated with total communication were predicted by their ability to comprehend sign language, not spoken language. (We define and discuss total communication below). These findings suggest that factors which promote the development of language comprehension in general, independent of sensory–motor modality, also promote reading development. In fact, the deaf children who showed the highest levels of reading and sign language comprehension tended to have parents who knew and used sign language with them from a very young age — 3 years or before. Parental use of sign language also meant that the deaf child was able to converse in signed language in nearly all domains of his or her life — both at home and school — which would mean that the child had abundant amounts of language input during childhood (Hoffmeister, 2000).

Other studies have also measured sign language skill in relation to reading development and found a positive relation between the two kinds of language. The sign language measures have included the following kinds of American Sign Language (ASL) knowledge: plural markers and synonyms/antonyms, ($r = +0.45$ to $+0.64$, Hoffmeister, 2000); comprehension of ASL classifiers, stories, and time markers (combined $r = +0.58$, Strong and Prinz, 2000); memory for ASL sentences, classifier production, and recognition of fingerspelling in ASL sentences ($r = +0.53$ to $+0.57$, Padden and Ramsey, 2000);

and comprehension of ASL stories and working memory for ASL sentences ($r = +0.49$ to 0.69 Chamberlain and Mayberry, 2000; Mayberry et al., 2003). One unique feature of these studies is that the high and positive correlation between sign language skill and English reading was found specifically for ASL, a natural sign language with a linguistic structure different from spoken English. These findings further show that the major impediment to deaf children's reading development is not simply an inability to speak English but rather impoverished language development, in any form, signed or spoken, as we discuss below.

Good and poor readers

The relation between ASL language ability and reading achievement was further investigated by Chamberlain (2002) who hypothesized that well developed reading skill is predicated on well developed language skill, even in sign language. To test the hypothesis, she measured the ASL and reading skills of a random sample of 31 deaf adults who reported using ASL as a primary language. Sign language skill was measured with two tasks, ASL grammatical judgement (Boudreault, 1999) and narrative comprehension in ASL and MCE, Manually Coded English described below (Mayberry et al., 2003). Reading skills were measured with two reading tests (the Gates–MacGinite and the Stanford). Performance distribution on the ASL and reading measures significantly overlapped. Half the adults performed at high levels on the sign language tasks, at near-native levels. These same individuals also could read well, reading at the 8th grade level or above. Most of the remaining participants performed at low levels on the sign language measures. These same individuals performed poorly on the reading tests, reading below grade 4 (Chamberlain, 2002) as Fig. 1 shows.

A few deaf adults read well but performed poorly on the sign language tasks. These individuals were, in actual fact, successful speakers of English. Although they considered sign language to be their primary mode of communication, they had successfully acquired spoken English in childhood and subsequently learned ASL as a second language in late adolescence. In other words, they had well-developed primary language skills. A few deaf adults performed at high levels on the sign language tasks but could not read well, constituting about 8.5% of the experimental sample. This figure is very similar to the proportion of the normally hearing population reported to have dyslexia, around 10%, that is, people who have good face-to-face language skills but cannot read (Chamberlain, 2002).

These results show that highly developed sign language skill is related to high levels of reading achievement in deaf individuals for whom sign language is a primary means of communication. Spoken language is not the only path to literacy development. These results also suggest that the low median reading levels of the deaf school-aged population are likely caused by low levels of primary language development, in sign language as well as in spoken language. Reading must be taught to deaf children, certainly. But in order to benefit from reading instruction, deaf children must have a well-developed primary language upon which to base the reading task.

Additional factors in reading achievement

Returning to the factor of socioeconomic status, Geers and Moog (1989) found in their sample of orally trained deaf students that those who achieved the highest reading levels were from middle class families. More specifically, they had parents who were college educated and professionally employed. They concluded that socioeconomic status predicts deaf children's reading achievement. This finding is supported by demographic data showing that Hispanic and Black deaf children show significantly lower levels of reading achievement than do White children (Allen, 1994). Socioeconomic status may have a greater impact on the academic attainment of deaf children than that of hearing children. This is because hearing children, no matter how poor, spontaneously acquire language by merely listening to family members who speak to them from infancy. By contrast, poor deaf children are at a high risk for not being exposed to accessible language at the right time in early childhood. This is because in most countries poverty translates into a lack of access to the educational and clinical services that expose deaf children to language at the appropriate age. These factors are early diagnosis of hearing loss, parent–infant and preschool programs, availability of hear-

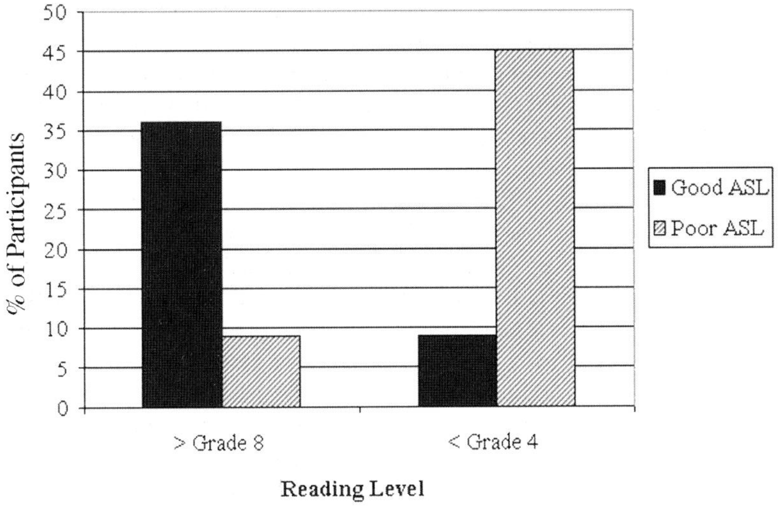

Fig. 1. The relation between English reading level and comprehension of American Sign Language (ASL) in a sample of 31 randomly selected deaf adults reporting ASL to be their primary language. *Good* ASL skills indicate nearly complete comprehension of ASL narratives and near-native control over ASL syntactic structures; *poor* ASL skills indicate minimal control of ASL syntactic structures and comprehension of less than half of an ASL narrative (extrapolated from Chamberlain, 2002).

ing aids, parent–infant programs that promote and teach sign language, parental sign language instruction, parent counseling, and so forth. This leads us directly to the question of why primary language skill is so difficult for deaf children to develop independent of socioeconomic status.

Language development

Because deaf children cannot hear the language spoken around them, they do not learn it spontaneously. In fact, one of the first signs that a child is deaf, aside from not responding to sound, is not beginning to talk at the expected age, 10–18 months (Meadow-Orlans, 1987). Making generalizations about the language development of deaf children is complex. This is due to the multiple sensory forms of linguistic input deaf children receive and the varying kinds and amounts of language input available to them during early childhood. For example, some deaf children receive no accessible language input of any kind (i.e., children who have severe to profound hearing losses that go undetected and thus receive no special intervention). Other deaf children receive incomplete spoken language input (incomplete because hearing aids and cochlear implants do not restore hearing to normal levels). Some other children receive sign language input in the form of MCE (Manually Coded English) or ASL. Signed language input is, in principle, fully accessible to deaf children due to its visual nature. Unfortunately, familial and educational circumstances often inadvertently conspire to yield both incomplete and reduced amounts of signed and spoken linguistic input throughout the deaf child's early life when normal language development occurs, as we discuss in detail below.

Speech

When considering deaf children's language development, it is important to distinguish the child's ability to speak from the child's ability to understand and produce language, that is, linguistic competence. The two factors of *speech* and *language* are clearly dissociable in deaf children's development. Indeed, intelligible speech is extremely difficult for deaf children to achieve. This is understandable for two reasons. First, deaf children either do not hear speech at all or hear it in a highly distorted fashion due to the sensori-neural nature of their hearing losses. Second, the visual facial movements people make when speaking provide only limited clues as to how speech is produced. Deaf children as a whole achieve low levels of speech intelligibility (for a review see

Seyfried and Kricos, 1989). Some proportion of deaf children learn to speak intelligibly. Such children typically have received special education at an early age (before preschool) with successful use of hearing aids, speech training, and very high levels of parental involvement in the child's speech and auditory development (Meadow-Orlans, 1987). Three other factors common to deaf children who successfully learn to speak are the following: (1) the ability to auditorily discriminate speech patterns, (2) higher than average nonverbal IQ, and (3) higher than average socioeconomic status (Geers and Moog, 1987).

Vocabulary

In a pioneering study of deaf children's cognitive development, Katheryn Meadow observed that, "The basic impoverishment of deafness is not lack of hearing, but lack of language. To illustrate this, we have only to compare the 4-year-old hearing child, with a working vocabulary of between two and three thousand words, to a child of the same age profoundly deaf since infancy, who may have only a few words at his command," (Meadow, 1968: 29).

The major developmental hurdle facing deaf children is not simply learning to speak intelligibly, but acquiring language — namely the lexicon, morphology, syntax, and semantics of language. Substantial delays in language development are the primary hallmark of childhood deafness without early and appropriate intervention. The reasons for this are simple. The average intensity of conversational speech by a male talker is around 60 dB. Even children with moderate hearing losses (i.e., 56–70 dB) show a 1-year delay in vocabulary development compared to age-matched children with no hearing loss. Children with severe hearing losses (71–90 dB) show a 3-year lag in vocabulary development (Davis, Elfenbein, Chum and Bentler, 1986). In turn, profound hearing loss (<91 dB) creates a significant delay in vocabulary development. One British study of 71 profoundly deaf children between the ages of 8 and 12 years showed their average comprehension of spoken vocabulary to be less than what would be expected of hearing 4-year-olds (Bishop, 1983). On a referential, mother–child communication task, a Canadian study found 8-year-old deaf children to show comprehension levels similar to 4-year-old hearing children (MacKay-Soroka, Trehub and Thorpe, 1988). Finally, an American study of 150 deaf children between the ages of 4 and 20 found severe delays in vocabulary comprehension. The deaf children tested showed little lexical development after 12–13 years (Moeller, Osberger and Eccarius, 1986), as shown in Fig. 2.

Delays in deaf children's vocabulary development are apparent from an early age. For example, one study reported that, during 15 months of intensive speech instruction, a 30 month old deaf child was able to learn *one* word a month (Lach, Ling and Ling, 1970). By contrast, hearing children spontaneously learn from 60–120 words a month between 30 and 48 months of age (Ingram, 1989). Lederberg and Everhart (1998) studied the early language of 20 deaf children and age-matched hearing children. They found that all the normally hearing children were producing two-word utterances at 22 months but half the deaf children were producing no language at this age. By 3 years of age, the normally hearing children were producing multi-word utterances but half the deaf children were producing only one-word utterances at an infrequent rate. This pattern of expressive language delay was constant across the different modes and types of early language intervention the deaf children received. This was true both in cases where the mothers and therapists used speech without sign and in cases where they used speech accompanied by sign (as in Total Communication, describe below). Despite their inability to hear their own voices and those of others, however, all the deaf children primarily used vocalizations to communicate with their hearing mothers. The mothers' use of signs did not prevent their deaf children from using speech (Lederberg and Everhart, 1998).

One accommodation the hearing mothers made to communicate with their deaf children was an increased use of body language and gesture between 22 months and 3 years (Lederberg and Everhart, 1998). This type of communicative accommodation was also observed in an earlier study. Hearing mothers of deaf infants between 12 and 18 months were observed to use similar amounts of vocalization and spoken language compared with mothers of age-matched hearing infants but they also used more gesture and tactile communication (Spencer, 1993).

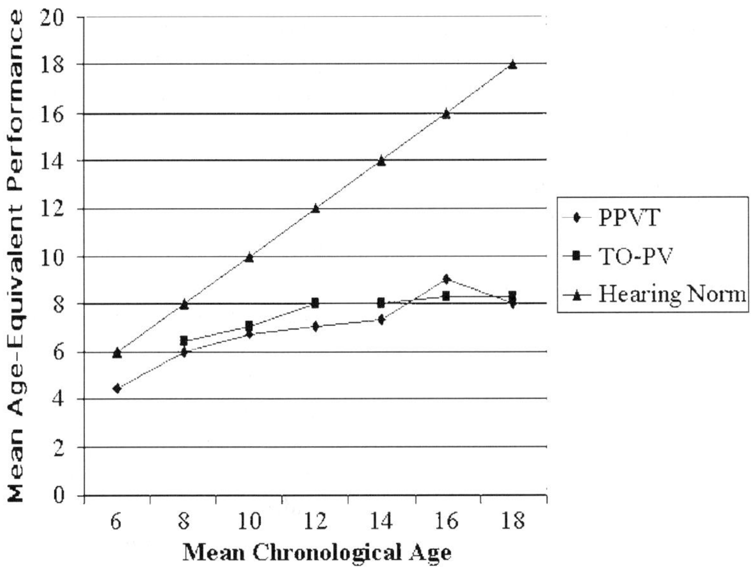

Fig. 2. The vocabulary comprehension test scores of 150 deaf children plotted as a function of expected performance for chronological age (with norms from hearing children added; redrawn from fig. 19, Moeller et al., 1986).

The striking delays in deaf children's vocabulary acquisition leads to the question of whether deafness affects the cognitive processes that underlie word learning. However, this appears not to be the case. Lederberg, Prezbindowski and Spencer (2000) found that overall vocabulary size, not age, predicted deaf children's word learning strategies. Young deaf children's ability to learn new words from context with minimal exposure was similar to that of hearing children, but only when vocabulary size was taken into account. This finding suggests that some kinds of language learning abilities emerge as a consequence of language development. Thus, deaf children whose language is very delayed may show learning patterns similar to younger hearing children, not due to deafness per se, but due instead to a significantly delayed rate of language growth. This is an important concept to which we return below.

Grammar

Given the highly delayed vocabulary acquisition of deaf children, it is not surprising to learn that their acquisition of syntax and grammatical morphology is also very delayed. In a study of orally-trained, 4–15-year-olds (75% of whom were 7 years and older), Geers and Moog (1978) found 50% of the children to have a level of expressive grammar lower than would be expected for hearing 3-year-olds (but with more mature content). In a study of 150 deaf children between the ages of 4 and 20, Moeller et al. (1986) found grammatical comprehension to be even more delayed than vocabulary comprehension. Few of the students tested achieved grammatical comprehension scores higher than would be expected for normally hearing 5–7-year-olds. Some researchers conclude that deaf children taught exclusively through spoken language appear to pass through the same general stages of language acquisition as their hearing peers but without reaching the same ultimate level of proficiency (Mogford, 1988).

Many similarities between deaf and hearing children's syntactic acquisition were documented in one of the most detailed investigations of deaf students' syntactic skills ever conducted. Quigley and his colleagues investigated the English syntactic skills of more than 400 deaf students on a variety of English grammatical structures including, for example, negation, conjunction, determiners, questions, pronominalization, relativization, and complementation, among others (for a review see Quigley and King, 1980). The research team first collected numerous samples of deaf children's writing to determine the most common types of grammatical errors they committed. In follow up studies, the team investigated the performance patterns of deaf students on a wide range of syntactic structures. The net result was both a screening test and a normed diagnostic test of grammatical skill, *Test of Syntactic Abilities* (Quigley, Steinkamp, Power and Jones, 1978).

These studies produced two main findings. First, deaf children's control of English syntax decreases with decreasing hearing levels. Second, the order of difficulty of English syntactic structures for deaf students, even those with profound hearing losses, is for the most part highly similar to those of English hearing students and second language learners of English (Quigley and King, 1980), as shown in Fig. 3. It is important to note, however, that this syntactic research was conducted solely through the modes of reading and writing. The extent to which these findings generalize to deaf children's face-to-face language in sign and/or speech is unclear. Nonetheless, these studies demonstrate the low level of control many deaf students have over English syntax when reading.

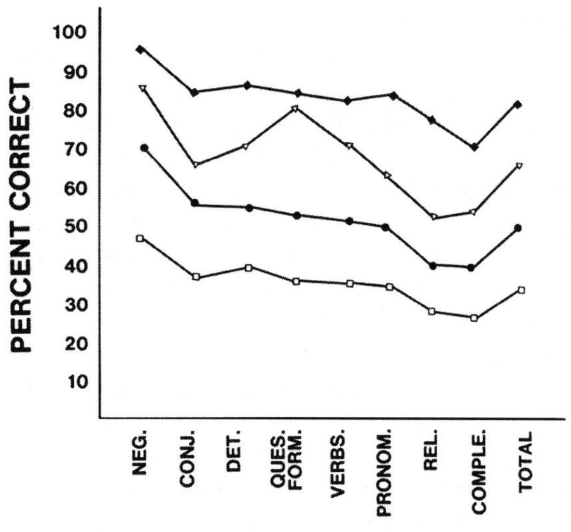

Fig. 3. Performance accuracy on selected English syntactic structures for 8–13-year-old hearing students, deaf students between the ages of 10–18 years in both the USA and Australia and deaf college students (fig. 7 from Quigley and King, 1980).

The achievement patterns deaf children show for spoken and written language indicate that they do not easily learn the grammar of a spoken language even in a visual form, i.e., reading and writing. Nearly a century of teaching and research with deaf children has also demonstrated that learning to read cannot serve as a primary language for deaf children for reasons we do not fully understand. Learning to read and learning a primary language are two different skills. We know now that learning to read is based upon the prior acquisition of a primary and dynamic 'face-to-face' language in either a signed or spoken form. Because primary language learning is often difficult and problematic for deaf children, educators have sought various means to facilitate language acquisition through the use of gesture and sign language. We now consider the gesture and sign language development of deaf children.

Gesture and homesign

Deaf children, who have not yet been exposed to sign language and have not yet acquired spoken language, often spontaneously create their own means of gesture communication for the purpose of self-expression. The phenomenon is known as *homesign*. 'Homesign' is an ASL term referring to the idiosyncratic gesture systems used by deaf individuals who were reared in isolation from other deaf signers. The phenomenon is that the deaf child makes statements and requests by combining points (to objects and people) with iconic gestures (called 'characterizing' gestures by Goldin-Meadow and Feldman, 1977) in an effort to communicate with hearing family members. For example, the child might point to an apple and then open and close his mouth around his fist to mean, "I eat an apple," (Goldin-Meadow, personal communication). All the young deaf children in hearing families observed by Goldin-Meadow and Mylander (1984) used gestures to communicate with their mothers with varying degrees of frequency.

In addition to creating a gesture lexicon, the deaf children combine their gestures into multi-gesture utterances in a rule-governed fashion. The children tend to gesture the patient (recipient of the action) followed by the action when the action is transitive (i.e., when the action acts on something as in 'eat, kick, twist,' etc.). However, when the action is intransitive (e.g., 'think, sleep, walk,' etc), the children tend to gesture the agent followed by the action (Goldin-Meadow and Feldman, 1977; Goldin-Meadow and Mylander, 1984).

In subsequent research these researchers found that the gesture lexicon and ordering rules of the gesture system originate from the deaf child and not their hearing parents. Indeed, the gestures of young deaf children differ from those of their hearing parents in frequency, complexity, and ordering patterns. The deaf child combines strings of gestures to convey ideas, or propositions (as the above example illustrates), similar to the way in which speakers combine strings of words to make statements. By contrast, the gestures produced by hearing people as they speak are much simpler. Speakers tend to produce only a single iconic gesture for each major idea they say (Mayberry and Nicholadis, 2000; McNeill, 1992). In homesign, gestures carry all of the meaning. In speech, spoken words carry all the meaning and gestures act as a supplement (McNeill, 1992). In young normally hearing children, gesture complexity increases with spoken language development from the earliest stages (Mayberry and Nicholadis, 2000). This means that gesture communication is linguistic for hearing children just as it is for deaf children.

The characteristics of homesign appear to be universal and transcend culture so far as is currently known. Goldin-Meadow and Mylander (1998) observed that Chinese deaf children produce homesign too. The homesign gestures and ordering patterns of the Chinese deaf children were very similar to those of American deaf children. Homesign may be a valuable diagnostic tool, although no research has yet documented the possibility. How often and how elaborately the young deaf child communicates via gesture prior to having learned any sign language or spoken language, or how frequently and complexly he or she gestures when speaking probably indicates increased symbolic sophistication (in either spoken or signed forms).

We now know that deaf children's gesture communication can be elaborate and shows some basic properties shared by all languages. How is homesign related to sign language? We turn now to this question.

Sign language origins

A common misconception about the origins of sign languages is that they were invented by hearing teachers. However, documents from some of the earliest teachers in the late 18th century show that they intentionally borrowed the signs and gestures their deaf pupils used in the classroom to communicate with one another and used them for instructional purposes (Lane, 1984). 20th century research in Nicaragua demonstrates how quickly sign languages emerge among communities of individuals who are deaf from birth.

After the Sandinista revolution, literacy and education became a national priority in Nicaragua, including the education of deaf children (Morford and Kegl, 2000). Before the revolution, individuals who were deaf did not attend school. Instead, they lived with their hearing families in isolation from one another. Like deaf children everywhere who are unable to communicate with spoken language, these isolated deaf individuals developed idiosyncratic gesture systems, or homesign, to communicate with their families. Their homesign systems had many of the properties described above (Morford and Kegl, 2000).

When the first school for deaf students was established in Nicaragua, linguists who were present at the time observed that the older students, namely adolescents and young adults, communicated with one another using their various homesign systems (Kegl, personal communication; Morford and Kegl, 2000). Recall that homesign consists of combinations of iconic and point gestures to create simple utterances, as described above. When the youngest deaf children arrived at the school (e.g., ages 4–5), they were exposed to the homesign used by the older deaf students for communication. Surprisingly, however, the younger children did not copy the homesign systems of the older students. Instead, they were observed to use a sign language! The signing of the youngest deaf students was quick, limited to the hands (i.e., the children did not use pantomime), constrained in space, and consisted of signs with sub-lexical structure (i.e., meaningless phonetic units). They ordered their signs in relation to one another with syntax and grammatical morphemes. In other words, these young deaf children had created a sign language, or

Idioma de Señas de Nicaragua, from homesign input (Morford and Kegl, 2000; Senghas, 1995; Senghas, Kegl, Senghas and Coppola, 1994).

The phenomenon of children creating linguistic structure from fragmented language input is by no means unique to sign language. The phenomenon, known as creolization, has often been observed in situations of language contact where adults speak a pidgin (vocabulary words of a foreign language strung together with little or no syntax or morphology as means of communication between groups of adults speaking different languages). Young children exposed to pidgins creolize them, that is, they create new syntax and morphology to fill the existing gaps in the pidgin to which they have been exposed (Bickterton, 1990). Indeed, some of the first linguists to study ASL initially hypothesized that the sign languages used by Deaf communities worldwide were analogous to spoken Creoles (Fischer, 1978).

The sudden appearance of *Idioma de Señas de Nicaraga* provides insights into how sign languages evolve. There are at least two necessary stages of sign language evolution. First, from the sparse, but accessible (i.e., visible), gesture input they receive from speaking people who gesture as they talk, deaf children create gesture communication — homesign. This homesign shows rudiments of linguistic structure, namely a limited lexicon and ordering rules (Goldin-Meadow and Mylander, 1998). Second, young deaf children exposed to the homesign of older deaf children, in turn, fill the grammatical gaps in this rudimentary, quasi-language input to create a sign language (Morford and Kegl, 2000). Sign language is thus a remarkable human adaptation to childhood deafness. Language capacity is such an integral part of the human endowment that when language expression in the auditory–oral form is blocked by profound deafness, it reappears one generation later in a readily accessible and expressible form that circumvents the spoken language barrier of deafness.

American Sign Language

Most Deaf communities in North America use a sign language known as American Sign Language, or ASL. ASL is a natural language that has evolved among deaf people in North America, probably in the manner described above. Because ASL is perceived by the eyes and expressed with the hands and arms (in addition to the face and torso), its grammatical structure (phonology, lexicon, morphology, syntax, and semantics) is highly spatial (Emmorey, 2002). ASL is not a version of English on the hands. However, ASL has rarely been used in classrooms for deaf children. In fact, ASL has historically been actively banned from classrooms for deaf children because the goal of educators has always been to teach spoken language. Most educators have traditionally believed that ASL impedes this goal (Baynton, 1996; Lou, 1988). Nonetheless, ASL is the native language of many deaf people who were exposed to sign at a young age, especially those with deaf parents. ASL is also the primary language of many deaf people who do not acquire spoken language, even though they often learn ASL at very late ages, as described below.

ASL acquisition

Deaf children exposed to ASL from birth by their deaf parents spontaneously acquire it in a fashion comparable to that of hearing children who spontaneously acquire spoken language. Beginning with a sign-babbling stage, the child begins with a one-word stage, moves to a two-word stage, and then begins to acquire the complex morphological system of ASL (Marentette and Mayberry, 2000; Newport and Meier, 1985; Petitto and Marentette, 1991; Schick, 1990). The child does not fully master ASL grammar until around 5–6 years of age or later (for recent research on sign language acquisition, see Chamberlain, Morford and Mayberry, 2000). The ease with which deaf children spontaneously acquire ASL unequivocally demonstrates that congenital deafness does not alter the child's ability to acquire grammar. Rather, the major problem congenital deafness poses for the young deaf child is accessibility to sufficient language input at the right age (Morford and Mayberry, 2000).

The age of exposure problem

One rationale behind early speech intervention programs for deaf children (and bilingual education for hearing children) is the idea that languages are best learned early in life (Scovel, 1989). People generally believe that spoken languages can only be learned spontaneously and perfectly in early childhood. This concept is referred to as the *critical period* for language acquisition. Critical periods are common in the development of living things and are defined as a time-bounded period during development when the developing system, such as vision, is most sensitive to environmental input. A well-studied human example in is the development of binocular vision (Greenough and Black, 1992). Although most researchers think that spoken language acquisition is guided by critical period learning, sign languages have traditionally been excluded from this principle. The prevailing conviction among many educators has been that proficiency in sign language can be readily attained by anyone at any age. However, recent research shows that the age constraints that guide the outcome of second language acquisition also apply to the ultimate outcome of sign language acquisition (Emmorey, Bellugi, Frederici and Horn, 1995; Newport, 1988).

In a series of studies, Mayberry and her colleagues (Mayberry, 1994; Mayberry and Eichen, 1991; Mayberry and Fischer, 1989) found numerous effects associated with age of sign language exposure. For example, overall accuracy decreased with later age of sign language acquisition. This was true for memory and comprehension of ASL sentences and stories as well as for sentences in a version of Pidgin Sign English (PSE), a simplified form of ASL with some English elements used between deaf and hearing people. Deaf participants who were not exposed to sign until late childhood and early adolescence, around 9–13 years, showed significant deficits in ASL comprehension, despite the fact that ASL was their primary means of communication and they had used ASL for all of their adult lives. Indeed, the performance of the deaf individuals who first learned ASL in adolescence was worse than what would be expected from second-language learners of a spoken language. Why might this be so?

Recall that the major consequence of childhood deafness is a significant delay in the development of spoken language. This means that when deaf adolescents are first exposed to sign language, it is often because they acquired insufficient spoken language to enable them to cope with everyday life. In other words, many deaf children are only allowed to use sign language after they prove that they are unable to acquire spoken language. For these deaf adolescents, then, sign language exposure occurs at an age well beyond early childhood. Importantly, these deaf students have often acquired very little functional spoken language prior to learning to sign. This situation is *not* second-language learning. This situation is akin to *first* language acquisition begun in adolescence. The important question then becomes whether these deaf students ever catch up with respect to their sign language skills. Do they ultimately use sign language as proficiently as second-language or native-language (i.e., acquired from birth) learners of ASL?

This question was investigated in another study (Mayberry, 1993). The ASL sentence comprehension skills of deaf adults with contrasting early language backgrounds were compared. One experimental group consisted of congenitally deaf adults who began to learn sign language between the ages of 9 and 13. They were exposed to sign language at this late age because their spoken language skills were not functional. Thus, their ASL acquisition was analogous to first-language learning. The comparison group consisted of deaf adults who were born with normal hearing which they suddenly lost between the ages of 9 and 11 due to various viral infections. After becoming deaf, these individuals were enrolled in schools for deaf children where sign language was used. Thus, one group acquired spoken English in early childhood (because they could hear) so ASL was clearly a *second* language for them. By contrast, the other group had acquired little language prior to learning ASL at the *same* older ages. The critical question was whether the two groups would show comparable ASL comprehension. The answer was no. The ASL skills of the two groups were very different. The second-language learners performed at near-native levels. By contrast, the late, first-language learners showed significant ASL comprehension deficits despite the fact that it was their primary language and they had been using it for many years (Mayberry, 1993), as Fig. 4 shows. Importantly, the late-language learners were as intelligent as the other groups in terms of non-verbal intelligence, as we discuss in detail below.

Thus, the postponement of first-language acquisition to ages beyond early childhood has permanent, deleterious effects on language comprehension in

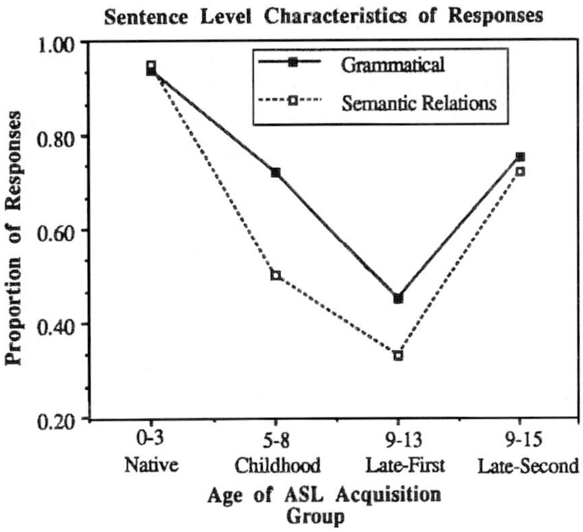

Fig. 4. ASL sentence comprehension and memory performance of deaf adults as a function of the age at which they were first began to learn ASL and whether it was their first or second language (fig. 4 from Mayberry, 1993).

later adulthood. This finding was replicated and extended in another study. Mayberry, Lock and Kazmi (2002) compared the English grammatical skills of two groups of second-language learners, one deaf and one hearing, to a group of late, first-language learners who were deaf. The deaf second-language learners of English acquired ASL from their deaf parents; they began to learn English as a second language in school between the ages of 5 and 7. The hearing second-language learners had a variety of native languages (Urdu, Italian, German, and French) and began to learn English as a second-language in school between the ages of 5 and 9. By contrast, the late first-language learners began to learn sign language and English at the same time between the ages of 5 and 9 when they enrolled in a school that used sign language; they had not acquired any language in early childhood. As predicted by previous research, there were no performance differences on the English syntax task for the two groups of second-language learners of English. The deaf, second-language learners and the hearing second-language learners performed similarly across all the English syntactic structures. However, the late-first language learners performed at low levels on all the English syntactic structures and tasks (Mayberry et al., 2002).

Together the results of these studies demonstrate that language exposure in early childhood is *necessary* for language to develop fully in any language, be it a first or second language. Deaf children exposed to accessible language in early life show second-language grammatical and reading skills comparable to hearing children, even though their first language was in sign rather than in speech. Thus, the unique risk congenital deafness poses for infants and children is that it prevents them from getting accessible language input at the right developmental stage. Deaf people who, for whatever reasons, are not exposed to accessible language during early childhood (in any form, spoken or signed), consequently suffer from two permanent handicaps: they cannot hear sound and they do not readily comprehend any language in any mode, be it in sign, speech, or writing. This second handicap, incomplete language comprehension, is completely preventable.

Educators have attempted to ameliorate the language problems common to deaf children through a variety of approaches. One commonly used educational method that combines the use of signs and speech is called Total Communication. We now turn to this means of classroom communication.

Total Communication

Two factors prompted a majority of American schools for deaf children to supplement a strictly vocal mode of instruction ('oralism') with signs. One factor was the dawning realization by linguists that the sign languages used by Deaf Communities worldwide were natural languages, such as American Sign Language, ASL, in North America (e.g., Klima and Bellugi, 1979; Stokoe, Casterline and Cronebeg, 1965). The second factor was widespread dissatisfaction with the academic achievement of deaf children taught exclusively through speech (Lou, 1988). The objective behind this philosophical change of heart, known as Total Communication, or TC, was to make the structure of spoken language visually accessible to deaf children. The hope was that deaf children would spontaneously acquire the grammar of spoken language by watching 'English in the air' in much the same fashion as hearing children acquire the grammar of spoken language by simply listening to 'English in the air' (Moores, 1982).[1]

Manually coded english

To implement TC, teachers and parents accompany their speech with a simultaneous rendition in sign. The sign portion is accomplished by borrowing vocabulary words/signs from ASL, signing them in English word order, and then using invented signs to represent grammatical English morphemes, such as determiners, plural and tense markers, and so forth. Several groups of educators began the task of inventing signed English morphology at the same time. Their various results are collectively known as Manually Coded English, or MCE (for a description, see Lou, 1988; Schick and Moeller, 1992; Wilbur, 1987).

Allen (1989) observed that, between 1974 and 1983, American deaf students showed gains in mean reading and mathematics achievement, especially at younger ages. Whether these gains were due to the widespread adoption of TC, the greater availability of services for families with deaf infants, or some combination of factors is, of course, impossible to say. The hope that TC would lead to vastly improved facility in English grammar for the majority of deaf children has not been fully realized, unfortunately. This is because 'mode' of communication is not the only factor that predicts deaf children's English learning and academic success, as we describe below.

Geers, Moog and Schick (1984) examined the ability of 327 profoundly deaf 5–8-year-olds to produce English sentences containing a variety of early developing grammatical structures. Half the children were orally trained and half were TC trained, i.e. speech plus MCE — manually coded English. Although there was considerable variation, the TC children as a group developed English grammar at a slower rate compared to the orally trained children. However, it is important to remember that orally trained children, as a group, are more likely to be privileged than TC children, especially with respect to hearing level and socioeconomic status, as described above. Leakey (1991) observed in one sample of TC trained children that they were correct less than half the time in their production of signed English grammatical morphemes, such as articles, prepositions, and auxiliary verbs and tense markers. These results seem to indicate that English grammar cannot be learned through a combined speech and sign mode. Factors other than communication mode may contribute to poorer than expected English language outcome, however. These factors constitute problems with respect to linguistic input and learnability. We consider these factors below.

The input problem

Even when English grammar is made visually accessible in classrooms through the use of simultaneous English and MCE, it is still often inaccessible to many deaf children for large portions of the day, especially at home. This is the situation for deaf children in day classes or schools when their hearing families make little effort to sign. For example, Mayberry et al. (2003) interviewed 24 severely and profoundly deaf 7–15-year-olds with hearing parents who attended TC day classes in a large city. One-third of the children reported that they could communicate with no one in their families because no family member knew or used any kind of signs or sign language with them. Another third reported that they could communicate with only one person in their family, typically the mother. Less than one-third of the children reported that they could communicate with family members through sign. These interview data suggest that the linguistic input many TC children receive, although visually accessible, is often restricted to class time in contrast to the speech overheard throughout the waking hours by hearing children.

Considerable success in learning English has been reported for TC educated children when their schools and families have made a concerted effort to provide consistent MCE input for the children in all aspects of their lives. Schick and Moeller (1992) investigated the English and reading skills of 13 profoundly deaf

[1] The signing used in Total Communication, commonly referred to as Manually Coded English (MCE), uses a grammar that is unlike ASL, the natural sign language used by deaf people in the United States and most of Canada. The grammar of ASL is dissimilar from English because it evolved independent of spoken English. ASL has evolved through generations of deaf children's minds. By contrast, MCE was invented by committees of educators to specifically mirror English grammar in sign. For a more detailed description of MCE, see Wilbur (1987).

children between the ages of 7 and 14. Unlike previous reports, all these deaf children read at levels within normal limits for hearing children. In addition, they performed at superior levels on a test of English grammar in comparison to norms based on orally trained deaf children (see Geers et al., 1984). Detailed analyses of the children's expressive English showed it to be very similar to that of matched normally hearing children in terms of complexity and grammatical intactness. There was a tendency for the deaf children to delete some types of grammatical morphology from their English expression, most notably those English morphemes that require a separate sign in MCE but are fused to the root word in spoken English (Schick and Moeller, 1992).[2] These findings show that the use of MCE can lead to high levels of functional language acquisition in a signed version of a spoken language, English in this case, and to literacy levels typical for hearing children. The key factor appears to be ensuring that the frequency and consistency of the child's signed language input is comparable in many ways to that of hearing children's spoken language input.

Other research shows that restricted language input may retard the development of signed language comprehension. Mayberry et al. (2003) studied 48 severely and profoundly deaf 7–15-year-olds. The children whose sign input was limited to classroom hours (that is, TC children with hearing, non-signing parents) understood stories given in sign language (both MCE and ASL) less well than children whose sign input was unlimited. The latter children had parents who signed with them at home, both deaf and hearing parents. The comprehension gap between the two groups, those with *limited* versus *abundant* sign input, became more marked with age (specifically, at 13–15 years as compared to 7–9 years). These findings suggest that the effects of restricted linguistic input on language development may be cumulative and hence not readily apparent in the young deaf child.

The facilitative effects of abundant sign input on language development via MCE were also found by Geers and Schick (1988). They compared the ability of two groups of TC children to produce a variety of early developing grammatical structures in English. One group of 50 profoundly deaf 5–8-year-olds had deaf parents who had used sign language with them from birth. The other group (matched for age, hearing level, and nonverbal IQ) had hearing parents whose sign skill varied considerably. The group with *abundant* sign input significantly outperformed the group with *limited* sign input on a test of English grammatical skill (given in simultaneously presented MCE and spoken English). Again, the differences between the two input groups with respect to production of English grammar became more marked with age. Indeed, the TC children who had received abundant sign input from birth produced English grammatical structures (in MCE with speech) at a level commensurate with a group of orally trained deaf children who were previously tested by the researchers (Geers and Schick, 1988).

To summarize, research results suggest that the crucial factor in deaf children's language development is not the sensory modality through which they perceive and produce language (i.e., speech without sign, speech with sign, or sign without speech). Instead, the abundance and richness of consistent linguistic input, accessible and available to the deaf child throughout early life and later schooling is a key factor in the child's cognitive outcome, both in terms of language development and educational achievement.

The learnability problem

Some researchers pose yet another version of the input problem, which we call the 'learnability problem.' Many linguists and educators criticize the use of MCE as the mode of instruction for deaf children because it is artificial, i.e., not a real language (Johnson, 1990; Johnson, Liddell and Erting, 1989). There are at least three linguistic and psychological consequences of this artificiality. By artificiality

[2] When using MCE, for example, the child would be likely to accompany both the morphemes of the verb, 'going' with two signs because each morpheme, 'go' and '-ing' are stressed syllables in speech. However, the same child would be less likely to accompany both the morphemes in the verb 'goes' with two signs because the English verb phrase is one syllable in speech. The verb 'goes' requires two signs, however, one sign for the root 'go' and another sign to mark the third-person singular, '-es'. Thus it should be clear that this type of sign morphological deletion in children's and adult's production of MCE is an adaptation to signing and speaking simultaneously when the syllabic and stress patterns of two modalities are in conflict with respect to stress patterns.

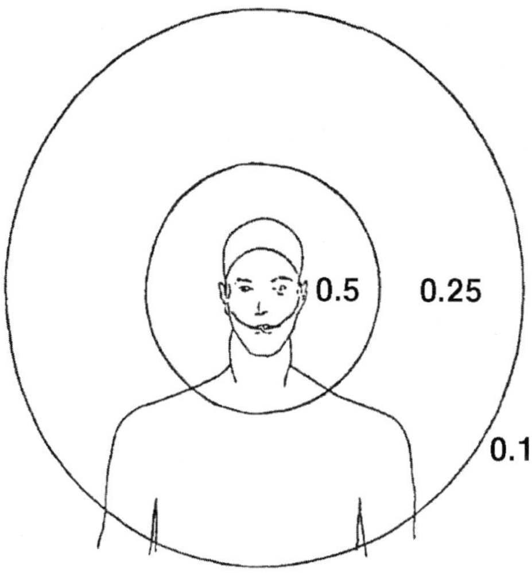

Fig. 5. Visual acuity is greatest at the face where signers focus during sign language perception. Visual acuity decreases sharply as a function of number of degrees from the focus point, ranging from 0.50 just beside the face to only 0.10 at the shoulder and chest. Areas of low visual acuity in the signer's visual focus rely on peripheral vision; peripheral vision, although poor in visual acuity, is adept at perception of movement trajectory and velocity (fig. 2 from Siple, 1978).

we mean using communication that has not evolved naturally through the minds of generations of young children, as have all natural languages, including signed languages.

The first consequences of using an artificial communication system are perceptual and phonological. Linguists now know that the signs of natural languages have sublexical structure, which means that all signs are constructed from a finite set of meaningless articulatory, or phonetic, units. One property of ASL phonological structure is that it evolved to fit the constraints of the human visual system. Siple (1978) first observed that ASL signers focus on one another's faces (and not on the hands and arms). This means that signs made around the face fall into the foveal area of the visual field, or central vision, as shown in Fig. 5. Central visual processes perceive form and shape. In fact, ASL signs made around the face use contrasts of small changes in handshape and location. Signs made away from the face fall into peripheral vision. Peripheral vision perceives the trajectory and velocity of movement. In fact, ASL signs made away from the face use contrasts of movement patterns.

Many of the invented MCE signs for English grammatical morphology violate the perceptual fit between central and peripheral visual processes and the articulatory structure of ASL signs. The poor fit between the visual processing and many MCE signs makes it impossible for the signer to see the form of many invented signs. For example, in some MCE systems the various forms of English verb auxiliary 'have, has, had' are created with handshape changes consisting of *V*, *S*, and *D* (finger spelled handshapes) made inward to the chest with two hands as a derivation of the root verb root 'have' in ASL. However, when looking at a signer's face, as all signers do, these handshape changes are invisible; only the movement and location of three invented signs can be detected, yielding only one sign rather than the three invented English grammatical auxiliary verbs. This observation was predicted by studies of sign identification in peripheral vision. Swisher, 1993 (Swisher, Christie and Miller, 1989) found that the handshapes of unfamiliar signs could not be recognized in peripheral vision. Supalla (1991) noted that the deaf children he observed who were educated with MCE tended to replace the invented pronouns of the MCE system they used with modifications to the movements of the signs, reminiscent of ASL grammatical inflections that indicate person, even though the children had never seen ASL.

The second and third consequences of the linguistic artificiality of MCE systems are morphological and prosodic. Linguists now know that sign languages have a strong tendency to produce grammatical morphology within various changes to movement trajectories through space; these grammatical morphemes are produced simultaneously with the sign root rather than through a sequence of signs. This creates visual intonation patterns through the air in which grammatical roots and morphemes are simultaneously combined. The linear, sign for morpheme, speech/sign expression of MCE systems destroys this visual intonation and significantly slows the pace of sign. In fact, many deaf adults remark that they cannot parse and grasp MCE signing.[3] Hearing adults do not have this problem because they listen to

[3] Patrick Boudreault, Pamela Witcher and Patricia Viens, personal communication.

the speech portion of MCE and thus are not required to perceive MCE solely through vision.

Summary

In asking how hearing affects the child's cognitive development, we have found that the primary deficit posed by deafness is a high risk for impoverished language acquisition in any form. We have seen that deaf children, as a group, show heterogeneous levels of language development related to both the developmental timing and accessibility of their language exposure. Some deaf children show high levels of language development (in signed or spoken language) commensurate with those of hearing peers but other deaf children show significantly delayed and depressed levels of language (in signed or spoken language). This state of affairs leads to two important questions. First, what are the consequences of this wide variation in language development (in signed or spoken language) for cognitive development? Second, does the sensory modality of the child's primary language (i.e., signed versus spoken language) have any specific effects on cognitive development? We begin our inquiry with a summary of IQ test performance followed by a look at memory, symbolic play, and conceptual development.

IQ test performance

Intelligence tests were originally devised to predict academic performance (Sternberg, 1989). Thus, one important question is whether the lower than average academic achievement of the deaf population (relative to the hearing population) is due to a lower than average IQ. Two issues related to the question have been studied in some detail. One question is how the nonverbal IQ performance of deaf students compares to the general population. Another issue is whether deaf children show unique performance patterns, that is, cognitive strengths or weaknesses that are atypical of normally hearing children. Our discussion of these issues will be facilitated if we first note which IQ tests are commonly administered to deaf students.

Mean nonverbal IQ

The office of Demographic Studies at Gallaudet University gathered IQ data on 41,000 deaf students enrolled in special education in the United States. 15,000 students had been given the performance scale of the WISC, the Leiter, and the Hiskey–Nebraska; the remaining students had been administered a variety of other nonverbal tests (Schildroth, 1976). Average performance IQ for the general hearing population is 100. Mean nonverbal IQ for deaf children with *no* additional handicap was 100.1. Deaf children with *one* additional handicap showed a lower mean nonverbal IQ of 86.5 (Schildroth, 1976).

Braden (1992) replicated these findings with a meta-analysis of 285 studies that together tested 171,517 deaf students from 1900–1988. Mean nonverbal performance IQ across the studies was 97.4 with a SD of 15.33. Braden discovered that mean nonverbal IQ increased as the study publication date increased. This improvement in IQ test scores may be due to better societal awareness of the special needs of deaf children in recent years. In addition, Braden (1992) noted that methods of IQ test administration have changed radically over the years. Studies that reported using a strictly oral means of test administration reported lower mean nonverbal IQ scores than those that used a combination of speech and signs. The finding is logical; children perform better on tests when they understand the directions.

On the performance scale of the WISC-R, deaf boys tend to perform at somewhat higher levels than deaf girls on subtests that are highly visual and spatial in nature (specifically, block design, object assembly, and picture completion). Deaf girls tend to outperform deaf boys on the coding subtest. Some psychologists think that the coding subtest, although nonverbal in nature, is related to language ability. Both the direction and magnitude of the reported sex differences among deaf students are identical to those reported for the general population, accounting for less than 1% of the variance (Phelps and Ensor, 1987).

Hearing preschoolers are often tested with The McCarthy Scales. Deaf preschoolers (2–5 years with no additional handicaps) perform similarly to hearing preschoolers on the McCarthy subtests that require *no* language, namely, block building, puzzle solving, and draw-a-design. The performance of deaf preschoolers on these nonverbal subtests is unrelated to the severity of their hearing loss, within a range of 65–110 dB (Bond, 1987).

Although the mean nonverbal IQ of the deaf population approximates that of the hearing population, some research suggests that the strengths and weakness of performance IQ in the deaf population are not identical to those of the normally hearing population. Such a finding would not be surprising, given the fact that deaf children must rely on vision to figure out the world to a much greater extent than do hearing children. As expected, then, analyses of performance IQ test items reveal that deaf children do not show the same hierarchy of item difficulty across various subtests as compared with hearing children (Maller, 1997; Zwiebel and Mertens, 1985).

Common IQ tests

The most frequently used test in North America is the Wechsler Intelligence Scale for Children (WISC). Typically the performance scale is administered; the verbal scale is infrequently administered (McQuaid and Alovisetti, 1981). In a review of 285 studies reporting measures of deaf children's IQ, Braden (1992) found that 14 different nonverbal tests have been used. Of these nonverbal IQ tests, five tests have norms for deaf children. Watson and Goldgar (1985) compared deaf children's performance on two of the tests, the WISC-R performance scale and the Hiskey–Nebraska Test of Learning Aptitude (H-NTLA). They found performance on the two tests to be highly correlated ($r = +0.85$). However, they also found that the H-NTLA showed greater kurtosis, that is, a distribution of scores in comparison to the WISC-R yielding many extreme scores, namely, scores < 70 and > 119, where 100 represents average performance. Braden (1992) found no significant differences for reported nonverbal IQ scores across studies that used norms for deaf children compared with studies that used norms developed for hearing children. This important comparison demonstrates, again, that the nonverbal IQ of deaf children does not differ from that of hearing children, as Table 1 shows. Indeed, this is a robust finding, as we discuss below.

Unique performance patterns

Verbal IQ

Verbal (i.e., language) tests or subtests are infrequently used to estimate the IQ of deaf children due to their pervasive language delay, as described in detail above. For example, Geers and Moog (1989) administered both the verbal and performance scales of the WISC-R to a group of profoundly deaf students who were educated orally. Despite their excellent spoken language skills however, the deaf students scored 22 points lower on the WISC-R verbal scale (with a mean of 89) than on the performance scale (with a mean of 111).

The verbal scale of the WISC-R has been administered experimentally in sign language (in several dialects) to deaf students. Mean verbal score in sign language was 96.3 when the digit span subtest was included in the overall score and 97.8 when it was excluded (Miller, 1985). Deaf students often show a reduced *sequential* short-term-memory span in comparison to hearing students for word lists (including digits) even when the stimuli are signs rather than written or spoken words, which we discuss in detail below (Hanson, 1982; Mayberry and Waters, 1991). Another study failed to replicate the finding of a normal verbal scale score and reported lower than average verbal scale scores on the WISC-R for a group of 27 deaf children when test administration was in various kinds of sign language (Chovan, James and Benfield, 1994). These conflicting results probably reflect real differences in the sign language skills of the deaf students tested in the two studies. Level of sign language development, and hence level of sign language comprehension and production, is heterogeneous in the deaf population and thus needs to be controlled in such studies, as explained above. Maller (2001) administered both the performance and verbal scales of the WISC-III to 110 deaf children ranging in age from 8–16 using "Pidgin Sign English that was mostly ASL" (Maller, 2001: 5). The deaf children with deaf parents significantly outperformed the deaf children with hearing parents on the verbal scale of the WISC-III with mean scores of 86.48 and 77.19 respectively. Note that the verbal scale performance of these deaf signing children was comparable to that of the orally educated deaf children discussed above reported by Geers and Moog (1989).

For the hearing population, verbal and performance scale scores on the WISC-R are correlated ($r = +0.50$). Verbal and performance IQ are also correlated for deaf students ($r = +0.45$, Craig and Gordon, 1988; Watson, Sullivan, Moeller and Jensen,

TABLE 1

Intelligence tests used to assess deaf and hard-of-hearing people [a]

Name of test	*N* studies	Mean IQ
Performance tests		
Chicago Non-Verbal Examination	5	97.25
Grace–Arthur Performance Scale	16	96.02
Hiskey–Nebraska Test of Learning Aptitude	17	97.53
Kaufman–Assessment Battery for Children	6	96.86
Leiter International Performance Scale	12	87.19
Ontario School Ability Examination	6	98.44
Snijers–Oomen Nonverbal Tests	5	96.71
WAIS-R Performance Scale	9	102.84
Wechsler–Bellevue Performance Scale	11	107.32
WISC Performance Scale	38	101.22
WISC-R Performance Scale	44	100.81
Motor-free nonverbal tests		
Draw-a-Man/Person	13	91.72
Pintner Non-Language Test	13	91.87
Ravens Progressive Matrices	17	97.56
Verbal tests		
WAIS-R Verbal Scale	5	84–36

[a] Published reports of IQ tests used during the past 50 years, table 1 from Braden, 1992.

1982). Performance on both the WISC-R and WAIS-R performance scales are also correlated with academic performance (Paal, Skinner and Reddig, 1988; Watson et al., 1982). Indeed, the correlation is impressive given the depressed language skills of most deaf students.

Uneducated deaf children

The assumption underlying the large-scale studies of IQ discussed above is that the deaf children under study are, or have been, enrolled in an educational program appropriate for deaf children from age 5 or 6 onwards as would be the case for normally developing hearing children. The expectation of normal, nonverbal IQ test performance clearly cannot be applied to deaf children who are educationally deprived. This is shown by case studies of deaf children who immigrated with their families to North America in late childhood or adolescence after having attended *no* school in their home country or a school for hearing children with no accommodations or interventions for their deafness. For example, Grimshaw and her colleagues (Grimshaw, Adelstein, Bryden and MacKinnon, 1998) investigated the development of a deaf boy raised in Mexico where he never attended school. His WISC-R and WAIS-R performance levels were 85 with above average performance on the Object Assembly subtest and very low performance on the Coding and Picture Arrangement subtests (specific scores were not given). Another case study of a 16-year-old deaf girl raised in Guatemala where she never attended school reported a nonverbal IQ level of "8 years" based on performance on the Leiter and unspecified subtests of the WAIS (Emmorey, Grant and Ewan, 1994). Morford (2001) reported the performance by two additional deaf students. One 13-year-old girl performed at the 5th percentile on the Ravens after having attended school for only 3 months. After 32 months of educational experience, she performed at the 50th percentile on the Ravens. Finally, a 12-year-old boy, who had attended a school for hearing children in his home country (but without any special consideration of his deafness), received a nonverbal IQ of 71 on the WISC-R after 19 months of being enrolled in a North American school for deaf children. After 31 months of special schooling he received a nonverbal IQ of 85 on the same test.

Together these case studies show that the average nonverbal IQ performance reported for the deaf school-aged population is a consequence of appropriate educational experiences at the appropriate young ages despite often severe language delay. Deaf children who suffer from educational deprivation do not show normal nonverbal IQ performance.

Higher than average nonverbal intelligence

Several investigators have observed that a subset of the deaf population shows higher than average performance on nonverbal IQ tests. In a study of more than 1000 deaf students, Sisco and Anderson (1980) observed that deaf students who had deaf parents outperformed their deaf peers who had hearing parents on every subtest of the WISC-R performance scale (with an overall mean performance IQ of 107 as compared to 96). Moreover, the deaf students raised in deaf families performed at higher mean levels compared to the hearing population mean on every subtest of the WISC-R performance scale (with a mean score of 107 as compared to 100).

Several explanations have been proposed to account for the higher than average nonverbal IQ shown by deaf children raised in deaf families. One hypothesis is that the performance difference reflects the fact that intelligence is, in part, inherited. This account, which we call the *genetic* hypothesis, argues that, because at least half of intelligence is inherited, deaf children who have deaf parents perform higher than average on nonverbal IQ tests because they have inherited genes for superior intelligence (for example, see Kusche, Greenberg and Garfield, 1983). Underlying this proposal is the idea that the deaf individuals who have been the most successful at reproducing over multiple generations are also the most intelligent.

The second explanation, which we call the *early learning* hypothesis, emphasizes the impact of the child's early environment on cognitive development. Some researchers speculate that early *language* exposure facilitates intellectual development in general (e.g., Vernon, 1968). Another version of this hypothesis is that deaf parents are better prepared than hearing parents to meet the early learning needs of the deaf child (e.g., Schlesinger and Meadow, 1972; Sisco and Anderson, 1980). Underlying both explanations is the premise that deaf children with deaf parents perform higher than average on nonverbal IQ tests because they have acquired language on schedule (in early childhood). In a third version of the hypothesis, other researchers propose that the effect relates to the physical form of the language being learned in early childhood. They posit that learning a visuospatial, or three-dimensional grammar, such as in ASL, boosts the child's visual and spatial abilities to higher than average levels (Bellugi et al., 1990).

The available data do not clearly adjudicate between the *genetic* and *early experience* hypotheses, although recent research has shed light on the question. As previously noted, Sisco and Anderson (1980) found that genetically deaf children (those with deaf parents) performed at *higher* mean levels on the WISC-R performance scale than the general population. However, Conrad and Weiskrantz (1981) only partially replicated the finding. They compared the performance of two groups of British deaf children whose deafness was genetic (those with deaf parents and those with hearing parents but deaf siblings) using norms from the British Ability Scales. Both deaf groups performed at higher than average levels than British hearing children. This finding is similar to the American results. Next they compared the performance of the two groups of deaf children with an age-matched group of hearing children from a private school. The performance of two deaf groups was indistinguishable from that of the hearing group on the Ravens' Progressive Matrices (a test of visual reasoning), Block Design, and a test of visual design recall (Conrad and Weiskrantz, 1981). However, Paquin (1992) argued that the hearing control group used by Conrad and Weiskrantz (1981) was not representative of the hearing British school-aged population but rather was a select sample from a small private school that probably selected students for above-average intelligence.

In a subsequent study, Kusche et al. (1983) replicated the original American findings (Sisco and Anderson, 1980). They compared the WISC-R performance scores of two groups of genetically deaf children (those with deaf parents and those with hearing parents but deaf siblings) to two matched groups of *nongenetically* deaf children (those with hearing parents and hearing siblings). The groups were matched on a number of factors including sex, age, hearing level, grade, and mother's educational level. The two groups of genetically deaf children had higher mean performance scores on the WISC-R than the hearing population mean (112 as compared to 100). The two genetically deaf groups also showed higher mean performance compared with the two *nongenetically* deaf groups (112 as compared to 101). These findings were partially replicated in another study (Craig and Gordon, 1988).

The higher than average performance IQ of the genetically deaf groups studied by Kusche et al. (1983) cannot be attributed to knowledge of sign language, because all the deaf groups, genetically deaf or not, knew and used sign language. This suggests that some portion of the higher than average nonverbal IQ of genetically deaf children may be inherited or that nongentic deafness can be associated with cognitive problems of some sort related to the cause of deafness. One way to test this hypothesis would be to test the performance IQ of the deaf children's parents and siblings.

Paquin (Paquin, 1992) investigated the genetic hypothesis by testing the nonverbal IQ of 31 families in which both the parents and the children were deaf. He obtained nonverbal IQ scores for both parents in 18 families, one parent in 13 families and 50 deaf children of the 31 families. He used either the WISC-R or the WAIS-R nonverbal performance scales. Performance on the two scales has been found to produce the same score (Braden and Paquin, 1985). Paquin found mean nonverbal performance to be 114.5 for the deaf parents and 114.0 for the deaf children. Replicating the previous American studies, the performance of the deaf parents and their deaf children was significantly above the mean of the hearing population (Paquin, 1992).

As Paquin (1992) notes, there are two possible mechanisms of genetic transmission of genes for deafness and nonverbal IQ; these mechanisms are assortative mating and pleiotropism. Assortative mating would produce higher nonverbal IQ among genetically deaf individuals if brighter deaf people have tended to marry other bright deaf people across generations. Pleiotropism would produce higher IQ among genetically deaf people if genes for both deafness and intelligence actually became linked over time and were expressed together. Such genetic linkage would predict that genetically deaf children would show higher than average nonverbal IQ but that their hearing siblings would not because the two genes are fused in expression (Paquin, 1992); this latter prediction has not been tested.

A major problem for the genetic explanation of the higher than average nonverbal IQ of deaf individuals with deaf parents, however, is that there over 100 different kinds of genetic deafness, both dominant and recessive (Boughman and Shaver, 1982). It is improbable that all genetic deafness is associated with higher than average performance IQ. However, this does not rule out the possibility that some types of genetic deafness may be linked with some types of intelligence.

Another possible explanation for the higher than average nonverbal IQ of genetically deaf individuals was investigated by Braden (1987). He tested both the manual reaction time and manual movement time of three groups of adolescents, genetically deaf, nongenetically deaf, and normally hearing; he also tested the groups' performance on the Ravens Progressive Matrices. The reaction time measure required participants to lift a finger in response to a given light; the movement time measure required participants to push a button below a given light. The deaf adolescents with deaf parents outperformed the other two groups on the reaction time measure. In addition, both deaf groups outperformed the normally hearing students on the movement time measure. The performance of the genetically deaf and hearing groups did not differ on the Ravens Progressive Matrices but the nongenetically deaf group performed at a lower level.

Factors related to language and early environment rather than to genetic background can explain these findings. First, it is important to know that the Ravens Progressive Matrices is an untimed reasoning test that has been found to be related to some aspects of language skill. In a study of 468 deaf students between the ages of 15 and 16, Conrad (1979) found that performance on the Ravens was highly correlated to measures of phonological decoding in memory for written words, i.e., to mental representations for vocabulary. Other research has found that performance on the Ravens is highly related to working memory (Carpenter, Just and Shell, 1990). Together these findings explain why the deaf children from deaf families performed similarly to the hearing group on the Ravens test. The deaf children from deaf families likely had a native sign language and hence developed mental language representations in addition to working memory (as we discuss in detail below). This would also explain why the deaf children from hearing families performed more poorly than the other two groups on the Ravens; they were likely to have experienced late and/or incomplete language exposure in sign or spoken language and thus have underdeveloped mental language representations and working memory. The finding that both the deaf groups outperformed the hearing group on the manual reaction time could be due to the fact that both groups used sign language as a primary language. They were highly practiced at moving their hands quickly. Finally, the finding that the deaf students from deaf families outperformed those from hearing families on reaction time to a visual stimulus could be due to the effects of exposure to a visual language in early childhood, something the deaf group from hearing families lacked. Research has found that exposure to sign in early life enhances some aspects of visual processing, as we discuss below.

Visuospatial skills and memory

Supernormal visual skills

Research investigating the visuospatial skills of deaf and hearing individuals has uncovered numerous positive effects of using sign language. For example, Bettger, Emmorey and Bellugi (1997) found that individuals who used ASL, native deaf signers, native hearing signers, and non-native deaf signers, all performed more accurately on the Benton Test of Facial Recognition than did hearing non-signers. The advantage was especially apparent on 'shadowed' faces, that is, stimuli that were harder to perceive. Other research has found that deaf children who know no sign language do not show performance advantages on the Benton Test of Facial Recognition (Parasnis, Samar, Bettger and Sathe, 1996). The positive effects of using sign language on face recognition are not limited to native signers. Non-native deaf signers and non-native hearing signers (teachers) were observed to require fewer trials to complete a face matching task compared with hearing non-signers (Arnold and Murray, 1998). As few as 2 years of sign language learning produced increased accuracy of facial expression identification in hearing individuals, especially of facial expressions that signal emotions of sadness and disgust. These facial expressions are harder for general population to identify (Goldstein and Feldman, 1995).

Learning and using sign language has also been found to sharpen the visuospatial abilities of recognizing movement patterns and generating and rotating mental images. For example, Chinese deaf children who use sign language were found to perform at higher mean levels than age-matched Chinese hearing children on memory for the movements of Chinese characters drawn in the air (Fok, Bellugi, Van Hoek and Klima, 1988). Both deaf and hearing native signers were found to generate and rotate visual images more quickly than hearing non-signers (Emmorey, Kosslyn and Bellugi, 1993). Moreover, deaf individuals who do not know sign language do not show these effects (Chamberlain and Mayberry, 1994). The degree to which these effects are contingent upon early sign exposure has not yet been fully explored (Emmorey, 1998). Also, it is important to note that the degree to which these effects interact with the well-documented, but small, differences in spatial processing between males and females has not been adequately investigated. In some studies, the differences between the experimental groups of hearing and deaf participants are more apparent for males than for females. Thus, future research needs to control for both age of sign language acquisition and sex. We discuss the brain correlates of these findings below after turning to memory skills.

Short-term memory

As early as 1917, Pintner and his associates found a considerable discrepancy between the digit spans of deaf and hearing children. The oldest deaf subjects in their studies had a mean digit span three digits less than the youngest hearing subjects. (For a review see Chamberlain and Mayberry, 2000). He concluded that deafness causes a delay in development which he called "mental retardation" (Pintner, 1928). Hoemann (1991) noted that more than four decades of research was required to refute this erroneous claim.

Recent investigations into the memory processes of deaf individuals explain Pintner's early findings, which have been consistently replicated. The digit span of hearing subjects typically exceeds the digit span of deaf subjects, even when the digits are given in a written or signed presentation. Research has found that auditory experience does influence STM span but indirectly, not directly. Audition affects STM span because it plays a major role in spoken language acquisition. Deaf children vary widely in their level of language development (spoken or signed), familiarity with written words, and in whether and how they use mental rehearsal as a strategy to facilitate recall.

Language development (or more simply, familiarity) determines how well words from a given language can be recalled. Individuals can recall more frequently occurring words than infrequent ones; individuals who speak two or more languages can recall more words from their native language than their second, or weaker, languages. Deaf children often show reduced STM spans for written words in comparison to age-matched hearing children simply because they are less familiar with English words. The STM spans of congenitally deaf children for written words are thus predicted by the dual factors of degree of hearing loss and degree of language development (Conrad, 1970, 1979; Hamilton and Holtzman, 1989; Novack and Bonvillian, 1996). When the linguistic element is removed from the STM task, and deaf children are asked to recall nonsense figures, their performance is equivalent to age-matched hearing children (Furth, 1966). When deaf children's visual strengths are tapped by asking them to recall the spatial array of a set of items, they often show equivalent (Logan, Mayberry and Fletcher, 1996) or superior performance in comparison to age-matched hearing children (Belmont and Karchmer, 1978). On spatial memory tasks, such as Corsi blocks, deaf children raised in deaf families have been found to outperform those from hearing families (Wilson, Bettger, Niculae and Klima, 1997).

Whether deaf children use rehearsal (mental repetition of the items to be recalled) as a strategy in memory processing is another important factor that explains observed STM span differences between deaf and hearing children. Bebko (1984) found that both orally and TC trained deaf children lagged several years behind hearing children in their development and use of spontaneous rehearsal strategies in serial STM tasks. Rehearsal development, in turn, was predicted by the child's language history. The probability that a deaf signing child would rehearse items during a STM task was thus related to the number of years he or she had used sign language (Bebko and McKinnon, 1990).

Even at the post-secondary level, STM discrepancies persist (Bellugi, Klima and Siple, 1975; Bonvillian, Rea, Orlansky and Slade, 1987) but the exact cause of these discrepancies is unclear. For example, deaf and hearing college students show similar STM spans when recall is free, or unordered (Hanson, 1982). When recall is serial, or ordered, the spans of deaf students are often, but not always, reduced with respect to hearing subjects (Hanson, 1990; Krakow and Hanson, 1985). This pattern has been reported several times in the literature (e.g., O'Connor and Hermelin, 1978) and has prompted some researchers to speculate that auditory experience is essential for temporal, or sequenced, processing. However, deaf and hearing adults show similar performance on temporal processing tasks when language is not involved, e.g., detection of flicker frequency (Poizner and Tallal, 1987). The most parsimonious explanation currently available, then, is that discrepancies between deaf and hearing students' STM spans for written words are related to real differences in cumulative linguistic experience.

Similar factors may account for the finding that deaf children's STM spans for signs and fingerspelling are also reduced in comparison to age-matched hearing children's span for spoken words. Deaf children vary widely in their developmental experience with sign language, which affects development of STM processes in at least three ways. Children who begin language acquisition at older ages and/or have limited language input during early childhood have underdeveloped sign language skill, which, in turn, affects their STM development (Mayberry and Waters, 1991). In addition, deaf children who are delayed in language acquisition are less likely to rehearse during STM tasks (Bebko and McKinnon, 1990). Finally, articulation differences between sign language and speech are also a factor. For example, sign duration as measured by the length of a given sign's movement trajectory has been found to influence STM span for signs in deaf signers (Wilson and Emmorey, 1998). This is analogous to the word length effect in memory for spoken words (Baddeley, Thomson and Buchanan, 1975) and has been found for fingerspelling memory in deaf children also (Mayberry and Waters, 1991).

Conceptual development

In asking how deafness affect the child's development, we have seen that, despite heterogeneity in primary language development and levels of reading and academic achievement, deaf children show normal performance levels on nonverbal IQ tests and above average performance on several types of visuospatial tasks. How might this pattern of cognitive strengths and weaknesses relate to the development of reasoning skills? Does childhood deafness impede the development of abstract and logical thought? The framework for this question has changed over time reflecting the theoretical shift that has occurred in developmental research with hearing children (Wellman and Gelman, 1992). Earlier research with deaf children investigated the question from the standpoint of general stages of cognitive development using Piaget's theory as a basis. Recent research has focused instead on domains of knowledge, such as the deaf child's understanding of people and the physical and biological worlds.

Symbolic play

In Piaget's theory of intellectual development, the child's early reasoning develops in stages through interactions with the physical world so that language is not initially essential to conceptual development. Children's play with objects and toys becomes increasingly complex and coincides with the onset of language in normally hearing children (McCune-Nicholich, 1981). Both early play and language are hypothesized to emerge from a unitary symbolic capacity (Bates, Benigni, Bretherton et al., 1979). One question with respect to deaf children has been whether their pervasive language delay affects their early play with objects. Another related question has been whether the disruption that deafness can pose for mother–child interactions impedes the deaf child's development of symbolic play. These questions have been addressed in some studies with conflicting results.

Spencer (1996) studied the play sophistication of 30 2-year-olds in three groups, deaf children with deaf mothers, deaf children with hearing mothers, and hearing children with hearing mothers. In addition to observing and coding the children's play, Spencer classified all the children as having one of three levels of language development, pre-word combinations, beginning word combinations, and frequent word combinations. She found that the frequency and duration of the children's abstract play, as well as ordered sequences, varied as a function of language development. A similar pattern held when she analyzed the play behavior of only the deaf children with hearing mothers; language development coincided with the frequency and duration of ordered play (Spencer, 1996).

In a follow-up study, Spencer and Meadow-Orlans (1996) found no play differences at 9 months of age across the same varying child–mother dyads, namely, deaf children with deaf mothers (13 pairs), deaf children with hearing mothers (15 pairs), and hearing children with hearing mothers (15 pairs). By 12 months of age, more of the hearing children showed sequenced play than did the deaf children; some of the deaf children showed developmental delays. At 18 months, all of the hearing children and all of the deaf children with deaf mothers showed pre-planned representational play but only half of the deaf children with hearing mothers did so. However, language development did not always coincide with the emergence of play. Some children at 12 months showed no language but nonetheless engaged in representational play. By 18 months, even the children with the lowest language levels showed some pre-planned representational play (Spencer and Meadow-Orlans, 1996). These results suggest that, although language and play may both emerge from the same symbolic capacity in young children, deafness primarily affects the emergence of the language portion of this capacity.

A large-scale study by Bornstein and his colleagues (Bornstein, Selmi, Haynes et al., 1999) found a complex relation between language development and the emergence of play. They assessed the language and play sophistication of 89 child/mother dyads of 4 contrasting types, hearing children with hearing mothers, hearing children with deaf mothers, deaf children with deaf mothers, and deaf children of hearing mothers. Few differences in the play sophistication between the hearing and deaf children were observed even though the hearing children, regardless of whether their mothers were hearing or deaf, had many more words than the deaf children. Independent of the hearing status of the child or mother, language and play was correlated for children younger than 22 months but not for children older than 22 months. Bornstein et al. (1999) interpreted these findings to mean that play and language constitute a unitary symbolic ability in the earliest stages of development that then bifurcates into two separate abilities with age.

Concept attainment

The ability of deaf children to form concepts despite delayed language was well illustrated in a study by Friedman (1987). She compared the performance of three groups of children on an object sorting task, (1) normally hearing children with normal language acquisition, (2) normally hearing children with specific language impairment, and (3) orally trained deaf children. In comparison to the hearing groups, the orally trained deaf children had delayed language acquisition and did not know the names of the categories they were being asked to classify. Nevertheless, the deaf children were able to sort objects by categories (such as tools and furniture) nearly as well as the hearing children with normal language acquisition. By contrast, the language disordered children, who could name all the objects and categories, had difficulty with all the sorting tasks.

Does deafness affect conceptual development beyond the child's early symbolic representations in play and object understanding? Using a Piagetian framework, Furth (Furth, 1966) and his colleagues studied the reasoning skills of deaf children in a large series of studies. Recall that in Piaget's theory, the child's early reasoning develops in stages through interactions with the physical world so that language is not initially essential to conceptual development. In his studies, Furth repeatedly found that deaf children, as a group, appear to follow the same stages of early conceptual development as their hearing peers despite pervasive language delay (Furth, 1991). For example, deaf children develop the concepts of sameness, symmetry, and part–whole relationships on schedule, but are slower to develop the concept of opposition (Furth, 1961, 1963). Opposition may be more difficult for deaf children with delayed language to understand simply because it is linguistically coded. Hearing children often acquire the vocabulary for opposites in tandem, as in 'hot/cold, little/big, dark/light,' and so forth (Ingram, 1989). It is important to note that the language skills (in sign or speech) of the children in these studies were not measured. Furth and his colleagues believed at the time that they were investigating cognitive development in children bereft of language. For this reason his book was titled, *Thinking Without Language*. However, it is important to remember that when these studies were conducted, next to nothing was known about sign language and it was not considered to be a language. Hence it was not acknowledged as such.

Reasoning ability

Reasoning skills in general

Studies of deaf children's more advanced conceptual and reasoning abilities are less common. This may be due in large part to the difficulty in studying the thought and reasoning processes of individuals who may not understand task instructions (and researchers who may not understand the individuals they test). For example, in a study of deaf children's development of the concept of conservation (of weight and liquid), French deaf children were found to lag behind hearing children by 4–8 years (Oleron and Herren, 1961). In a replication study, Furth (1966) noted that American deaf children used labels in the experimental tasks in what appeared to be an opposite fashion compared to hearing children. The deaf children consistently signed the word 'more' over the container that had least liquid in response to the question, "Are these the same?" He surmised that what the deaf children actually meant was that the container with the least amount of liquid required *more* liquid in order to be equivalent with the other container, not that they lacked the ability to discern equivalence, or conserve (Furth, 1966). After training on the task, the deaf children tested showed the ability to conserve at about a 2-year lag with respect to hearing children.

The ability of deaf children and adults to discover and use abstract symbols and follow rules of logic shows some lag in development but no atypical patterns. For example, Youniss, Furth and Ross (1971) studied the ability of high and low achieving deaf and hearing adolescents to acquire and use logic symbols. After 1 week of training, most of the hearing participants could perform the task but few of the deaf participants could. With additional training, most of the deaf participants performed as well as the hearing participants. Like minority or educationally underachieving groups, the deaf participants required more training than did the hearing participants. The analogy was demonstrated by Furth (1964) who found that deaf and hearing adult participants showed comparable performance on a logic task when they were matched on the basis of academic achievement and socioeconomic status. Note that academic achievement would likely reflect language skills of the deaf participants as well.

Theory of mind

We turn now from general stages of cognitive development to the deaf child's acquisition of knowledge in specific cognitive domains. Does deafness affect the child's ability to learn about the worlds of objects, biology, and people? The cognitive domain that has received the most attention is deaf children's understanding of other peoples' behavior, the concept referred to as 'theory of mind.' In order to achieve this understanding, the child needs to learn that other people have desires and beliefs that are different from her or his own and that these desires and beliefs can explain the behavior of others (Wellman and Gelman, 1992). Understanding the mental states of other people is rooted in the infant's recognition of the facial expression and later identification of emotional states in others. Theory of mind also arises from young child's understanding that ideas about objects and actions are not the same as real objects and actions. The question for deaf children has been whether the fact that they have fewer interactions with other people during early life and/or delayed language development affects this important cognitive achievement.

In a series of studies, Peterson and Siegal (1995, 1997, 1999) investigated the performance of deaf children on theory of mind tasks. In the first study, they tested the performance of 26 Australian deaf children with hearing parents between the ages of 8 and 13 on a false-belief task. In this task, the child is shown a story enacted by two puppets. One puppet, Sally Ann, hides a marble in a basket and leaves. A second puppet appears and then moves the marble to a covered box and leaves. When the first puppet returns, the child is asked where Sally Ann will look for the marble. This question is followed by control questions, namely, where is the marble actually located and where did Sally Ann put the marble in the first place? Previous research has found that 4-year-old normally developing, hearing children can perform this task. However, Peterson and Siegal (1995) found that only 35% of the deaf children they tested could perform the task. Success on the task was unrelated to the deaf children's age or nonverbal IQ (Draw-a-Man or Ravens).

Peterson and Siegal (1995) next compared the performance of the deaf children to published data available from 14 children with Downs' syndrome and 20 children with autism (Baron-Cohen, Leslie and Frith, 1985). The performance of the deaf children was below that of the children with Downs' syndrome but comparable to that of the autistic children. These results suggest that language development is a key factor in theory of mind development, although the deaf children's language skill was not measured in this study.

In a second study, Peterson and Siegal (1997) replicated and extended their findings. They tested 4 groups of children: deaf children with deaf parents (native signers who were 9 years old), deaf children between the ages of 4 and 13 with hearing parents, autistic children between the ages of 4 and 14, and hearing, normally developing 4-year-olds. The children were asked to perform false-belief tasks, as described above. In addition, the children performed tasks requiring biological knowledge, such as whether a baby cat adopted by a family of giraffes would grow up to be a giraffe or a cat, and object knowledge, such as whether a photograph and drawing of a object represented the same thing. On the false-belief tasks, the deaf children with deaf parents (native signers) performed as well as the hearing preschoolers. By contrast, the deaf children with hearing parents and the autistic children performed at similar and lower levels. These findings were further replicated in a third study assessing performance on false-belief tasks with the addition of an orally trained deaf group. The orally trained deaf children performed at similar levels to the deaf children with deaf parents. It is important to note that the orally trained children had better hearing than both the other deaf groups (deaf of deaf and deaf of hearing, Peterson and Siegal, 1999). The net results of these studies suggest that language development plays a key role in children's ability to understand the behavior of others. Language appears to be less important to the development of other core domains of knowledge, as shown by the fact that the hearing and deaf groups did not differ on tests of object and biological knowledge.

What is it about language development that fosters the conceptual development known as 'theory of mind?' Peterson and Siegal surmised that the important factor was the number of conversations children are able to have with proficient language users. Two subsequent studies suggest that not only are conversations important, but that overall level of language development is key as well. Courtin and Melot (1998) replicated these findings and added important controls to their investigation of theory of mind in deaf children. First, they eliminated any deaf child who could not follow the instructions. Second, they tested only children with profound hearing losses. Next, they tested five groups of French children. Two groups were hearing children, 4-year-olds and 5-year-olds. Three groups were deaf: one group were 5-year-olds with deaf parents, and two groups were both 7-year-old with hearing parents; one group used sign language and the other was orally trained. The 5-year-old deaf children with deaf parents passed more false-belief tasks than did either the 4- or 5-year-old hearing children or the two groups of deaf children with hearing parents. In turn, the 5-year-old hearing children passed more false-belief tasks children than did the 7-year-old deaf children with hearing parents.

Similar results were found in a large-scale study of deaf children where, unlike the previous studies, their language skills were tested in detail (deVilliers, deVilliers, Hoffmeister and Schick, 2000). Measures of vocabulary and complex grammatical structures in either ASL or spoken English, such as complements and relative clauses, correlated with the deaf children's ability to perform false-belief tasks. This finding suggests that both the ability to name others' motivations via language, which requires a well-developed vocabulary, and the ability to express one's thoughts about others' motivations, which requires complex sentence structure, or syntax, enable children to understand and predict the behavior of others. Deaf children whose language is impoverished show clear and substantial delays in the development of this conceptual domain. The key factor is clearly not deafness. The key factor is well-developed language.

We have seen that childhood deafness has diverse effects on children's cognitive development as a function of early access to language and family and educational environments. Significant numbers of deaf children show very delayed and depressed language development but other deaf children do not. Some deaf children show supernormal visuospatial skills, apparently due to using sign language, but other children do not. How are these diverse patterns of cognitive development related to brain development? Does childhood deafness affect how the brain organizes itself to perform language and non-language cognitive tasks? Researchers have investigated three versions of this question. One line of research asks if there are brain correlates of auditory deprivation and/or sensory compensation. A related line of inquiry asks what regions of the brain process sign language and whether these are the same as those that process spoken language. A third, but little investigated, line of research asks whether and how impoverished language skills affect overall brain organization.

Neuropsychological function

Sensory compensation

A common belief about people who are blind or deaf is that they develop 'extra' perceptual skill in the intact sense to compensate for the impaired sense. In other words, blind people are thought to 'hear' better than sighted people and deaf people are thought to 'see' better than hearing people (Niemeyer and Starlinger, 1981). Recent research has found some evidence in support of this folk wisdom from the standpoint of childhood deafness.

In a series of studies, Neville and her colleagues asked groups of deaf and hearing adults to perform an experimental task requiring detection of movement presented to peripheral vision. They found that congenitally deaf adults who used sign language showed ERPs (event-related brain potentials) that were 5–6 times larger than those of hearing adults over both the left and right occipital regions. These brain regions are normally responsible for visual analysis (Neville and Lawson, 1987a,b,c). In addition, when performing the movement detection task, the deaf adults showed ERPs 2–3 times larger than those of hearing participants over the left temporal and parietal regions (typically responsible for linguistic processing). The greater and more widespread brain activity in response to visual stimuli by the deaf adults as compared to the hearing adults was also apparent behaviorally. The deaf adults were faster and more accurate at detecting movements in peripheral vision than were the hearing adults (Neville and Lawson, 1987a).

In subsequent experiments, Neville and Lawson (Neville and Lawson, 1987b) found that the heightened cortical response to visual stimuli shown by congenitally deaf adults is due in part to knowing and using sign language and not solely due to deafness. They compared the ERPs and behavioral responses of three groups of participants: congenitally deaf adults who used ASL, hearing adults who acquired ASL as a native language from deaf parents, and hearing adults who were unfamiliar with sign language. The three groups responded differently to the movement detection task in the following fashion.

Hearing adults unfamiliar with ASL responded as expected; they showed larger ERPs over the right hemisphere (both the temporal and parietal regions) than the left hemisphere. The right hemisphere is typically involved in spatial processing. By contrast, both the deaf and hearing groups who used ASL showed larger ERPs over the *left* than right hemisphere (Neville and Lawson, 1987a). For people who sign, movement is linguistically salient; ASL grammatical morphemes are made with varying movement trajectories; also signers signal in peripheral vision when they wish to take conversational turns (Swisher, 1993). Because movement patterns are grammatical and pragmatic for people who sign, their brains responded appropriately, i.e., with the language left-hemisphere. Finally, there were also differences in cortical processing between the hearing and deaf groups who used ASL that could then be interpreted as effects specifically related to childhood deafness. The congenitally deaf adults who knew sign language showed larger ERPs over the occipital regions than did the hearing adults who knew sign language (Neville and Lawson, 1987a).

Bosworth and Dobbins (1999) replicated these results by finding strong right-visual field effects (i.e., left hemisphere) for deaf adult signers (who learned by age 6) in a motion detection task when the stimuli were presented to peripheral vision. By contrast, hearing adults unfamiliar with ASL showed strong left-visual effects (right hemisphere). In another study, Bavelier, Corina and Neville (1998) asked deaf native ASL signers and hearing adults unfamiliar with ASL to monitor changes in the luminance of displays of moving dots presented to either central or peripheral vision. Using fMRI (functional magnetic resonance imaging), they found that the deaf native ASL signers showed greater neural responses to motion in peripheral vision than did hearing adults who were non-signers. The greater responses of the deaf native signers were in the motion analysis area of the occipital lobe, namely the MT/MST pathway at the temporal-occipital junction near the anterior and lateral occipital sulci.

What do these findings reveal about the effects of childhood deafness on brain organization? Neville (1993) has interpreted these results to mean that there are separate neurocortical effects for (1) sensory compensation and (2) acquiring a spatial grammar. Childhood deafness produces visual (sensory) compensation in regions of the cortex normally responsible for the visual processing of motion. These cortical areas of the brain respond with significantly more vigor in deaf adults who use ASL than in hearing adults (regardless of whether the hearing adults know sign language or not). In addition, learning and using a spatial grammar and relying on visual pragmatics both prompt the left (language) hemisphere to respond to visual motion patterns, independent of hearing ability. Because the left hemisphere processes language, it treats movement patterns as linguistic stimuli in people who sign. This theoretical interpretation has been supported by the results of two other lines of research, as we described below.

Cortical correlates of sign language processing

Studies of sign language processing allow us to ask the critical question as to whether the language centers of the left hemisphere are specifically specialized for the auditory and oral aspects of language. The alternative possibility is that the left hemisphere language centers of the brain are abstractly specialized for language, independent of sensory–motor modality. One way to answer this question is to investigate individual cases of left- and right-hemisphere brain damage in adult deaf signers. A second way to answer the question is to neuroimage the sign language processing of deaf and hearing signers. Recent research has used both approaches.

Using case studies of brain damage, researchers have asked whether the spatial grammar of ASL is processed by the left hemisphere language centers or by the space/form, motion, and face processing centers of the right hemisphere (for a review see Corina, 1998). Like hearing speakers, deaf signers who suffer lesions to the left posterior temporal region show serious ASL expressive language deficits (Corina, Kritchevsky and Bellugi, 1996). Also comparable to hearing speakers, left anterior temporal lesions in deaf signers result in ASL articulation deficits (Poizner, Klima and Bellugi, 1987). At the same time, these left-hemisphere lesions do not produce visuospatial deficits. In other words, deaf signers show difficulty expressing and articulating ASL as a consequence of left-hemisphere damage but do not show difficulties in recognizing pictures or performing block design or face recognition tasks. By contrast, subsequent to right-hemisphere lesions, deaf signers show marked deficits performing visuospatial tasks, such as picture and face recognition and block design, but no or few deficits in ASL expression and articulation (Corina, 1998; Corina et al., 1996; Poizner et al., 1987). Together these case studies demonstrate a marked dissociation between language and non-language processes in terms of left and right hemisphere function. This is so despite the commonality in visuospatial surface forms for both sign language and non-language tasks such as block design or picture identification. This means that the brain organizes its work by abstract cognitive function and not surface sensory form.

Neuroimaging studies have both corroborated and complicated the overall picture presented by case studies of brain damage in deaf signers. Although case studies find ASL expressive and articulation deficits subsequent to left- but not right-hemisphere lesions, neuroimaging studies conducted to date show both left- and right-hemisphere activation in sign language processing. Some of the conflicting results between these two research paradigms may be due in part to confounding factors related to experimental design, language tasks, and participant controls. However, it is important to know that a similar situation of conflicting results characterizes neuroimaging studies of spoken language (Poeppel, 1996).

In a fMRI study using ASL and English sentences, Neville and her colleagues (Neville, Bavelier, Corina et al., 1998) found that deaf and hearing native ASL signers showed activation in the classic language areas of the left hemisphere, Broca's and Wernicke's areas, when processing ASL sentences. Hearing, native English speakers unfamiliar with ASL showed similar activation patterns in the left-hemisphere when reading English sentences. However, in the ASL task, both the deaf and hearing native ASL signers showed additional activation in the right hemisphere in the areas of superior temporal lobe, the angular region, and the inferior prefontal cortex. When reading English sentences, the deaf ASL natives showed right hemisphere activation, as did the hearing ASL natives but to a lesser extent. The hearing, native English speakers unfamiliar with ASL did not show this pattern of right-hemisphere activation when reading the English sentences.

Right hemisphere activation for sign tasks was also found in a rCBF (regional cerebral blood flow) study by Rönneberg, Söderfeldt and Risberg (1998). Using semantic classification and episodic memory tasks, they found deaf signers to show activation in the right visual association areas, i.e., temporal–occipital. However, the hearing speakers showed activation in the left temporal area when performing the task in speech. Unfortunately, the sign language acquisition histories of the deaf adults were not described in this study, nor were any measures taken of the deaf adults' sign language proficiency. It is thus unclear whether the deaf participants in this study were 'native' or non-native learners of sign.

As previously described, non-native learning of ASL produces substantial differences in ASL comprehension in comparison to native learning (Mayberry and Eichen, 1991; Mayberry et al., 2002). It is not clear what activation patterns should be expected for second- versus first-language ASL learners. For example, some PET studies using various tasks requiring lexical search have found identical activation patterns for the first and second spoken language (Klein, Milner, Zatorrre et al., 1995, 1999). By contrast, one ERP study examining the processing of closed class (grammatical) words showed different activation patterns for first as compared to second-languages as a function of age of second-language acquisition (Weber-Fox and Neville, 1996).

Finallly, Petitto and her colleagues (Petitto, Zatorre, Guana et al., 2000) conducted a PET study of hearing adult speakers and adult deaf signers. The deaf adults were native or early learners of either ASL or LSQ (Langue des signes québeçoise, the sign language used among culturally French deaf people in Québec and Ontario). The deaf participants watched either ASL or LSQ syllables, watched ASL or LSQ signs, copied ASL or LSQ signs, and generated ASL or LSQ verbs in response to signed nouns. The hearing adults were native speakers of English and watched the same signed syllables and signed words as the deaf participants; the hearing participants additionally read English nouns and spoke verbs in response. On the verb generation task both the deaf and hearing participants showed activation in the left inferior frontal cortex. When watching the signed syllables and single signs, the deaf participants showed bilateral activation of the superior temporal gyrus but the hearing non-signers did not because the sign stimuli was not linguistic for them.

To summarize, the neuroimaging studies of sign language conducted to date have all found left hemisphere activation in the classical Wernicke and Broca's areas for a variety of sign language tasks in deaf and hearing native signers. As such, the findings corroborate the available case studies of brain damage in deaf signers. Left hemisphere lesions lead to ASL deficits, as has been found to be the case for hearing people who use spoken languages. However, some neuroimaging studies have found varying degrees of right hemisphere activation associated with sign language processing for which no satisfactory explanation has been offered to date. These conflicting results could be due to a variety of factors including different imaging methods and linguistic tasks in addition to possible differences in the early language histories of the participants. Also, it is important to note that the case studies of left- and right-hemisphere lesions are primarily studies of ASL expression whereas the neuroimaging studies are mostly studies of ASL comprehension. Considerably more research is required to determine what the right hemisphere contributes to sign language processing (and/or reading) and how a late age of acquisition affects this pattern. This will be a complex endeavor because, on the one hand, the right hemisphere processes aspects of language in hearing people including features of prosody and discourse. In addition, the right hemisphere also processes non-language, visuospatial information as in recognizing objects and faces in hearing and deaf people.

Although significant progress has been made in understanding the neurocortical correlates of auditory deprivation and sign language processing, we still know very little about how the severe language delay and deprivation that can accompany childhood deafness affects cortical organization. We now turn to this question.

Congenital deafness and hemispheric dominance

Using EEG patterns to create topographical maps of cortical function, Wolff and Thatcher (1990) studied 79 deaf children and a matched group of hearing children 6–16-years-old. Half the deaf children were genetically deaf and the other half were exogenously deaf (whom the researchers classified as 'neurologically at risk'). Based on the assumptions of their EEG coherence model, both deaf groups showed more neuronal differentiation (maturation) over the occipital (visual) regions than did the hearing children. The deaf groups also showed greater differentiation over the right hemisphere than the hearing children. These findings corroborate Neville's research showing that childhood deafness produces sensory compensation, or enhancement, in the areas of the cortex normally responsible for visual and spatial processing, described above.

Wolff and Thatcher (1990) observed another difference between the deaf and hearing children.

Again, based on the assumptions of their EEG model, the deaf children showed less neuronal differentiation (maturation) over the left and right frontal lobes than the hearing children. Reduced frontal lobe differentiation was also related to the groups' behavior. Both the genetically and exogenously deaf children scored one standard deviation higher than the matched group of hearing children on a hyperactivity measure. Finally, they observed that both deaf groups showed less neuronal differentiation (maturation) over the left (language) hemisphere than did the hearing children. They reported that this finding was consistent with several previous studies reporting reduced left-hemisphere dominance for language among deaf children as compared to hearing children (see for example, Ashton and Beasley, 1982; Gibson and Bryden, 1984; Marcotte and LaBarba, 1985, 1987). The repeated finding that, as a group, deaf children show reduced left-hemisphere dominance for language is likely due to their delayed and fragmentary exposure to language in early childhood. The sign language skills of the deaf children who participated in these studies were not tested, however. Another of Wolf and Thatcher's (1990) findings supports this interpretation. They found that the deaf children with deaf parents, i.e., native ASL signers, showed greater differentiation (maturation) over the left hemisphere than did the deaf children with hearing parents (both genetically and exogenously deaf). Clearly, future research investigating the effects of childhood deafness on cortical organization with other neuroimaging paradigms is required and must carefully measure and describe the sign language skills of the participants under study.

Other research has reported a higher incidence of left-handedness among deaf children. This may be related to the reduced left-hemispheric dominance for linguistic processing among deaf children, as a group, as a consequence of their pervasive language delay and deprivation. For example, in a study of 226 deaf high school and college students and 226 hearing students, Bonvillian, Orlansky and Garfield (1982) found 15% of the deaf students to be left-handed but only 10% of the hearing students to be left-handed. Approximately 10% of the hearing population is left-handed. Conrad (1979) reported a similar incidence of sinistrality among deaf British high schoolers — 17%. A higher incidence of sinistrality for deaf as compared to hearing children has also been found for deaf children in India (Ittyerah and Sharma, 1997). Bonvillian et al. (1982) noted that over 85% of the deaf left-handers in their study first learned to sign at 8 years of age or later. They speculated that delayed language acquisition contributes to left-handedness. In a study of children acquiring ASL from their deaf parents, Bonvillian, Richards and Dooley (1997) observed that the 24 preschoolers showed a marked right-hand preference when signing as compared to when they were performing non-language tasks. They further found that hand dominance among the ASL learning children was related to measures of motor development rather than language acquisition. Finally, there are other possible explanations for the higher incidence of left-handedness in the deaf school-aged population. For example, the left-handers identified in the Bonvillian et al. study also had a greater incidence of exogenous deafness than the right handers. This factor is important because the incidence of left-handedness is greater for brain-damaged individuals than for the general population. In addition, these deaf children may have experienced less pressure to be right-handed than is typical for hearing children.

In sum, we know little about the effects delayed and impoverished language acquisition on brain organization, although it is common phenomenon among children born deaf. Much more research is required to tease apart the cortical correlates of sensory compensation, sign language acquisition and use, and language deprivation in early life.

Summary

Now we return to the question with which we started. What does hearing contribute to the child's cognitive development? We have seen that children who are born deaf frequently experience severely delayed and impoverished language development regardless of mode of expression, that is, spoken language or sign language. The delayed and depressed language development of deaf children, as a group, is not caused by, and does not cause, general intellectual deficiencies in cognitive domains that function independent of language. This fact demonstrates that language and non-language cognitive development is dissociable to a large degree. Deaf children show normal early play behavior and conceptual development in comparison to hearing children. Deaf children also show normal performance on nonverbal IQ tests. Deaf children and adults who use sign language often show above average performance on several kinds of visuospatial tasks, including face recognition, block design, movement detection, and spatial memory, although the degree to which these effects are dependent upon age of sign language acquisition is currently unknown.

The language difficulties endemic to the population of children who are born deaf are completely preventable and caused by a lack of exposure to accessible linguistic input at the right time in human development, namely infancy and early childhood. The language difficulties caused by postponing exposure to accessible language until late childhood and adolescence are permanent and not ameliorated by substituting sign language for spoken language at an older age. Deaf children's significantly delayed language development, in sign or speech, leads to poor reading achievement; on average it is lower than literate levels. However, many deaf children read as well as their normally hearing peers; successful reading achievement can be based on either successful spoken language development or successful sign language development. Deaf children's incomplete language development also delays their ability to understand the motivations and actions of other people. The possible negative ramifications of the all too common language problems of deaf children on complex cognitive action in adulthood are unknown. However, it is clear that deaf people as a group are remarkably adept and clever at leading independent lives despite stupendous obstacles, more so than most other disadvantaged groups (Jacobs, 1989; Schein and Delk, 1974).

The study of deaf children has given us numerous insights into the nature of neurocognitive development of all children. Deaf children have shown us that the human mind is characterized by enormous linguistic creativity. When language is unavailable, the child's mind invents one (home sign). When groups of people are cut off from auditory language, they spontaneously use a visual one (sign language). Deaf children have also shown us that the human brain is remarkably flexible and not fooled by superficial differences in sensory form. The brain allocates labor by abstract function, not sensory perception. Whether the left or right hemisphere processes spatial information depends upon whether the information serves a linguistic function or not. The left hemisphere processes language even when it is visual and spatial. Finally, the young brain is very plastic and works to capacity. When auditory information is unavailable, the brain allocates more of its resources to the processing of peripheral visual information.

Although deaf children have taught us a great deal, numerous questions remain. Little is known about the neurocognitive development of deaf children who mature in linguistic and/or social isolation. Little is known about how deaf children learn to read. Little is known about how poverty affects the development of deaf children. Little is known about the emotional development of deaf children in relation to their language development or lack thereof. How does congenital deafness affect human development? Both profoundly and not at all.

Acknowledgements

Preparation of this chapter was supported by grants from the Natural Sciences and Engineering Research Council of Canada (171239) and the Social Sciences and Humanities Research Council of Canada (410–98-0803 and 410–2001-0621). I am grateful to Pamela Witcher for voluminous library research, Daphne Ducharme and Elizabeth Lock for carefully reading an earlier version of the paper and Carl Vonderau for his critical eye. I also thank S. Sigalowitcz and I. Rapin for the opportunity to delve into the disparate fields that contribute to our understanding of childhood deafness.

References

Allen TE: Patterns of academic achievement among hearing impaired students: 1974 and 1983. In Schildroth A, Karchmer M (Eds), Deaf Children in America. San Diego: College Hill Press, pp. 161–206, 1989.

Allen TE: Who are the deaf and hard-of-hearing students leaving high school and entering postsecondary education? Washington, DC: Gallaudet University, 1994.

Allen TE, Schoem SR: Educating deaf and hear-of-hearing youth: What works best? Paper presented at the Combined

Otolaryngological Spring Meetings of the American Academy of Otolaryngology, Scottsdale, AZ, May 1997.
Arnold P, Murray C: Memory for faces and objects by deaf and hearing signers and hearing nonsigners. Journal of Psycholinguistics Research: 27; 481–497, 1998.
Ashton R, Beasley M: Cerebral laterality in deaf and hearing children. Developmental Psychology: 18; 294–300, 1982.
Baddeley A, Thomson N, Buchanan M: Word length and the structure of short-term memory. Journal of Verbal Learning and Verbal Behavior: 14; 1975.
Baron-Cohen S, Leslie AM, Frith U: Does the autistic child have theory of mind? Cognition: 21; 1985.
Bates E, Benigni L, Bretherton I, Camaioni L, Volterra V: The Emergence of Symbols, Cognition, and Communication in Infancy. New York: Academic Press, 1979.
Bavelier D, Corina DP, Neville HJ: Brain and language: A perspective from sign language. Neuron: 21; 275–278, 1998.
Baynton DC: Forbidden Signs: American Culture and the Campaign Against Sign Language. Chicago: The University of Chicago Press, 1996.
Bebko JM: Memory and rehearsal characteristics of profoundly deaf children. Journal of Experimental Child Psychology: 38; 415–428, 1984.
Bebko JM, McKinnon EE: The language experience of deaf children: Its relation to spontaneous rehearsal in a memory task. Child Development: 61; 1744–1752, 1990.
Bellugi U, Klima E, Siple P: Remembering in signs. Cognition: 3; 93–125, 1975.
Bellugi U, O'Grady L, Lillo-Martin D, Hynes MO, Van Hoek, Corina D: Enhancement of spatial cognition in deaf children. In Volterra V, Erting CJ (Eds), From Gesture to Language in Hearing and Deaf Children. New York: Springer-Verlag, pp. 278–298, 1990.
Belmont JM, Karchmer MA: Deaf people's memory: There are problems testing special populations. In Gruneberg M, Morris P, Sykes R (Eds), Practical Aspects of Memory. London: Academic Press, pp. 581–588, 1978.
Bettger JG, Emmorey K, Bellugi U: Enhanced facial discrimination: Effects of experience with American Sign Language. Journal of Deaf Studies and Deaf Education: 2; 223–233, 1997.
Bickterton D: Language and Species. Chicago: The University of Chicago Press, 1990.
Bishop DVM: Comprehension of English syntax by profoundly deaf children. Journal of Child Psychology and Psychiatry: 24; 415–434, 1983.
Bond GG: An assessment of cognitive abilities in hearing and hearing-impaired preschool children. Journal of Speech and Hearing Disorders: 52; 319–323, 1987.
Bonvillian JD, Orlansky MD, Garland JB: Handedness patterns in deaf persons. Brain and Cognition, 1: 141–157, 1982.
Bonvillian JD, Rea CA, Orlansky MD, Slade LA: The effect of sign language rehearsal on deaf subjects' immediate and delayed recall of English word lists. Applied Psycholinguistics, 8: 33–54, 1987.
Bonvillian JD, Richards HC, Dooley TT: Early sign language acquisition and the development of hand preference in young children. Brain and Language, 58: 1–22, 1997.
Bornstein MH, Selmi AM, Haynes OM, Painter KM, Marx ES: Representational abilities and the hearing status of child/mother dyads. Child Development: 70; 1999.
Bosworth R, Dobbins K: Left hemisphere dominance for motion processing in deaf signers. Psychological Science: 10; 256–262, 1999.
Boudreault P: Grammatical processing in American Sign Language: Effects of Age of Acquisition and Syntactic Complexity. Unpublished masters thesis, McGill University, Montreal, 1998.
Boughman JA, Shaver KA: Genetic aspects of deafness: Understanding the counseling process. American Annals of the Deaf: 127; 393–400, 1982.
Braden JP: An explanation of the superior performance IQs of deaf children of deaf parents. American Annals of the Deaf: 132; 263–266, 1987.
Braden JP: Intellectual assessment of deaf and hard-of-hearing people: A quantitative and qualitative research synthesis. School Psychology: 21; 82–94, 1992.
Braden JP, Paquin MM: A comparison of the WISC-R and WAIS-R performance scales in deaf adolescents. Journal of Psychoeducational Assessment: 3; 285–290, 1985.
Carpenter PA, Just MA, Shell P: What one intelligence test measures: A theoretical account of the processing in the Raven Progressive Matrices test. Psychological Review: 97; 404–431, 1990.
Chamberlain C: Reading skills of deaf adults who sign: Good and Poor readers compared. Unpublished doctoral dissertation. McGill University, Montreal, 2002.
Chamberlain C, Mayberry RI: Do the deaf 'see' better? Effects of deafness on visuospatial skills. Poster presented at TENNET V, Montreal, May 1994.
Chamberlain C, Mayberry RI: Theorizing about the relationship between ASL and reading. In Chamberlain C, Morford JP, Mayberry RI (Eds), Language Acquisition by Eye. Mahwah, NJ: Lawrence Erlbaum and Associates, pp. 221–260, 2000.
Chamberlain C, Morford JP, Mayberry RI (Eds): Language Acquisition by Eye. Mahwah, NJ: Lawrence Erlbaum and Associates, 2000.
Chovan W, James R, Benfield J: Varied sign language systems and their mediating effects on WISC-R verbal subtests of profoundly deaf student: A replication. Perceptual and Motor Skills: 78; 61–62, 1994.
Conrad R: Short-term memory processes in the deaf. British Journal of Psychology: 61; 179–195, 1970.
Conrad R: The Deaf School Child. London: Harper and Row, 1979.
Conrad R, Weiskrantz BC: On the cognitive ability of deaf children with deaf parents. American Annals of the Deaf: 126; 995–1003, 1981.
Corina DP: Studies of neural processing in deaf signers: Toward a neurocognitive model of language processing in the deaf. Journal of Deaf Studies and Deaf Education: 3; 35–48, 1998.
Corina DP, Kritchevsky M, Bellugi U: Visual language pro-

cessing and unilateral neglect: Evidence from American Sign Language. Cognitive Neuropsychology: 13; 321–351, 1996.

Courtin C, Melot AM: Development of theories of mind in deaf children. In Marschark M, Clark D (Eds), Psychological Perspectives on Deafness, Vol. 2. Mahwah, NJ: Lawrence Erlbaum Associates, pp. 79–101, 1998.

Craig HB, Gordon HW: Specialized cognitive function and reading achievement in hearing-impaired adolescents. Journal of Speech and Hearing Disorders: 53; 30–41, 1988.

Davis JM, Elfenbein JL, Chum RS, Bentler R: Effects of mild and moderate hearing impairments on language, educational, and psychosocial behavior of children. Journal of Speech and Hearing Disorders; 51: 1986.

Emmorey K: The impact of sign language use on visuospatial cognition. In Marschark M, Clark D (Eds), Psychological Perspectives on Deafness. Mahwaw NJ: Lawrence Erlbaum and Associates, 1998.

Emmorey K: Language, cognition, and the brain: Insights from sign language research. Mahwah, NJ: Lawrence Erlbaum Associates, 2002.

Emmorey K, Bellugi U, Frederici A, Horn P: Effects of age of acquisition on grammatical sensitivity: Evidence from on-line and off-line tasks. Applied Psycholinguistics: 16; 1995.

Emmorey K, Grant R, Ewan B: A new case of linguistic isolation: Preliminary report. Paper presented at the Boston University Conference on Language Development, Boston, Nov. 1994.

Emmorey K, Kosslyn SM, Bellugi U: Visual imagery and visual-spatial language: Enhanced imagery abilities in deaf and hearing ASL signers. Cognition: 46; 139–181, 1993.

Fischer SD: Sign language and Creoles. In Siple P (Ed), Understanding Language Through Sign Language Research. New York: Academic Press, pp. 309–331, 1978.

Fok A, Bellugi U, Van Hoek K, Klima ES: The formal properties of Chinese languages in space. In Liu I, Chen H, Chen M (Eds), Cognitive Aspects of the Chinese Language. Hong Kong: Asian Research Service, pp. 117–205, 1988.

Friedman J: Classification skills in normally hearing and oral deaf preschoolers: A study in language and conceptual thought. In Martin DC (Ed), Cognition, Education and Deafness. Washington: Gallaudet College Press, 1987.

Furth HG: The influence of language on the development of concept formation in deaf children. Journal of Abnormal and Social Psychology: 63; 386–389, 1961.

Furth HG: Conceptual discovery and control on a pictorial part-whole task as a function of age, intelligence and language. Journal of Educational Psychology: 54; 191–196, 1963.

Furth HG: Conceptual performance in deaf adults. Journal of Abnormal and Social Psychology: 69; 676–681, 1964.

Furth HG: Thinking Without Language: Psychological Implications of Deafness. New York: The Free Press, 1966.

Furth HG: Thinking without language: A perspective and review of research with deaf people. In Keating KP, Rosen H (Eds), Constructivist Perspectives on Developmental Psychopathology and Atypical Development. Hillsdale, N.J.: Erlbaum Associates, pp. 203–227, 1991.

Geers A, Moog J: Syntactic maturity of spontaneous speech and elicited imitations of hearing-impaired children. Journal of Speech and Hearing Research: 43; 380–391, 1978.

Geers AE, Moog JS: Predicting spoken language acquisition of profoundly hearing-impaired children. Journal of Speech and Hearing Disorders: 52; 84–94, 1987.

Geers A, Moog J: Factors predictive of the development of literacy in profoundly hearing-impaired adolescents. The Volta Review: Feb/Mar; 69–86, 1989.

Geers A, Moog G, Schick B: Acquisition of spoken and signed English by profoundly deaf children. Journal of Speech and Hearing Disorders: 49; 378–388, 1984.

Geers A, Schick B: Acquisition of spoken and signed English by hearing-impaired children of hearing-impaired or hearing parents. Journal of Speech and Hearing Disorders: 53; 136–143, 1988.

Gibson CJ, Bryden MP: Cerebral laterality in deaf and hearing children. Brain and Language: 23; 1–12, 1984.

Goldin-Meadow S, Feldman H: The development of language-like communication without a language model. Science: 197; 1977.

Goldin-Meadow S, Mylander C: Gestural communication in deaf children: The effects and noneffects of parental input on early language development. Monographs of the Society for Research in Child Development: 49; 1984.

Goldin-Meadow S, Mylander C: Spontaneous sign systems created by deaf children in two cultures. Nature: 391; 279–281, 1998.

Goldstein N, Feldman RS: Knowledge of American Sign Language and the ability of hearing individuals to decode facial expressions of emotion. Nonverbal Behavior: 20; 111–122, 1995.

Greenough WT, Black JE: Induction of brain structure by experience: Substrates for cognitive development. In Gunna MR, Nelson CA (Eds), Developmental Behavioral Neuroscience. Minnesota Symposia on Child Psychology, Vol. 24, pp. 155–200, 1992.

Grimshaw GM, Adelstein A, Bryden MP, MacKinnon GE: First-language acquisition in adolescence: Evidence for a critical period for verbal language development. Brain and Language: 63; 237–255, 1998.

Hamilton H, Holtzman T: Linguistic encoding in short-term memory as a function of stimulus type. Memory and Language: 17; 541–550, 1989.

Hanson VL: Short-term recall by deaf signers of American Sign Language: Implications for encoding strategy to order recall. Journal of Experimental Psychology, Learning, Memory and Cognitio: 8; 572–583, 1982.

Hanson VL: Recall of order information by deaf signers: Phonetic coding in temporal order recall. Memory and Cognition: 18; 604–610, 1990.

Hoemann HW: Piagetian perspectives on research with deaf students. In Keating DP, Rosen H (Eds), Constructivist perspectives on developmental psychopathology and atypical development. Hillsdale, NJ: Erlbaum, 1991.

Hoffmeister R: A piece of the puzzle: ASL and reading comprehension in deaf children. In Chamberlain C, Morford JP,

Mayberry RI (Eds), Language Acquisition by Eye. Mahwah, NJ: Lawrence Erlbaum Associates, pp. 143–164, 2000.

Ingram D: First Language Acquisition: Method, Description, and Explanation. New York: Cambridge University Press, 1989.

Ittyerah M, Sharma R: The performance of hearing-impaired children on handedness and perceptual motor tasks. Genetic, Social, and General Psychology Monographs: 123; 285–302, 1997.

Jacobs LM: A Deaf Adult Speaks Out. Washington, DC: Gallaudet University Press, 3rd Edition, 1989.

Johnson RC: The publication and early aftermath of unlocking the curriculum. Sign Language Studies: 69; 295–325, 1990.

Johnson RE, Liddell S, Erting C: Unlocking the curriculum: Principles for achieving access in Deaf education. Washington, DC: Gallaudet Research Institute, 1989.

Klein D, Milner B, Zatorrre RJ, Meyer E, Evans AC: The neural substrates of underlying word generation: A bilingual functional-imaging study. Proceedings of the National Academy of Sciences: 92; 2899–2903, 1995.

Klein D, Milner B, Zatorre RJ, Zhao V, Nikelski J: Cerebral organization in bilinguals: A PET study of Chinese-English verb generation. NeuroReport: 10; 2841–2846, 1999.

Klima ES, Bellugi U: The Signs of Language. Cambridge: Harvard University Press, 1979.

Krakow RA, Hanson VL: Deaf signers and serial recall in the visual modality: Memory for signs, fingerspelling, and print. Memory and Cognition: 13; 265–272, 1985.

Kusche CA, Greenberg MT, Garfield TS: Nonverbal intelligence and verbal achievement in deaf adolescents: An examination of heredity and environment. American Annals of the Deaf: 127; 458–466, 1983.

Lach RD, Ling D, Ling AH: Early speech development in deaf infants. American Annals of the Deaf: 115; 522–526, 1970.

Lane H: When the Mind Hears: A History of the Deaf. New York: Random House, 1984.

Leakey TA: Signed English: The acquisition of morphology in deaf children. Unpublished Honors Thesis, Chicago, The University of Chicago, 1991.

Lederberg AR, Everhart VS: Communication between deaf children and their hearing mothers: The role of language, gesture, and vocalizations. Journal of Speech, Language, and Hearing Research: 41; 887–899, 1998.

Lederberg AR, Prezbindowski AK, Spencer PE: Word-learning skills of deaf preschoolers: The development of novel mapping and rapid word learning strategies. Child Development. 71, 1571–1585, 2000.

Lichtenstein EH: The relationship between reading processes and English skills of deaf college students. Rochester, NY: National Technical Institute for the Deaf, 1983.

Logan K, Mayberry M, Fletcher J: The short-term memory of profoundly deaf people for words, signs, and abstract spatial stimuli. Applied Cognitive Psychology: 10; 105–119, 1996.

Lou MW: The history of language use in the education of the Deaf in the United States. In Strong M (Ed), Language, Learning and Deafness. New York: Cambridge University Press, pp. 75–98, 1988.

MacKay-Soroka S, Trehub SE, Thorpe LA: Reception of mothers' referential messages by deaf and hearing children. Developmental Psychology: 24; 227–285, 1988.

Maller SJ: Deafness and WISC-III item difficulty: Invariance and fit. Journal of School Psychology: 35; 299–314, 1997.

Maller SJ: The validity of WISC-III subtest analysis for deaf children. Unpublished ms. 2001.

Marentette PF, Mayberry RI: Principles for an emerging phonological system: A case study of early ASL acquisition. In Chamberlain C, Morford JP, Mayberry RI, Language Acquisition by Eye. Mahwah, NJ: Lawrence Erlbaum, pp. 71–90, 2000.

Marcotte AC, LaBarba RC: Cerebral lateralization for speech in deaf and normal children. Brain and Language: 26; 244–258, 1985.

Marcotte AC, LaBarba RC: The effects of linguistic experience on cerebral lateralization for speech production in normal hearing and deaf adolescents. Brain and Language: 31; 276–300, 1987.

Mayberry RI: First-language acquisition after childhood differs from second-language acquisition: The case of American Sign Language. Journal of Speech and Hearing Research: 36; 1258–1270, 1993.

Mayberry RI: The importance of childhood to language acquisition: Insights from American Sign Language. In Goodman JC, Nusbaum HC (Eds), The Development of Speech Perception: The Transition from Speech Sounds to Words. Cambridge: MIT Press, pp. 57–90, 1994.

Mayberry RI, Chamberlain C, Waters G, Doehring D: Reading development in relation to sign language structure and input. Manuscript in preparation, 2003.

Mayberry RI, Eichen EB: The long-lasting advantage of learning sign language in childhood: Another look at the critical period for language acquisition. Journal of Memory and Language: 30; 486–512, 1991.

Mayberry RI, Fischer SD: Looking through phonological shape to lexical meaning: The bottleneck of non-native sign language processing. Memory and Cognition: 17; 740–754, 1989.

Mayberry RI, Lock E, Kazmi H: Linguistic ability and early language exposure. Nature: 417; 38, 2002.

Mayberry RI, Nicholadis E: Gesture reflects language development: Evidence from bilingual children. Current Directions in Psychological Science: 9; 192–196, 2000.

Mayberry RI, Waters G: Children's memory for sign and fingerspelling in relation to production rate and sign language input. In Siple P, Fischer S (Eds), Theoretical Issues in Sign Language Research, Vol. 2: Psychology. Chicago: University of Chicago Press, pp. 211–229, 1991.

Mayer C, Wells G: Can the linguistic interdependence theory support a bilingual–bicultural model of literacy education for deaf students? Journal of Deaf Studies and Deaf Education: 1; 93–107, 1996.

McCune-Nicholich L: Toward symbolic functioning: Structure of early pretend games and potential parallels with language. Child Development: 52; 785–797, 1981.

McNeill D: Hand and Mind: What Gestures Reveal about Thought. Chicago: The University of Chicago Press, 1992.

McQuaid F, Alovisetti M: School psychological services for

hearing-impaired children in New York and New England area. American Annals of the Deaf: 126; 37–43, 1981.

Meadow KP: Early manual communication in relation to the deaf child's intellectual, social, and communicative functioning. American Annals of the Deaf: 113; 29–41, 1968.

Meadow-Orlans KP: An analysis of the effectiveness of early intervention programs for hearing-impaired children. In Guralnick MJ, Bennett FC (Eds), The Effectiveness of Early Intervention for At-Risk and Handicapped Children. New York: Academic Press, pp. 325–362, 1987.

Miller MS: Experimental use of signed presentations of the verbal scale of the WISC-R with profoundly deaf children: A preliminary report. In Martin DS (Ed), Cognition, Education and Deafness. Washington, DC: Gallaudet College Press, pp. 134–136, 1985.

Moeller MP, Osberger MJ, Eccarius M: Receptive language skills. Language and Learning Skills of Hearing Impaired Students. Asha Monographs: 23; 41–54, 1986.

Mogford K: Oral language acquisition in the prelinguistically deaf. In Bishop D, Mogford K (Eds), Language Development in Exceptional Circumstances. Edinburgh: Churchill Livingstone, pp. 110–131, 1988.

Moores D: Educating the deaf: Psychology, Principles and Practices (2nd ed.). Boston: Houghton Mifflin, 1982.

Moores DF, Sweet C: Relationships of English grammar and communicative fluency to reading in deaf adolescents. Exceptionality: 1; 191–210, 1990.

Morford JP: A longitudinal study of grammatical production and comprehension in two adolescent first language learners. Under review, 2001.

Morford JP, Kegl JA: Gestural precursors to linguistic constructs: How input shapes the form of language. In McNeill D (Ed), Language and Gesture. Cambridge UK: Cambridge University Press, pp. 358–387, 2000.

Morford JP, Mayberry RI: A reexamination of 'early exposure' and its implications for language acquisition by eye. In Chamberlain C, Morford JP, Mayberry RI (Eds), Language Acquisition by Eye. Mahwah, NJ: Lawrence Erlbaum and Associates, pp. 111–128, 2000.

Neville HJ: Neurobiology of cognitive and language processing: Effects of early experience. In Johnson MH (Ed), Brain Development and Cognition. Cambridge: Blackwell, pp. 424–447, 1993.

Neville HJ, Bavelier D, Corina D, Rauschecker J, Karni A, Lalwani A, Braun A, Clark V, Jezzard P, Turner R: Cerebral organization for language in deaf and hearing subjects: Biological constraints and effects of experience. Proceedings of National Academy Sciences: 95; 922–929, 1998.

Neville HJ, Lawson D: Attention to central and peripheral visual space in a movement detection task: An event-related potential and behavioral study. I. Normal hearing adults. Brain Research: 405; 253–267, 1987a.

Neville HJ, Lawson D: Attention to central and peripheral visual space in a movement detection task: An event-related potential and behavioral study. II. Congenitally deaf adults. Brain Research: 405; 268–283, 1987b.

Neville HJ, Lawson D: Attention to central and peripheral visual space in a movement detection task. III. Separate effects of auditory deprivation and acquisition of a visual language. Brain Research: 405; 284–294, 1987c.

Newport E: Constraints on learning and their role in language acquisition: Studies of the acquisition of American Sign Language. Language Sciences: 10; 147–172, 1988.

Newport E, Meier R: The acquisition of American Sign Language. In Slobin DI (Ed), The Crosslinguistic Study of Language Acquisition: Vol. 1. The Data. Hillsdale, NJ: Lawrence Erlbaum and Associates, pp. 881–939, 1985.

Niemeyer W, Starlinger I: Do the blind hear better? Investigations on auditory processing in congenital or early acquired blindness. II. Central functions. Audiology: 20; 510–515, 1981.

Novack LL, Bonvillian JD: Word recall in deaf students: The effects of different coding srategies. Perceptual and Motor Skills: 83; 627–639, 1996.

O'Connor N, Hermelin B: Seeing and Hearing and Space and Time. London: Academic Press, 1978.

Oleron P, Herren H: L'acquisition des conservations et le langage: Etude comparative sur des enfants sourds et entendants. Enfance: 14; 203–219, 1961.

Paal N, Skinner S, Reddig C: The relationship of non-verbal intelligence measures to academic achievement among deaf adolescents. Journal of Rehabilitation of the Deaf: 21; 8–11, 1988.

Padden C, Ramsey C: American Sign Language and reading ability in deaf children. In Chamberlain C, Morford JP, Mayberry RI (Eds), Language Acquisition by Eye. Mahwah, NJ: Lawrence Erlbaum Associates, pp. 165–189, 2000.

Paquin MM: The superior nonverbal intellectual performance of deaf children of deaf parents: An investigation of the genetic hypothesis. Unpublished doctoral dissertation, The California School of Professional Psychology, Berkeley/Alameda, 1992.

Parasnis I, Samar VJ, Bettger JG, Sathe K: Does deafness lead to enhancement of visual spatial cognition in children? Negative evidence from deaf nonsigners. Journal of Deaf Studies and Deaf Education: 1; 145–152, 1996.

Peterson CC, Siegal M: Deafness, conversation and theory of mind. Journal of Child Psychology and Psychiatry: 36; 459–474, 1995.

Peterson CC, Siegal M: Domain specificity and everyday biological, physical, and psychological thinking in normal, autistic, and deaf children. New Directions for Child Development: 75; 55–70, 1997.

Peterson CC, Siegal M: Representing inner worlds: Theory of mind in autistic, deaf, and normal hearing children. Psychological Science: 10; 126–129, 1999.

Petitto LA, Marentette PF: Babbling in the manual mode: Evidence for the ontogeny of language. Science; 251: 1493–1495, 1991.

Petitto LA, Zatorre RJ, Guana K, Nikelski EJ, Dostie D, Evans AC: Speech-like cerebral activity in profoundly deaf people while processing signed languages: Implications for the neural basis of human language. Proceedings of the National Academy of Science: 97; 13961–13966, 2000.

Phelps L, Ensor A: The comparison of performance by sex of

deaf children on the WISC-R. Psychology in the Schools: 24; 209–214, 1987.

Pintner R: A mental survey of the deaf. Journal of Educational Psychology: 19; 145–151, 1928.

Pintner R, Patterson DG: A comparison of deaf and hearing children in visual memory for digits. Journal of Experimental Psychology: 2; 76–88, 1917.

Poeppel D: A critical review of PET studies of phonological processing. Brain and Language: 55; 317–351, 1996.

Poizner J, Klima ES, Bellugi U: What the Hands Reveal About the Brain. Cambridge, MA: MIT Press, 1987.

Poizner H, Tallal P: Temporal processing in deaf signers. Brain and Language: 30; 52–62, 1987.

Quigley SP, King CM: Syntactic performance of hearing impaired and normal hearing individuals. Applied Psycholinguistics: 1; 329–356, 1980.

Quigley S, Steinkamp M, Power D, Jones B: Test of Syntactic Abilities. Beaverton, OR: Dormac, 1978.

Rönneberg J, Söderfeldt B, Risberg J: Regional cerebral blood flow during signed and heard episodic and semantic memory tasks. Applied Neuropsychology: 5; 132–138, 1998.

Schein JD, Delk MT: The deaf population of the United States. Silver Spring, MD: National Association of the Deaf, 1974.

Schick B: The effects of morphological complexity on phonological simplification in ASL. Sign Language Studies: 66; 25–41, 1990.

Schick B, Moeller MP: What is learnable in manually coded English sign systems? Applied Psycholinguistics: 3; 313–340, 1992.

Schildroth A: The relationship of nonverbal intelligence test scores to selected characteristics of hearing impaired students. Washington, DC: Gallaudet College: Office of Demographic Studies, 1976.

Schlesinger HS, Meadow KP: Sound and Sign: Childhood Deafness and Mental Health. Berkley: University of California Press, 1972.

Scovel T: A Time to Speak: A Psycholinguistic Inquiry into the Critical Period for Human Speech. Cambridge: Newbury House, 1989.

Senghas A: Children's contribution to the birth of Nicaraguan Sign Language. Unpublished doctoral dissertation, MIT, Cambridge, 1995.

Senghas A, Kegl J, Senghas RJ, Coppola M: Sign language emergence and sign language change: Children's contribution to the birth of a language. Poster presented at the Winter Meeting of the Linguistics Society of America, Boston, Jan. 1994.

Seyfried DH, Kricos PB: Language and speech of the deaf and hard of hearing. In Schow RL, Nerbonne MA (Eds), Introduction to Audiologic Rehabilitation. Boston: Allyn and Bacon, pp. 168–228, 1989.

Siple P: Visual constraints for sign language communication. Sign Language Studies: 19; 95–110, 1978.

Sisco FH, Anderson RJ: Deaf children's performance on the WISC-R relative to hearing status of parents and child-rearing experiences. American Annals of the Deaf, Oct: 923–930, 1980.

Spencer PE: Communication behaviors of infants with hearing loss and their hearing mothers. Journal of Speech and Hearing Research: 36; 311–321, 1993.

Spencer PE: The association between language and symbolic play at two years: Evidence from deaf toddlers. Child Development: 67; 867–876, 1996.

Spencer PE, Meadow-Orlans KP: Play, language and maternal responsiveness: A longitudinal study of deaf and hearing infants. Child Development: 67; 3176–3191, 1996.

Sternberg RJ: The Triarchic Mind: A New Theory of Human Intelligence. New York: Penguin, 1989.

Stokoe WC, Casterline D, Cronebeg C: A Dictionary of American Sign Language. Washington, DC: Gallaudet College Press, 1965.

Strong M, Prinz P: Is American Sign Language skill related to English literacy? In Chamberlain C, Morford JP, Mayberry RI (Eds), Language Acquisition by Eye. Mahwah, NJ: Lawrence Erlbaum Associates, pp. 131–141, 2000.

Supalla SJ: Manually Coded English: The modality question in signed language development. In Siple P, Fischer SD (Eds), Theoretical Issues in Sign Language Research, Vol. 2: Psychology. Chicago: The University of Chicago Press, pp. 85–109, 1991.

Swisher MV: Perceptual and cognitive aspects of recognition of signs in peripheral vision. In Marschark M, Clark D (Eds), Psychological Perspectives on Deafness. Hillsdale, NJ: Lawrence Erlbaum, pp. 209–227, 1993.

Swisher MV, Christie K, Miller SL: The reception of signs in peripheral vision by deaf persons. Sign Language Studies: 63; 1989.

Vernon M: Fifty years research. Journal of Rehabilitation of the Deaf: 1; 1968.

deVilliers PA, deVilliers JG, Hoffmeister R, Schick B: Theory of mind development in signing and non-signing Deaf children: The impact of sign language on social-cognition. Paper presented at the 7th International Conference on Theoretical Issues in Sign Language Research, Amsterdam, July 2000.

Watson BU, Goldgar DE: A note on the use of the Hiskey–Nebraska Test of Learning Aptitude with deaf children. Language, Speech, and Hearing Services in Schools: 16; 53–57, 1985.

Watson BU, Sullivan PM, Moeller MP, Jensen JK: Nonverbal intelligence and English language ability in deaf children. Journal of Speech and Hearing Disorders: 47; 199–204, 1982.

Weber-Fox CM, Neville HJ: Maturational constraints on functional specializations for language processing: ERP and behavioral evidence in bilingual speakers. Journal of Cognitive Neuroscience: 8; 231–256, 1996.

Wellman HM, Gelman SA: Cognitive development: Foundational theories of core domains. Annual Review of Psychology: 43; 337–375, 1992.

Wilbur RB: American Sign Language: Linguistic and Applied Dimensions. Boston: College-Hill Press/Little, Brown and Company, 1987.

Wilson M, Bettger JG, Niculae I, Klima ES: Modality of language shapes working memory: Evidence from digit span and spatial span in ASL signers. Journal of Deaf Studies ad Deaf Education: 2; 150–160, 1997.

Wilson M, Emmorey K: A 'word length effect' for sign language: Further evidence for the role of language in structuring working memory. Memory and Cognition: 26; 584–590, 1998.

Wolff AB, Thatcher RW: Cortical reorganization in deaf children. Journal of Clinical and Experimental Neuropsychology: 12; 209–221, 1990.

Youniss J, Furth HG, Ross B: Logical symbol use in deaf and hearing children and adolescents. Developmental Psychology: 5; 511–517, 1971.

Zwiebel A, Mertens DM: A comparison of intellectual structure in deaf and hearing children. American Annals of the Deaf: 130; 27–31, 1985.

© 2003 Published by Elsevier Science B.V.
Handbook of Neuropsychology, 2nd Edition, Vol. 8, Part II
S.J. Segalowitz and I. Rapin (Eds)

CHAPTER 21

Early language development and its neural correlates

Elizabeth Bates [a,*], Donna Thal [a], Barbara Finlay [b] and Barbara Clancy [b]

[a] *Center for Research in Language, University of California, San Diego, 9500 Gilman Drive, La Jolla, CA 92093-0526, USA*
[b] *Department of Psychology, 248 Uris Hall, Cornell University, Ithaca, NY 14853, USA*

Introduction

Most children master the basic structures of their native language by the age of four, together with an array of cognitive and social accomplishments that appear to be necessary for language learning to take place. As a result of all this rapid development, the 4-year-old is a very sophisticated being: indeed, we have met children as young as three who can use their new linguistic tools to engage in dialogues about life after death, and the existence or non-existence of God. How does all this happen in such a short time, in all normal children, in every culture? It is difficult to escape the conclusion that language is part of our biological heritage, an achievement that depends upon the unique characteristics of the human brain. To the extent that this is true, developmental psychology and cognitive neuroscience are faced with a great opportunity: by studying the co-development of brain and language in the first few years of life, we may be able to identify some of the neural mechanisms that permit the emergence of language in our species.

Unfortunately, this is easier said than done. There is a discouraging disparity between our knowledge of language development and our knowledge of the brain mechanisms that support it in humans, a disparity so great that it is difficult to formulate a coherent theory of the neural events that make language possible. In fact, as we will point out later, current evidence suggests that the relationship between brain and language development is far more complex than previously believed, with causation running in both directions — including effects of learning itself on the developing nervous system.

On the behavioral side, a vast and detailed body of information about language acquisition has been gathered in the 40 years since Roger Brown and his contemporaries launched modern research in this field (Kessel, 1988). This includes information from dozens of different languages (Slobin, 1985–1997), in situations of poverty and privilege (Hart and Risley, 1995; Wells, 1985), in normal children and in a range of clinical populations (Beeghly and Cicchetti, 1987; Bishop and Mogford, 1993; Broman and Fletcher, 1999; Broman and Grafman, 1994; Leonard, 1998; Tager-Flusberg, 1994, 1999; Thal and Reilly, 1997). Although the process of data collection and transcription is tedious and expensive, a computerized archive of child language data has been established that puts these hard-won products at the disposal of interested researchers around the world (MacWhinney, 1992, 1995; MacWhinney and Snow, 1985, 1990). As a result, detailed records of language acquisition are now available to linguists, computer scientists, neuroscientists and other investigators who do not have the necessary time or expertise to gather such data for themselves. To be sure, controversies abound in this field, and there is no consensus about the nature of language learning or the amount of innate knowledge that is necessary for such learning to take place. There are still many proponents of a strong nativist view, in which language

* Corresponding author. E-mail: bates@crl.ucsd.edu

is viewed as an 'instinct' (Pinker, 1994) or a special-purpose 'mental organ' (Fodor, 1983), with its own neural architecture and its own genetic program (Gopnik, 1997; Rice, 1996). However, evidence and arguments have mounted for a more epigenetic perspective, in which the human capacity for language emerges, phylogenetically and ontogenetically, from quantitative changes in mental/neural systems that humans share with other species (Bates, Bretherton and Snyder, 1988; Bates, Thal and Marchman, 1991; Deacon, 1997; Elman, Bates, Johnson et al., 1996; Lieberman, 1998; MacWhinney, 1999; Quartz and Sejnowski, 1997; Tomasello and Call, 1997). Some of these controversies could be resolved if we had a better understanding of the relationship between brain and behavior during the language-learning years. The comparative study of language and brain development has been held back not by a lack of information about behavioral change, but by a paucity of information about the changes that take place in the human brain during the years in which most children acquire their first language. There are two related explanations for this disparity.

First, for ethical reasons many of the most important tools of modern neuroscience (e.g. single-cell recording) cannot be used with human beings of any age. A handful of non-invasive methods can be applied in the study of human adults (e.g. magnetic resonance imaging; positron emission tomography; event-related brain potentials), but there are additional ethical and/or practical constraints that limit the use of these methods with human children. In other areas of cognition (e.g. memory, attention, visual perception), some of these ethical and practical constraints can be circumvented through the use of animal models. For obvious reasons, we cannot build a convincing animal model of language use or language learning — although, as we will outline in more detail below, it may be possible to formulate useful animal models of the non-linguistic mechanisms on which our capacity for language is built. [1]

The second problem follows from the first. Much of our information about the neural bases of language has come from studies of brain-damaged adults, based on well-known correlations between site of lesion and forms of language breakdown (i.e. aphasia). However, these brain–behavior correlations are far from perfect, and there are a number of serious logical and empirical problems that limit the interpretability of lesion data (Bates, McDonald, MacWhinney and Appelbaum, 1991; Caramazza, 1986; Shallice, 1988). These problems multiply when the lesion method is extended to studies of brain-injured children, because the effects of focal brain injury in childhood are much less severe and even less consistent than the effects of a homologous injury in an adult. Although this plasticity is not total, and some residual effects of early damage can be seen in young victims of either left- or right-hemisphere injury (Aram, 1988; Aram, Ekelman, Rose and Whitaker, 1985; Aram, Ekelman and Whitaker, 1985; Dennis and Whitaker, 1976; Eisele and Aram, 1995; Vargha-Khadem, Isaacs and Muter, 1994; Vargha-Khadem, Isaacs, Watkins and Mishkin, 2000), it seems clear that the human brain can organize or reorganize in ways that we do not yet understand. In fact, *most* children with early focal brain injury achieve what appear (on the basis of current measures) to be normal or near-normal levels of language ability, despite damage to regions of cerebral cortex that are thought to be crucial for normal language functioning in an adult. This phenomenon provides an interesting and important challenge to neurolinguistic research. As we will point out later, our understanding of the effects of early focal brain injury has improved markedly in the last few years, as researchers move their focus from retrospective studies (looking at the sequelae of early injury, long past the period in which language is normally acquired) to prospective studies (following children with congenital injuries from the very beginning of language development, observing the plastic reorganization for language for which these children are famous *as it occurs*).

[1] The ongoing debate about 'ape language' remains unresolved. On the one side, it is claimed that chimpanzees are merely skilled imitators, and that none of their signs are symbolic (Seidenberg and Petitto, 1979). Yet work with the pygmy chimpanzee (*Pan paniscus*, Savage-Rumbaugh, 1986) has provided support for linguistic abilities in that species. She has reported generative use of signs and convincing evidence of comprehension of spoken English.

Despite these positive signs, many aphasiologists believe that research on language development in brain-injured children is too complex, and should be postponed until we make more progress in understanding aphasia in the adult 'steady state'.[2] Is research on the brain bases of language development too difficult to undertake at this time? Although this concern is understandable, we propose a more optimistic view, dubbed the *structure-from-motion principle*: The outer boundaries and internal structure of a physical object are often easier to see when that object starts to move; so too, the relationship between brain and language may emerge more clearly when we observe its construction over time, under a range of normal and abnormal conditions.

Our goal in this chapter is to promote much-needed research on the neural substrates of language development, by describing milestones and variations in the behavioral domain that parallel developments in the human brain. We should stress from the outset that such correlations do not imply *any* simple form of cause and effect. Language development necessarily reflects a complex bidirectional interplay of maturation and experience: although some level of brain organization is necessary for learning to take place, it is now clear that experience helps to shape the architecture of the brain throughout development (Elman et al., 1996). Hopefully the correlations that we will point out here will ultimately be replaced by a more subtle theory of the brain and the mechanisms responsible for language learning in our species, one that can accommodate the bidirectional cascade of causes that are responsible for these events.

The remainder of this chapter is organized as follows:

Component parts of language. In this section we will define those linguistic terms (e.g. phonology, semantics, grammar, pragmatics) that are typically used in studies of language and language development.

Adult aphasia. Traditionally, neuropsychological research with adults is used as the starting point for neuropsychological studies of children. In this section, we will review efforts in the adult aphasia literature to establish a one-to-one mapping between components of language and components of the brain. We will show why this effort has failed, and why most aphasiologists are searching for a new framework to characterize language breakdown in adults. We end this section by suggesting a reversal of the traditional approach: developmental research may help adult aphasiology to shape the new framework by providing a new view of brain/mind architecture based on the mechanisms that are used to get language off the ground in the first place.

Prerequisites to language. This section offers a summary of the developments in the first year of life that lead up to the emergence of meaningful speech. The summary is divided into five areas of cognition and communication that come together in the child's first efforts to map sound onto meaning around 8–10 months of age, including (1) the ability to analyze and produce speech sounds, (2) the ability to recognize and categorize objects (the obvious prerequisite to naming), (3) the development of imitation (i.e. the ability to translate auditory and/or visual input into a motor analogue), (4) the development of those forms of intentionality (including social intentions and means-end analysis) that are necessary for the deliberate use of sound to express meaning, (5) basic changes in memory that make it possible to store and reproduce sound-meaning pairs.

Language milestones. Here we will describe basic milestones within 'language proper', including first signs of word comprehension (9–10 months), first signs of word production (12–13 months), first word combinations (20 months), and the burst of grammatical development that follows soon thereafter (20–30 months). We will also characterize some relatively late changes in linguistic ability, from 3 years of age through puberty.

Variations and dissociations. This section is a supplement and corrective to **Prerequisites to language** and **Language milestones**, focusing on the range of variations that are possible at each of these developmental milestones: variations in rate and style that have been observed within a single language, variations that occur across drastically different language types, and certain robust

[2] The term 'steady state' is used here because it is a commonly used term to describe the asymptotic levels that are reached in many structural and functional systems by adulthood. However, we do not mean to imply that there are no changes in the adult brain.

dissociations between linguistic milestones that have been reported in normal and abnormal populations. This will include a survey of dissociations (or lack thereof) in children with congenital lesions to the left or right hemisphere, an important contrast to our review of adult aphasia in **Adult aphasia**.

Neural correlates of language development. After our survey of milestones and variations in language development, this section will contain an overview of current information about pre- and postnatal development in the human brain, focusing on similarities and differences between those events in humans and other species, with the hope of deriving some neural factors that may play a role in the emergence of language in our species. If our reader is hoping for a neat match between linguistic milestones and maturational events in the human brain, s/he will be very disappointed. We will show instead that the search for simple one-to-one correlations between neural and behavioral events must be abandoned in favor of dynamic theories that can encompass the complex bidirectional interplay of brain and behavior that occurs during development.

The component parts of language

The study of speech sounds (phonetics and phonology)

The study of speech sounds can be divided into two subfields: *phonetics* and *phonology*. Phonetics is the study of speech sounds as physical and psychophysical events. This includes a huge body of research on the acoustic properties of speech, and the relationship between acoustic features and speech perception (Ohala and Jaeger, 1986; Pickett, 1985). It also includes the detailed study of speech as a motor system, with a combined emphasis on the anatomy and physiology of speech production (Levelt, 1989; Levelt, Roelofs and Meyer, 1999). Within the field of phonetics, linguists work side by side with acoustical engineers, experimental psychologists, computer scientists and biomedical researchers (Blumstein and Stevens, 1981; Jakobson, Fant, Gunnar and Halle, 1952; Kent, Weismer, Kent et al., 1999; Perkell et al., 1997).

Phonology is a very different discipline, focused on the abstract representations that underlie speech perception and production, within and across human languages. For example, a phonologist may concentrate on the rules that govern the voiced/voiceless contrast in English grammar, e.g. the contrast between the unvoiced '-s' in 'cats' and the voiced '-s' in 'dogs'. This contrast in plural formation bears an uncanny resemblance to the voiced/unvoiced contrast in English past-tense formation, e.g. the contrast between an unvoiced '-ed' in 'walked' and a voiced '-ed' in 'wagged'. Phonologists seek a maximally general set of rules or principles that can explain similarities of this sort, and generalize to new cases of word formation in a particular language. Hence phonology lies at the interface between phonetics and the other regularities that constitute a human language, one step removed from sound as a physical event.

Some have argued that phonology should not exist as a separate discipline, and that the generalizations discovered by phonologists will ultimately be explained entirely in physical and psychophysical terms. Others maintain that phonology is a completely independent level of analysis, whose laws cannot be reduced to any combination of physical events. A unification of these two disciplines is limited by the fact that training in phonology takes place entirely within the field of linguistics while training in phonetics usually takes place in departments of psychology, cognitive science, computer science or acoustic engineering. As a result, phonologists and phoneticians are rarely active consumers of each other's research. Nevertheless, there are reasons for optimism. First, there have been a number of theoretical advances in phonology, including 'autosegmental phonology' and 'optimality theory' (Menn and Stoel-Gammon, 1995; Stemberger and Bernhardt, 1999) that bring the field closer to an understanding of the physical substrates of the sound system. Second, there is a complementary trend within experimental phonetics, as researchers make use of ideas and methods from computer science and neural network modeling (Dell, Schwartz, Martin et al., 1997; Plaut, 1994) that are much more compatible with these new phonological theories. These new ideas have just begun to appear in research on phonetic and phonological development, with great promise for the future.

The study of meaning (semantics)

The study of linguistic meaning takes place within a subfield of linguistics called *semantics*. Semantics is also a subdiscipline within philosophy, where the relationship between meaning and formal logic is emphasized. Semantics can be divided into two areas: *lexical semantics*, focused on the meanings associated with individual lexical items (i.e. words), and *propositional* or *relational semantics*, focused on those relational meanings that we typically express with a whole sentence.

Lexical semantics has been studied by linguists from many different schools, ranging from the heavily descriptive work of lexicographers (i.e. 'dictionary writers') to theoretical research on lexical meaning and lexical form in widely different schools of formal linguistics and generative grammar (Fauconnier, 1985; Goldberg, 1995; Jackendoff, 1983; Lakoff, 1987; Langacker, 1987; Newmeyer, 1998; Tomasello, 1998). Some of these theorists emphasize the intimate relationship between semantics and grammar, using a combination of lexical and propositional semantics to explain grammar; others argue for the structural independence of these linguistic domains.

The study of lexical processing is one of the busiest subfields in psycholinguistics, because it is now possible to study the 'temporal microstructure' of word comprehension and word production, in and out of context, using computer-controlled, 'on-line' techniques (both behavioral and electrophysiological) that can track these events with 1–10-ms sensitivity (Gernsbacher, 1994; Grosjean and Frauenfelder, 1996; Kutas and Van Petten, 1994; Marslen-Wilson, 1989; Small, Cottrell and Tanenhaus, 1988). The major issues of concern within this field are similar to the ones that divide linguists: some view lexical access as an independent mental activity, a kind of reflex that is not influenced by higher levels of knowledge (although the products of lexical access are rapidly passed on to these higher mental processes — Friederici and Frazier, 1992; Levelt et al., 1999; O'Seaghdha, 1997; Swinney, 1979); others view lexical access as a process that is deeply penetrated by sentence meaning and other sources of information, a process that may actually begin before the very first portion of a target word is presented (Allopenna, Magnuson and Tanenhaus, 1998; Altmann, Van Nice, Garnham and Henstra, 1998; Elman, 1990; Elman and McClelland, 1986; Grosjean, 1980; MacDonald, Pearlmutter and Seidenberg, 1994; MacWhinney and Bates, 1989; Marslen-Wilson and Tyler, 1981, 1987; McRae, Spivey-Knowlton and Tanenhaus, 1998; Spivey-Knowlton, Tanenhaus, Eberhard and Sedivy, 1998; Van Petten, Coulson, Rubin et al., 1999; Vu, Kellas, Metcalf and Herman, 2000; Vu, Kellas and Paul, 1998). This split in psycholinguistics between 'modularists' and 'interactionists' reflects the split in theoretical linguistics between proponents of 'linguistic autonomy' (e.g. Chomsky, 1982) and cognitive linguists who emphasize the interactions between grammar and semantics (e.g. Bates and Goodman, 1997; Langacker, 1987).

In contrast to the feverish empirical work on lexical semantics and lexical processing in the field of psycholinguistics, propositional semantics has been dominated primarily by philosophers of language. The primary issues here revolve around the relationship between the 'natural logic' that underlies natural language, and the range of possible logical systems that have been uncovered in the last two centuries of research on formal reasoning. A *proposition* is defined as a statement that can be judged true or false. The internal structure of a proposition consists of a *predicate* and one or more *arguments* of that predicate. An argument is an entity or 'thing' that we would like to make some point about. A one-place predicate is a state, activity or identity that we attribute to a single entity (e.g. we attribute beauty to Mary in the sentence "Mary is beautiful", or we attribute 'engineerness' to a particular individual in the sentence "John is an engineer"); an n-place predicate is a relationship that we attribute to two or more entities or things (e.g. we predicate an asymmetric relationship of 'kissing' to two entities in the sentence "John kisses Mary", or we predicate an asymmetric relationship of 'giving' to three entities in the sentence "John gives Mary a book"). Philosophers tend to worry about how to determine the truth or falsity of propositions, and how we convey (or hide) truth in natural language and/or in artificial languages. Linguists worry about how to characterize or taxonomize the propositional forms that are used in natural language. Psychologists tend instead to worry about the shape and nature of the mental representations that encode propositional knowledge, with developmental psychologists emphasizing the process by which children attain the ability to express this propositional knowledge.

The study of how signals are combined (grammar)

The subfield of linguistics that studies how individual words and other sounds are combined to express meaning is called *grammar*. The study of grammar is traditionally divided into two parts: *morphology* and *syntax*.

Morphology refers to the principles governing the construction of complex words and phrases, for lexical and/or grammatical purposes. This field is further divided into two subtypes: *derivational morphology* and *inflectional morphology*. Derivational morphology deals with the construction of complex content words from simpler components, e.g. derivation of the word 'government' from the verb 'to govern' and the derivational morpheme '-ment'. Some have argued that derivational morphology actually belongs within lexical semantics, and should not be treated within the grammar at all. However, such an alignment between derivational morphology and semantics describes a language like English better than it does richly inflected languages like Greenlandic Eskimo, where a whole sentence may consist of one word with many different derivational and inflectional morphemes. Inflectional morphology refers to modulations of word structure that have grammatical consequences, modulations that are achieved by *inflection* (e.g. adding an '-ed' to a verb to form the past tense, as in 'walked') or by *suppletion* (e.g. substituting the irregular past tense 'went' for the present tense 'go'). Some linguists would also include within inflectional morphology the study of how free-standing function words (like 'have', 'by', or 'the', for example) are added to individual verbs or nouns to build up complex verb or noun phrases, e.g. the process that expands a verb like 'run' into 'has been running' or the process that expands a noun like 'dog' into a noun phrase like 'the dog' or prepositional phrase like 'by the dog'.

Syntax is defined as the set of principles that govern how words and other morphemes are ordered to form a possible sentence in a given language. For example, the syntax of English contains principles that explain why "John is kissing Mary" is a possible sentence while "John is Mary kissing" sounds quite strange. Note that both these sentences would be acceptable in German, so to some extent these rules and constraints are arbitrary. Syntax may also contain principles that describe the relationship between different forms of the same sentence (e.g. the active sentence "John hit Bill" and the passive form "Bill was hit by John"), and ways to nest one sentence inside another (e.g. "The boy that was hit by John hit Bill").

Languages vary a great deal in the degree to which they rely on syntax or morphology to express basic propositional meanings. A particularly good example is the cross-linguistic variation we find in means of expressing a propositional relation called *transitivity* (loosely defined as "who did what to whom"). For example, English uses word order as a regular and reliable cue to sentence meaning (e.g. in the sentence "John kissed a girl", we immediately know that "John" is the actor and "girl" is the receiver of that action). At the same time, English makes relatively little use of inflectional morphology to indicate transitivity or (for that matter) any other important aspect of sentence meaning. For example, there are no markers on "John" or "girl" to tell us who kissed whom, nor are there any clues to transitivity marked on the verb "kissed". The opposite is true in Hungarian, which has an extremely rich morphological system but a high degree of word order variability. Sentences like "John kissed a girl" can be expressed in almost every possible order in Hungarian, without loss of meaning, for at least two reasons. First, the Hungarian language provides case suffixes on each noun that unambiguously indicate who did what to whom. In addition, Hungarian puts special markers on the verb that agree with the object in definiteness. Hence the Hungarian translation of our English example would be equivalent to "John-actor indefinite-girl-receiver-of-action kissed-indefinite".

Some theoretical linguists are interested in developing a theory of Universal Grammar, defined as a set of innate constraints on the forms that a grammar can take in any natural language. Proponents of linguistic autonomy (e.g. Bickerton, 1981; Chomsky, 1980, 1988, 1995; Lightfoot, 1989) or 'linguistic modularity' (Fodor, 1983; Levelt, 1989) believe that this Universal Grammar will prove to be quite arbitrary in form, based on innate principles that evolved for grammar and nothing else — a kind of 'linguistic algebra' (Marcus, 1999; Pinker, 1997, 1999). These theorists further argue that human beings have evolved a 'mental organ' for grammar, an innate and hard-wired neural system that is unique to our species, in the same way that echo location may be unique to bats (Pinker, 1994; Pinker and Bloom, 1990). Others believe that grammars look the way they do for a reason, and that any universals we might discover across natural languages will ultimately prove to reflect universal meanings and/or universal constraints on information processing. Members of the second school (called 'functional grammar' or 'cognitive grammar') believe that grammar is a way of solving communication problems that takes a particularly well-developed form in our species; nevertheless, the mechanisms used for grammar have their roots in more ancient neural and cognitive systems that we share with other species (Bates and MacWhinney, 1989; Bates et al., 1991). This controversy has colored a great deal of research in linguistics and psycholinguistics, and has played a major role in modern research on aphasia, as we will see shortly.

The study of language as a communicative system (pragmatics)

The various subdisciplines that we have reviewed so far reflect one or more aspects of linguistic form, i.e. the set of signals that human beings use to convey meaning. *Pragmatics* is defined as the study of language in context, a field within linguistics and philosophy that concentrates instead on language as a form of communication, a tool that we use to accomplish certain social ends (Birner and Ward, 1998; Cole, 1981; Givón, 1989; Prince, 1981). Pragmatics is not a well-defined discipline; indeed, some have called it the wastebasket of linguistic theory. It includes the study of *speech acts* (a taxonomy of the socially recognized acts of communication that we carry out when we declare, command, question, baptize, curse, promise, marry, etc.), *presuppositions* (the background information that is necessary for a given speech act to work, e.g. the subtext that underlies a pernicious question like "Have you stopped beating your wife?"), and *conversational postulates* (principles governing conversation as a social activity, e.g. the set of signals that regulate turn-taking, and tacit knowledge of whether we have said too much or too little to make a particular point).

Pragmatics also contains the study of *discourse*. This includes the comparative study of discourse types (e.g. how to construct a paragraph, a story, or a joke), and the study of *text cohesion,* i.e. the way we use individual linguistic devices like conjunctions ('and', 'so'), pronouns ('he', 'she', 'that one there'), definite articles ('the' versus 'a') and even whole phrases or clauses (e.g. "The man that I told you about. . . ") to tie sentences together, differentiate between old and new information, and maintain the identity of individual elements from one part of a story to another (i.e. *coreference relations*). Within a new and growing branch of linguistics called *information structure*, linguists are analyzing the relationship between specific grammatical forms and the discourse functions that they serve. From this point of view, the traditional boundary between grammar and pragmatics (treated as different kinds of content) is giving way to a unified view in which pragmatic factors serve as the motivation for grammatical form (Lambrecht, 1994; Langacker, 1987; Newmeyer, 1998; Tomasello, 1998).

It should be obvious that pragmatics is a heterogeneous domain without firm boundaries. Among other things, mastery of linguistic pragmatics entails a great deal of sociocultural information: information about feelings and internal states, knowledge of how the discourse looks from the listener's point of view, and the relationships of power and intimacy between speakers that go into calculations of how polite and/or how explicit we need to be in trying to make a conversational point. This is one area where social–emotional disabilities could have a devastating effect on language development and language use (Butterworth, Harris, Leslie and Wellman, 1991; Cicchetti and Carlson, 1989; Gopnik and Meltzoff, 1997; O'Connell and Bretherton, 1984; Sodian, Taylor, Harris and Perner, 1991; Tomasello and Call, 1997).

Adult aphasia

The term 'aphasia' refers to the breakdown of language in adults following an acquired insult to the brain. This is one of the oldest fields in cognitive neuroscience (extending back as far as 3000 B.C. in the first Egyptian Surgical Papyrus), and one of the most interesting, because it is clear that language can break down in a variety of different ways depending on the nature and location of the injury. The problem is, however, that there is still no consensus about the nature or location of the mechanisms responsible for different kinds of aphasia. We can distinguish three periods in the history of the field, starting with relatively simple accounts and moving forward to the grand confusion that characterizes our understanding of aphasia today.

Sensorimotor accounts of aphasia

When the basic aphasic syndromes were first outlined by Broca, Wernicke and their colleagues, differences among forms of linguistic breakdown were explained along sensorimotor lines, rooted in rudimentary principles of neuroanatomy. For example, the symptoms associated with damage to a region called Broca's area were referred to collectively as *motor aphasia*: slow and effortful speech, with a reduction in grammatical complexity, despite the apparent preservation of speech comprehension at a clinical level. This definition made sense when we consider the fact that Broca's area lies near the motor strip. Conversely, the symptoms associated with damage to Wernicke's area were defined collectively as a *sensory aphasia*: fluent but empty speech, marked by moderate to severe word-finding problems, in patients with serious problems in speech comprehension. This characterization also made good neuroanatomical sense, because Wernicke's area lies at the interface between auditory cortex and the various association areas that were presumed to mediate or contain word meaning. Isolated problems with repetition were further ascribed to fibers that link Broca's and Wernicke's area (resulting, if lesioned, in Conduction aphasia); still other syndromes involving the selective sparing or impairment of reading or writing were proposed, with speculations about the fibers that connect visual cortex with the classical language areas (for an influential and highly critical historical review, see Head, 1926). This sensorimotor characterization of the various aphasias is appealing in its simplicity and its correspondence to known facts about the sensorimotor organization of the brain. Indeed, it is the account that we still find in some medical school textbooks. Unfortunately, it does not account for detailed facts about the sparing and impairment of language in different forms of aphasia, which brings us to the next phase.

Linguistic accounts of aphasia

In the period between 1960 and 1980, a revision of the sensorimotor account was proposed (summarized in Kean, 1985). Psychologists and linguists who were strongly influenced by generative grammar sought an account of language breakdown in aphasia that followed the componential analysis of the human language faculty proposed by Chomsky and his colleagues. This effort was fueled by the discovery that Broca's aphasics do indeed suffer from comprehension deficits: specifically, these patients display problems in the interpretation of sentences when they are forced to rely entirely on grammatical rather than semantic or pragmatic cues (e.g. they successfully interpret a sentence like "The apple was eaten by the girl", where semantic information is available in the knowledge that girls, but not apples, are capable of eating, but fail on a sentence like "The boy was pushed by the girl", where either noun can perform the action). Because those aspects of grammar that appear to be impaired in Broca's aphasia are precisely the same aspects that are impaired in the patients' expressive speech (namely, morphology and complex syntax), the idea was put forth that Broca's aphasia may represent a selective impairment of grammar (in all modalities), in patients who still have spared comprehension and production of lexical and propositional semantics. This led to the proposal that Broca's area may be the neural home of a modular 'grammar processor' (Caplan and Hildebrandt, 1988; Zurif and Caramazza, 1976).

From the same point of view, the problems associated with Wernicke's aphasia were reinterpreted to reflect a selective impairment of semantics (resulting in comprehension breakdown and in word-finding deficits in expressive speech), accompanied by a selective sparing of grammar (evidenced by the patients' fluent but empty speech). Hence Wernicke's area could be viewed as a 'lexical semantic processor' (Ullman et al., 1997). Similar reinterpretations were made of Conduction aphasia, with researchers noting that (in addition to problems with repetition) these patients display a host of phonological problems that could be explained if we assumed that Conduction aphasia arises from damage to a separate 'phonological processor'.

Finally, other investigators working within this 'linguistic module' approach to brain and language pointed out that right-hemisphere damage seems to lead to specific deficits in understanding the point of a joke, or telling a good story, which could mean that the right hemisphere is the natural home of some kind of 'pragmatics processor'. For example, Gardner and his colleagues have presented some evidence to suggest that aspects of linguistic pragmatics are selectively impaired in patients with right-hemisphere damage. These patients reportedly demonstrate difficulties in following the point of a joke, telling a coherent story (Gardner, Brownell, Wapner and Michelow, 1983) and interpreting idioms (VanLancker and Kempler, 1986) — all domains that require the ability to relate a sentence to its verbal or non-verbal context. They also demonstrate problems with some of the paralinguistic skills that are sometimes ascribed to pragmatics (i.e. prosody or tone-of-voice phenomena that convey emotion and distinguish one speech act from another (Ross, 1981; Ross and Mesulam, 1979).

By the mid-1980s, many investigators were convinced that the brain is organized into separate and dissociable modules, one for each major component of language. It was never entirely obvious how or why the brain ought to be organized in just this way (e.g. why Broca's area, the supposed seat of grammar, ought to be located near the motor strip), but the lack of a compelling link between neurology and neurolinguistics was more than compensated for by the apparent isomorphism between aphasic syndromes and the components predicted by linguistic theory. It looked for a while as if Nature had provided a cunning fit between the components described by linguists and the spatial representation of language in the brain. Unfortunately, evidence against this attractive theory has accumulated in the last 15 years, leaving most aphasiologists in search of a third alternative to both the original modality-based account (i.e. motor vs. sensory aphasia) and to the linguistic account (i.e. grammatical vs. lexical deficits).

The current crisis in aphasiology

To understand why the linguistic approach to aphasia has fallen on hard times, consider the following arguments against the neural separation of words and sentences (for more extensive reviews, see Bates and Goodman, 1997; Bates and Wulfeck, 1989).

(1) Deficits in word finding (called 'anomia') are observed in all forms of aphasia, including Broca's aphasia (Goodglass, 1993). This means that there can never be a full-fledged double dissociation between grammar and the lexicon, weakening claims that the two domains are mediated by separate brain systems. In fact, it now looks as though lexical deficits accompany any and all linguistic symptoms, including the mild naming deficits that accompany normal aging and those that afflict young normals under stress (Bates and Goodman, 1997).

(2) Deficits in expressive grammar are not unique to agrammatic Broca's aphasia, or to any other clinical group. English-speaking Wernicke's aphasics produce relatively few grammatical errors, compared with English-speaking Broca's aphasics. However, this fact turns out to be an artifact of English! Non-fluent Broca's aphasics tend to err by omission (i.e. leaving out grammatical function words and dropping inflections), while Wernicke's err by substitution (producing the wrong inflection). Because English has so little grammatical morphology, it provides few opportunities for errors of substitution, but it does provide opportunities for function word omission. As a result, Broca's seem to have more severe problems in grammar. However, the grammatical problems of fluent aphasia are easy to detect, and very striking, in richly inflected languages like Italian, German or Hungarian. This is not a new discovery; it was pointed out long ago by Arnold Pick, the first investigator to use the term 'agrammatism' (Pick, 1913/1973).

(3) Deficits in receptive grammar are even more pervasive, showing up in Broca's aphasia, Wernicke's aphasia, and in many patient groups who show no signs of grammatical impairment in their speech output (Bates, 1991; Dick, Bates, Wulfeck et al., 1999). In fact, it is possible to demonstrate grammatical symptoms very similar to those observed in aphasia in normal college students who are forced to process sentences under various kinds of stress (e.g. perceptual degradation, time-compressed speech, or cognitive overload — Blackwell and Bates, 1995; Dick et al., 1999; Kilborn, 1991). Under such conditions, listeners find it especially difficult to process inflections and grammatical function words, and they also tend to make errors on complex sentence structures like the passive (e.g. "The girl was pushed by the boy") or the object relative (e.g. "It was the girl who the boy pushed"). These aspects of grammar turn out to be the weakest links in the chain of language processing, and for that reason, they are the first to suffer when anything goes wrong.

(4) One might argue that Broca's aphasia is the only 'true' form of agrammatism, because these patients show such clear deficits in both expressive and receptive grammar. However, numerous studies have shown that these patients retain knowledge of their grammar, even though they cannot use it efficiently for comprehension or production. For example, Broca's aphasics perform well above chance when they are asked to detect subtle errors of grammar in someone else's speech (Devescovi, Bates, D'Amico et al., 1997; Linebarger, Schwartz and Saffran, 1983; Lu, Bates, Li et al., 2000; Wulfeck and Bates, 1991). It is hard to understand how a patient who has lost her 'grammar organ' would perform so well in detecting detailed and language-specific grammatical mistakes.

In the wake of all this evidence, we must reject the appealing idea that language breaks down along the lines laid out by linguists (and reviewed in **Component parts of language**). The effects of brain injury appear to cut across traditional linguistic boundaries, and although there are indeed qualitative differences in the symptom patterns associated with particular aphasic syndromes (i.e. fluent Wernicke's aphasia and non-fluent Broca's aphasia), a characterization of the mental/neural mechanisms responsible for these patterns still eludes us. Aphasiologists are hard at work on alternative accounts of the different forms of language breakdown that have been observed to date. For example, many investigators are now pursuing the idea that fluent and non-fluent aphasia represent differential disruption of *strategic* or *slow* components of language processing (impaired in fluent aphasia) versus *automatic* or *fast* components (impaired in non-fluent aphasia) — a difference that may cut across phonetic, semantic and grammatic boundaries (Milberg, Blumstein and Dworetzky, 1988; Zurif, Swinney and Garrett, 1990). Other investigators still seek an account that honors the structural details of generative grammar, although their proposals are much more subtle and restricted in scope than the original notion of 'central agrammatism' (Caplan and Waters, 1999; Grodzinsky, 2000). Still others have rejected any attempt at all to map linguistic symptoms onto separate components of the brain (for a critical review, see Shallice, 1988). At the moment, there is absolutely no consensus regarding the nature of the neural mechanisms that are responsible for linguistic symptoms in brain-injured adults.

Given the current disarray in research on adult aphasia, it seems most unwise to apply the same well-worn taxonomies to research on the neural bases of language development in children. If adult language does not break down along traditional linguistic lines, we should not expect it to build up along those lines either. The linguistic terms that we have introduced here are still useful, but they apparently do not stand in a one-to-one relationship to brain organization. For example, although children babble before they speak, and they produce single words before they produce sentences, such parallels do not go beyond this broad description. The developmental literature reveals lexical effects on phonology and vice-versa in the first stages of word production (Locke, 1983; Menn and Stoel-Gammon, 1995; Vihman, Ferguson and Elbert, 1986; Vihman and Greenlee, 1987), semantic effects on grammar and vice-versa that begin even before the child is able to produce a single sentence (Bates and Goodman, 1997; Caselli, Bates, Casadio et al., 1995; Caselli, Casadio and Bates, 1999), and pragmatic effects on the entire process of language learning (Bamberg, 1988; Bates, 1976; Berman and Slobin, 1994; Ochs and Schieffelin, 1979). To account for basic milestones of language learning in neural terms, we need a more dynamic model, based on the skills that a small child needs to break into language during the first few years of life — which brings us at last to normal language development and its cognitive, perceptual and social prerequisites.

Prespeech and prerequisites to language across the first year

An overview and quick summary of the many behavioral developments in the first year of life that prepare children for language can be found in Table 1.

Perception and production of the speech signal

Research on the development of speech sounds can be divided into two parts: perception and production. Considerable progress has been made in both these areas in the last 30 years, particularly in the domain of speech perception.

Speech perception

A series of clever techniques has been developed to determine the set of phonetic/phonemic contrasts that are perceived by preverbal infants. These include High-Amplitude Sucking (capitalizing on the fact that infants tend to suck vigorously when they are attending to an interesting or novel stimulus), habituation and dishabituation (relying on the tendency for small infants to 'orient' or re-attend when they perceive an interesting change in auditory or visual input), and operant generalization (e.g. training an infant to turn her head to the sounds from one speech category but not another, a technique that permits the investigator to map out the boundaries between categories from the infant's point of view). For reviews of research using these techniques, see Aslin, Jusczyk and Pisoni (1998), Eimas, Miller and Jusczyk (1987), Haith and Benson (1998), Kellman and Banks (1998) and Kuhl (1986).

After many years of experience with these procedures, it now seems clear that human infants are capable of perceiving virtually all of the speech contrasts used in natural language, at birth and/or within the first few weeks of life. There is even a certain amount of (controversial) evidence suggesting that infants may acquire a preference for the speech sounds of their native language during the last few weeks in utero (DeCasper and Fifer, 1980; Jusczyk, Friederici, Wessels et al., 1993; Mehler, Jusczyk, Lambertz et al., 1988). Because the acoustic ability of human infants is so impressive, some investigators have argued that we possess an innate and highly specialized 'speech detector', an ability that is unique to our species (Eimas, 1985). Alas, current research on speech perception in other species suggests that this conclusion was premature (Kuhl, 1986). The capacity to perceive speech contrasts has now been found in several different species, including evidence that chinchillas and other mammals perceive consonant boundaries in a categorial fashion! The mammalian auditory system is a splendid device that is capable of many fine-grained auditory discriminations; these discriminations apparently include speech, whether or not the species in question will need the particular auditory contrasts used by human language.

Of course human infants do a number of things that we are very unlikely to observe in a chinchilla. For example, Kuhl and Meltzoff (1988) have presented 2–3-month-old infants with visual displays of mouths making different speech sounds (e.g. a face making the sound "eeeee" on the left screen; the same face making the sound "ooooo" on the right screen). When one of these two sounds is played from a speaker located midway between the two visual displays, infants look significantly longer at the display that matches the speech sound, suggesting that they are capable of a very early form of 'lip reading'. Not only that, these infants also struggle to reproduce the sound themselves — but only when the sound and visual display are presented together (i.e. they do not make the same mouth movements to either the sound or the visual image presented alone).

Assuming that no one observes a similar result in chinchillas (a most unlikely prospect), should we conclude from this result that human babies have an innate and domain-specific device for mapping speech sounds onto mouths? Although we cannot rule this out at present, this possibility has to be balanced against recent evidence that human infants are

TABLE 1

Preverbal to verbal development

Age in months	Sound (Perception)	Sound (Production)	Meaning (Conceptual content)	Intentionality (Social and non-social)	Coding capacity (Imitation and memory)
0	All speech contrasts can be heard	Vegetative sounds	Object detection	Innate signals (smiles, cries, etc.)	
1					
2					'Pseudo-imitation'
3	Vocal/facial matching	Cooing, babbling without consonants		Passive anticipation of actions by others	Anticipates position of object in a moving visual display
4					
5			Changes in complexity of pattern detection and pattern anticipation	Joint attention to objects; objects and people are familiar goals achieved with familiar means	
6	Language-specific vowel prototypes				Ability to retrieve a hidden object at zero delay, if obstacle can be easily removed
7		Canonical or reduplicative babble with consonants			
8					
9	Loss of sensitivity to non-native speech contrasts begins	Word-like sounds	Object categorization	First signs of tool use; novel means to familiar ends; humans as tools to objects; objects as tools to human interaction	True imitation. Ability to retrieve a hidden object after delay of up to 15 s
10					

extraordinarily fast learners. For example, Saffran, Aslin and Newport (1996) exposed 8-month-old infants to a series of drab and uninteresting speech sounds, presented by a disembodied artificial voice that was played in the room in which the infants were happily playing with toys on the floor. The sounds were made up of strings of meaningless syllables like "BA DI CO RA BI" in which some syllables were presented in random combinations while others were always presented together, as if they represent the ordered components of a word (e.g. "BADICO"). After only two minutes of exposure to these unattended sounds, the infants were given an opportunity to listen to the same stimuli, or to exactly the same syllables played in different orders (breaking up the statistical structure of the original 'word-like sounds'). In this 'preferential listening task' (in which infants displayed their preferences by turning to the relevant speaker), the 8-month-olds showed a reliable preference for the 'new and unusual' strings. In other words, two minutes of exposure to a boring and repetitive stimulus were sufficient for these babies to induce the statistical regularities in the input, without reinforcement and without paying much attention. When this result first appeared, some investigators suggested that it was only possible because humans have a 'special-purpose speech acquisition device.' However, the same result has now been demonstrated with auditory tones, and with visual stimuli that have no speech content of any kind. The bottom line is that human babies are very good at statistical induction, with minimal exposure. Furthermore (as we will point out in more detail below), they also have a very strong interest in social stimuli, coupled with the ability and the drive to reproduce those actions for themselves. Hence it is entirely possible that they have learned the mapping between speech sounds and mouth movements in the first days or weeks of life.

In fact, the major message from the speech perception literature in the last few years has been the extraordinary speed and power of learning. In addition to the finding that some learning has taken place in utero, Kuhl and colleagues have shown that infants rapidly acquire a preference for language-specific vowels (called 'vowel magnets'), with clear differentiation evident by 6 months of age among Japanese, English and Swedish infants (Kuhl, 1993; Kuhl, Williams, Lacerda et al., 1992). Jusczyk and his colleagues have published a comprehensive series of studies showing how and when English children acquire a host of language-specific phonological regularities (called 'phonotactics' — Jusczyk, 1997; Jusczyk and Houston, 1999; Santelmann and Jusczyk, 1998; Tincoff and Jusczyk, 1999). For example, between 6 and 10 months of age, English-learning infants seem to be tuned into the statistical fact that English words tend to have stress on the first syllable (in contrast with languages like French in which stress is more likely to occur on the final syllable).

In view of all this evidence for language-specific learning, research on infant speech perception has shifted in a new direction, attempting to identify when infants *lose* the ability to hear all the phonetic/phonemic contrasts that are used in languages other than their own. For example, Japanese adults find it very difficult to hear the English contrast between "ra" and "la"; Japanese infants can hear the same contrast perfectly well. When does the child begin to 'shut down' or inhibit unnecessary contrasts? Current studies suggest that the selective loss or inhibition of non-native consonants is already underway by 10–12 months of age (Lalonde and Werker, 1990; Werker and Tees, 1984). This is the point at which children begin to understand meaningful speech (see below), to recognize the intonational contours that are typical of their own language (Hirsh-Pasek, Kemler Nelson, Jusczyk et al., 1987), and to produce the particular sounds of their native language in their own prespeech babble (Boysson-Bardies, Sagart and Durand, 1984). In other words, children begin to inhibit perception of sounds that are *not* in their native language at the same point that they begin to understand and produce the sounds that *are* in their language. Hence, even though children may start out as 'citizens of the world' (Kuhl, 1985), ready to learn any human language, they swim upstream against the flood of sound coming toward them from the very beginning, working doggedly, persistently and successfully to carve up all those sounds into the ones that they will need. This is an impressive accomplishment.

Speech production

The literature on speech production is considerably older than the literature on speech perception, per-

TABLE 2

Language milestones and nonlinguistic correlates

Language milestone	Age of onset	Nonlinguistic correlates	Variations in style
Word comprehension	8–10 months	Tool use, deictic gestures, gestural routines, causal understanding, shifts in categorization	Word vs. intonation
Word production	11–13 months	Recognitory gestures in symbolic play, deferred imitation	Referential vs. expressive
Word combinations	20–24 months	Gestural combinations in symbolic play, shifts in categorization, changes in patterns of block building, gestural combinations in motor and social play	Nominal vs. pronominal
Grammar	28 months	Active sequencing in spontaneous symbolic play	Noun lovers vs. noun leavers

haps because the study of speech output is less dependent on new technologies. Nevertheless, the pace of research on phonological development has increased markedly in the last few years. We will restrict ourselves here to an overview of the basic milestones summarized in Table 2 (for details see Locke, 1983; Menn, 1985).

In the first two months, the sounds produced by human infants are reflexive in nature, 'vegetative sounds' that are tied to specific internal states (e.g. crying). Between 2–6 months, infants begin to produce vowel sounds (i.e. cooing and sound play). So-called canonical or reduplicative babbling starts between 6–8 months in most children: babbling in short segments or in longer strings that are now punctuated by consonants (e.g. "dadada"). Research by Boysson-Bardies et al. (1984) and others suggests that babbling 'drifts' toward the particular sound patterns of the child's native language between 6 and 10 months; that is, native speakers are able to discriminate at above-chance levels between the babbling produced by Chinese, Arabic, English or French infants. However, we still do not know what features of the infants' babble lead to this discrimination (i.e. whether it is based on consonants, syllable structure and/or the intonational characteristics of infant speech sounds). In fact, several investigators have argued that there are hard maturational limits on the infant's ability to control the detailed gestures required for speech production. Hence, even though intonation may 'drift' in language-specific directions, the production of consonants seems to be relatively immune to language-specific effects until the second year of life (Eilers, Oller, Levine et al., 1993; Oller, 1980; Roug, Landberg and Lundberg, 1989.

Whether or not their consonants match the specifics of their native language, most children begin to produce 'word-like sounds' around 10 months of age, used in relatively consistent ways in particular contexts (e.g. "nana" as a sound made in requests; "bam!" pronounced in games of knocking over toys). From this point on (if not before), infant phonological development is strongly influenced by other aspects of language learning (i.e. grammar and the lexicon). There is considerable variability between infants in the particular speech sounds that they prefer. However, there is clear continuity from prespeech babble to first words in an individual infant's 'favorite sounds' (Vihman, 1985). This finding contradicts a prediction by Jakobson (1968), who believed that prespeech babble and meaningful speech are discontinuous. Phonological development has a strong influence on the first words that children try to produce (i.e. they will avoid the use of words that they cannot pronounce, and collect new words as soon as they develop an appropriate 'phonological template' for those words, Schwartz, 1978). Conversely, lexical development has a strong influence on the sounds that a child produces; specifically, the child's 'favorite phonemes' tend to derive from the sounds that are present in his first and favorite words. In fact, children appear to treat these lexical/phonological prototypes like a kind of basecamp, exploring the world of sound in various directions without losing sight of home (Leonard, Newhoff and Mesulam, 1980).

Phonological development interacts with lexical and grammatical development for at least 2 years beyond this point (Vihman, 1985). For example, children who have difficulty with a particular sound (e.g. the sibilant "-s") appear to postpone productive use of grammatical inflections that contain that sound (e.g. the plural, Camarata and Gandour, 1985). A rather different lexical/phonological interaction is illustrated by many cases in which the 'same' speech sound is produced correctly in one word context but incorrectly in another (e.g. the child may say "guck" for "duck", but have no trouble pronouncing the "d" in "doll").

After 3 years of age, when lexical and grammatical development have 'settled down', phonology also becomes more stable and systematic: either the child produces no obvious errors at all, or s/he may persist in the same phonological error (e.g. a difficulty pronouncing "r" and "l") regardless of lexical context, for many more years. The remainder of lexical development from 3 years to adulthood can generally be summarized as an increase in fluency, including a phenomenon called 'coarticulation', in which those sounds that will be produced later on in an utterance are anticipated by moving the mouth into position on an earlier speech sound (hence the "b" in "bee" is qualitatively different from the "b" in "boat").

The basic facts of speech production and its development have not changed very much in the last 10–15 years. However, there have been some major changes in the theoretical frameworks used to describe and explain these events. This includes proposals couched in phonological theories like Autosegmental Phonology and Optimality Theory (Menn and Stoel-Gammon, 1995; Stemberger and Bernhardt, 1999), as well as proposals based on connectionist or 'neural network' models of acoustic and articulatory learning (Plaut, 1994). Because this is a relatively 'hard' physical domain, permitting a clear and unambiguous test of competing hypotheses, phonological/phonetic development is an area in which it may be possible to make serious progress regarding the interplay of maturation and learning during the first 3 years of life.

To summarize so far, the development of speech as a sound system begins at or perhaps before birth (in speech perception), and continues into the adult years (e.g. with an increase in fluency and coarticulation). However, there is one point in phonetic and phonological development that can be viewed as a kind of watershed: 8–10 months, marked by phonological drift, the onset of canonical babbling, the first signs that non-native speech sounds have been inhibited, and the first signs of word comprehension — which brings us to the next domain.

Object recognition and categorization

To understand the idea that things have names (i.e. *reference*), a human child must be able to recognize and categorize objects and events (Case, 1998; Haith and Benson, 1998; Mareschal and Quinn, 2001; Rogoff, 1998). There has been a real explosion in our knowledge of object recognition and categorization in infancy, using some of the same techniques described in the section on speech perception (high-amplitude sucking, habituation and dishabituation, operant generalization), together with techniques that are unique to the visual modality (i.e. preferential looking, eye movement monitoring — for detailed reviews, see Bertenthal and Clifton, 1998; Gibson and Spelke, 1983; Haith, 1990; Osofsky, 1987). It is now clear that infants under 6 months of age are much more competent than we previously believed, capable of surprisingly fine-grained discriminations of object boundaries and three-dimensional space. This includes at least some ability to perceive the cross-modal characteristics of objects and events. One example will suffice (Meltzoff and Borton, 1979): very young infants are placed before a two-choice visual array, with a nubbly-textured nonsense form on one side and a display with smooth contours on the other. If a nubbly-textured pacifier is placed in the infant's mouth, s/he tends to look longer at the nubbly display; if a smooth-textured pacifier is placed in the infant's mouth, more visual attention is directed to the display with smooth contours. It appears that pioneers like Piaget (1954, 1962) underestimated the extent of the infant's innate preparation for visual exploration of the physical and social world — innate skills that also help to prepare the child for those cognitive categories that lie at the core of every natural language.

However, it is also clear that the child's ability to form concepts and categories undergoes marked development from 0–9 months of age. These include changes between 2 and 5 months in the infant's ability to predict or anticipate changes in a moving display (Haith, 1990), changes between 3 and 9 months in the ability to synthesize a whole pattern out of local details (Bertenthal, Campos and Haith, 1980; Bertenthal, Proffitt, Spetner and Thomas, 1985; Spitz, Stiles and Siegel, 1989), and changes between 6 and 10 months in the ability to recognize objects as members of a category (Cohen and Younger, 1983; Reznick and Kagan, 1983). If we were asked to choose a point at which object categories are clearly established, with sufficient stability and flexibility to serve as the basis for acts of labelling or reference (e.g. "Where's the doggie?"), we would (again) choose 8–10 months of age as a watershed.

Imitation

The development of speech production presupposes a well-developed capacity to imitate, i.e. the ability to transform an auditory input into a motor output. Piaget's original stage model of sensorimotor development postulated six stages in the development of imitation: from no imitation at all (Stage 1, 0–2 months), through various levels of 'pseudo-imitation' (repetition of adult models that are already present in the child's own motor repertoire — Stages 2–4, 2–8 months), to the first signs of 'true imitation' (reproduction of novel motor patterns — Stage 5, 9–18 months), to a final stage of 'deferred imitation' (reproduction of novel motor patterns from memory — Stage 6, beginning somewhere between 12 and 18 months). Current evidence suggests that Piaget was wrong about at least two of these points. First, human neonates apparently can reproduce a small set of innate motor patterns in response to an adult model (e.g. sticking out the tongue, Meltzoff and Moore, 1979). Hence 'pseudo-imitation' is present at Stage 1. Second, deferred imitation has now been demonstrated in children as young as 9 months of age (Meltzoff, 1988). However, Piaget's observations about the transition from pseudo-imitation to true imitation appear to be correct. Furthermore, the ability to reproduce novel vocal and gestural patterns appears around the now-familiar 8–10-month turning point (e.g. the onset of gestures like "bye-bye" and "pattycake", and the onset of prosodic contours and consonant-vowel babbling sounds that start to approximate patterns present in the child's linguistic input).

Imitation is an aspect of early cognitive development in which human infants are real 'stars', outperforming any other primate by orders of magnitude. In fact, as Tomasello and Call (1997) note in their book on primate cognition, there is so little evidence for systematic imitation of novel models in other primates that expressions like "monkey see, monkey do" or the verb "to ape" are quite misleading. However, the bare beginnings of a capacity for imitation are visible in the primate line, and recent discoveries in primate neurophysiology have led to some tentative conclusions about the neural basis of imitation (Rizzolatti, Fadiga, Gallese and Fogassi, 1996). Rizzolatti and his colleagues have uncovered regions of monkey prefrontal cortex in which neurons tend to fire when the animal is planning a particular hand movement, or a movement of the arm in a particular direction. Interestingly, the same neurons also fire when the monkey observes a human being making the same movements! These 'mirror neurons' constitute a powerful demonstration of 'analysis by synthesis', in which the actions of another animal are analyzed by internally reproducing a version of the same act. Because human infants outperform all other primates in imitation of novel acts, it seems quite likely that this kind of process has undergone powerful selection in our species.

Joint reference and intentionality

Language acquisition is an active process. No child would ever crack the code that maps meaning onto sound without the will and the ability to try those mappings out for herself. First, the child needs a strong motivation to communicate with others, and to be like (sound like) other people. Without this motivation, it is unlikely that any child would ever spend the necessary hours attending, imitating, practicing and contemplating the linguistic input. Second, every human child must understand the means-end relationship between sound and meaning. Symbols constitute a form of tool use: we use them as instruments for social interchange, and, through the use of symbols, other human beings can be moved to act on our behalf. There are important changes in both these aspects of intentionality across the first 8 months of life, developments that prepare the child for entry into a linguistic system.

Social motivation, at least in some form, is innate in our species. However, there are also important changes in the nature and complexity of social intentions across the first year. The newborn infant is responsive to touch, and s/he can differentiate the human voice and face from other auditory and visual stimuli, showing an early preference for these species-specific patterns. Face-to-face interaction begins in the first hours of life, and increases in complexity across the next few weeks. Back and forth games of 'vocal tennis' are also common by three months. By five months of age, infants have learned to follow the parent's line of visual regard, resulting in a 'joint reference' to the same objects and events in the world (Butterworth, 1990; Butterworth and Jarrett, 1991). However, infants do not take an active role in the establishment of joint reference until 8–9 months of age, when they begin to show, give and eventually point to objects as a form of social exchange.

This 8–9-month transition toward the active use of objects in social exchange occurs in two directions: use of objects as a means of obtaining adult attention (e.g. giving, showing, pointing), and use of adults as a means of obtaining a desired object (e.g. reaching, eye contact, pointing and request sounds used interchangeably in a deliberate and persistent request sequence). Bates, Camaioni and Volterra (1975) have referred to these two forms of human tool use as 'proto-declaratives' and 'proto-imperatives'. Interestingly, these two forms of 'human tool use' coincide with a third, non-social form of tool use: the use of one object as a means of obtaining another (e.g. pulling on a cloth support to bring a desired toy within reach). All three forms of tool use (object-to-object, object-to-person, person-to-object) are highly correlated in a sample of 9-month-old children (Bates, Benigni, Bretherton et al., 1979); and all three forms are also correlated with the subsequent emergence of meaningful speech (see below).

Tomasello and Call have pointed out that joint reference is another arena in which human infants excel, outperforming other primates of any age. It is perhaps for this reason that human infants go on to achieve 'secondary reasoning', computing the intentions of other human beings and acting on them. Hence joint reference can be viewed as the basis of what has been called 'theory of mind', referring to our ability to reason about the contents of other people's minds (Baron-Cohen, Riviere, Fukushima et al., 1996; Charman and Baron-Cohen, 1995; Leslie, 1994). This kind of ability is crucial for the computations that are involved in telling a good story, or getting one's point across by taking the other person's point of view into account (e.g. the difference between "He hit me" vs. "That boy I told you about yesterday hit me again!"). Hence joint reference (established in the first year) and secondary reasoning (established a year or so later) can be viewed as critical phylogenetic and ontogenetic inputs into our ability to acquire and use a grammar (Tomasello, 1998; Tomasello and Call, 1997).

Memory

Finally, to achieve mastery of a system that maps meaning onto sound, human children must have the ability to store, recognize, and recall signals in the appropriate context. This will necessarily involve advances in memory, including recognition memory for speech comprehension, recall for speech production, and the working or planning memory required to stage a novel utterance. This is yet another area where infancy researchers have made a great deal of progress (Haith and Benson, 1998; Harris, 1983; Mandler, 1998; Schneider and Bjorklund, 1998). For example, we now know that 2-month-old infants can learn to recognize a sequence of simple events (e.g. moving lights) well enough to anticipate the next move (Haith, Benson, Roberts and Pennington, 1994). There are also marked shifts in the ability to remember and/or retrieve a hidden object after a short delay between 7 and 10 months of age (Baillargeon and Graber, 1988; Piaget, 1954), as well as the length of time the location of the object can be held in memory (Diamond, 1985). Therefore there is considerable evidence for some forms of visual recognition memory very early in life (see Rovee-Collier, 1984; Rovee-Collier, Lipsitt and Hayne, 1998). Some form of recall memory has also been shown in infants as young as 9 months. For example, 9-month-old infants are capable of reproducing a novel action after a 24-hour (Meltzoff, 1988) and a 1-month delay (Bauer and Hertsgaard, 1993; Bauer and Wewerka, 1995), suggesting that at least one form of recall is also available within the same 8–10-month window (see *Imitation* above).

Putting this evidence together, we may conclude that 9-month-old infants have some aspects of memory that are necessary to hold in mind a sound or word while retrieving from memory an object category (word comprehension). They may also have the ability to retrieve and produce a sound from memory in the presence of an associated class of objects or events (word production).

In all of the cognitive and communicative domains that we have just reviewed, important changes take place between 8 and 10 months of age, providing the child with the basic skills required to initiate language learning. Language acquisition cannot get underway until some threshold level is reached in all these domains, and maturational changes in any of these domains may influence the nature and timing of language acquisition beyond the first stage. In addition, we propose that limitations in one or more of these areas may be responsible for the array of developmental language pathologies described in this volume (see chapters by Nass, 2002; Rapin, Allen and Dunn, 2003; Van Hout, 2003). In the next three sections, we will use this framework to analyze basic milestones in language development, from babbling to the acquisition of complex discourse skills.

Milestones of language development

We have reviewed the early stages of normal language development in a number of different places, to make a number of different points: on the role of language within the broader framework of infant development (Bates, O'Connell and Shore, 1987), on individual differences in style and rate of development across the normal range (Bates et al., 1988), on continuity of individual differences from infancy to the childhood years (Bates, Dale and Thal, 1995; Thal and Bates, 1989), on the cognitive correlates of language learning (Bates and Snyder, 1987), on relations between linguistic and gestural development (Bates, Thal, Whitesell et al., 1989; Iverson and Thal, 1997; Shore, Bates, Bretherton et al., 1990; Thal and Bates, 1990; Thal and Tobias, 1992, 1994; Thal, Tobias and Morrison, 1991), on relations between language development and language evolution (Bates et al., 1979, 1991), on similarities and dissimilarities between adult aphasia and the dissociations observed in normal and abnormal language development (Bates and Thal, 1991; Reilly, Bates and Marchman, 1998), and on norms of language development from a practitioner's point of view (Thal and Bates, 1989; Thal and Katich, 1996; Thal et al., 1991b). Readers are referred to those sources for details. Here we will restrict ourselves to a brief review of major events in language, in enough detail to support claims about (a) how things come together (basic milestones and their cognitive correlates), and (b) how things come apart (variations and disociations under normal and abnormal conditions), providing enough information to consider how milestones and variations in language acquisition map onto major events in human brain development.

Word comprehension

The first systematic evidence for word comprehension is generally found between 8 and 10 months, usually in response to specific, contextually supported sounds (e.g. responding appropriately to "no no", to his/her own name, or to a few routines such as patty-cake or waving bye-bye). However, many children display a rapid spurt in comprehension after this point. Indeed, most parents can no longer keep track of their child's receptive vocabulary beyond 16 months of age, because it has become too large. For example, in a recent study of approximately 1800 children in San Diego, Seattle, and New Haven (Fenson, Dale, Reznick et al., 1994), parents estimated that their children comprehended an average of 67 words at 10 months, 86 words at 12 months, 156 words at 14 months, and 191 words at 16 months.

Word production

True word production typically begins between 11 and 13 months. As with comprehension, it usually starts with a few contextually supported vocal routines such as producing animal sounds in a ritualized game, or consistently using a specific sound when requesting an object or activity. Those ritualized 'words' turn into what looks like true naming of objects by 12–13 months in most children, but the words remain limited in scope, and they are unstable (coming and going from the child's repertoire) until the child has established a repertoire of about 10 consistently produced words. From that point, stable new words are added gradually until the child has a production vocabulary of approximately 50–75 words (Goldfield and Reznick, 1990). In the first part of the 'one-word stage', single words are used primarily to label and/or to ask for objects and people. That is, except for a few idiosyncratic non-nominal terms like "bye-bye" and "up", they are used to communicate referential rather than predicative information.

For many children the 50–75-word point is pivotal in development, as it coincides with what has been called the 'vocabulary burst', i.e. a rapid acceleration in the rate at which new words are learned. In our recent tri-city norming study (Fenson et al., 1994), parents reported that their children produced an average of 10 words at 12 months, and 64 words at 16 months. By 24 months, the average production vocabulary has reached 312 words, and by 30 months it is 534 words. In many individual cases it is even larger (see *Variations*, below). This vocabulary burst is accompanied by changes in vocabulary composition; specifically, there is a *proportional* increase in verbs, adjectives and other words that serve as predicates (i.e. relational terms) in the adult language. For example, verbs typically comprise less than 2% of the first 50 words produced by English-speaking children; by the time cumulative vocabulary reaches 100 words, verb ratios have risen to 10–12%. It is tempting to conclude that there has been a qualitative shift in the way that words are acquired and used, a shift from reference (single-word meaning) to predication (relational meaning). This shift may be implicated in the next major milestone, the onset of word combinations.

Word combinations

Word combinations typically emerge between 18 and 20 months. However, the correlation between word combinations and vocabulary size tends to be considerably stronger than the correlation between word combinations and age. In fact, most children begin to combine words when their cumulative vocabulary falls between 50 and 100 words (Bates et al., 1988; Fenson, Dale, Reznick et al., 1993; Fenson et al., 1994). Interestingly, this is also the point at which children begin to produce verbs, adjectives and other predicate terms, suggesting that the move into 'sentencehood' does depend (at least in part) on the emergence of predicative or relational meanings.

The form and content of first word combinations have been studied in detail in many languages (e.g. Braine, 1976). Although there is considerable variability from one language to another in the forms that children use to communicate relational meanings (see **Prerequisites to language**), these studies show that the same basic stock of relational meanings are encoded by 20-month-olds all around the world. Those meanings revolve around existence (e.g. appearance, disappearance and reappearance of interesting objects or events), desires (refusal, denial, requests), basic event relations (agent–action–object, possession, change of state or change of location), and attribution ('hot', 'pretty', etc.).

Grammatical development

A rapid 'burst' of grammatical development typically occurs between 20 and 36 months of age, a kind of high-level repetition of the vocabulary burst that occurred earlier in the second year. At this point we see rapid growth in the language-specific means available to encode the stock of meanings which have previously been encoded with single words. At the same time, children also produce language-specific contrasts whose meanings may be quite opaque. For example, take the issue of gender marking in German: what child *or* adult can make sense of the fact that the word for 'bottle' in German is feminine, but the word for 'little girl' is neuter? And yet before age 3–4, normal children manage to acquire most of their grammar, including many apparently arbitrary and abstract contrasts (e.g. grammatical gender), together with some fairly complex syntactic devices (e.g. passives, relatives). This is why most 3-year-olds sound like competent speakers of their native language, despite serious limits in vocabulary and continuing limits in speech fluency.

Changes after 3 years of age

Although the basic structures of grammar are laid down before 4 years of age in most languages (see *Cross-linguistic variation*, **Prerequisites to language** below), there are still some significant changes in the nature of language use after this point (besides, of course, changes in the content of vocabulary that continue across the life span).

First, there are changes in the extent to which children use language for *discourse cohesion* purposes. Indeed, Karmiloff-Smith (1979) has suggested that there is a complete reorganization of language between 4 and 6 years of age, from 'intrasentential grammar' (grammar that is used to express simple single-sentence meanings) to 'intersentential grammar' (use of the same basic grammatical contrasts to express the relationship between sentences). Returning to the terminology we introduced earlier, this means that children are learning to use grammar for discourse and/or text cohesion purposes. For example, the child learns that use of a pronoun 'he' requires prior establishment of the referent (i.e. the entity to which 'he' refers) in the information shared by speaker and listener. It should be obvious why this is not a purely linguistic skill: it requires considerable knowledge of the listener, a 'theory of mind' that takes many years to construct. It is also likely that this move from sentence-level grammar to discourse-level grammar is encouraged by entry into the school system, where children receive much more experience with connected discourse, in oral and written forms.

Second, there are changes in the *accessibility* of forms that have been there for a considerable period of time. This point is perhaps best illustrated by a recent study in our laboratories examining changes in the probability and nature of grammatical passives in children between 3 and 18 years of age (Marchman, Bates, Burkhardt and Good, 1991). We set up a situation that could be viewed as the 'ecological niche' for passive forms: presented with a series of short cartoons in which one animal acts on another (e.g. a horse bites a goat), children were asked to describe the scene from the point of view of the receiver-of-the-action (e.g. "Tell me about the goat" or "What happened to the goat?"). In this situation, adults produce a passive form more than 80% of the time (e.g. "The goat was bitten by the horse"). In the same situation, most children are capable of producing at least one passive by 3 years of age. However, it is also clear that small children prefer not to produce the passive at all, using a range of alternative forms that avoid the difficult passive form but accomplish the 'discourse goal' of focusing on the object (e.g. "The goat was sitting there and then the horse bit him"). In other words, even though almost all the children in the study possess knowledge of how to produce at least one passive (the top line in Fig. 1), there is consistent growth in the accessibility of passives in real-time language use (the bottom line in Fig. 1). There are also gradual changes in the nature of the passive forms that children prefer to produce (e.g. a gradual shift from 'get' passives, as in "The goat got bitten" to 'be' passives, as in "The goat was bitten", even though both forms co-exist within individual children for many years). For obvious reasons, it would be inappropriate to choose any single point in development from 3–18 years as 'the moment' at which adult-like use of the passive is acquired. Many of the other late-onset language functions that we have investigated in our laboratories show a similar linear shift from age 3–4 to adolescence. For these reasons, we are persuaded that grammatical performance changes gradually over time from 3 years to adulthood. There is very little evidence for sudden or discontinuous change in linguistic abilities after 4 years of age. We will return to this point later, when we discuss aspects of brain development that parallel major milestones in the development of language.

Are these milestones specific to language? Probably not, at least not the early ones. At each of the early stages noted above, researchers have found correlates in non-linguistic cognition. These include intentional communication and means-end understanding between 9 and 11 months (Bates et al., 1979), production of single words and 'recognitory gestures' or 'enactive names' around 12–13 months (Bates et al., 1979; Escalona, 1973; Werner and Kaplan, 1963), and a correlation between word combinations and gesture combinations around 20 months of age (Brownell, 1988; Fenson and Ramsay, 1981; McCune-Nicolich, 1981; McCune-Nicolich and Bruskin, 1982; O'Connell and Gerard, 1985; Shore, 1986; Shore, O'Connell and Bates, 1984) (see Table 2). There is also evidence for a link between later grammatical development (around 28 months of age) and the ability to reproduce arbitrary sequences of 5 gestures (Bauer, Hertsgaard, Dropik and Daly, 1998). Interestingly, this grammar/gesture link is not observed if only 3 gestures are used, or if the sequence that binds these gestures is causal

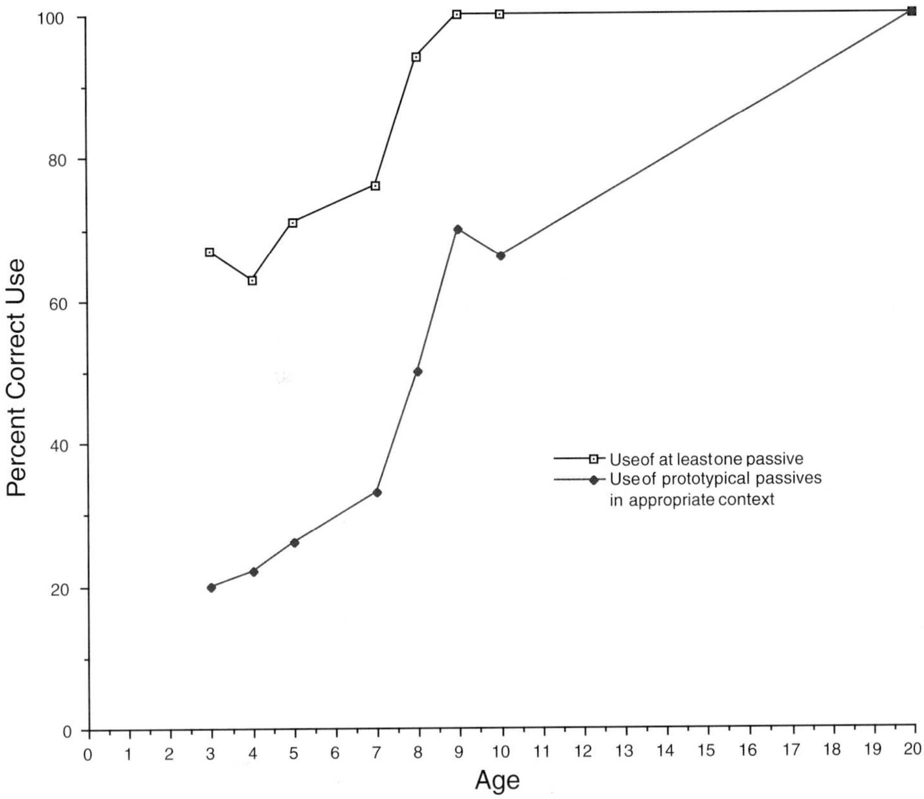

Fig. 1. Knowledge versus accessibility of passive forms.

and meaningful. Hence the later link seems to have something to do with memory demands that language shares with non-linguistic systems. All of these language/cognition correlations are interesting, because they suggest that language development is paced by mechanisms outside of language proper. However, our interpretation of these results must be tempered by the variations documented below.

Variations and dissociations in language development

Variations

We can divide our discussion of variations in normal language development into three parts: cross-linguistic variations, variations in rate of development within a single language (in this case, English), and a new and puzzling literature on variations in 'style' of language learning.

Cross-linguistic variations

There are marked variations from one language to another in the nature and timing of all language milestones. For example, contrary to an influential 'universalist' theory of phonological development proposed years ago by Roman Jakobson (1968), recent cross-linguistic studies of phonological development by Ferguson, Vihman and their colleagues (Vihman, 1985; Vihman et al., 1986; Vihman and Greenlee, 1987) have shown that the content and nature of babbling varies a great deal from language to language. Although there are some consistent tendencies (e.g. fricatives tend to develop late in every language), there is little evidence for the kind of lawful unfolding of phonological contrasts that Jakobson envisioned. Jakobson also suggested that there is a 'silent period' between babble and speech, and discontinuity in the forms that children use in babble and speech. Current evidence suggests instead that there is a great deal of continuity in the forms that children use in their prespeech babble and their first words. Because these 'favorite sounds' vary from one language to another, this suggests that cross-language differences in the content of phonology begin by 8–10 months of age! Furthermore, rare forms like clicks in Bantu, vowel harmony in Turkish or Hungarian, or tones in Chinese come in surprisingly early. Hence cross-linguistic differences in 'markedness' (a continuum from common to rare forms) fail to predict the order in which children acquire the speech contrasts in their language.

With regard to cross-language variation at the one-word stage, it is fair to say that acquisition starts with something like a one-word stage in every language. But there are variations in the form of this 'one-at-a-time' phase of development. For example, 1-year-old infants may start out by producing little pieces of a complex word in languages like Greenlandic Eskimo (where many whole sentences consist of a single word plus many inflections). And in languages with a very rich and salient morphological system (e.g. Turkish), children sometimes begin to produce verb or noun inflections late in the one-word stage, i.e. before they have produced any word combinations (Slobin, 1985–1997).

These variations are now uncontroversial, but there are others that have been hotly debated in the last few years. For example, Gentner (1982) wrote a very influential paper arguing that nouns must always precede verbs in early development, in every language in the world, for several reasons: because verbs convey more complex and evanescent concepts (compared with the solid and bounded simplicity of the objects conveyed by common nouns), and because verbs tend to carve up reality in much more variable ways from language to language. In contrast, Choi and Gopnik (1995) and Tardif (1996) presented evidence from Korean and Chinese, respectively, suggesting that nouns do not always appear before verbs. They argued that verbs are acquired earlier in these languages because they are more salient (e.g. Korean is an SOV language where verbs appear at the end, in an easily remembered position, and Korean and Chinese are both languages that permit extensive omission of nouns, so that a sentence is often composed of a single naked verb!). Indeed, Gopnik and Choi even went so far as to suggest that these language differences feed back on non-linguistic cognition, and as a result, Korean children perform better on means-end tasks (which are more verb related) while English children perform better on object permanence tasks (which are more noun related). This was an exciting idea, and it set off a lively round of research. However, in the end the issue has come down to one of methodology. When researchers use diary or parental report methods that provide a comprehensive estimate of all the words in the child's vocabulary, then the familiar pattern of 'nouns before verbs' seems to be the rule in every language, including Korean (Pae, 1993; for a review, see Caselli et al., 1995). Furthermore, when 1-year-old Korean and American children were exposed to novel nonsense nouns and verbs in the same experimental task, nouns were learned more easily than verbs in both groups (Au, Dapretto and Song, 1994). Hence when we use methods that tap into what the child knows, the noun–verb sequence seems to be a cross-linguistic universal. However, when we look at free speech records that tell us what forms children prefer to use (statistically speaking), cross-linguistic differences in the proportional use of nouns and verbs may be observed.

The idea that language-specific variations can change the way we think (including non-verbal cognition) is an old one in linguistics, proposed in its strongest form by the 20th-century linguist Benjamin Whorf. According to the 'Whorf hypothesis', languages cut up reality in a variety of ways, and native speakers of those languages will tend to view reality in ways that are predictable from their language. So, for example, in languages that have noun classifiers marking the shape of objects, children are (or so it was proposed) more sensitive to variations in shape at a very young age. Evidence in favor of this interesting hypothesis has been largely disappointing. However, there has been a recent surge of interest in a modified version of the Whorf hypothesis, in which language does not change basic perceptual and cognitive processes, but it can draw our attention to aspects of reality that we might not have noticed without it. As a case in point, Choi and Bowerman (1991) have built on another difference between English and Korean: both languages have prepositions to contrast 'in' and 'out', but Korean also makes a contrast between 'in-close-fitting' and 'in-loose-fit'.

Young Korean children seem to pick this up quite easily. Furthermore, McDonough, Choi, Bowerman and Mandler find that English- and Korean-speaking children begin to be responsive to terms for containment and support by about 18 months, and respond appropriately to the distinctions their own language makes (McDonough, Choi, Bowerman and Mandler, 2002). If more evidence of this kind can be found, it will provide strong support for a strongly interactive theory of the development of language and cognition in the first years of life.

The most compelling evidence for cross-language variation begins after 20 months of age, when grammatical development is well underway. Here we see so much variation as a function of linguistic input that it is difficult to maintain the belief in one 'universal stage' of grammatical learning (Bates and Marchman, 1988). For example, the whole system of case morphology appears to be completely mastered in Turkish by 2 years of age; this early mastery reflects the fact that Turkish morphology is exceptionally regular (i.e. very few exceptions) and phonologically salient (with clear stress-bearing inflections occurring at the end of every noun). By contrast, Russian and Serbo-Croatian children take much longer to learn their 'messy' case system (i.e. systems which involve a large number of irregular forms and several arbitrary contrasts, including gender). There are also large variations from one language to another in the acquisition of word order: from very early display of word order regularities in a 'rigid' language like English, to a near-absence of word order regularity in a flexible language like Turkish. Finally, many so-called complex forms appear quite early in a few languages, if they are very frequent and used for common pragmatic purposes (e.g. relative clauses in Italian, which are five times as common in Italian 3-year-olds than they are in their English counterparts, Bates and Devescovi, 1989; passives in Sesotho, used very frequently by adults and acquired before 3 years of age by Sesotho children, Demuth, 1989).

There is a sense in which this had to be true. For example, adult native speakers of Italian have to produce approximately three times more morphological contrasts than English speakers to convey the same idea. Consider, for example, the sentence "Wolves eat sheep", which contains three words (wolf, eat, sheep) and four morphemes (where wolves = wolf + plural marker). In Italian, the corresponding sentence would be "I lupi mangiano le pecore", in which articles are obligatory, both the article and the noun are marked for number and gender, and the verb is obligatorily marked for third person plural. For all these reasons, the Italian sentence contains five words, and fourteen morphological contrasts! This leads to two logical possibilities for cross-linguistic differences in grammatical development: (1) Italian children will take three times as long to acquire their language, or (2) Italian and English children acquire their language at the same rate, but at any given point in development, Italians will produce roughly three times as much morphology as their English counterparts. Evidence to date suggests that the latter hypothesis is correct.

Individual differences within English: variations in rate

Even if we restrict ourselves to the acquisition of English, we find marked variations in rate of development among normal children throughout the first stages of language learning, as follows.

Babbling

Individual children vary markedly in the content (i.e. preferred sounds) and onset of prespeech babble (Cruttenden, 1970; Ferguson, 1984; Kent and Miolo, 1995; Locke, 1983, 1988; Vihman et al., 1986; Vihman and Greenlee, 1987). Normal children typically begin to produce canonical babble somewhere between 6 and 10 months — a substantial range of variation, considering how many changes occur in the first year of life. There is also variation in the course of phonological development after this point. Some children stick with a very small set of phonetic contrasts for a number of weeks or months while others attempt a much larger array from the very beginning.

Word comprehension

Although systematic evidence of word comprehension is usually available by 8–10 months, there is enormous variability after this point in the rate at which receptive vocabulary grows (Bates et al., 1988; Benedict, 1979; Reznick, 1990). For example, in the tri-city norming study for the MacArthur Communicative Development Inventories (Fenson et al., 1994), parents reported a mean comprehension vocabulary of 67 words at 10 months of age; but the standard deviation was very large (60.19), with a range from 2–280 words. At 12, 14 and 16 months, scores varied similarly: a mean of 86 at 12 months (SD 49.23, range 7–242), a mean of 156 at 14 months (SD 77.95, range 11–343), and a mean of 191 at 16 months (SD 87.58, range 40–396). Of course one can always question whether the outer extremes are valid in a study based on parental report (especially for comprehension, which may be more difficult for some parents to assess, Tomasello and Mervis, 1994), but there are good reasons to believe (based on laboratory validations of the CDI — Bates and Goodman, 1997; Jahn-Samilo, Goodman, Bates et al., 2000; Reznick, 1990; Ring, 1999; Thal, O'Hanlon, Clemmons and Frailin, 1999) that the means and standard deviations are a faithful reflection of reality.

Word production

There is also large variation in the age of onset and course of development of expressive vocabulary. In our tri-city study, parents reported vocabulary onset in individual children from as early as 8 months. As with comprehension, production vocabularies across individual children varied widely. Some examples follow: at 12 months mean production vocabulary was reported as 10 (SD 11.20, range 0–52), at 16 months mean production was 64 words (SD 70.27, range 0–347), at 24 months the mean number of words produced was 312 (SD 173.67, range 7–668) and at 30 months the mean was 534 (SD 116.65, range 208–675). The impressive array of variation that can be observed from 8–30 months is illustrated in Fig. 2 (redrawn from Fenson et al., 1993, using percentiles rather than standard deviations).

We reported above that many children show a vocabulary burst at the point where cumulative vocabulary falls between 50 and 75 words. However, in a longitudinal study of language development in the second year, Goldfield and Reznick (1990) were the first to report that there are also individual differences in the shape of vocabulary change over time. Some children did show the typical 'burst', but others showed a more even rate of change at every point. Yet another group appeared to develop in a series of small bursts, each followed by a small plateau. In a recent longitudinal study by Goodman and colleagues (Goodman, Bates, Jahn et al., 1999; Goodman and Bauman, 1995), 28 children were followed monthly from 8–30 months of age; parents filled out the CDI monthly, and children came into the laboratory to participate in language assessments monthly from 12–30 months. There were strong positive correlations between laboratory and CDI assessments of language growth, not only in vocabulary size but also in the shape of the growth curves that individual children display across this period of development. We may conclude with confidence that the variation in rate of vocabulary growth illustrated in Fig. 2 is real, and can be observed in both cross-sectional and longitudinal designs, in both parent report and laboratory observations. The fact that this much variation is observed within the normal range provides an important lesson for clinicians: risk for language disorders must be evaluated against the full range of variation that we can expect to see in perfectly healthy, normal children.

Word combinations

Although 20 months is reported as the mean age for production of novel word combinations, the range of normal variation around this milestone is wide. Novel combinations have been reported as early as 14 months of age (Bates et al., 1988). At the same time, many normal children do not produce combinations of any kind before 24 months. There is also a certain amount of variation in the relationship between word combinations and vocabulary size: approximately 20% of the sample in our tri-city norming study were reported to produce at least a few word combinations with vocabularies under 50 words; and another 15% with vocabularies between 100 and 300 words were still not producing any word combinations at all. Hence, although the relationship between lexical development and word combinations is very strong (see 'dissociations' below), the appearance of first word combinations is not locked to a single vocabulary size.

Early grammar

A widely used index of early grammatical development in English is Mean Length of Utterance in

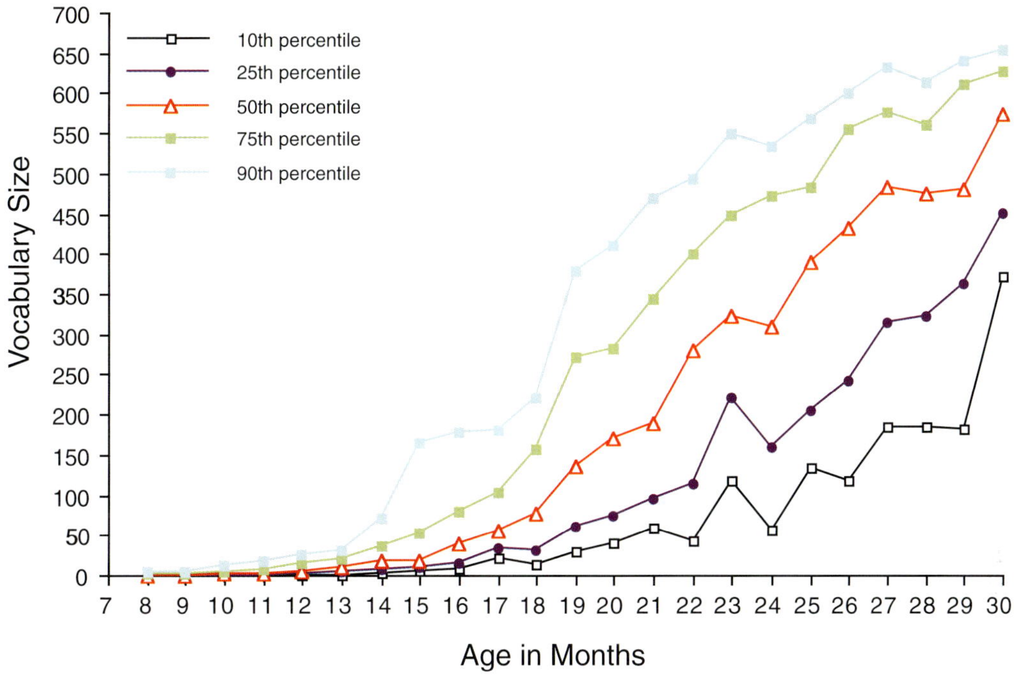

Fig. 2. Variation in the development of expressive vocabulary from 8–30 months.

morphemes (MLU). This is a count that includes content words, function words, and inflections like the plural '-s' or the past tense '-ed'. Brown (1973) used MLU to break development down into epochs: MLU ranges from 1.05–1.50 in Early Stage I (single words to first combinations), from 1.5–2.0 in Late Stage I (first inflections), from 2.0–2.5 in Stage II (productive control over grammar begins), 2.5–3.0 in Stage III (grammatical development well underway), from 3.0–3.5 in Stage IV (complex sentences begin), and so on. Chapman (1981) has provided norms for middle-class children using Brown's stages, and they are expressed as ranges: 19.1–23 months is the average for Early Stage I, 23.8–26.9 months for Late Stage I, 27.7–30.8 months for Stage II, 31.6–34.8 months for Stage III, and 35.6–38.7 months for Stage IV. However, in videotaped laboratory sessions, Bates et al. (1988) found cases across the full range from Stages I to IV in a sample of 27 healthy middle-class children at 28 months of age.

In the tri-city norming study for the MacArthur Communicative Development Inventories, parents were asked to provide three written examples of the longest sentences they had heard their child say recently (Fenson et al., 1994). A mean was computed from these three utterances, providing a measure that we have called maximum sentence length (MSL). Although this is an upper limit measure (rather than a mean length) and it is calculated from three examples (rather than the typical 50–100) used for MLU calculations (Miller, 1981), MSL correlated highly and significantly ($r = 0.77$ and 0.74, $p < 0.01$, for 20- and 24-month-old children, respectively) with MLU (Fenson et al.). Like MLU, we also found wide variation across individual children. Examples at selected ages follow: at 16 months mean MSL was 1.48 (SD 0.88, range 1–4.7), at 20 months mean MSL was 2.78 (SD 1.59, range 1–77), at 24 months mean MSL was 4.69 (SD 2.66, range 1–12.3), and at 30 months mean MSL was 8.18 (SD 3.45, range 3–19). It is fair to conclude, then, that the variation in grammatical development is substantial.

Individual differences within English: variations in style

In addition to these well-documented variations in rate, there is also a sizeable literature on variations in 'style' of language learning (Bates et al., 1988; Bloom, Lightbown and Hood, 1975; Dore, 1974; Horgan, 1979, 1981; Nelson, 1973; Peters, 1977, 1983) that has shown an interesting dissociation within language. Briefly summarized, children may be described as using 'analytic' versus 'holistic' learning styles. So-called 'analytic children' enter into language development by breaking the input down into small units, and struggling to understand those units before attempting a synthesis. This pattern shows up at every level of development: from babbling (where short and consistent consonant–vowel segments predominate), to first words (where the child concentrates on object naming), to first word combinations (telegraphic speech with function words and inflections eliminated). In contrast, so-called 'holistic children' seem to enter into language development from the opposite extreme: they start by using relatively large, global chunks of speech in familiar contexts, giving their speech a more adult-like sound while they gradually break speech units down into their component parts. This style can also be found at every level of language development: from babbling (where sporadic consonants are nested within long streams of sentence-like intonation), to first words (with heterogeneous vocabularies that often include formulaic expressions like 'wannit'), to first word combinations (where inflections, pronouns, and other function words may be present from the beginning, in frozen expressions and/or in formulae with limited productivity).

Because these variations cut across age levels and content domains (from babbling through grammar), most investigators agree that individual differences in 'linguistic style' reflect the differential operation of two fairly general learning mechanisms: an analytic mechanism that serves to break linguistic input down into smaller segments, and a holistic mechanism that makes it possible for the child to remember and reproduce relatively large segments of speech before those segments have been fully analyzed or understood (Bates et al., 1988; Nelson, 1973; Peters, 1977; Thal, Bates, Zappia and Oroz, 1996). Both mechanisms are necessary for normal language learning to take place, but children may differ in the degree to which they rely on one or the other. The causes of such a differential preference are still unknown, and there is considerable controversy concerning the relative contribution of environmental factors (e.g. maternal style), child temperament (e.g. reflective vs. impulsive approaches to solving a problem), and/or individual differences in the rate at which the different neural mechanisms responsible for language start to mature (see below). In fact, these explanations are not mutually exclusive: any and all of them may serve to encourage differential reliance on analytic/segmenting vs. holistic/suprasegmental mechanisms in language learning. Later we will look at recent evidence from children with focal brain injuries, suggesting that the differential contribution of left- vs. right-hemisphere processes may play some role in the determination of stylistic variation.

Having described milestones and variations in the way that language 'comes together' in normally developing children, we can now turn to the ways that language can 'come apart'. We will start by looking at dissociations within the normal range, and then present a summary of variations and dissociations in children with congenital injury to the left or right side of the brain. Taken together, these associations and dissociations provide clues to the component parts (linguistic or non-linguistic) that constitute our faculty for language learning, with implications for how and where these various aspects of language are acquired and mediated in the brain.

Dissociations within the normal range

Comprehension and production

One of the most striking disparities in the second year is that found between comprehension and production. In the lexical domain, comprehension almost always exceeds production; furthermore, comprehension appears to mark an *upper limit* on the number of words a child can produce. For example, children with receptive vocabularies under 50 words rarely produce more than 10 words, those with receptive vocabularies under 100 words usually have production vocabularies in the 0- to 50-word range. Very large expressive vocabularies are rarely seen in children with reported comprehension vocabularies under 150 words. However, comprehension clearly does not set a *lower limit* on word production: at every point across the comprehension range from 0–200 words, we have found at least a few children who produce little or no meaningful speech.

As described by Thal and her colleagues (Thal and Bates, 1989; Thal, Marchman and Stiles et al., 1991), these dissociations are particularly marked in a population of 'late talkers', i.e. children between 18 and 24 months of age who are in the bottom tenth percentile for expressive vocabulary. Some of these children are equally delayed in comprehension and production, but others appear to be normal for their age in receptive language despite their expressive delays (as established by laboratory testing as well as parental report). In a follow-up study of the same children (Thal et al., 1991b), spared comprehension discriminated between those children who ultimately caught up with their peers in expressive language (i.e. so-called 'late bloomers'), while the children with both receptive and expressive delays between 18 and 24 months fell even farther behind their age mates, qualifying for a clinical diagnosis of specific language impairment. Similar results were found for children classified at a younger age. Specifically, Thal (1999) used the MacArthur Communicative Development inventory (CDI) to identify children with delays in production but normal comprehension, and those with delays in both comprehension and production, at 16 months of age. At 28 months, vocabulary production and grammatical complexity scores on the CDI were well within the normal range for the late producers who had normal comprehension at 16 months. Scores for the children with delays in both comprehension and production, on the other hand, were in or close to the delayed range on both measures of expressive language. These results could lead one to conclude that a dissociation between comprehension and production is associated with positive outcomes. However, such a conclusion requires qualification. In a study focused on the effects of intervention on language learning in language-delayed toddlers, Olswang and Bain (1996) examined children who were delayed in both comprehension and production who had varying degrees of difference between comprehension and production. In that study, the children with greater comprehension/production gaps were least likely to make the transition from single- to multiword speech during the period of intervention. Thus, a dissociation between comprehension and production, with production lower than comprehension, is associated with a positive outcome when comprehension is in the normal range, and with a more negative outcome when comprehension is delayed.

Comprehension/production disparities are also observed at the other end of the developmental spectrum, i.e. in children who are 'early talkers' (in the top tenth percentile for expressive vocabulary between 12 and 21 months of age). Many of these children are equally advanced in comprehension and production, but we also find children who meet our 'early talker' criterion despite receptive vocabularies in the normal range (i.e. within one standard deviation of the mean). At first glance, this seems like a startling finding: how can a child move into the front ranks in word production without achieving comparable status in word comprehension? The reason is that most individuals (children and adults) typically produce only a small proportion of their receptive vocabulary (think of the words that you produce in everyday conversation, compared with all the words that you recognize when filling out a crossword puzzle). The early talkers who display a Production > Comprehension profile apparently do so by producing an abnormally large *proportion* of their receptive vocabularies; in essence, they are trying to tell us everything they know! These cases prove that comprehension and production can be dissociated in either direction, a double dissociation which most neuropsychologists would accept as evidence for the existence of two distinct mental/neural mechanisms (e.g. Shallice, 1988).

Analytic/holistic style

The comprehension/production dissociation is also related (albeit indirectly) to the analytic/holistic style distinction described earlier. Within the second year of life, children at the analytic extreme tend to be high comprehenders, and more precocious overall; children at the holistic end tend to be less advanced in comprehension, and slower to develop overall. However, our recent work with early talkers suggests that this association is not necessary. This can be seen best in a case study of two children who were extraordinarily precocious in early expressive language. SW was 21 months old and had an expressive vocabulary of 627 words; MW was 17 months old and had an expressive vocabulary of 596 words. Both children also produced a wide array of verbs and adjectives as well as nouns, a development that typically signals the onset of grammar. And both had begun to master the rudiments of English grammatical morphology, producing contrasting endings on at least a few nouns and verbs (e.g. 'walk' vs 'walking'). The one clear difference between these two exceptional children revolves around sentence length: MW had a Mean Length of Utterance (MLU) in morphemes of 2.39, equivalent to a 30-month-old child; SW had just begun to combine words, with an MLU of 1.19, within the range of what we would expect for a child of her age. Because these children are not measurably different in their mastery of noun and verb endings, we would not want to conclude that they demonstrate a dissociation between vocabulary and grammar. Nor would we want to conclude that MW is advanced in syntax, since her long sentences contain very little evidence for transformation, extraction, inversion, or any of the operations that define and characterize the syntactic component of grammar. We suggest, instead, that SW and MW vary markedly in the size of the unit that they are able to store and produce at any given time. This interpretation is supported by the fact that MW had a repertoire of idioms like "No way, José!" and "You little monkey!". Her ability to manipulate, and even blend, these large units is illustrated by the expression "No way, you monkey!", which she produced for the first time in our lab. In other words, we suggest that SW and MW represent an analytic-holistic dissociation in two children who are both quite advanced, but without differences in levels of comprehension and/or expressive vocabulary.

Grammar vs. vocabulary

Inspired by claims in the adult neurolinguistic literature, we have also looked carefully for a third type of dissociation, between grammar and semantics (with special reference to vocabulary development). To our surprise, the relationship between grammar and vocabulary development has turned out to be one of the strongest associations that has ever been observed in any aspect of human development (with the possible exception of height and weight!). Fig. 3 (from Bates and Goodman, 1997) illustrates the powerful non-linear developmental function that governs the relationship between grammatical complexity and vocabulary size. These data are taken from the MacArthur parent report forms, but several studies in our laboratory have shown the same strong relationship in laboratory measures as well. Notice that the relationship holds at every point from 50–600 words (covering the period from 16–30 months of age). One certainly might have expected a relationship at the lower end of the distribution, simply because one cannot combine words until there is something to combine. We might also have expected some kind of 'trigger' or 'threshold' relationship between vocabulary and grammar, e.g. a critical number of words that need to be acquired for grammar to get off the ground. What we find instead is a continuous and accelerating function that holds at every point across this period of development. To be sure, there is some variation around this curve, but we do not find extreme dissociations of the sort that clearly are observed for comprehension and production (e.g. children who understand more than 200 words but produce virtually nothing). This powerful relationship holds for very late talkers, and very early talkers as well.

In short, we have found very little evidence to support the idea that grammar and lexical semantics can 'come apart' in the early years of language learning (Bates et al., 1988). There is some evidence for a *temporary* dissociation between vocabulary size and the onset of word combinations in a small number of children (e.g. the cases of SW and MW, described above), but as we have just noted, these observations may be a by-product of analytic vs. holistic style (i.e. the ability to extract, store and reproduce relatively short units, vs. the ability to record and reproduce long but underanalyzed phrases). For the moment, we conclude that the comprehension/production and analytic/holistic dissociations observed in our work to date represent the most robust and natural 'fault lines' in the human language processor. By contrast, dissociations between grammar and vocabulary are not observed in healthy, normal children, suggesting that these two aspects of language are governed and acquired by the same mental/neural mechanisms. This brings us to our final consideration in this section: variations and dissociations among linguistic milestones children with congenital brain injury.

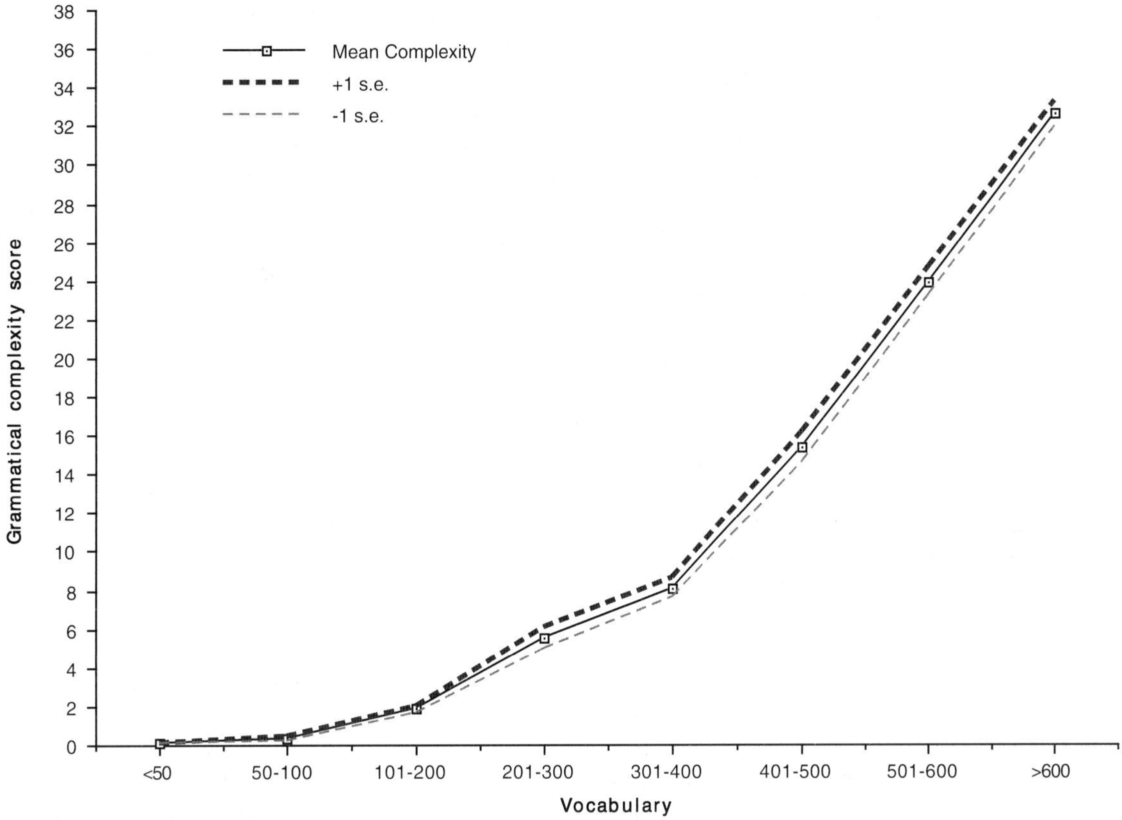

Fig. 3. Mean and standard errors for grammatical complexity in children at different age levels.

Variations and dissociations in infants with focal brain injury

The neural bases of the dissociations we have just described are still unknown, but our research on early language development in infants with focal brain injury has provided a few clues, permitting us to reject some of the more obvious hypotheses suggested by the adult aphasia literature.

All of our studies to date have focused on infants with unilateral injuries sustained before 6 months of age. There has been a great deal of controversy about this population since the 1930s. Early studies suggested that early unilateral injuries have no effect at all on long-term language outcomes, and that the two hemispheres of the brain are equipotential for language at the beginning of life (Basser, 1962; Lenneberg, 1967). Later studies (in the 1970s and 1980s) reported subtle deficits in language in left-hemisphere-damaged children (e.g. Aram, 1988; Dennis and Whitaker, 1976; Riva and Cazzaniga, 1986; Riva, Cazzaniga, Pantaleoni et al., 1986), and concluded that the left hemisphere is innately and irreversibly specialized for language. However, it is important to point out that none of these later studies actually conducted a direct statistical comparison of children with left- vs. right-hemisphere injury (for a critical review, see Bishop, 1997), nor did they provide evidence for anything like a true childhood aphasia following early unilateral injury.

More recent reviews of the literature suggest a compromise between equipotentiality and irreversible determinism (Bates, Vicari and Trauner, 1999; Eisele and Aram, 1995; Stiles, Bates, Thal et al., 1998; Vargha-Khadem et al., 1994, 2000). First, it is now widely agreed that early unilateral injury does not lead to clinically significant language disorders in the vast majority of cases, if children with extraneous complications are excluded from the sample. To be sure, children with a history of brain injury tend to perform below neurologically intact age-matched controls on a host of linguistic and non-linguistic measures, but their performance is usually in the normal to low-normal range, corresponding to an average drop in verbal and non-verbal IQ of about 5–7 points. Second, when left- and right-hemisphere-damaged children are compared directly (with sample sizes large enough and sufficiently well matched to permit a statistical test), and measured after 5–6 years of age (when language acquisition is virtually complete), there is no evidence to date for a difference in long-term language outcomes as a function of lesion side (left vs. right), lesion site (e.g. anterior vs. posterior) or even lesion size (large vs. small).

In contrast with the results of retrospective studies, prospective studies of development prior to 4–5 years of age in this population demonstrate moderate to severe delays in all the early language milestones. These include delays in the onset of babbling and preverbal communication (Marchman, Miller and Bates, 1991), and delays between 1 and 5 years of age in lexical development and grammar (Bates et al., 1997; Reilly et al., 1998; Thal et al., 1991a; Vicari, Albertoni, Chilosi et al., 2000). Most important for our purposes here, we find more dissociations than we would expect by chance in this period of development, and we find correlations between these dissociations and specific lesion sites.

Comprehension vs. production

Based on the adult aphasia literature, we might expect a profile of delayed production with normal comprehension to occur more often in children with left anterior involvement (by analogy to adult Broca's aphasia). Conversely (by analogy to adult Wernicke's aphasia), we might expect children with left posterior damage to display a profile in which comprehension vocabularies fall below the levels that are normally observed in children at the same level of production. This issue has been investigated by Thal et al. (1991) and more recently by Bates et al. (1997). Results of both studies were quite surprising: it seems that the development of word comprehension is *not* selectively affected by lesions to left posterior cortex. Instead, the Wernicke-like profile was actually more common in children with right-hemisphere damage, a finding that has no obvious parallel in the adult aphasia literature. However, this finding is compatible with electrophysiological studies of normally developing children (Mills, Coffey and Neville, 1993; Mills, Coffey-Corina and Neville, 1997), which show that the difference in the brain's response to familiar vs. unfamiliar words is bilateral (but somewhat larger on the right) prior to approximately 18 months of age. After that point (and strongly correlated with the 'vocabulary burst'), there seems to be a reorganization in the brain's response to familiar words, with a larger difference between familiar and unfamiliar words observed in the left hemisphere, primarily across frontal and temporal sites. To explain these findings, Bates et al. (1997) suggest that the right hemisphere plays a larger role in the first stages of word comprehension because that hemisphere appears to be particularly important for integration of information across multiple sources (Stiles et al., 1998). For adults who already know their language (and also for older infants), this kind of multi-modal integration may not be necessary in order to understand a familiar word. But for infants who are struggling to 'crack the code', right-hemisphere resources may play a particularly important role.

Analytic vs. holistic style

As we noted earlier (see *Variations in style*), children who are acquiring English tend to deal initially with pronouns and other function words in one of two ways: analytic/referential style children tend to leave those forms out of their speech altogether; holistic/pronominal style children tend to produce those forms from the very beginning, but only in rote, 'frozen' expressions. Applying these definitions to our focal lesion sample, Thal et al. reported a significantly higher incidence of holistic/pronominal style across the sample as a whole than we would expect if the sample were drawn randomly from the normal population (based on norms from Fenson et al., 1993). This finding is reminiscent of a report by Johnston and Kamhi (1984), showing that language-impaired children tend to 'pad' their utterances by extensive use of a handful of grammatical function words. There were, however, several cases of extreme referential style in the focal lesion data as well. These contrasting extremes provide us with an opportunity to examine two different hypotheses that have been offered to explain the analytic/holistic dissociations observed in normal children (see Bates et al., 1988, for a discussion).

The interhemispheric hypothesis is based on the claim that the left hemisphere is specialized for fine-grained analytic operations, while the right hemisphere is specialized for holistic/configurational operations (e.g. Bradshaw and Nettleson, 1981). By this argument, an analytic/segmenting approach to language learning should be blocked if the left hemisphere is damaged, while a holistic/configurational approach should be blocked if the right hemisphere is damaged. This prediction is reasonable, but it is not borne out by our studies of infants with focal brain injury. In fact, Thal et al. report a significantly *higher* incidence of pronominal/expressive style in children with right-hemisphere damage, with proportionally more referential/telegraphic speech in children with left-hemisphere damage. This finding suggests that left-hemisphere processes may play an important role in the early production of pronouns and other function words — even when those words are used in rote or 'formulaic' expressions. In short, although the right-hemisphere account of holistic style in normal children is an appealing one, it receives no support from the patterns observed in children with focal brain injury.

The intrahemispheric hypothesis is based on an analogy between Broca's aphasia and analytic/referential style (i.e. telegraphic speech with a high proportion of content words, especially nouns), and on an analogy between Wernicke's aphasia and holistic/pronominal style (i.e. fluent but 'empty' speech with a high proportion of pronouns and other function words). By this logic, analytic style should be more common in children with left anterior damage, while holistic style should occur more often in children with left posterior injuries. This hypothesis is also disconfirmed by the Thal et al. findings. In fact, the holistic/pronominal pattern was significantly less common in children with left posterior injuries, suggesting that regions of left posterior cortex may play a particularly important role in the production of pronouns and other grammatical function words — even when (or particularly when) those forms are largely restricted to memorized fragments of speech.

There is a third possibility which could account for all these findings, although it has not been explored in the literature on individual differences in normal children. We know from research on visual–spatial pattern analysis by Stiles and others (see below) that children and adults with LH damage demonstrate deficits in the *extraction of local detail*, while children and adults with RH damage experience difficulty with *overall configuration*. The interhemispheric hypothesis described above assumes an equation between formulaic speech (including unanalyzed use of grammatical function words) and holistic/configurational analysis. However, this assumption may be incorrect. Instead, it is possible that 'expressive style' children produce a relatively high proportion of pronouns and function words in their first word combinations because they have extracted a higher-than-normal proportion of 'local detail' from their linguistic input; they reproduce these 'little words' in a rote fashion, and may be slightly delayed in the long-term mastery of the rules that govern those forms (see Bates et al., 1988, for a discussion) because they have failed to integrate those forms into the larger semantic–grammatic framework that motivates use of pronouns and other function words in the adult language.

This local-detail hypothesis has several advantages for our purposes here. First, it suggests that 'expressive style' should be minimal in children with left posterior damage — the same lesion type that is associated with problems in extraction of local detail in our visual–spatial tasks (see below). Second, this proposal could account for the other expressive language problems displayed by infants with left posterior damage, from babbling through onset of grammar. By analogy with the adult literature, we tend to equate comprehension with sensory processing, and production with motor abilities. However, during the period in which children are learning to produce speech, they have to analyze the speech stream in sufficient detail to permit the construction of a motor analogue. It is possible that the selectively greater problems in expressive language displayed by children with left posterior damage derive not from motor problems but from limitations on the kind of sensory analysis that is required for precise sensory-to-motor mapping. Once that phase of learning is over, there may be a corresponding reduction in the role played by left posterior cortex in expressive language — particularly for 'overlearned' aspects of production, i.e. phonology and grammar.

So which hypothesis is correct? Bates et al. obtained a rather clear conclusion in their investigation of children between 19–30 months of age: expressive/holistic style was significantly more common in children with right-hemisphere damage. In other words, the pattern of 'running off at the mouth' that is characteristic of expressive/holistic style seems to be more common when the right hemisphere is unable to perform its modulating/integrative role in early language learning.

Grammar vs. vocabulary

In the same study by Bates et al., it was also possible to ask whether grammar and vocabulary dissociate at any point during the first stages of language learning. The answer was very clear: they do not dissociate, at least not in this period of development. Bates et al. do report that some lesions have a greater effect on expressive language development than others, but these lesions have equally serious effects on both vocabulary and grammar. Specifically, children whose lesions involved the left temporal lobe tend to suffer greater delays in both vocabulary and grammar across the first years of language learning, an effect that is still visible as late as 5 years of age (but not beyond that point). In addition, they report that children who have frontal damage to *either* the left *or* right hemisphere also tend to move more slowly in expressive language development. However, this bilateral effect only reached statistical significance between 19 and 30 months of age (the most intensive period of language development, encompassing both the vocabulary burst and the first wave of grammaticization in normally developing children). Most important for our purposes here, the delaying effects of frontal involvement were equally evident in grammar and vocabulary. It appears that the same laws that govern co-development of grammar and vocabulary in children who are neurologically intact are also operating in the focal lesion sample, suggesting that the acquisition of grammar and vocabulary may be mediated by the same neural mechanisms during this period of development.

Are there any populations in which we do see a dissociation between grammar and vocabulary? Selectively greater delays in grammar (compared with vocabulary and other aspects of pragmatics and semantics) have been reported for much older children in several different populations, including Specific Language Impairment (Johnston and Kamhi, 1984; Leonard, 1998), Down Syndrome (Chapman, 1995; Fowler, 1993; Singer Harris, Bellugi, Bates et al., 1997; Vicari, Caselli and Tonucci, 2000) and even in deaf children who are trying to acquire an oral language (Volterra and Bates, 1989). The reasons for the selective vulnerability of grammar have been hotly debated (Bishop, 1992, 1994; Rice and Wexler, 1995; Rice, Wexler and Cleave, 1995). Some investigators attribute this selective delay to deficits in an innate grammar module, controlled by a specific gene that is deficient in children with Specific Language Delay. Other investigators have argued instead that children with SLI suffer from some kind of perceptual impairment (Bishop, 1994, 1997; Tallal, Stark, Kallman and Mellits, 1980, 1981; Tallal, Stark and Mellits, 1985a,b), one which has greater effects on grammatical morphology than any other aspect of language precisely because those 'little words' and endings are low in perceptual salience.

We are sympathetic to the latter position, for two reasons. First, studies in our laboratory have shown that selective deficits in grammatical morphology can be induced in perfectly normal college students when they are forced to process sentences under perceptually degraded conditions, through compression, low-pass filtering, or some combination of the two (Blackwell and Bates, 1995; Dick et al., 1999; Dick, Bates, Wulfeck and Dronkers, 1998; Kilborn, 1991; see also Miyake, Carpenter and Just, 1994). This result lends plausibility to the hypothesis that a subtle congenital deficit at the perceptual level could have serious repercussions for language development in general, but for grammatical development in particular. Second, the fact that this profile of grammatical delay is also observed in deaf children and in children with Down Syndrome lends support to the idea that such a delay reflects weaknesses in auditory processing (an area that is known to be especially vulnerable in Down Syndrome — Chapman, 1995). In this regard, a recent study by Singer Harris et al. (1997) compared the first stages of vocabulary and grammar in children with Down Syndrome (for whom auditory deficits are a frequent problem) and a matched sample of children with Williams Syndrome (who are known to have particularly acute hearing). Both groups of children were equally and massively delayed in early vocabulary, suggesting that language cannot get off the ground until children reach the same cognitive level (or mental age) at which language appears in normal children. Indeed, there were no significant differences between the Down and Williams populations — until the point at which grammar begins to flourish. At this point, a significant difference emerged. For children with Williams Syndrome, the growth of grammar was tied quite closely to vocabulary size (following the curve in Fig. 3), but children with Down Syndrome displayed levels of grammar below what we would expect for their vocabulary size. It is worth noting that there were strong correlations between grammar and vocabulary in both groups (i.e. the two domains do not completely dissociate), but the slope of the function for Down children was very low, as we would expect if grammar had to be acquired through some kind of noise filter.

Returning for the moment to evidence from the focal lesion population, a comparison between the substantial delays observed in infancy and the normal to low-normal performance in older children leads to a hypothesized 'window of recovery' between 1 and 5–6 years of age, a period in which children with focal brain injury find alternative ways to solve the problem of language acquisition. This finding permits us to cast the old problem of brain/behavior correlations in a different light, and provide a solution to the debate between proponents of equipotentiality and proponents of irreversible determinism. On this compromise view, there are initial biases in the regions of the brain that are likely to take over the language task, such that lesions to these areas create specific patterns of delay during language acquisition. However, these biases can be overcome, and alternative forms of brain organization for language can emerge across the course of language learning. Of course much more evidence is necessary before we can draw firm conclusions about the neural factors that underlie normal and abnormal variations in language learning. Only one conclusion seems clear so far: The brain regions that mediate language acquisition in the first years of life are not necessarily the same regions that mediate processing and maintenance of language in the adult. This brings us to the next and final section, on human brain development and its relationship to the language milestones and variations that we have discussed in such detail.

The neural correlates of language milestones

We have shown that the course of language development is exceedingly complex, characterized by massive variability across children, and by multiple bursts and plateaus within individual children. We have also seen that learning plays an extremely important role throughout this process, starting as early as the third trimester of pregnancy. Children start to pick up language-specific preferences *in utero*, and they continue to 'tune' the language processor in various directions depending on the nature of their input. This is not the view of language development that Lenneberg (1967) had in mind when he laid down a series of observations and predictions about the maturation of language. Lenneberg paid more attention to means than variations in language acquisition by English-speaking children, and he proposed that these milestones may be timed by a biological clock that also governs motor milestones like crawling and walking. In his 1967 book, he provided a famous table comparing milestones in language and motor development (e.g. first steps and first words around the first birthday) in defense of this maturational view. This oft-cited table is based on average onset times across different samples of children, but it implies a set of correlations that ought to hold within individual children as well. As it turns out, there is little evidence for such a lockstep process when milestones are compared within the same sample of healthy, normal children. For example, Bates et al. (1979) looked for such correlations in their longitudinal study of language and communication from 9–13 months. There were no significant links between motor and language milestones, and if anything the non-significant correlation between walking and talking seemed to run in the wrong direction, as if there were a slight tendency for children to make some kind of choice about where to invest their energies among the various skills that are starting to emerge around this time. And yet we know that the nervous system continues to develop after birth in our species. Surely it ought to be possible to find neural correlates (and perhaps neural causes?) for the dramatic changes that characterize language development in the first few years of human life.

In an earlier version of this chapter (Bates, Thal and Janowsky, 1992), we joined the search for neural correlates of language development, and pointed out two likely candidates for such a relationship. First, we noted (see above) that the period between 8 and 10 months of postnatal life is a behavioral watershed, characterized by marked changes and reorganizations in many different domains including speech perception and production, memory and categorization, imitation, joint reference and intentional communication, and of course word comprehension. We speculated that this set of correlated changes (and they are correlated within individual children) may be related to the achievement of adult-like patterns of connectivity and brain metabolism, with particular reference to changes involving the frontal lobes. Second, we noted (see above) that the period between 16 and 30 months encases a series of sharp non-linear increases in expressive language, including exponential increases in both vocabulary and grammar. We pointed out a possible link between this series of behavioral 'bursts' and a marked increase in synaptic density and brain metabolism that was estimated to take place around the same time. We produced our own table comparing estimated/average onset times for behavioral and neural events across the human lifetime, and we speculated (based on average onset times across different children) that some kind of causal relationship may be involved. That table was very popular, and has been cited frequently since the 1992 chapter appeared (though not as frequently as its ancestor in the Lenneberg volume). Hence some readers may be disappointed to find that the table has disappeared, replaced by a much more complex and challenging story. It is undoubtedly the case that brain maturation plays a causal role in language learning and in many other aspects of behavior development. But we have learned a number of lessons that mitigate this claim, and make us wary of summary tables that imply any simple form of cause and effect. Here are three lessons that have led us to remove the old table of correlations.

First, it has become increasingly clear that learning plays a massive role in language development. Of course this has to be true in some trivial sense, because we know that English children learn English and Chinese children learn Chinese. However, there has been a long tradition of skepticism about learning in the child language literature, because language development is characterized by so many 'funny looking' events, including long plateaus interrupted by exponential shifts, with occasional steps backward (e.g. the child who produces error-free versions of the past tense for several weeks or months, and then suddenly starts to make mistakes like 'goed' and 'stooded-up'). These non-linearities and non-monotonicities have led many investigators to underplay the role of garden-variety learning in favor of a maturational view in which apparent discontinuities at the behavioral level are caused by discontinuities in the nervous system (Pinker, 1994; Wexler, 1996). Although this is a plausible scenario, and it might be true for some subset of events, it rests on a mistaken assumption: that 'garden-variety learning' is a simple linear process, and cannot produce non-linear and especially non-monotonic functions of the kind that are so often observed in language development. As it turns out, that simply isn't true. In the last decade, we have seen many examples of non-linear and non-monotonic learning in artificial neural networks (Elman et al., 1996). These multi-layered networks are relatively simple in their structure (and certainly must be viewed as abstract toys, in comparison with real nervous systems at any level of phylogeny), but they are very good at pattern perception and learning, and they have been used to simulate in considerable detail many of the 'funny looking' learning functions that characterize language development. They are able to do this because, despite their simplicity, they constitute non-linear dynamical systems, which are notorious for their unpredictability and for the wide range of growth functions that they can display. In other words, the linear view of 'garden-variety learning' is wrong. At the same time that we have learned to appreciate the emergence of complex learning in simple systems, evidence has also mounted showing that very young infants are capable of rapid and powerful forms of statistical learning, inside and outside of the linguistic domain (e.g. Bates and Elman, 1996; Elman and Bates, 1997; Saffran et al., 1996). Putting these trends together, we can no longer assume that all discontinuities in behavior reflect discontinuities in the developing nervous system. Even within a structurally stable learning device, funny-looking things can happen — including the discontinuities that characterize language and communicative development at the 8–10-month watershed, and the exponential bursts that are observed in vocabulary and grammar between 16 and 30 months.

Second, we know much more than we knew 10 years ago about human brain development, before and after birth. Ten years ago there was an appealing story in the air that we incorporated into our chapter on language and its neural correlates: prenatal development is characterized primarily by 'additive events' (e.g. neural tube formation, cell proliferation and migration, and the first wave of connectivity); postnatal development does include some further additive events (especially synaptogenesis and myelination), but it is characterized primarily by 'subtractive events', including the whittling away or subtraction of cells, axons and (above all) synapses under the careful guidance of experience. This general view of exuberant growth in the first wave (more cells, axons and synapses than the organism will ever need) followed by subtraction is still true, but not in the two-stage form in which we presented it the first time around. Instead, our current view of brain development acknowledges a host of both additive and subtractive events, before and after birth, in multiple dimensions with multiple gradients. In fact, the picture of human brain development that we will try to present here is one that is quite compatible with the burgeoning literature on early (even prenatal) learning, because so many of the events required to create a learning machine take place within the first two trimesters of prenatal human life. Everything that happens after that is really a matter of degree — maturational changes at every level of the system, in multiple overlapping gradients. These postnatal changes do have interesting computational consequences, but one is hard pressed to find anything that changes in a punctate fashion. Above all, there is little evidence for the old-fashioned notion of modular brain systems that 'turn on' at a particular time, like successive levels in a computer game.

Third, it has become increasingly clear that the relationship between brain development and behavior is bidirectional. That insight was already present in our earlier chapter, where we underscored the role of experience in synaptic elimination and other subtractive events, yielding the metaphor of experience as a sculptor working away in the studio of life. However, recent research in developmental neurobiology has shown that the bidirectional dance between brain development and experience occurs at many more levels of the system, including additive events throughout the lifetime of the organism. To be sure, a huge wave of synaptogenesis that takes place in the first year of postnatal life is never seen again, and the early waves of neurogenesis and migration have no postnatal parallels. Nevertheless, it is now known that complex learning in adulthood induces synaptogenesis and other striking morphological changes in brain regions related to the challenging new task (Kleim, Lussnig, Schwarz et al., 1996; Kleim, Swain, Czerlanis et al., 1997). In a few privileged areas of the brain, like the dentate gyrus of the hippocampus, new brain cells can be formed throughout life and the rate can be modified depending on experience (Kempermann, Brandon and Gage, 1998; Kornack and Rakic, 1999). As a result of all this new information, it is no longer advisable to assume (without further evidence) that correlated changes in brain and behavior reflect a causal flow in one direction. It could just as easily be the other way around.

With these lessons in mind, we will provide an overview of basic events in human brain development that precede, prepare, parallel and (perhaps) participate in the language-learning process. We will review neural events globally, concentrating mainly, but not exclusively, on the *isocortex* (a synonym for *neocortex* that neuroanatomists prefer because it does not make false assumptions about how 'new' in phylogeny the cortex is), and not only on those areas conventionally viewed as 'language areas' in the adult. Unquestionably, neurological disturbances in these areas will produce language-related deficits (at least in the adult), but it may be more accurate to think of language acquisition and production as an interactive process involving auditory, visual, somatosensory, motor, memory, emotional and associative functions. The neural areas governing these functions are located in widespread regions of temporal, parietal, frontal, and prefrontal cortices, and do not develop in isolation.

We will address attention to three issues.

(1) *Prenatal Neural Events: Fundamental Brain Scaffolding.* What is the state of the brain at or before birth when the rudiments of language learning begin?

(2) *Postnatal Neural Events.* What types of neurodevelopmental events take place after birth and across the period in which languages are learned? We will focus here on synaptogenesis, the process through which neurons receive their connections, as the key changing component of brain organization during this period, and on the postnatal elaboration of gradients of various maturational processes initiated prenatally.

(3) *Interactions of Neural Patterns and Events with Language Learning.* Do any neurodevelopmental events seem placed or ordered in such a way as to constrain when events in language learning might occur? Alternately, does language learning itself alter the course of brain development?

Prenatal events: fundamental brain scaffolding

Fixing the timing of events

There are no experimental studies directly relating language and cognitive development to brain maturation, and there are only a handful of studies that have tried to relate disorders of brain and behavioral development to fundamental cellular processes. As a result, our estimates of maturational timing in the human brain must be based on correlational and comparative approaches. Fortunately, the literature on perinatal brain development in other mammals has grown so rich in the past decade that our basis for correlation and inference is extremely strong. We are also aided by recent investigations showing that the schedule of human brain development can be mapped with some precision onto the maturational schedules of other animals (Clancy, Darlington and Finlay, 2001; Darlington, Dunlop and Finlay, 1999; Finlay and Darlington, 1995). In fact, the order and relative spacing of early neural events is remarkably stable across all mammalian species, permitting use of a log/linear equation to generate a sequence of predicted dates for corresponding developmental events in humans. This model captures the statistical relationships among 92 mammalian developmental events obtained from 9 different mammalian species, including some from humans. With a model that is initially derived from non-humans, we are able to predict known dates of human developmental events with considerable precision, and as a result we can also predict the dates for events that have not yet been empirically measured in our species. Although there are many striking similarities across species, this approach has also shown that primates (including humans) differ systematically from other mammals in the timing of neurogenesis (which refers to the process in which new neurons are produced) in two key neural regions, the limbic system and the isocortex. The limbic system is a circuit of widely distributed neural structures that includes the hippocampal formation, associated with memory and spatial learning, as well as neural regions associated with olfaction and emotion. Neurogenesis of the limbic regions is abbreviated in primates, resulting in uniformly smaller limbic structures when compared to similar areas in non-primates. In contrast, the isocortex in primates has a relatively protracted neurogenesis, and a consequently increased relative size (Clancy et al., 2001; Finlay and Darlington, 1995). A very simple principle underlies this difference in the relative size and shape of brain systems: if a species gains extra cycles of neurogenesis across the course of evolution, the greatest relative enlargement occurs in the parts of the brain that develop relatively late.

With this fact about primate variability factored into the Finlay and Darlington (1995) statistical model we are able to produce reliable predictions for the dates of a number of uninvestigated human neural developmental events, including aspects of neurogenesis, pathway formation, and various regressive events across functional brain systems which would typically require invasive procedures for accurate determination (discussed in more detail in Clancy et al., 2001). Unless indicated, all statements in the following text about the time of occurrence of maturational events in human neural development are drawn from data produced using this comparative mammalian model.

First trimester. It is startling to realize how much of fundamental brain morphology and organization is already laid down by the end of the first three months of life (before many mothers even know that they are pregnant). Approximately 10 days after conception, the developing embryo, as yet without much tissue differentiation, has implanted itself into the uterine wall. There it quickly flattens into three distinct layers (ectoderm, mesoderm and endoderm); the skin, sense organs and the rest of the central nervous system will all develop out of the ectodermal layer. Within the ectoderm, rapid proliferation of cells on either side of the midline along the length of the entire embryo pushes up edges of tissue which meet and form the neural tube, enclosing a fluid-filled ventricle. The neural tube gives rise to the entire brain, forebrain at one end, and spinal cord at the other. All neurons in the brain are generated from stem cells on the inside of the tube, called either the ventricular zone because it adjoins the ventricle, or the proliferative zone. Neurons migrate out from the ventricular zone to the overlying mantle along radial glial guides, with some number of their mature neuronal features already specified and others to be picked up as they migrate and settle into their terminal regions by communication with other cells and the general cellular environment. By six weeks, the form of a human embryo is recognizable.

Virtually every neuron in the nervous system is generated in the first trimester, with the exception of the tail of the distribution of the last layer of the isocortex, and the external granular layer of the cerebellum. Two other exceptions are the hippocampal dentate gyrus and the olfactory bulb, which are (as far as we now know) the only regions in which neurons are generated throughout life (albeit at a very low rate) in all mammals studied, including primates (Bayer, 1982, 1983; Kornack and Rakic, 1999; Kuhn, Dickinson-Anson and Gage, 1996; Luskin, 1998). The first activity the early-generated neurons engage in is to lay down the basic axonal pathways of the brainstem (Easter, Ross and Frankfurter, 1993). An interesting point to note here is how variable (in different parts of the nervous system) the sequence of neural differentiation can be — there is no simple lockstep plan for all neurons like "Migrate; become electrically excitable; produce axon; produce dendrites; make neurotransmitter, fire away." To take the case of axons alone, axons can be produced while neurons are migrating; not produced until the terminal site is reached; may show growth of multiple stages and types (branching or not, for example); may be produced and then retracted; or may show prolonged periods of no growth ('waiting periods').

Two more critical processes are virtually complete by the end of the first trimester: the differentiation of cells into different subtypes (also called 'cell specification') and the migration of cells from their birthplace in the ventricular zone to their ultimate destinations in cortical sites. In fact, these two events (specification and migration) are functionally intertwined. The 'type' of a neuron includes many aspects — what shape it has, what information it receives, what transmitters and receptors it produces, and so forth. Some of these features can be specified by location, so that the path taken by a cell as it migrates and its ultimate arrival in a certain brain region will fix some aspects of its 'type' while others are set on, or immediately after, generation in the ventricular zone (Cepko, 1999). For example, cells begin to express various complements of signaling chemicals (neurotransmitters and neuromodulators) before migration, as soon as they are born in the ventricular zone (Lidow and Rakic, 1995). The neurotransmitters and neuromodulators that any particular class of cells exhibits (including both receptors and the metabolic machinery for making and degrading these substances) continue to develop in the following months. Although there are many different kinds of neurochemicals within and across cell types, there seems to be a general developmental principle at work: in early stages of development, neurons will often co-express multiple transmitters and modulators whereas single cells in the mature brain exhibit much less diversity.

Second trimester. This is the period in which the basic wiring of the brain takes place, i.e. the large patterns of connectivity develop between neural regions, including the isocortex. This picture is confirmed in humans by looking for molecular markers that reflect the activity of building axonal and dendritic arbors (Honig, Herrmann and Shatz, 1996). From a developmental point of view, one of the most important events is the establishment of connections from the thalamus to all regions of the isocortex. The thalamus is a subcortical structure that transmits virtually all sensory input from the body surface and special sense organs (except olfaction) to the isocortex. Developmentally, the thalamus maintains the 'packaging' that separates one kind of input from another (e.g. visual, auditory, somatosensory). These connections are set up in the second trimester in a pattern that very much resembles the adult pattern from the start, with animal studies showing that visual, somatosensory, auditory and limbic areas of cortex all receive projections fairly exclusively from those thalamic nuclei that will project to them in adulthood (Miller, Chou and Finlay, 1993; Molnar, Adams and Blakemore, 1998; O'Leary, Schlaggar and Tuttle, 1994). This is particularly important for theories of development, because it means that the brain is 'colonized' by the body long before birth, with boundaries between major brain regions determined by their input well before the outside world has a chance to instruct the brain. Intracortical pathways (i.e. connections from one cortical region to another) also begin to establish their mature connectivity patterns in the second trimester. The corpus callosum makes its first appearance around postconceptional day 90 and lays down a pattern of homotopic connections over the following month, that is, connections between the area of cortex and its corresponding cortex on the other side (reviewed in Innocenti, 1991). The long-range axonal connections start to produce synapses in their target structures in short order, although the bulk of synaptogenesis will occur later (Antonini and Shatz, 1990; Bourgeois and Rakic, 1993).

As we noted earlier, neural development is characterized at many levels and at many points in time by exuberance or overproduction of elements (an additive event), followed by a large-scale 'shake-down' or elimination of the same elements (a subtractive or regressive event). A particular kind of regressive event called apoptotic neuronal death occurs in the second trimester ('apoptosis' is a morphologically distinct kind of cell death associated with an orchestrated death program, not a disorganized dissolution of the cell). This kind of developmental cell death usually occurs in close association with the establishment of major axon pathways between regions, and can contribute to removal of errors in axonal connections and numerical matching of connecting populations of cells (Finlay, 1992). Apoptosis can be quite extensive and rapid, often resulting in the loss of the majority of the neurons originally generated. For example, the retina establishes its connections with subcortical targets in the third month post conception in humans, and reaches the peak number of axons in the optic nerve about a month later. By the end of month 5, retinal ganglion cell loss is over, removing as much as 80% of the originally generated cell population (a process that has been directly demonstrated in humans — Provis and Penfold, 1988; Provis, Van Driel, Billson and Russell, 1985). Such cell loss also occurs in the isocortex, particularly in the subplate and the upper cortical layers (Shatz, Chun and Luskin, 1988; Woo, Beale and Finlay, 1991). Though subplate loss is prenatal, isocortical death in the upper layers may extend into the first couple of postnatal months (O'Kusky and Colonnier, 1982). Overall, early neuronal death seems to serve to grossly fix cell numbers in interconnecting populations and to fine-tune topographic projections between structures, but does not contribute to the kind of fine-tuning of connectional anatomy associated with learning from the extrauterine environment in the isocortex.

The second trimester is also the period in which something akin to learning or 'self-instruction' begins, a process of activity-dependent self-organization of the nervous system. While the physiological and cellular consequences of this phenomenon have been best studied in the visual system, it seems like such a useful developmental mechanism for organizing spatially distributed systems that it is likely it will be discovered elsewhere. For example, the first motor activity of the fetus begins at 2–3 months post conception and continues through intrauterine life, and although the neuroanatomical consequences of this activity are not known, the pattern of activity that it generates in the nervous system is structured and phasic (Robertson, Dierker, Sorokin and Rosen, 1982). In the retina, 'waves' of activity begin to be propagated across the retinal surface, generated by amacrine cells, beginning (in cats and ferrets) after basic connectivity is established and stopping before eye opening, corresponding to second trimester in human development (reviewed in Wong, 1999). This organized activity can be the basis for a kind of primitive categorization, a process in which similar (correlated) inputs hang together while dissimilar (uncorrelated) inputs dissociate. An important example can be found in the establishment of ocular dominance columns, a stripe-like pattern of left-right alternation in primary visual cortex which seems to reflect the brain's solution to competing (unlike) waves of input from the two eyes that feed into overlapping regions. Because retinal waves produce a hypercorrelation of the activity of spatially adjacent cells in the retina, this information can also be used to fine-tune topographically mapped projections, and it could also produce more detailed spatial structures like orientation sensitivity in visual cortical neurons. This self-organizing process has some very interesting theoretical implications for developmental psychologists: activity-dependent organization occupies a middle ground in the nature-nurture debate, where some of the same mechanisms that will be used later for learning from the outside world (i.e. response to correlations in the input) are used in utero to set up the basic functional architecture of the brain. In utero, some of this organizing activity may be imposed by the activity of the body itself, or by the intrinsic circuitry of the nervous system.

Third trimester. By the beginning of the seventh month of gestation, a remarkably large number of neural events are complete. The human fetus has matured to the point where the eyes move and remain open for measurable periods of time (though there isn't much to see — more on this below). Reciprocal connectivity from higher-order cortical areas to primary areas has also begun (Burkhalter, 1993). Pathways exhibit the initial process of myelination (Yakovlev and Lecours, 1967). Large descending pathways from the cortex are also in the process of development. Aside from the more obvious role of descending pathways in motor control, the appearance of descending pathways also means that the brain has started to 'talk back' to its input regions, a form of interaction found in all sensory as well as motor systems. The nature and function of this 'top-down' connectivity within sensory systems are still poorly understood (the term 'top- down' is preferred to 'feedback' since it does not prejudge the region of initiation), but it is now clear that simple bottom-up processing sequences are not sufficient to explain many behavioral phenomena. Upon maturity, some top-down projections will actually be many times more robust than their 'bottom-up' counterparts (see Churchland, Ramachandran and Sejnowski, 1994). These descending projections are believed to be involved in the dynamic processing strategies that are tied to attention and learning (Cauller, 1995; see collection in Koch and Davis, 1994) and so it is quite interesting in this regard that they continue to develop well after birth.

In the eighth and ninth month, a massive and coordinated birth of synaptic connections begins in the isocortex and related structures, as we will discuss in detail in the next section. In general, however, it is fair to say that the infant arrives in the world with a nervous system whose working components are in place and organized. All cells are generated, all major incoming sensory pathways are in place and have already gone through a period of refinement of their total number of cells, connections, and topographic organization. Intracortical and connectional pathways are well developed, though output pathways lag behind. The microstructure of such features as motion and orientation selectivity in the visual system is already present, though more remains to be elaborated. The 'big' cortical regions — primary sensory and motor regions — have their adult input and topography, though we do not know yet if all of the multiple subareas described for the primate cortex have sorted themselves out (Felleman and Van Essen, 1991). This brain is up and running at birth, ready to learn. In fact, it has been capable of learning for several weeks, a neurophysiological fact that complements and supports surprising new evidence for prenatal learning of at least some aspects of speech (see **Prerequisites to language** above).

Postnatal neural events

Now we turn to a consideration of events that extend past birth, with special emphasis on the neural events that surround language learning. As we have already pointed out, the search for punctate and lockstep correlations between neural and behavioral milestones has proven fruitless. However, we can draw some interesting lessons about behavior from the shifting neural landscape that characterizes postnatal brain development in humans.

Myelination

Myelination refers to an increase in the fatty sheath that surrounds neuronal pathways, a process that increases the efficiency of information transmission. In the central nervous system, sensory areas tend to myelinate earlier than motor areas — a fact that has been cited as a possible contributor to the comprehension/production disparity observed in some children. Intracortical association areas are known to myelinate last, and continue to myelinate at least into the second decade of life. Myelination of some callosal and associational cortical regions may continue well into maturity, extending throughout the third and even fourth decade (Yakovlev and Lecours, 1967).

Speculations about the brain basis of behavioral development have often revolved around the process of myelination because it continues for so many years after birth (Parmelee and Sigman, 1983; Volpe, 1987). However, interest in the causal role of myelination has waned. First, because this is such a protracted process, there are no clear-cut transitions that might provide a basis for major reorganizations in the behavioral domain. Second, we know that 'under-myelinated' connections in the young human brain are still capable of transmitting information; additions to the myelin sheath may increase efficiency, but they cannot be the primary causal factor in brain organization of language or any other higher cognitive process. Third, the discovery of other large-scale progressive and regressive events in early brain development that are influenced by interactions of maturation and experience are more appealing candidates as the sculptors of behavioral development — which brings us to a consideration of synaptogenesis.

Synaptogenesis

None of the neural events we have discussed so far span the dramatic events that define early language development. The production and placement of neurons is complete before birth in all structures that do not continue neurogenesis throughout life. Regional connectivity of the isocortex begins in the second trimester and, although completed postnatally, it bears no obvious relationship to changes in language ability except in a permissive sense. A mature reciprocal pattern from secondary to primary visual cortex (although not the mature density) is accomplished somewhere between 4 months and 2 years in developing humans (Burkhalter, 1993). Myelination 'brackets' language acquisition only in the most global sense, i.e. it takes place somewhere between gestation and adulthood. Synaptogenesis, however, is an event that occurs in the critical time window for early language development, and seems optimally placed for the rapid statistical learning infants show in both the visual and auditory realms during this time (Saffran et al., 1996).

Synaptogenesis and synapse elimination co-occur over most of early postnatal development, and they co-occur throughout life. However, there are some interesting features to synaptogenesis and elimination within the perinatal period that seem quite closely related to early language acquisition. Because this is such an appealing candidate for a correlational and (perhaps) causal role in language development, we need to provide some important details about the methods used to calculate synaptic growth, and the problems that are encountered in the measurement of this moving target.

The word 'synapse' is often used loosely to designate an elemental functional connection between neurons, but anatomists use it more specifically, and look for specific features of synaptic form associated with particular functions. Synapses are chemical junctions between neurons, visible as described here with electron microscopy. Axonal or presynaptic processes contain the metabolic machinery to produce neurotransmitters and package them, often in recognizable packages of vesicles, and a 'presynaptic specialization', a thickening of the cellular membrane that can transfer the contents of the synaptic vesicle to the synaptic cleft between neurons in response to activity of the presynaptic neuron. There is also a visible thickening of the membrane of the postsynaptic neuron, on the opposite side of the synaptic cleft, with the machinery to take up, and perhaps degrade, the neurotransmitter released by the postsynaptic cell, and to cause depolarization or hyperpolarization of the postsynaptic cell. Most, but not all, excitatory synapses have 'asymmetric' synapses, in which the presynaptic specialization is thicker and denser than the postsynaptic one; most inhibitory synapses are 'symmetric', with pre- and postsynaptic thickenings of equal density. The location of the synapse is significant to its function — a synapse can be located on the cell body of the neuron itself, on the shafts of dendrites, or on small spikes appropriately called dendritic spines, which will have consequences for how effectively the presynaptic input can induce changes in the postsynaptic cell. For each neuron, a single synapse usually only contributes a tiny fraction of its input — according to Kandel, Schwartz and Jessell (1991), morphological data indicate an average neuron can receive 10,000–>150,000 contacts postsynaptically. A record 200,000 spines on Purkinje cells of the cerebellum have been estimated, but 15,000 is average on layer V cells of the isocortex (Koch and Zador, 1993). It is important to note that chemical synapses are only one part of the total number of ways neurons may communicate — there can be direct electrical coupling between cells (this is particularly prominent in early development), cells can communicate through the release of gases, notably nitric oxide, and by altering — through any means — the extracellular milieu of the neurons surrounding them. Chemical synapses, however, are easily recognizable, countable and are a central component of neuronal signalling, and hence have been much studied.

A primary mode of learning in the nervous system (though not the only mode) takes place when the juncture is formed or modified as a function of experience, a 'strengthening' or 'weakening' referred to as Hebbian learning. If we ask ourselves where the nervous system stores its 'knowledge' (assuming that this term is useful at all), most neuroscientists would agree that synaptic connectivity is the primary means by which knowledge is represented in the brain (Elman et al., 1996), whether that knowledge is innate (set up independent of experience), learned (set up by experience) or somewhere in between (as in the above-mentioned case of prenatal activity dependence). This is why there is so much interest in the role of synaptogenesis and synaptic connectivity in behavioral development.

In cognitive science, the number of synapses is often thought of as an index for the amount and complexity of information transfer in a structure. Even though synaptic number might be used as such a metric in some comparisons [for example, after certain kinds of experience (Greenough, 1984)], it is misleading to understand synaptic numbers in development in this way. 'More' in development does not necessarily mean better, more complex, or more mature. To take an extreme case, sudden infant death syndrome (SIDS) is associated with an excess number of persisting synapses in the medulla (O'Kusky and Norman, 1994, 1995). This point is important for understanding a high-profile controversy about synaptogenesis and the peak of synaptic numbers in the isocortex of primates and humans. Briefly, in work with rhesus macaques, Rakic and colleagues described a rapid increase in the number of synapses that seemed to take place almost simultaneously across a number of cortical areas, reaching a peak at around the same time in frontal, cingulate, somatosensory and visual cortical areas (Bourgeois, Goldman-Rakic and Rakic, 1994; Granger, Tekaia, Lesourd et al., 1995; Rakic, Bourgeois, Eckenhoff et al., 1986; Zecevic, Bourgeois and Rakic, 1989; Zecevic and Rakic, 1991). In contrast, Huttenlocher, working with human material, showed that the peak of synaptic density varies between visual, auditory and somatosensory regions, with the frontal regions not reaching their peak until 3–4 years after birth, while the visual and auditory regions peak more closely to birth (Huttenlocher and Dabholkar, 1997). A closer examination proves that the story these two investigators tell is not very different after all. Part of the confusion lies in mistakenly identifying peak of synaptogenesis with all other aspects of maturational change in different cortical areas.

In order to understand this literature, some of the methodological issues involved in the counting of synapses must be addressed. The most useful information about synaptic growth would be the documentation of a change in absolute number of synapses within a single structure, or perhaps the average number of synapses per neuron within an identified structure. The latter is currently the preferred method of analysis in studies investigating the effects of experience on synaptic changes in adult animals (Jones, Klintsova, Kilman et al., 1997). However, this is not the measure used in developmental studies like those of Huttenlocher or Rakic, for a very simple reason: while synapses are growing, the rest of the brain in a young animal is changing as well. It is difficult to calculate a ratio of 'synapses per unit' when the nominator and the denominator are both moving targets. In fact, with the exception of primary visual cortex and a few other areas, the borders of most cortical areas are not well-defined enough in early development to assess a change in volume of a cortical area, let alone the number of synapses in that area.

An alternative would be to measure the absolute number of synapses per neuron. To obtain the absolute number of synapses per neuron with confidence, a stereological method of relatively recent invention can be used to eliminate the problems involved in counting synapses and neurons of massively different sizes and shapes in very thin sections (discussed in Guillery and Herrup, 1997). This requires a particular method of tissue preparation and analysis that was not used when the initial (and very valuable) samples of macaque and human brain tissue were gathered. Therefore, to analyze the available tissue, 'assumption-based' stereology is used, which means that certain assumptions are made about the shape and distribution of the things that we are going to count. Different assumptions (all of them very plausible) produce absolute estimates of synaptic density that can vary by factors of 3–4, as the papers themselves demonstrate. Even so, we can get a reasonable idea of how the number of synapses changes in the cortex in a relative sense if not an absolute one (taken with several grains of salt).

Both Rakic and Huttenlocher counted the number of visible synapses in a thin section of cortical tissue, expressed as a fraction of the area of the 'neuropil' (which we will define in a moment), and then stereologically or otherwise correct their counts to get the number of synapses in a volume of tissue. The neuropil is defined by exclusion — it is that area of tissue in the brain in cell-dense areas like the cortex that remains after large, 'non-synaptic' chunks of tissue are excluded, such as neural and glial cell bodies, myelinated axons and blood vessels. To show that synaptic density per volume of neuropil rises or falls during development is not particularly informative, because both the numerator and denominator of the fraction can be expected to change significantly and independently of each other in early development. In the numerator, the absolute synapse number can rise or fall. In the denominator (the volume of neuropil), the size and number of spines, varicosities, dendritic inclusions (e.g. vesicles) can also change with age. Moreover, artifactual deviations could be caused by tissue shrinkage (a common event in brain tissue prepared for microscopic analysis). One possible outcome could be that the synapses/neuropil ratio might stay constant, with an increase in synapse number simply mirrored by an increase in its support structure, the neuropil.

Now, back to the question of development: Rakic and Huttenlocher have both shown that the ratio of synapses to neuropil accelerates wildly beginning just before birth, in both the macaque and the human, and across a wide variety of cortical areas. In macaques, the peak of synaptic density across cortical areas is reached two to four months after birth (Fig. 4a, replotted from Bourgeois et al., 1994; Granger et al., 1995; Rakic et al., 1986; Zecevic et al., 1989; Zecevic and Rakic, 1991). In humans, the curves are very similar, with a marked perinatal increase in synaptic density that begins around birth and flattens postnatally across all cortical areas (Fig. 4b). It should be noted that synapse counts may, or may not, vary across different cortical regions. In the graph, for example, synapse counts in human auditory cortex appear to outnumber those in other human and macaque cortical regions. However, for the technical reasons noted above, and for other methodological considerations, including a possible variability based on the cause of death, absolute values of synapse counts should be considered somewhat conditional, especially in human tissue. Moreover, we have attempted to normalize the data by plotting synapse numbers as a percent of the total at puberty, which we arbitrarily defined as 12 years in human and 3 years in macaque. The 'take home' message from the graph lies not in the absolute numbers, but rather in the pattern of *relative* changes. Huttenlocher's claim that synaptogenesis in prefrontal cortex does not reach its peak in humans until approximately 3–4 years of age rests on the accuracy of a single observation of frontal cortex at 3.5 years of age. However, the macaque data show similar variability, with primary visual cortex peaking latest. In other words, there simply are not enough data available at this time to settle the matter. Even if the Huttenlocher pattern does prove true, this is not the most interesting aspect of these events. The most interesting feature in both the macaque and the human data lies in the strikingly similar timing of acceleration and deceleration, not in the peak. To see why, let's look more closely at the broader schedule of synaptogenesis, before and after birth.

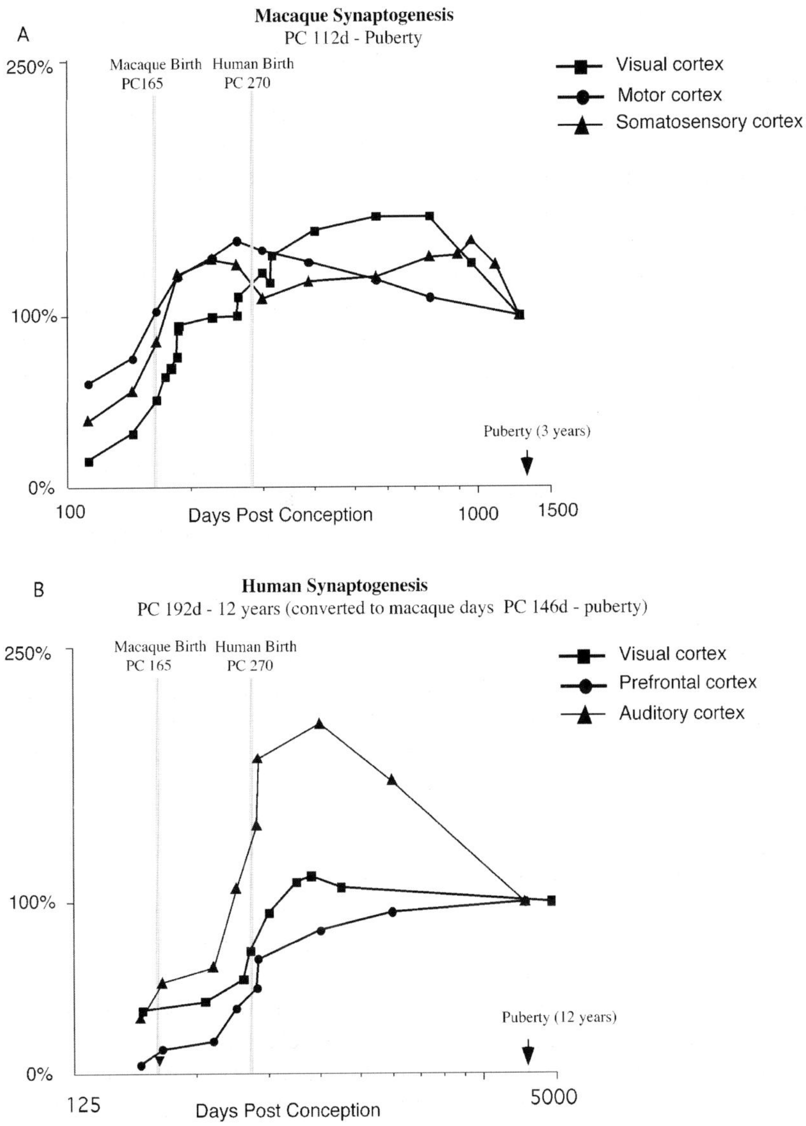

Fig. 4. Re-plotted synaptogenesis data from macaque and human depict coordinated perinatal increases in cortical synapses. Note that peaks of synaptic density in both primates vary across the different cortical regions. (A) In macaques, the peaks of synaptic density are reached two to four months following birth. (B) Human synaptogenesis curves are similar to macaque curves, with a marked increase in synaptic density that begins around birth and flattens postnatally across all cortical areas. For this graph, human days were converted into macaque days using the comparative model of Finlay and Darlington (1995). As the converted data indicate, if humans underwent an accelerated period of synaptogenesis at the maturational stage of macaques at birth (when macaques show rapid synaptogenesis), peaking would occur several weeks prior to any opportunity for environmental stimuli.

Remember that the ratio of synapses to neuropil is a ratio of moving targets. So to understand the development of synaptic connectivity, we need to understand what the denominator of the synaptic ratio (the amount of neuropil) is doing during this same period. Data are not available for humans, but in monkey cortex the relative proportion of neuropil soars from initially insignificant values around PC 50 (50 days post conception) to very high values at PC 100. This prenatal explosion in monkeys corresponds (according to the Finlay/Darlington/Clancy model) to PC 62–127 in humans, still well before birth. After that, the amount of neuropil remains constant at about 70–75% per section until about 1 year of life, followed by a long slow decline to a value of about 50% that is reached at some point well past puberty. Meanwhile, the whole brain is getting bigger. In macaques and marmosets, the volume of visual cortex (with comparable increases in both depth and surface area) overshoots its adult size by about 45% at 6 months of postnatal age, and then regresses to its adult volume. Overall brain volume increases from birth to adulthood by about a factor of two in monkeys, and by a factor of almost four in humans. Because we know that the size of some components like primary visual cortex declines across the same period, the overall increase in brain size must be due to increases in the size of secondary and tertiary visual areas, non-visual areas, as well as in the number of supporting elements and myelinated fibers in the brain. We can safely conclude that the generation of synapses in the entire isocortex of humans accelerates around birth, overshoots by a substantial proportion in the first 6 months or so, and then declines to its adult value. Although fewer data are available for non-cortical regions, a similarly timed burst and decline of synaptogenesis occurs in the striatum (Brand and Rakic, 1984). Where the exact 'peak' lies is probably not too important, as it will be influenced by any number of co-occurring additive and subtractive events. The important point is that the brain suddenly starts to generate massive numbers of synapses just before environmental experience, in all of its regions associated with sensory, motor, motivational, and linguistic ability.

What causes the dramatic perinatal acceleration of synaptogenesis? Using visual cortex as a test case, Rakic and colleagues looked into the possibility that this marked increase is actually caused by the barrage of experience that occurs around birth (Bourgeois and Rakic, 1996).

However, when monkeys were deprived of visual input, the initial acceleration of synaptogenesis was unchanged, though later changes in arrival at final synaptic number, proportions of synaptic types, the laminar arrangement of synapses and so forth, were observed, as has been demonstrated in many investigations of the effects of experience on synaptic organization. O'Kusky (1985) tried a similar experiment with dark-reared cats, and also found no changes in the acceleration of synaptogenesis. However, one could argue that this kind of deprivation experiment is misleading, because the deprivation might induce a host of compensatory changes in other parts of the system. To control for this possibility, a second, 'mirror image' experiment was conducted in which monkeys were delivered three weeks prematurely, so that the hypothetical barrage of experience would begin much sooner than it would normally occur (Bourgeois, Jastreboff and Rakic, 1989). Again, there was no effect on the timing of synapse acceleration and peak — it occurred precisely when it should occur, based on the monkey's anticipated gestational birthdate, not the prematurely induced one. Secondary effects on types and distributions of synapses were also seen in this study, so experience does matter. However, experience doesn't seem to be responsible for the burst in synaptogenesis.

Humans present an evolutionary experiment that is the opposite of the premature delivery manipulation, because we are born late with respect to organizational neural milestones like neurogenesis. Although we think of human infants as being behaviorally quite immature at birth, (making the mental comparison to infant monkeys, for example) there are many aspects in which the human brain is unusually 'mature' at birth, at least in terms of the absolute duration from initial neuron and process formation to birth. For example, the last layers of human cortex are generated around postconceptional day 100, but birth doesn't occur until 6 months later. Monkeys have less of an interval — the last layers of cortex come up around postconceptional day 80, but birth is at 165, a little less than three months later. Eye opening in all mammals is coordinated with neural events, but is not well predicted by birth, and can occur weeks after birth, or weeks before, *in utero*. If human infants were born at the same 'neural maturational age' as macaques, by our formula (Clancy et al., 2001), they would be born at about 7 months post conception. [It is somatic growth, not brain growth, in human infants that is relatively retarded (Sacher, 1980)]. When we look at the relationship between synaptogenesis and birth in humans, we find a rare and rather exciting exception to the general laws of neural development that create such orderly similarities between humans and other mammals: synaptogenesis seems to occur much later in humans than it occurs in other primates, jumping forward several weeks ahead of the point where it would occur in 'macaque time.' Why should this be? If humans underwent an accelerated period of synaptogenesis at the maturational stage corresponding to the stage when macaques show rapid synaptogenesis, it would occur several weeks prior to birth (Fig. 4b). And if this occurred, the human fetus would be in possession of a large reservoir of synaptic plasticity to contemplate the uterine wall! Which would of course be a terrible waste of resources. Timing of peak synaptogenesis to just precede the onset of experience can be seen in other primates (marmoset) (Missler, Eins, Merker et al., 1993; Missler, Wolff, Merker and Wolff, 1993), and in animals such as rats (Blue and Parnavelas, 1983), where eye opening occurs after birth (which essentially marks a similar transition from a dark, burrow-restricted environment to the external world). The peaking of synaptogenesis is the first instance we have found of a neural maturational event tied explicitly to birth, rather than to the intrinsic developmental timetable of the brain which can be quite dissociated from birth (Darlington et al., 1999). Recent work has shown that it is a signal from the fetus that initiates labor, coordinating maturation in the fetus with physiology in the mother. It would be interesting if this same signal might also initiate wholesale neuroanatomical changes in the fetus itself (Nathanielsz, 1998). In any case, the bottom line for present purposes is this: experience does not cause the burst in synaptogenesis, but evolution has coordinated synapse production with birth. Why? Perhaps to guarantee a large reservoir of resources for all the learning that is about to occur. By providing a reservoir of already-formed synapses at the onset of experience in every part of the isocortex, the brain prepares itself for both expected and unexpected learning opportunities.

In fact, the number of synapses present are in excess of the eventual adult number (Zecevic and Rakic, 1991), and we spoke before about how the immediate postnatal phase of development is distinguished by regressive events like axon retraction and synaptic elimination. It has become clear, however, that it would be a mistake to view early development as a solely 'regressive' period. In both intermediately aged and mature nervous systems, additive and subtractive events co-occur and overlap (Quartz and Sejnowski, 1997). Perhaps the developing nervous system is simply allowing itself the possibility of both additive and subtractive events, rather than simply additive ones, by the installation of large numbers of synapses just prior to experience. This initial 'overproduction' of synapses may be a way of producing continuity in mechanisms of synaptic stabilization from initial development to adulthood.

Why on earth does nature bother to produce so many elements just to throw them away? The massive overproduction and subsequent pruning of synapses is an expensive neural tactic in terms of neural components and energy cost. Between ages 2 and 5, it has been estimated that 5000 synapses are disappearing each second in the visual cortex alone (Bourgeois, 1997), and similar recessions are most likely occurring in all cortical areas that participate in language. What purpose could this steady decline serve, especially occurring as it does in a period when details of language (including complex grammar) are mastered? The strategy of excess production followed by pruning has been documented in other neural areas, notably in callosal axonal connectivity, where it has been proposed to permit the neural adjustments that favor evolutionary changes (Innocenti, 1995). Certainly flexibility is a primary outcome of such a system, but refinement, defined in terms of accuracy and speed despite complexity, may be another important consequence of these regressive stages. Empirical studies are limited to observed descriptions of gross synapse counts, but computer simulations have been run that yield interesting information about the computational consequences of this peculiar strategy of overproduction and pruning (Elman et al., 1996). For one thing, in adaptively constructed neural networks that employ overproduction and removal of synapses, input information is more reliably preserved than it is in simple feed-forward networks (Adelsberger-Mangan and Levy, 1993, 1994). Networks constructed using adaptive synaptogenesis also manage to 'sculpt' connections that permit quicker transformations of complex data when compared to networks constructed with conventional non-adjustable connective mechanisms. Moving away from machines back to humans, it is true that the net numbers of synapses are decreasing during adolescence; however, new ones are still sprouting, resulting in a constant and co-occurring process of production and trimming that could also serve to adjust and improve on initial connections.

So now let's take a closer look at the various kinds of synaptogenesis that occur before and after birth, and also consider some of the local and global events that affect the learning potential (and perhaps the learning style) within and across brain regions. A summary of the timetable of synaptic stages can be found in Fig. 5, in which milestones of language acquisition and production are mapped alongside sequences of some of the human neural events that are discussed in this section.

Developmental differences in synapse morphology and distribution. The sequence of synaptogenesis can be classified into five stages (reviewed in Bourgeois, 1997). In the initial stage, synapses are present in the preplate (later subplate and marginal zone) which comprises the earliest-generated cortical neurons. This is followed by a secondary stage in which synapses are generated in the cortical plate itself, initially following a gradient corresponding to that of the developing cortical neurons. Phase III of synaptogenesis is the synchronized global perinatal burst phase described above; at its peak in the infant macaque, it is estimated that 40,000 synapses are formed each second in the visual cortex alone (Bourgeois, 1997). Phase IV is a stabilized high level that lasts from late infancy until puberty, while in the last phase, which extends from puberty to adulthood, synapses steadily decline in density and absolute number.

Variations in morphological characteristics of the third stage of proliferating synapses make it clear that the complexities of the synaptogenic peak extend beyond sheer numbers. There are also interesting development changes in the kinds of synaptic connections that are being made. This includes a change in the ratio of asymmetric to symmetric synapses during the perinatal period — recall that asymmetric synapses are more likely to be excitatory and symmetric inhibitory. During Phase III of synaptogenesis, the asymmetric (putative excitatory) connections decline in number while the numbers of symmetric (putative inhibitory) synapses remain about the same (Bourgeois and Rakic, 1993; Zecevic and Rakic, 1991). Functionally, this means that there may be a developmental shift from a high proportion of excitatory activation toward a more tempered balance between excitation and inhibition, which seems a plausible account of the increasingly better coordination of perception and action.

The sites of synaptic innervation are also altered over development (Zecevic and Rakic, 1991). Early in development (in the more exuberant phase), large numbers of connections are made (or attempted) on the shafts (the trunks and branches) of dendrites. Later there is a shift in contact site, with more connections on dendritic spines. Because spine contact may allow depolarization and associated neurotransmitter release to be localized with more specificity than shaft contact (Harris and Stevens, 1989), this shift in site might reflect an increase in connectional efficiency during the early learning process. Theoretical models, as well as imaging experiments which can track ion flow in single cells, also support the role of spine contact in the induction of the plasticity associated with learning (reviewed in Koch and Zador, 1993). Overall, the significance of these changes in the constellations of the types and forms of synaptic interaction is just beginning to be understood. In the future, we may be able to track the changing functions and relative maturity of cortical areas by looking at constellations of varying synaptic morphology alone. Right now, we know that it is these kinds of things that are changing as function matures, without a very direct structure/function link.

So let us leave synaptogenesis and move on to other, larger-scale changes in brain structure and function that start prenatally but extend well into the postnatal period. We will return to the prenatal genesis of some of the patterns that will set up maturational gradients of different features of the cortex, and relate them to postnatal synaptogenesis. If we are looking for the developmental counterpart of 'mental organs' somewhere in the brain, this is where we need to look.

Maturational gradients of the isocortex in the early postnatal period. Anyone hoping for fundamental simplicity in patterning of the early maturation of the cortex will be disappointed, but we will argue here

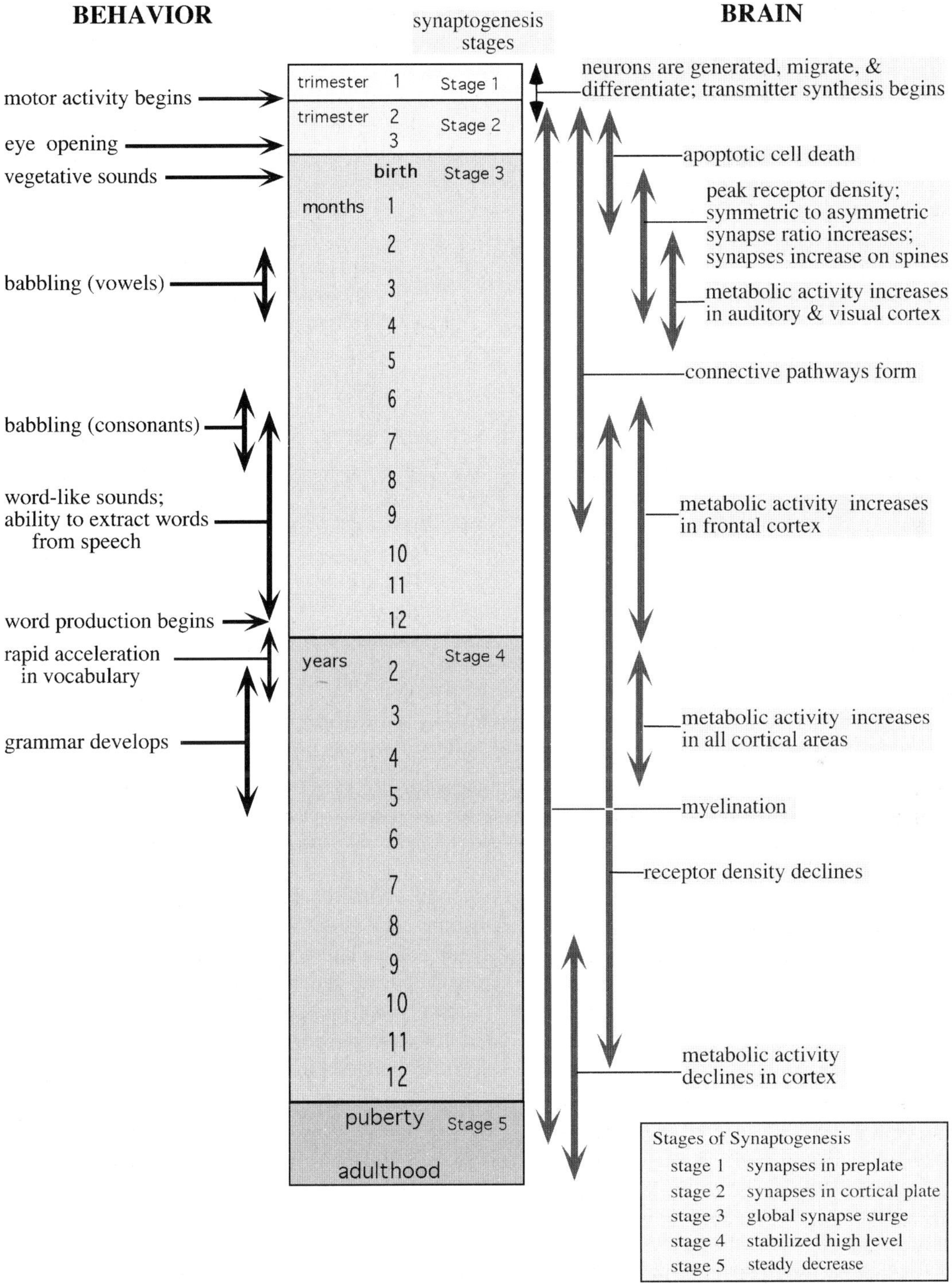

Fig. 5. Milestones of language acquisition and production are mapped alongside overlapping sequences of neural events occurring in the developing human brain.

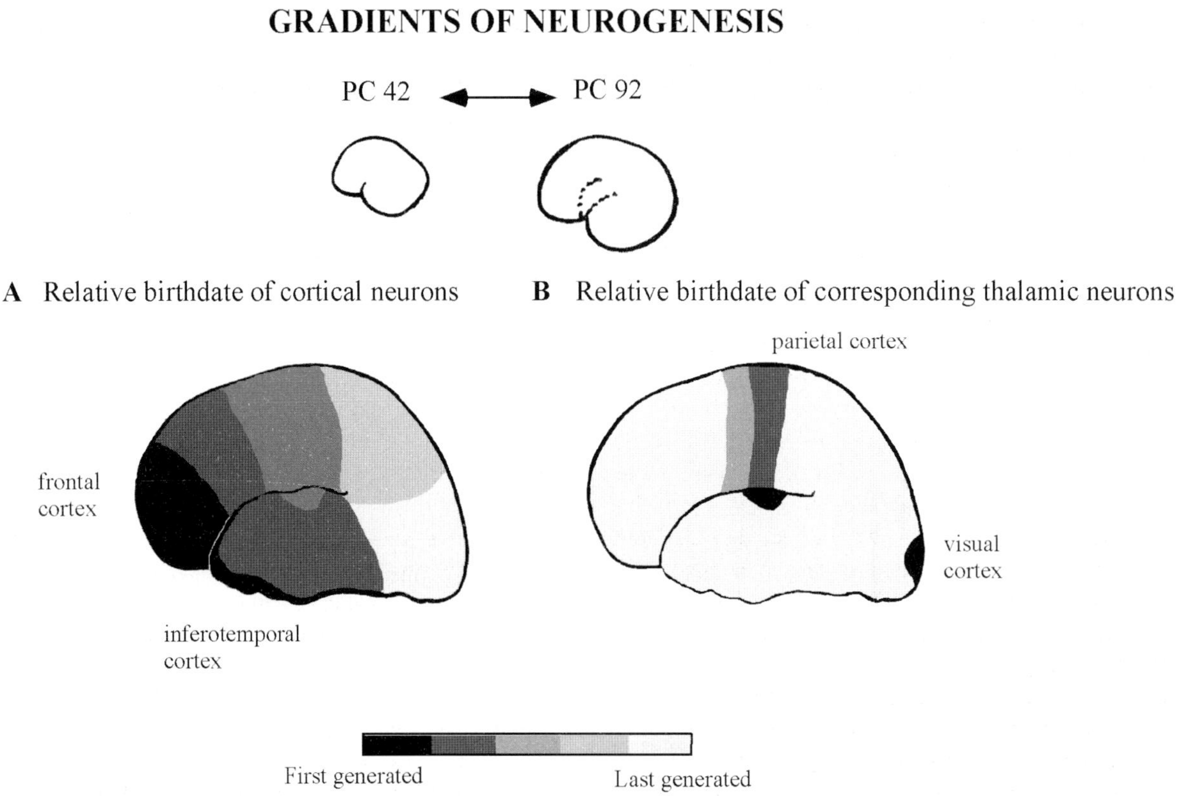

Fig. 6. Maturational gradients in early postnatal development superimposed on a lateral view of the human cortex on the day of birth (PC270). (A) Neurogenesis of cortical neurons begins at the rostrolateral margin of the cortex, where frontal cortex abuts inferotemporal cortex, and proceeds posteriorly through parietal cortex to primary visual cortex, framing a period of genesis of about 50 days (PC day 42 to PC 92). (B) Neurogenesis of corresponding thalamic neurons begins with the medial geniculate body (auditory cortex), the lateral geniculate body (visual cortex) and the ventrobasal complex (somatosensory cortex), followed by neurons that innervate motor cortex. The last thalamic neurons to be produced are located in the nuclei that innervate the frontal, parietal and inferotemporal cortex.

that complexity is the message, and that each cortical area can be viewed as a point in a multidimensional space of various maturational gradients which could well provide the reason for later local functional specializations. There is not a single dimension called 'maturational state' that any area of the isocortex can be retarded or advanced on (which makes it less likely there could be a moment when a region 'turns on'). Rather, each isocortical area is best viewed an assembly of different features, including neurogenesis, process and axon extension, neurotransmitter inclusion, type and rate of synaptogenesis. The simultaneous peaking of synaptogenesis across all cortical areas, supporting the notion of a global signaling process, is an exception to this general rule. Because different areas of the brain follow maturational gradients that don't match in order, interesting temporal asynchronies are produced — for example, in some areas, intracortical connections will be relatively more mature than thalamic connections (the frontal cortex), and in others, the reverse will hold (primary visual cortex). Fig. 6 contrasts the gradients that are observed in two critically different aspects of cortical development: the timing of peak neurogenesis in different cortical areas compared to peak neurogenesis of their corresponding thalamic nuclei, both superimposed on the cortex of a schematized human brain.

Intrinsic cortical gradients

The isocortex has its own gradient of maturation that affects the entire isocortical sheet (because that is what the cortex really is, despite its folds) and is quite conserved across all mammals. Bayer, Altman and colleagues have produced detailed studies of the timing of neurogenesis in rodents (Altman and Bayer, 1979a,b, 1988; Bayer, Altman, Russo and Zhang, 1993) and we are able to apply the comparative mammalian model of Finlay and Darlington (1995) to predict a similar time sequence for humans. Neurogenesis begins at the front edge of the cortex where frontal cortex abuts inferotemporal cortex and proceeds back to primary visual cortex, framing a period of genesis that can last over 30 days in primates from front to back; in humans, this would lead us to expect a neurogenesis window of about 50 days extending from approximately PC day 42 to PC 92. The limbic cingulate cortices also get an early start, in humans beginning genesis about PC 43. The maturational edge then possessed by frontal and limbic cortex would then be expected to continue in various aspects of the intrinsic development of those parts of isocortex. More mature neurons begin to elaborate neuropil, and extend local and long-range connections, but there is little direct association between the time of a neuron's genesis and when it makes its connections as this also depends heavily on the maturational/trophic status of the regions it must connect to. As depicted in the maturational gradient in Fig. 6a paradoxically, the frontal cortex, viewed in hierarchical models as the last maturing cortical area, is in fact one of the first to be produced and thus quite 'mature' in some features. This is one more example of the limits of the traditional hierarchical view of brain development, in which the frontal regions are mistakenly viewed as 'late' on every dimension.

Imposed thalamic gradients

Each area of cortex receives a thalamic input by maturity, but the order of thalamic development in no way resembles the intrinsic cortical gradient (Fig. 6b). This is very important, because as we noted earlier, it is the thalamus that carries instructions to the cortex from the sensory and motor periphery, dividing the cortical sheet into specific regions with specific jobs. If intrinsic cortical gradients and imposed thalamic gradients occur in different orders, then we have a dissociation with potentially very interesting consequences. In general, the primary sensory nuclei in the thalamus, including the ventrobasal complex (somatosensory), parts of the medial geniculate body (auditory), and the lateral geniculate body (visual) are generated first, and establish their axonal connections to the cortex first. Various other nuclei, motor and cingulate are intermediate in their timing, and the last to be produced are the nuclei that innnervate the frontal, parietal and part of the inferotemporal cortex. It is the thalamic order of neurogenesis that gives rise to the hierarchical notion of cortical development (e.g. "visual matures early; frontal matures late"), although this gradient is really not a general rule. So what might this mean for frontal cortex, the area that bears so much weight in speculation about human evolution (e.g. Deacon, 1997)? No one actually knows for sure (because the necessary electrophysiological data are not available), but the fact that frontal cortex matures relatively early (intrinsic gradient) but receives its input from the thalamus relatively late (thalamic gradient) might mean that frontal cortex specializes in intracortical communication (through working connections to other cortical regions). In other words, this difference in developmental gradients might mean that frontal cortex is primed for higher-order associative function from the start, not by virtue of being 'out of the circuit' early on.

General modulatory cortical input

What we have talked about so far has revolved around the construction and interconnectivity of cortical and thalamic regions, i.e. the basic wiring diagram for passage of explicit information. There is another set of subcortical structures that project to the cortex that are deeply implicated in systems of arousal, attention and emotion in adulthood, and in modulation of plasticity and growth in development. Innervation across the different brain areas by the axonal fibers of these systems terminates in patterns specific to each area of the isocortex, but the axons originate from a relatively small number of neurons in common subcortical structures (for review see Role and Kelly, 1991). Cholinergic fibers arise from the basal forebrain (nucleus basalis), norpinepherine fibers from the locus coeruleus and the lateral tegmentum, serotonin fibers from the raphe nuclei, and dopamine fibers originate in the cells of the substantia nigra and ventral tegmental area, although some connections also originate from neurons intrinsic to the cortex (Parnavelas, Kelly,

Franke and Eckenstein, 1986; Parnavelas, Moises and Speciale, 1985). During development, the long-range transmitter/modulatory systems are focused throughout the entire isocortex with the exception of the less diffuse dopamine system which focuses more specifically on limbic and prefrontal cortical regions. Unlike the precocious thalamic afferents, cholinergic and aminergic innervation begins relatively late in development, elaborating after birth, although there is some transient embryonic innervation (Dori and Parnavelas, 1989; Kalsbeek, Voorn, Buijs et al., 1988) at a time corresponding to the second trimester in humans. We really don't know what these systems are 'for' developmentally, except that disturbing them affects normal development. The whole picture of cortical development will have to include these systems in due course; we will briefly review what is known.

In rats, permanent cholinergic innervation begins around eye-opening, reaching adult levels by 1 month postnatal (Dori and Parnavelas, 1989); the serotonergic and noradrenergic timetables are similar (Lidov and Molliver, 1982). Dopamine innervation also begins postnatally but does not achieve mature patterns until full adulthood (2 months postnatal, Kalsbeek et al., 1988). Because we can reasonably conclude that the timing of this innervation, like other neural events, is conserved across species, we can extrapolate these innnervation dates to begin in the second or third trimesters of human gestation, likely extending well into the first postnatal year and, for dopamine innervation, into the adolescent years.

What might the protracted and largely postnatal innervation of these neural fibers mean to a human infant or toddler in the process of learning so many behaviors, including language? We know that these transmitters are implicated in mechanisms of arousal and reward, but that they also have multiple functions in many distributed systems, so that it is probably as unlikely in development that each transmitter will have just one function as it is in adulthood. For example, acetylcholine, a deficit of which is associated with Alzheimer's disease, can have both excitatory and inhibitory functions in the brain. Norepinephrine is conventionally believed to increase activity and attention, but it too can have inhibitory effects. Serotonin is well known for its role in abating depression, but functions vary; low levels of serotonin have been implicated in aggression and it may also be a factor in the perception of pain. The dopamine system, highly concentrated in the prefrontal cortex, is believed to participate in aspects of cognition and is also a primary factor in many drug actions, including amphetamines. It is also associated with schizophrenia and Parkinson's disease. It would seem that the progressive innervation of these substances into the developing brain is timed so that they can optimally influence learning behaviors, but much additional research will be needed to tease out a distinct role for each.

Neurochemicals and receptors. The transmitters used in the systems described above are just a small number of the chemicals that can be set in motion from the presynaptic (or launching) side of the synapse. About 20 neurotransmitters (which have rather strict classification criteria) have already been identified (glutamate and GABA are high-profile examples) and many more are under investigation. These include neuromodulatory peptides such as cholecystokinin (CCK) as well as the compound nitric oxide (NO), highly implicated in development. Upon maturity, the neural areas subserving functions associated with language will contain unique combinations of neural transmitters and modulators in distribution patterns distinctive to each area, a form of neural 'fingerprint'. Some substances arrive from cells located outside the cortex; some are synthesized 'on site.' Unlike fingerprints, however, synthesis and distributions of these neural substances change over the course of maturity (Goldman-Rakic and Brown, 1982; Hayashi, Yamashita, Shimizu and Oshima, 1989; Hornung and Fritschy, 1996) making them strong candidates for roles in development. Although much research remains to be done, it is certainly likely — given the timing of the fluctuations and combinations — that these variations in neural substances may play a functional role in maturing behaviors such as language learning.

Neural receptors are the other side of the synapse — the gating (or docking) portion of the postsynaptic complex where neurotransmitters and modulators can exert influence on the cells they contact. One developmental alteration has been consistently documented regardless of the species, the cortical area under investigation, or the related neurosubstance:

there is a dramatic overproduction of virtually every type of receptor which occurs around the time of birth (Gremo, Palomba, Marchisio et al., 1987; Herrmann, 1996; Hornung and Fritschy, 1996; Lidow, Goldman-Rakic and Rakic, 1991), similar to, and simultaneous with, the perinatal surge of synaptogenesis. The receptor surge greatly supports the notion that the perinatal burst of synapse construction described by morphological criteria produces functional synapses, since appropriate transmitters and receptor sites (which are recognized by labeling of specific proteins and amino acids and not synaptic morphology) are produced concurrently. One receptor type in particular, the *N*-methyl-D-asparate (NMDA) receptor, routinely implicated in learning and development, may actually influence formation of new synapses (Aoki, 1997; Brooks, Petit, LeBoutillier and Lo, 1991). The appearance of an NMDA subunit, as well as some other transmitter-related substances, even precedes initial phases of synaptogenesis (Aoki, 1997; Zecevic and Milosevic, 1997). Interestingly, not all receptors are located on the postsynaptic cell. Neurons also employ an apparent self-monitoring tactic; they contact themselves, so some receptors are located on the cell body of origin. Similar to the many other events we have described in the developing brain, interactions between receptor formation, neurosubstance synthesis, and synaptogenesis are likely to be more complicated than any simple cause-and-effect mechanism.

Interactions of neural events and language learning

The picture of human brain development that we have provided here leaves little room for a lockstep table of correlates between language milestones and neural events, but it does provide some useful constraints on how we should conceive of this complex bidirectional relationship, with implications for both normal and abnormal development. In an effort to integrate these ideas about neural development with the behavioral events reviewed earlier in this chapter, we close with four conclusions, or better yet, four working hypotheses to guide future research in this area: (1) readiness for learning, (2) experience-driven change, (3) rethinking two specific postnatal correlates of language, and (4) sensitive periods.

Readiness for learning

There was a period in developmental psychology when the capacities of the newborn infant for perception and learning were vastly underestimated. Much-needed correctives to this misunderstanding have come in two waves: research demonstrating rich perceptual skills in the first few weeks of life (e.g. Bertenthal and Clifton, 1998; Johnson, 1998; Kellman and Banks, 1998), and research demonstrating at least some learning *in utero*, as well as a capacity for rapid learning of arbitrary statistical patterns (including language-specific phonetic details) in the first months of life. With the first wave, there was extensive speculation in the literature on infant development regarding the stock of innate knowledge that infants must possess in order to perform so well in (for example) tasks that require response to complex transformation of objects, including their disappearance and reappearance (Spelke, 1994; Spelke, Breinlinger, Macomber and Jacobson, 1992; Spelke and Newport, 1998). With the second wave, it has become increasingly evident that we have underestimated the power and speed of learning even in very young infants, forcing a revaluation of the extent to which infant performance is influenced by learning vs. innate perceptual, motor and perhaps even conceptual biases about the nature of the physical and social world (Elman and Bates, 1997; Seidenberg, 1997; Thelen and Smith, 1994, 1998). The material that we have reviewed in this chapter provides support for the idea that the infant brain is up and running at or before birth. The fundamental scaffolding is already in place for learning, and the newborn brain is capable of enough thalamocortical and intracortical communication to permit the acquisition of distributed patterns within and across modalities (e.g. visual–auditory mapping, visual–tactile mapping, auditory–motor mapping, and so forth). Nor do we see any evidence for the hypothesis that whole bounded regions of the brain are 'pre-functional', quiescent, inactive, waiting for some key maturational event before they can 'turn on' in the postnatal period.

Of course the newborn still has a lot to learn. It will take weeks or months before she has cracked the speech code for her particular language, and even longer before that code can be mapped in a systematic and productive way to extract and express meaning. Postnatal changes in the brain may make learning more efficient (or less efficient, see *Sensitive periods*, below), and these events will certainly have computational consequences for the kinds of learning and reasoning that the child can carry out. But the capacity for learning is there from the beginning of postnatal life. Future studies of brain and behavioral development may want to focus on postnatal changes in neuroanatomy and neurophysiology as they relate to the nature and efficiency of language learning and language use, including the kinds of planning the child can carry out, and the amount and kinds of memory and attention that a child can deploy in a given task. All the relevant neural systems may be in place and ready to work from the beginning, but that does not mean that they are being used in an adult manner, nor that they are being used in all the tasks for which they will eventually be relevant. An area may 'turn on' at some point in postnatal development not because it has finally attained the necessary wiring, or the necessary ratio of neurochemicals, but because the child has finally figured out how that area can and should be employed within a given task. A reorganization in the way that the brain is used (as a result of learning) is not the same thing as a reorganization that is caused by the sudden appearance of a new player. Most classic 'insight' experiments make this assumption; if a chimpanzee seems to stack boxes to get bananas, it is not usually assumed a new box-stacking–banana area has suddenly turned on, but, rather, that existing elements have been recombined to solve the task. In language development, we might ask how such a process could occur at a non-conscious level. Recent neural imaging studies of human adults have shown that the configuration of highly active areas changes markedly across a 20-min period as the subject attains expertise in a new task (Petersen, Van Mier, Fiez and Raichle, 1998). If that is true for mature and sophisticated adults, over a very short period of time, it will undoubtedly prove true for children who are in the process of acquiring language for the first time.

Experience-driven changes

It is now clear that learning itself contributes to the structure of the developing brain, in infants and in adults. Any number of studies have shown that various aspects of the experience presented to an animal will profoundly alter the time course of synapse elimination, and that experience will also produce increases in synapse numbers (although it does not seem to affect the first fast phase of synaptogenesis, which appears to be locked in to coincide with birth). Particular clear examples of an experience-dependent increase can be found in a series of experiments by Greenough and colleagues examining the effects of enriched housing and/or skill learning on morphological changes in rodent brain. These studies have consistently documented significant increases in dendritic fields and in the ratio of synapses per neurons in rats exposed to complex environments or involved in learning tasks when measured against handled controls (Black, Isaacs, Anderson et al., 1990; Greenough, Hwang and Gorman, 1985; Turner and Greenough, 1985). Experience-based synaptogenesis is also accompanied by increases in populations of supporting cells such as astrocytes and oligodendrocytes (Sirevaag and Greenough, 1987), as well as by increases in metabolic activity as measured by mitochondria volume (Sirevaag and Greenough, 1987) and vasculature branching (Sirevaag, Black, Shafron and Greenough, 1988). We may reasonably conclude that similar reactive neural changes accompany learning in the developing human brain — indeed, although existing human data must be interpreted with caution, post mortem analysis of human adult brains indicates a correlation between high levels of education and increased dendritic branching in Wernicke's area (Jacobs, Schall and Scheibel, 1993).

Hence, if we do eventually find evidence for neuroanatomical and neurophysiological events that correlate with milestones in language development, we must be open to the possibility that these correlations are the product rather than the cause of language learning. In the same vein, if we find evidence of neuroanatomical and/or neurophysiological differences between children who are developing normally and children who are substantially delayed in language learning, we should not assume that this neural indicator has caused a language delay. It is equally possible (in the absence of evidence to the contrary) that a particular neural correlate of language impairment reflects the behavioral state of the system. That is, the brain may still be in a relatively immature state because the relevant experience-driven events have not yet taken place. This insight certainly applies to the burgeoning literature on neural correlates of Specific Language Impairment and/or congenital dyslexia, and it may apply to other disorders as well.

Rethinking two postnatal correlates of language

In our earlier review of early language development and its neural correlates, we underscored two potentially interesting postnatal correlates of major language milestones: changes in frontal lobe activity that seemed to coincide with the 8–10-month watershed in comprehension, communication, imitation and reasoning, and changes in synaptic density that seemed to coincide with bursts in vocabulary and grammar between 16 and 30 months. We would now like to put these correlates in a different light.

The idea that behavioral events late in the first year of life are correlated with changes in frontal lobe function rested primarily on two sources of evidence. The first (cited earlier) is a positron emission study (PET) of human infants suggesting that there is a marked increase in frontal lobe metabolism starting between 9 and 12 months postnatal age (Chugani, Phelps and Mazziotta, 1987). Because these studies were taken in a resting state (when infants were sedated or asleep), and not in response to any particular stimulus or task, Chugani suggested that the sharp increase in glucose metabolism might be caused by a burst in synaptogenesis of the sort postulated by Huttenlocher and Rakic, reflecting a structure-to-function gradient (i.e. more synapses = more glucose metabolism). The second source of evidence comes from lesion studies showing that infant monkeys with bilateral frontal lobe lesions behave very much like age-matched normal controls until a critical point in development (roughly equivalent to 8–12 months in postnatal human life) when normal animals learn to solve short-term memory tasks that are failed by the lesioned animals and by adults with frontal lobe pathology (Diamond and Goldman-Rakic, 1989; Goldman-Rakic, 1987; Pennington, 1994). Findings like these have led to the hypothesis that the frontal lobes 'come on line' around 9 months of age, coinciding in humans with dramatic changes in many aspects of language, cognition and social interaction. However, it now seems very clear that the frontal lobes are functional (though still immature) by the end of the second trimester, and may actually be *more* mature than other areas in terms of their intracortical connectivity.

How can we reconcile these apparently contradictory claims? The resolution may lie in the difference between *absolute functionality* (i.e. whether or not an area is working at all) and *task-specific functionality* (i.e. whether the organism has reached a state in which that area is recruited and activated for a given task). Evidence for the latter view comes from another finding by Jacobs, Chugani and colleagues (Jacobs, Chugani, Allada et al., 1995), a positron emission tomography study of infant monkeys that shows high levels of frontal lobe metabolism at birth, well before the point at which monkeys solve the short-term memory tasks that have been associated with frontal lobe function. These authors do find a further increase in metabolism later on, in many regions of the brain including the frontal lobes, compatible with the idea that metabolism and synaptogenesis increase together after birth. However, the amount of activity seen in the frontal lobes of newborn monkeys is not compatible with the standard view that frontal lobes develop especially late. If Goldman-Rakic's classic findings are not 'caused' by the sudden appearance of mature frontal cortex, how can we explain the sudden relevance of frontal lesions for memory tasks around the human equivalent of 8–10 months of postnatal age? We suggest that these results can be reinterpreted within the bidirectional framework that we have recommended here, in which areas are *recruited* into complex tasks across the course of learning. On this argument, normal infants (humans and monkeys) cannot succeed in so-called frontal lobe tasks until they have made enough progress (perceptual, motor, mnemonic) to realize that a new set of strategies is required — strategies that are, in turn, only possible with the involvement of the frontal lobes. We tentatively suggest that the 8–10-month behavioral watershed in human infants may involve a learning-dependent change in social and cognitive systems that have developed in parallel because they began in parallel (at or before birth), are roughly similar in complexity, and may also be in communication with each other. As a result, all of these systems reach a certain critical level of organization around the same time (approximately 8–10 months). At this point, in each of these behavioral domains, frontal lobe regions that are particularly well suited for short-term memory and planning are recruited. Individuals with damage to the relevant frontal regions may be at a significant disadvantage at this point (particularly if the lesions are bilateral), resulting either in developmental arrest or in a significant slowing of progress in language, cognition and communication.

The hypothesized parallel between synaptogenesis and the correlated burst in vocabulary and grammar that are observed from 16–30 months requires more recharacterization still. It is now reasonably clear that the initial burst in synaptogenesis itself is independent of experience, arranged to coincide with the barrage of experience that will arrive at birth. Debates about the timing and location of the peak (or peaks) in synaptogenesis might continue to rage, but they are based on too few samples for us to reach any kind of empirical resolution. Predictions based on cross-species modelling suggest that the human peak is probably reached around 6 months after birth, holding at a plateau for an undetermined period of time and declining slowly into the second decade of life. At this point, that is about all that we can say about this particular set of events. It is intriguing that the peak and plateau of synaptogenesis in humans brackets the primary events in early language development (from word comprehension at 8 months to the mastery of fundamental aspects of grammar, including complex syntax, by 3–4 years). Whether the perinatal burst of synaptogenesis represents an uninstructed, generic set of neural possibilities, such as a neural net set up with random connections, or a richly patterned, prescriptive set of connections, we simply do not know at this point — the reader is asked to project his/her own biases onto this reasonably neutral fact.

Is there any possibility that we should rule out? In our view, it would be wise to rule out the idea that the 'vocabulary burst' and the 'grammar burst' depend entirely on synaptogenesis for their shape and size, because such bursts are also observed when learning occurs in a non-linear dynamical system with a stable architecture (Elman et al., 1996). Such exponential bursts are characteristic of learning, and are observed whether or not they are superimposed on a burgeoning brain. Hence the compelling parallel between the 'language burst' and the 'synapse burst' may represent a mutually beneficial relationship, but not a crucial and direct relationship of cause and effect.

Sensitive periods

The term 'sensitive period' is preferred by neurobiologists over the widely used and widely misunderstood term 'critical period', because the former term implies a softer and more plastic set of developmental constraints and transitions. The term 'critical period' is still used in the literature on language development, and it is often used to imply hard boundaries and a crisp dissociation in the mechanisms that are responsible for language learning in children vs. adults (for discussions, see Bates, 1999; Bialystok and Hakuta, 1994; Elman et al., 1996; Johnson and Newport, 1989; Oyama, 1992; Weber-Fox and Neville, 1996). The notion of a critical period for language has been invoked to explain differences between first- and second-language learning, and to account for age-related changes in recovery of language abilities following left-hemisphere injury. It has been shown that adults and children perform at similar levels in the early stages of second-language learning when learning conditions are controlled (Snow and Hoefnagel-Hohle, 1978). The one compelling exception to this general rule is the ability to learn a second language without an accent, which seems to elude all but a very rare subgroup of talented adults. However, studies that focus on the later stages of language learning have shown that adults tend to 'fossilize' at a level below native speakers, while children generally go on to acquire full competence (Johnson and Newport, 1989). Results like these provide support for the idea that there is an age-related decrease in plasticity for language learning, but there is no consensus about the shape of this function or its cause. For one thing, the shape of the drop-off in second-language learning seems to vary markedly depending on the aspect of language that is measured (with declines that start in periods varying from 2 years of age to late adulthood). This is true not only across domains (e.g. an earlier decline for accent-free phonetic production than for various measures of grammar), but within domains as well (e.g. a different age-related decline for each and every rule of the grammar, Johnson and Newport, 1989). Results like these have led many investigators to conclude that there is no 'single moment' when the window of linguistic opportunity slams shut, but rather, a series of gradients that vary with task difficulty and other poorly understood parameters.

A similar story has emerged for the age-related decline in recovery from unilateral brain injury. For example, Goodman and Yude, 1996 (see also Bates et al., 1999) have compared performance on verbal and non-verbal IQ tests for adults who suffered from unilateral injuries to the right or left hemisphere at different points from birth to adolescence. To their surprise, both of their outcome measures showed a significant U-shaped relationship to age of lesion onset: the worst outcomes were observed in patients whose lesions occurred between 1 and 5 years of age; for patients with congenital lesions and for patients whose lesions occurred between approximately 6 and 12 years, verbal and non-verbal IQ were both within the low-normal range. This kind of non-monotonic relationship between age and outcome is not predicted by anybody's theory of critical periods.

Does the literature on brain development shed light on this issue? In the well-studied primate visual system, multiple overlapping sensitive periods have been identified (Harwerth, Smith, Duncan et al., 1986) and it is likely that human language acquisition is affected by similar complex receptive intervals. Although these learning periods were once thought to be fixed in time, it is now clear that the temporal windows when adequate experience is necessary for proper development are more flexible than previously assumed, and may be retarded or advanced by natural or empirical means. For example, the sensitive vocal learning period for songbirds can be extended or delayed by environmental factors (Kroodsma and Pickert, 1980). Songbirds that hatch in the beginning of the summer normally learn their songs in a restricted 2–3-month period following birth, during which they are exposed to a number of adult song types and long daylight hours, but birds born late in the summer experience shorter daylight periods and greatly reduced song-learning opportunities. Kroodsma found that a reduction of either the length of the photoperiod or the amount of song exposure could delay the critical song-learning period — adaptively, the delay lasts until the following spring when the later-born birds have another opportunity to learn adult songs. Sensitive periods in mammals are also affected by activity; dark-rearing will extend visual sensitive periods in cats (Stryker and Harris, 1986).

Links between cortical architecture and plasticity during these sensitive periods have been tested in mammalian cortex by Shatz and colleagues who investigated the distribution patterns of the NMDA R1 subunit, which varies during normal visual cortical development in correlation with the periods of axonal growth that form ocular dominance columns (Catalano, Chang and Shatz, 1997). Interestingly, visual deprivation through dark-rearing did not alter the developmental time course or normal laminar distribution pattern of the NMDA R1 subunit in visual, auditory or somatosensory cortices. The failure of visual experience to modify the normal time course of this receptor is similar to the synaptogenesis surge that is also unaffected by lack of visual experience (Bourgeois and Rakic, 1996). However, when all visual activity was blocked with the sodium channel blocker tetrodotoxin (dark-rearing does not block spontaneous firing of retinal ganglion cells), the distribution of the NMDA R1 subunit was drastically altered, implying that activity during sensitive periods is related to underlying physical changes in the developing neural architecture.

We must also be prepared for the possibility that learning itself affects the subsequent ability of the brain to learn something new. We noted that infants have developed a preference for the vowel contrasts in their language by 6 months of age; around 10 months of age, they start to suppress phonemic contrasts that are not in their native language. In order for the child to 'tune in' to the contrasts that she will need, it seems that she must 'tune out' contrasts that play no clear predictive role. We know that a similar process is played out on the neural level: like inputs are sorted together, unlike inputs are pushed apart, and unsuccessful connections are eliminated or drafted into some other task. Now, consider the following statistics: assuming a taciturn family in which an English-speaking child hears approximately 5 hours of speech input per day (from himself or others), at a mean rate of 225 words per minute, the average 10-year-old child has heard 1,034,775,000 English phonemes (at an average of 25,869, 375 trials per phoneme). She has heard just under 250 million words (including 17,246,250 renditions of the most common function word) and 28 million sentences, with more than 6 million past-tense verbs and 12 million plural nouns. In short, she has had many opportunities to entrench the most frequent elements of her native language. The numbers double by 20 years of age (assuming this child does not develop a predilection for the telephone during adolescence). Under these conditions, we should not be surprised that it is hard to reorient the entire system and acquire a similar level of competence in a second language. Brain maturation affects experience, but experience returns the favor, altering the very structure of the brain. Hence the putative critical period for language (which really comprises many overlapping sensitive periods) may be one more example of the bidirectional events that have been the focus of this chapter.

The search for a neuroanatomical basis for language learning has, at this time, no unequivocal conclusion. We have noted here some neural developmental alterations that accompany language milestones. These neural events may drive, or alternatively, reflect developmental behaviors such as language learning — although the complexity of the interactions remains to be researched. What is clear is that timetables for human neural developmental events cannot be simply mapped onto sequences of language acquisition and production. As depicted schematically in Fig. 5, the human brain develops as an overlapping and interconnected series of multimodal additive and regressive neural events, many of which are completed prior to birth. Although certain cortical events, especially developmental modifications in the numbers, components, and locations of synapses, may contribute somewhat more directly, all pre- and post-natal events should perhaps be considered essential to the language-learning process.

Acknowledgements

Support for Elizabeth Bates and Donna Thal was provided by NIH/NINDS P50 NS22343 (Center for the Study of the Neurological Basis of Language and Learning), NIH/NIDCD Program Project P50 DC01289–0351 (Origins of Communication Disorders), by RO1 DC00216 to Elizabeth Bates, and by RO1 DC00482 to Donna Thal. Support for Barbara Finlay was provided by NIH Grant R01 19245 and NSF/INT grant 96–04599, and for Barbara Clancy by NIMH postdoctoral research fellowship T32 MN19389.

References

Adelsberger-Mangan DM, Levy WB: Adaptive synaptogenesis constructs networks that maintain information and reduce statistical dependence. Biological Cybernetics: 70(1); 81–87, 1993.

Adelsberger-Mangan DM, Levy WB: The influence of limited presynaptic growth and synapse removal on adaptive synaptogenesis. Biological Cybernetics: 71(5); 461–468, 1994.

Allopenna PD, Magnuson JS, Tanenhaus MK: Tracking the time course of spoken word recognition using eye movements: Evidence for continuous mapping models. Journal of Memory and Language: 38; 419–439, 1998.

Altman J, Bayer SA: Development of the diencephalon in the rat. IV. Quantitative study of the time of origin of neurons and the internuclear chronological gradients in the thalamus. Journal of Comparative Neurology: 188(3); 455–471, 1979a.

Altman J, Bayer SA: Development of the diencephalon in the rat. VI. Re-evaluation of the embryonic development of the thalamus on the basis of thymidine- radiographic datings. Journal of Comparative Neurology: 188(3); 501–524, 1979b.

Altman J, Bayer SA: Development of the rat thalamus: II. Time and site of origin and settling pattern of neurons derived from the anterior lobule of the thalamic neuroepithelium. Journal of Comparative Neurology: 275(3); 378–405, 1988.

Altmann GTM, Van Nice KY, Garnham A, Henstra J-A: Late closure in context. Journal of Memory and Language: 38; 459–484, 1998.

Antonini A, Shatz CJ: Relationship between putative neurotransmitter phenotypes and connectivity of subplate neurons during cerebral cortical development. European Journal of Neuroscience: 2; 744–761, 1990.

Aoki C: Postnatal changes in the laminar and subcellular distribution of NMDA-R1 subunits in the cat visual cortex as revealed by immuno-electron microscopy. Developmental Brain Research: 98(1); 41–59, 1997.

Aram D: Language sequelae of unilateral brain lesions in children. In Plum F (Ed), Language, Communication, and the Brain. New York: Raven Press, 1988.

Aram D, Ekelman B, Rose D, Whitaker H: Verbal and cognitive sequelae following unilateral lesions acquired in early childhood. Journal of Clinical and Experimental Neuropsychology: 7; 55–78, 1985.

Aram D, Ekelman B, Whitaker H: Lexical retrieval in left and right brain-lesioned children. Brain and Language: 28; 61–87, 1985.

Aslin RN, Jusczyk PW, Pisoni DB: Speech and auditory processing during infancy: Constraints on and precursors to language. In Damon W (Series Ed) and Kuhn D, Siegler R (Vol. Eds), Handbook of Child Psychology: Vol. 2 Cognition, Perception and Language, 5th ed. New York: Wiley, pp. 147–198, 1998.

Au T, Dapretto M, Song Y-K: Input vs. constraints: Early word acquisition in Korean and English. Journal of Memory and Language: 33(5); 567–582, 1994.

Baillargeon R, Graber M: Evidence of location memory in 8-month-old infants in a nonsearch AB task. Developmental Psychology: 24(4); 502–511, 1988.

Bamberg MGW: Form and Function in the Construction of Narratives: Developmental Perspectives. Berlin: Mouton de Gruyter, 1988.

Baron-Cohen S, Riviere A, Fukushima M, French D et al.: Reading the mind in the face: A cross-cultural and developmental study. Visual Cognition: 3(1); 39–59, 1996.

Basser L: Hemiplegia of early onset and the faculty of speech with special reference to the effects of hemispherectomy. Brain: 85; 427–460, 1962.

Bauer PJ, Hertsgaard LA: Increasing steps in recall of events: Factors facilitating immediate and long-term memory in 13.5-month-old and 16.5-month-old children. Child Development: 4(10); 443–450, 1993.

Bauer PJ, Wewerka SS: One- to two-year-olds recall of events: The more expressed, the more impressed. Journal of Experimental Child Psychology: 59(3); 475–469, 1995.

Bates E: Language and Context: Studies in the Acquisition of Pragmatics. New York: Academic Press, 1976.

Bates E (Ed): Special issue: Cross-linguistic studies of aphasia. Brain and Language: 41(2); 1991.

Bates E: Plasticity, localization and language development. In Broman S, Fletcher JM (Eds), The Changing Nervous System: Neurobehavioral Consequences of Early Brain Disorders. New York: Oxford University Press, pp. 214–253, 1999.

Bates E, Benigni L, Bretherton I, Camaioni L, Volterra V: The Emergence of Symbols: Cognition and Communication in Infancy. New York: Academic Press, 1979.

Bates E, Bretherton I, Snyder L: From First words to Grammar: Individual Differences and Dissociable mechanisms. New York: Cambridge University Press, 1988.

Bates E, Camaioni L, Volterra V: The acquisition of performatives prior to speech. Merrill-Palmer Quarterly: 21; 205–226, 1975.

Bates E, Dale P, Thal D: Individual differences and their implications for theories of language development. In Fletcher P, MacWhinney B (Eds), Handbook of Child Language. Oxford: Blackwell, 1995.

Bates E, Devescovi A: A cross-linguistic approach to sentence production. In MacWhinney B, Bates E (Eds), The Crosslinguistic Study of Sentence Processing. New York: Cambridge University Press, pp. 225–256, 1989.

Bates E, Elman J: Learning rediscovered. Science: 274; 1849–1850, 1996.

Bates E, Goodman J: On the inseparability of grammar and the lexicon: Evidence from acquisition, aphasia and real-time processing. Language and Cognitive Processes: 12(5/6); 507–586, 1997.

Bates E, MacWhinney B: Functionalism and the competition model. In MacWhinney B, Bates E (Eds), The Crosslinguistic Study of Sentence Processing. New York: Cambridge University Press, 1989.

Bates E, Marchman V: What is and is not universal in language acquisition. In Plum F (Ed), Language, Communication and the Brain. New York: Raven Press, 1988.

Bates E, McDonald J, MacWhinney B, Appelbaum M: Maximum likelihood procedures for group and individual data in aphasia research. Brain and Language: 40; 231–265, 1991.

Bates E, O'Connell B, Shore C: Language and communication in infancy. In Osofsky J (Ed), Handbook of Infant Development, 2nd ed. New York: Wiley and Sons, 1987.

Bates E, Snyder L: The cognitive hypothesis in language development. In Uzgiris I, McV. Hunt J (Eds), Research with Scales of Psychological Development in Infancy. Champaign-Urbana: University of Illinois Press, 1987.

Bates E, Thal D: Associations and dissociations in child language development. In Miller J (Ed), Research on Child Language Disorders: A Decade of Progress. Austin, TX: Pro-Ed, 1991.

Bates E, Thal D, Janowsky J: Early language development and its neural correlates. In Segalowitz S, Rapin I (Eds), Handbook of Neuropsychology, Vol. 7: Child Neuropsychology. Amsterdam: Elsevier, pp. 69–110, 1992.

Bates E, Thal D, Marchman V: Symbols and syntax: A Darwinian approach to language development. In Krasnegor N, Rumbaugh D, Schiefelbusch R, Studdert-Kennedy M (Eds), Biological and Behavioral Determinants of Language Development. Hillsdale, NJ: Erlbaum, pp. 29–65, 1991.

Bates E, Thal D, Trauner D, Fenson J, Aram D, Eisele J, Nass, R: From first words to grammar in children with focal brain injury. In Thal D, Reilly J, (Eds), Developmental Neuropsychology: 13(3); 447–476, 1997.

Bates E, Thal D, Whitesell K, Fenson L, Oakes L: Integrating language and gesture in infancy. Developmental Psychology: 25(6); 1004–1019, 1989.

Bates E, Vicari S, Trauner D: Neural mediation of language development: Perspectives from lesion studies of infants and children. In Tager-Flusberg H (Ed), Neurodevelopmental Disorders. Cambridge, MA: MIT Press, pp. 533–581, 1999.

Bates E, Wulfeck B: Comparative aphasiology: A cross-linguistic approach to language breakdown. Aphasiology: 3; 111–142 and 161–168, 1989.

Bauer P, Hertsgaard L, Dropik P, Daly B: When even arbitrary order becomes important: developments in reliable temporal sequencing of arbitrarily ordered events. Memory: 6(2); 165–198, 1998.

Bayer SA: Changes in the total number of dentate granule cells in juvenile and adult rats: a correlated volumetric and 3H-thymidine autoradiographic study. Experimental Brain Research: 46(3); 315–323, 1982.

Bayer SA: 3H-thymidine-radiographic studies of neurogenesis in the rat olfactory bulb. Experimental Brain Research: 50(2–3); 329–340, 1983.

Bayer SA, Altman J, Russo RJ, Zhang X: Timetables of neurogenesis in the human brain based on experimentally determined patterns in the rat. Neurotoxicology: 14(1); 83–144, 1993.

Beeghly M, Cicchetti D: An organizational approach to symbolic development in children with Down syndrome. In Cicchetti D, Beeghly M (Eds), Atypical Symbolic Development. San Francisco: Jossey-Bass, 1987.

Benedict H: Early lexical development: Comprehension and production. Journal of Child Language: 6; 183–200, 1979.

Berman RA, Slobin DI: Relating Events in Narrative: A Crosslinguistic Developmental Study [in collaboration with Ayhan Aksu-Koc et al.]. Hillsdale, NJ: Erlbaum, 1994.

Bertenthal BI, Campos JJ, Haith MM: Development of visual organization: The perception of subjective contours. Child Development: 51; 1072–1080, 1980.

Bertenthal BI, Clifton RK: Perception and action. In Damon W (Series Ed.) and Kuhn D, Siegler R (Vol. Eds), Handbook of Child Psychology: Vol. 2. Cognition, Perception and Language, 5th ed. New York: Wiley, pp. 51–102, 1998.

Bertenthal BI, Proffitt DR, Spetner NB, Thomas MA: The development of infant sensitivity to biomechanical motions. Child Development: 56; 531–543, 1985.

Bialystok E, Hakuta K: In Other Words: The Science and Psychology of Second-Language Acquisition. New York: BasicBooks, 1994.

Bickerton D: The Roots of Language. Ann Arbor, MI: Karoma, 1981.

Birner BJ, Ward G: Information Status and Noncanonical Word order in English. Amsterdam; Philadelphia: J. Benjamins, 1998.

Bishop D: The underlying nature of specific language impairment. Journal of Child Psychology and Psychiatry: 33; 3–66, 1992.

Bishop D: Grammatical errors in specific language impairment: Competence or performance limitations? Applied Psycholinguistics: 15; 507–550, 1994.

Bishop D: Uncommon Understanding: Development and Disorders of Comprehension in Children. Hove, UK: Psychology Press, 1997.

Bishop D, Mogford K. (Eds) : Language Development in Exceptional Circumstances. Hillsdale, NJ: Erlbaum, 1993.

Black JE, Isaacs KR, Anderson BJ, Alcantara AA, Greenough WT: Learning causes synaptogenesis, whereas motor activity causes angiogenesis, in cerebellar cortex of adult rats. Proceedings of the National Academy of Sciences USA: 87(14); 5568–5572, 1990.

Blackwell A, Bates E: Inducing agrammatic profiles in normals: Evidence for the selective vulnerability of morphology under cognitive resource limitation. Journal of Cognitive Neuroscience: 7(2); 228–257, 1995.

Bloom L, Lightbown L, Hood L: Structure and variation in child language. Monographs for the Society for Research in Child Development: 40; Serial #160, 1975.

Blue ME, Parnavelas JG: The formation and maturation of synapses in the visual cortex of the rat. I. Qualitative analysis. Journal of Neurocytology: 12(4); 599–616, 1983.

Blumstein SE, Stevens KN: Phonetic features and acoustic invariance in speech. Cognition: 10 (1-sup-3); 25–32, 1981.

Bourgeois JP: Synaptogenesis, heterochrony and epigenesis in the mammalian neocortex. Acta Paediatrica Supplement: 422; 27–33, 1997.

Bourgeois JP, Goldman-Rakic PS, Rakic P: Synaptogenesis in the prefrontal cortex of rhesus monkeys. Cerebral Cortex: 4(1); 78–96, 1994.

Bourgeois JP, Jastreboff PJ, Rakic P: Synaptogenesis in visual cortex of normal and preterm monkeys: Evidence for intrinsic regulation of synaptic overproduction. Proceedings of the National Academy of Sciences USA: 86(11); 4297–4301, 1989.

Bourgeois JP, Rakic P: Changes of synaptic density in the primary visual cortex of the macaque monkey from fetal to adult stage. Journal of Neuroscience: 13(7); 2801–2820, 1993.

Bourgeois JP, Rakic P: Synaptogenesis in the occipital cortex of macaque monkey devoid of retinal input from early embryonic stages. European Journal of Neuroscience: 8(5); 942–950, 1996.

Boysson-Bardies B, Sagart L, Durand C: Discernible differences in the babbling of infants according to target language. Journal of Child Language: 11; 1–15, 1984.

Bradshaw J, Nettleson N: The nature of hemispheric specialization in man. Behavioral and Brain Sciences 4: 51–91; 1981.

Braine MDS: Children's first word combinations. Monographs of the Society for Research in Child Development. Serial No. 164, Vol. 41:1, 1976.

Brand S, Rakic P: Cytodifferentiation and synaptogenesis in the neostriatum of fetal and neonatal rhesus monkeys. Anatomy and Embryology: 169(1); 21–34, 1984.

Broman S, Fletcher JM (Eds) (1999) : The Changing Nervous System: Neurobehavioral Consequences of Early Brain Disorders. New York: Oxford University Press, 1999.

Broman S, Grafman J (Eds): Atypical Cognitive Deficits in Developmental Disorders: Implications for Brain Function. Hillsdale, NJ: Erlbaum, 1994.

Brooks WJ, Petit TL, LeBoutillier JC, Lo R: Rapid alteration of synaptic number and postsynaptic thickening length by NMDA: An electron microscopic study in the occipital cortex of postnatal rats. Synapse: 8(1); 41–48, 1991.

Brown R: A First Language: The Early Stages. Cambridge, MA: Harvard University Press, 1973.

Brownell C: Combinatorial skills: Converging developments over the second year. Child Development: 59; 675–685, 1988.

Burkhalter A: Development of forward and feedback connections between areas V1 and V2 of human visual cortex. Cerebral Cortex: 3(5); 476–487, 1993.

Butterworth B: Self-perception in infancy. In Cicchetti D, Beeghly M (Eds), The Self in Transition: Infancy to Childhood. Chicago: University of Chicago Press, pp. 199–137, 1990.

Butterworth G, Harris P, Leslie A, Wellman H: Perspectives on the child's theory of mind. 2. Preface. Special issue, British Journal of Developmental Psychology: 9; 190, 1991.

Butterworth G, Jarrett N: What minds have in common is space: Spatial mechanisms serving joint visual attention in infancy. British Journal of Developmental Psychology: 9; 55–72, 1991.

Camarata S, Gandour J: Rule invention in the acquisition of morphology by a language-impaired child. Journal of Speech and Hearing Disorders: 50; 40–45, 1985.

Caplan D, Hildebrandt N: Disorders of Syntactic Comprehension. Cambridge, MA: MIT Press, 1988.

Caplan D, Waters GS: Verbal working memory and sentence comprehension. Behavioral and Brain Sciences: 22(1); 77–94, 122–126, 1999.

Caramazza A: On drawing inferences about the structure of normal cognitive systems from the analysis of patterns of impaired performance: The case for single-patient studies. Brain and Cognition: 5; 41–66, 1986.

Case R: The development of conceptual structures. In Damon W (Series Ed.) and Kuhn D, Siegler R (Vol. Eds), Handbook of Child Psychology: Vol. 2. Cognition, Perception and Language, 5th ed. New York: Wiley, pp. 745–800, 1998.

Caselli MC, Bates E, Casadio P, Fenson J, Fenson L, Sanderl L, Weir J: A cross-linguistic study of early lexical development. Cognitive Development: 10; 159–199, 1995.

Caselli MC, Casadio P, Bates E: A comparison of the transition from first words to grammar in English and Italian. Journal of Child Language: 26; 69–111, 1999.

Catalano SM, Chang CK, Shatz CJ: Activity-dependent regulation of NMDAR1 immunoreactivity in the developing visual cortex. Journal of Neuroscience: 17(21); 8376–8390, 1997.

Cauller L: Layer I of primary sensory neocortex: Where topdown converges upon bottom-up. Behavioral Brain Research: 71(1–2); 163–170, 1995.

Cepko CL: The roles of intrinsic and extrinsic cues and bHLH genes in the determination of retinal cell fates. Current Opinion in Neurobiology: 9(1); 37–46, 1999.

Chapman RS: Computing mean length of utterance in morphemes. In Miller JF (Ed), Assessing Language Production in Children: Experimental Procedures. Baltimore: University Park Press, 1981.

Chapman RS: Language development in children and adolescents with Down Syndrome. In Fletcher P, MacWhinney B (Eds), Handbook of Child Language. Oxford: Basil Blackwell, pp. 641–663, 1995.

Charman T, Baron-Cohen S: Understanding photos, models, and beliefs: A test of the modularity thesis of theory of mind. Cognitive Development: 10(2); 287–298, 1995.

Choi S, Bowerman M: Learning to express motion events in English and Korean: The influence of language-specific lexicalization patterns. Cognition: 41(1–3); 83–121, 1991.

Choi S, Gopnik S: Early acquisition of verbs in Korean: A cross-linguistic study. Journal of Child Language: 22(3); 497–525, 1995.

Chomsky N: Rules and Representations. New York: Columbia University Press, 1980.

Chomsky N: Lectures on Government and Binding. New York: Foris, 1982.

Chomsky N: Language and Problems of Knowledge: The Managua Lectures. Cambridge, MA: MIT Press, 1988.

Chomsky N: The Minimalist Program. Cambridge, MA: MIT Press, 1995.

Chugani HT, Phelps ME, Mazziotta JC: Positron emission tomography study of human brain functional development. Annals of Neurology: 22; 487–497, 1987.

Churchland PS, Ramachandran VC, Sejnowski TJ: A critique of pure vision. In Koch C, Davis JL (Eds), Large-Scale Neuronal Theories of the Brain. Cambridge, MA: MIT Press, 1994.

Cicchetti D, Carlson V (Ed): Child Maltreatment: Theory and Research on the Causes and Consequences of Child Abuse and Neglect. New York: Cambridge University Press, 1989.

Clancy B, Darlington RB, Finlay BL: Translating developmental time across mammalian species. Neuroscience: 105; 7–17, 2001.

Cohen LB, Younger BA: Perceptual categorization in the infant. In Scholnick EK (Ed), New Trends in Conceptual Representation: Challenges to Piaget's Theory? Hillsdale, NJ: Erlbaum, 1983.

Cole P (Ed): Radical Pragmatics. Cambridge University Press, 1981.

Cruttenden A: A phonetic study of babbling. British Journal of Communication: 5; 110–117, 1970.

Darlington RB, Dunlop SA, Finlay BL: Commentary: Neural development in metatherian and eutherian mammals: Variation and constraint. Journal of Comparative Neurology: 411(3); 359–368, 1999.

Deacon T: The Symbolic Species: The Co-Evolution of Language and the Brain. New York: Norton, 1997.

DeCasper AJ, Fifer WP: Of human bonding: Newborns prefer their mothers' voices. Science: 208; 1174–1176, 1980.

Dell GS, Schwartz MF, Martin N, Saffran EM, Gagnon DA: Lexical access in aphasic and nonaphasic speakers. Psychological Review: 104(4); 801–838, 1997.

Demuth K: Subject, topic and Sesotho passive. Journal of Child Language: 17; 67–84, 1989.

Dennis M, Whitaker H: Language acquisition following hemidecortication: Linguistic superiority of the left over the right hemisphere. Brain and Language: 3; 404–433, 1976.

Devescovi A, Bates E, D'Amico S, Hernandez A, Marangolo P, Pizzamiglio L, Razzano C: An on-line study of grammaticality judgments in normal and aphasic speakers of Italian. In Menn L (Ed), Special issue on cross-linguistic aphasia. Aphasiology: 11(6); 543–579, 1997.

Diamond A: Development of the ability to use recall to guide action, as indicated by infants' performance on $A^{\overline{B}}$. Child Development: 56(4); 868–883, 1985.

Diamond A, Goldman-Rakic PS: Comparison of human infants and rhesus monkeys on Piaget's AB task: Evidence for dependence on dorsolateral prefrontal cortex. Experimental Brain Research: 74; 24–40, 1989.

Dick F, Bates E, Wulfeck B, Utman J, Dronkers N: Language deficits, localization, and grammar: Evidence for a distributed model of language breakdown in aphasics and normals. Manuscript submitted for publication, 1999.

Dick F, Bates E, Wulfeck B, Dronkers N: Simulating deficits in the interpretation of complex sentences in normals under adverse processing conditions (Abstract). Brain and Language: 65(1); 57–59, 1998.

Dore J: A pragmatic description of early language development. Journal of Psycholinguistic Research: 4; 423–430, 1974.

Dori I, Parnavelas JG: The cholinergic innervation of the rat cerebral cortex shows two distinct phases in development. Experimental Brain Research: 76(2); 417–423, 1989.

Easter SS Jr, Ross LS, Frankfurter A: Initial tract formation in the mouse brain. Journal of Neuroscience: 13(1); 285–299, 1993.

Eilers R, Oller DK, Levine S, Basinger O, Lynch M, Urbano R: The role of prematurity and socioeconomic status in the onset of canonical babbling in infants. Infant Behavior and Development: 16; 297–316, 1993.

Eimas PD: The equivalence of cues for the perception of speech by infants. Infant Behavior and Development: 8; 125–138, 1985.

Eimas PD, Miller JL, Jusczyk PW: On infant speech perception and the acquisition of language. In Harnad S (Ed), Categorical Perception. New York: Cambridge University Press, 1987.

Eisele J, Aram D: Lexical and grammatical development in children with early hemisphere damage: A cross-sectional view from birth to adolescence. In Fletcher P, MacWhinney B (Eds), The Handbook of Child Language. Oxford: Basil Blackwell, pp. 664–689, 1995.

Elman JL: Finding structure in time. Cognitive Science: 14; 179–211, 1990.

Elman JL, Bates E: Letters, Science: 276; 1180, 1997.

Elman JL, Bates E, Johnson M, Karmiloff-Smith A, Parisi D, Plunkett K: Rethinking Innateness: A Connectionist Perspective on Development. Cambridge, MA: MIT Press/Bradford Books, 1996.

Elman JL, McClelland J: Interactive processes in speech perception: The TRACE model. In Rumelhart D, McClelland JL (Eds), Parallel Distributed Processing: Explorations in the Microstructure of Cognition. Cambridge, MA: MIT Press, 1986.

Escalona S: Basic modes of social interaction: Their emergence and patterning during the first two years of life. Merrill-Palmer Quarterly: 19; 205–232, 1973.

Fauconnier G: Aspects of Meaning Construction in Natural Language. Cambridge, MA: MIT Press, 1985.

Felleman DJ, Van Essen DC: Distributed hierarchical processing in the primate cerebral cortex. Cerebral Cortex: 1(1); 1–47, 1991.

Fenson L, Ramsay D: Effects of modelling action sequences on the play of twelve, fifteen, and nineteen-month-old children. Child Development: 32; 1028–1036, 1981.

Fenson L, Dale P, Reznick JS, Thal D, Bates E, Hartung J, Pethick S, Reilly J: The MacArthur Communicative Development Inventories: User's Guide and Technical Manual. San Diego: Singular Publishing Group, 1993.

Fenson L, Dale PA, Reznick JS, Bates E, Thal D, Pethick SJ: Variability in early communicative development. Monographs of the Society for Research in Child Development, Serial No. 242, Vol. 59, No. 5, 1994.

Ferguson C: From babbling to speech. Invited address to the International Conference on Infant Studies, New York, April, 1984.

Finlay BL: Cell death and the creation of regional differences in neuronal numbers. Journal of Neurobiology: 23(9); 1159–1171, 1992.

Finlay BL, Darlington RB: Linked regularities in the development and evolution of mammalian brains. Science: 268(5217); 1578–1584, 1995.

Fodor J: The Modularity of Mind. Cambridge, MA: MIT Press, 1983.

Fowler AE: Language abilities in children with Down syndrome: Evidence for a specific delay. In Cicchetti D, Beeghley M (Eds), Children with Down syndrome: A Developmental Perspective. Cambridge, UK: Cambridge University Press, pp. 302–328, 1993.

Friederici AD, Frazier L: Thematic analysis in agrammatic comprehension: Syntactic structures and task demands. Brain and Language: 42; 1–29, 1992.

Gardner H, Brownell HH, Wapner W, Michelow D: Missing the point. The role of the right hemisphere in the processing of complex linguistic materials. In Perceman E (Ed), Cognitive Processing in the Right Hemisphere. New York: Academic Press, 1983.

Gentner D: Why are nouns learned before verbs: Linguistic relativity versus natural partitioning. In Kuczaj II SA (Ed), Language Development, Vol. 2: Language, Thought and Culture. Hillsdale, NJ: Erlbaum, 1982.

Gernsbacher MA: Handbook of Psycholinguistics. San Diego: Academic Press, 1994.

Gibson EJ, Spelke ES: The development of perception. In Flavell JH, Markman EM (Eds), Cognitive Development: Vol. 3. Handbook of Child Psychology, 4th ed. New York: Wiley, 1983.

Givón T: Mind, Code and Context: Essays in Pragmatics. New York: Academic Press, 1989.

Goldberg AE: Constructions: A Construction Grammar Approach to Argument Structure. Chicago: University of Chicago Press, 1995.

Goldfield B, Reznick JS: Early lexical acquisition: Rate, content, and the vocabulary spurt. Journal of Child Language: 17(1); 171–184, 1990.

Goldman-Rakic PS: Development of cortical circuitry and cognitive function. Child Development: 58; 601–622, 1987.

Goldman-Rakic PS, Brown RM: Postnatal development of monoamine content and synthesis in the cerebral cortex of rhesus monkeys. Brain Research: 256(3); 339–349, 1982.

Goodglass H: Understanding Aphasia. San Diego: Academic Press, 1993.

Goodman JC, Bauman A: Group uniformity and individual differences in the rate and shape of language development. Society for Research in Child Development Abstracts: 10; 112, 1995.

Goodman J, Bates E, Jahn J, Appelbaum M, Elman J, Carnevale G: Early lexical development and the dynamics of change. Paper presented at the VIIIth International Congress for the Study of Child Language, San Sebastian, Spain (Basque Country), 1999, July.

Goodman R, Yude C: IQ and its predictors in childhood hemiplegia. Developmental Medicine and Child Neurology: 38; 881–890, 1996.

Gopnik A, Meltzoff AN: Words, Thoughts, and Theories. Cambridge, MA: MIT Press, 1997.

Gopnik M (Ed): The Inheritance and Innateness of Grammars. New York: Oxford University Press, 1997.

Granger B, Tekaia F, Le Sourd AM, Rakic P, Bourgeois JP: Tempo of neurogenesis and synaptogenesis in the primate cingulate mesocortex: Comparison with the neocortex. Journal of Comparative Neurology: 360(2); 363–376, 1995.

Greenough WT: Structural correlates of information storage in the mammalian brain: A review and hypothesis. Trends in Neurosciences: 7; 229–233, 1984.

Greenough WT, Hwang HM, Gorman C: Evidence for active synapse formation or altered postsynaptic metabolism in visual cortex of rats reared in complex environments. Proceedings of the National Academy of Sciences USA: 82(13); 4549–4552, 1985.

Gremo F, Palomba M, Marchisio AM, Marcello C, Mulas ML, Torelli S: Heterogeneity of muscarinic cholinergic receptors in the developing human fetal brain: Regional distribution and characterization. Early Human Development: 15(3); 165–177, 1987.

Grodzinsky Y: The neurology of syntax: language use without Broca's area. Behavorial and Brain Sciences: 23(1); 1–21, 64–71, 2000.

Grosjean F: Spoken word recognition processes and the gating paradigm. Perception and Psychophysics: 28; 267–283, 1980.

Grosjean F, Frauenfelder U (Eds): A Guide to Spoken Word Recognition Paradigms. Special issue of Language and Cognitive Processes. Hove, England: Psychology Press, 1996.

Guillery RW, Herrup K: Quantification without pontification: Choosing a method for counting objects in sectioned tissues [comment]. Journal of Comparative Neurology: 386(1); 2–7, 1997.

Haith MM: The formation of visual expectations in early infancy: How infants anticipate the future. In Rovee-Collier C (Ed), Abstracts of papers presented at the Seventh International Conference on Infant Studies. Special issue of Infant Behavior and Development, Vol. 13, p. 11. Norwood, NJ: Ablex, 1990, April.

Haith MM, Benson JB: Infant cognition. In Damon W (Series Ed.) and Kuhn D, Siegler R (Vol. Eds), Handbook of Child Psychology: Vol. 2. Cognition, Perception and Language, 5th ed. New York: Wiley, pp. 199–254, 1998.

Haith M, Benson J, Roberts R, Pennington B (Eds): The Development of Future-Oriented processes. Chicago: The University of Chicago Press, 1994.

Harris KM, Stevens JK: Dendritic spines of CA 1 pyramidal cells in the rat hippocampus: Serial electron microscopy with reference to their biophysical characteristics. Journal of Neuroscience: 9(8); 2982–2997, 1989.

Harris PL: Infant cognition. In Haith MM, Campos JJ (Eds), Infancy and the Biology of Development: Vol. 2. Handbook of Child Psychology. New York: Wiley, 1983.

Hart B, Risley T: Meaningful Differences in the Everyday Experience of Young American Children. Baltimore, MD: Brookes, 1995.

Harwerth RS, Smith EL, Duncan GC, Crawford ML, Von Noorden GK: Multiple sensitive periods in the development of the primate visual system. Science: 232(4747); 235–238, 1986.

Hayashi M, Yamashita A, Shimizu K, Oshima K: Ontogeny of cholecystokinin-8 and glutamic acid decarboxylase in cerebral neocortex of macaque monkey. Experimental Brain Research: 74(2); 249–255, 1989.

Head H: Aphasia and Kindred Disorders of Speech. Cambridge: Cambridge University Press, 1926.

Herrmann K: Differential distribution of AMPA receptors and glutamate during pre- and postnatal development in the visual cortex of ferrets. Journal of Comparative Neurology: 375(1); 1–17, 1996.

Hirsh-Pasek K, Kemler Nelson D, Jusczyk PW, Cassidy K, Druss B, Kennedy L: Clauses are perceptual units for young infants. Cognition: 26; 269–286, 1987.

Honig LS, Herrmann K, Shatz CJ: Developmental changes revealed by immunohistochemical markers in human cerebral cortex. Cerebral Cortex: 6(6); 794–806, 1996.

Horgan D: Nouns: Love 'em or leave 'em. Address to the New York Academy of Sciences, 1979, May.

Horgan D: Rate of language acquisition and noun emphasis. Journal of Psycholinguistic Research: 10; 629–640, 1981.

Hornung JP, Fritschy JM: Developmental profile of GABAA-receptors in the marmoset monkey: Expression of distinct subtypes in pre- and postnatal brain. Journal of Comparative Neurology: 367(3); 413–430, 1996.

Huttenlocher PR, Dabholkar AS: Regional differences in synaptogenesis in human cerebral cortex. Journal of Comparative Neurology: 387(2); 167–178, 1997.

Innocenti GM: The development of projections from cerebral cortex. Progress in Sensory Physiology: 12; 65–114, 1991.

Innocenti GM: Exuberant development of connections, and its possible permissive role in cortical evolution. Trends in Neurosciences: 18(9); 397–402, 1995.

Iverson J, Thal D: Communicative transitions: There's more to the hand than meets the eye. In Weatherby A, Warren S, Reichle J (Eds), Transitions in Prelinguistic Communication: Pre-Intentional to Intentional and Pre-Symbolic to Symbolic. Baltimore: Brookes, 1997.

Jackendoff RS: Semantics and Cognition. Cambridge, MA: MIT Press, 1983.

Jacobs B, Chugani HT, Allada V, Chen S, Phelps ME, Pollack DB, Raleigh MJ: Developmental changes in brain metabolism in sedated rhesus macaques and vervet monkeys revealed by positon emission tomography. Cerebral Cortex: 3; 222–233, 1995.

Jacobs B, Schall M, Scheibel AB: A quantitative dendritic analysis of Wernicke's area in humans. II. Gender, hemispheric, and environmental factors. Journal of Comparative Neurology: 327(1); 97–111, 1993.

Jahn-Samilo J, Goodman JC, Bates E, Appelbaum M, Sweet M: Vocabulary learning in children from 8 to 30 months of age: A comparison of parental report and laboratory measures. Project in Cognitive and Neural Development Technical Report #00-06. La Jolla: University of California, San Diego, 2000.

Jakobson R: Child Language Aphasia and Phonological Universals. Paris: Mouton, 1968.

Jakobson R, Fant C, Gunnar M, Halle M: Preliminaries to speech analysis: The distinctive features and their correlates (Tech. Rep. No. 13). Acoustics Laboratory, Massachusetts Institute of Technology, Cambridge, MA, viii, 58 pp, 1952.

Johnson J, Newport E: Critical period effects in second language learning: the influence of maturational state on the acquisition of English as a second language. Cognitive Psychology: 21; 60–99, 1989.

Johnson MH: The neural basis of cognitive development. In

Damon W (Series Ed.) and Kuhn D, Siegler R (Vol. Eds), Handbook of Child Psychology: Vol. 2 Cognition, Perception and Language, 5th ed. New York: Wiley, pp. 1–50, 1998.

Johnston JR, Kamhi AG: Syntactic and semantic aspects of the utterances of language-impaired children: The same can be less. Merrill-Palmer Quarterly: 30; 65–85, 1984.

Jones TA, Klintsova AY, Kilman VL, Sirevaag AM, Greenough WT: Induction of multiple synapses by experience in the visual cortex of adult rats. Neurobiology and Learning Memory: 68(1); 13–20, 1997.

Jusczyk PW: Finding and remembering words: Some beginnings by English-learning infants. Current Directions in Psychological Science: 6(6); 170–174, 1997.

Jusczyk PW, Friederici AD, Wessels JMI, Svenkerud V, Jusczyk AM: Infants' sensitivity to the sound pattern of native-language words. Journal of Memory and Language: 32; 402–420, 1993.

Jusczyk PW, Houston DM: The beginnings of word segmentation in English-learning infants. Cognitive Psychology: 39(3-4-); 159–207, 1999.

Kalsbeek A, Voorn P, Buijs RM, Pool CW, Uylings HB: Development of the dopaminergic innervation in the prefrontal cortex of the rat. Journal of Comparative Neurology: 269(1); 58–72, 1988.

Kandel ER, Schwartz JH, Jessell TM: Principles of Neural Science (3rd ed.). Norwalk, CT: Appleton and Lange, 1991.

Karmiloff-Smith A: A Functional Approach to Child Language. Cambridge University Press, 1979.

Kean ML (Ed): Agrammatism. New York: Academic Press, 1985.

Kellman PJ, Banks MS: Infant visual perception. In Damon W (Series Ed.) and Kuhn D, Siegler R (Vol. Eds), Handbook of Child Psychology: Vol. 2 Cognition, Perception and Language, 5th ed. New York: Wiley, pp. 103–146, 1998.

Kempermann G, Brandon E, Gage F: Environmental stimulation of 129/SvJ mice causes increased cell proliferation and neurogenesis in the adult dentate gyrus. Current Biology: 8; 939–942, 1998.

Kent RD, Miolo G: Phonetic abilities in the first year of life. In Fletcher P, MacWhinney B (Eds), Handbook of Child language. Oxford: Basil Blackwell, pp. 303–334, 1995.

Kent RD, Weismer G, Kent JF, Vorperian HK, Duffy JR: Acoustic studies of dysarthric speech: Methods, progress, and potential. Journal of Communication Disorders: 32(3); 141–186, 1999.

Kessel F (Ed): The Development of Language and Language Researchers: Essays in Honor of Roger Brown. Hillsdale, NJ: Erlbaum, 1988.

Kilborn K: Selective impairment of grammatical morphology due to induced stress in normal listeners: Implications for aphasia. Brain and Language: 41; 275–288, 1991.

Kleim JA, Lussnig E, Schwarz ER, Comery TA, Greenough WT: Synaptogenesis and Fos expression in the motor cortex of the adult rat following motor skill learning. Journal of Neuroscience: 16; 4529–4535, 1996.

Kleim JA, Swain RA, Czerlanis CM, Kelly JL, Pipitone MA, Greenough WT: Learning-dependent dendritic hypertrophy of cerebellarstellate neurons: Plasticity of local circuit neurons. Neurobiology of Learning and Memory: 67; 29–33, 1997.

Koch C, Davis JL: Large-Scale Neuronal Theories of the Brain. Cambridge, MA: MIT Press, 1994.

Koch C, Zador A: The function of dendritic spines: Devices subserving biochemical rather than electrical compartmentalization. Journal of Neuroscience: 13(2); 413–422, 1993.

Kornack DR, Rakic P: Continuation of neurogenesis in the hippocampus of the adult macaque monkey. Proceedings of the National Academy of Sciences USA: 96(10); 5768–5773, 1999.

Kroodsma DE, Pickert R: Environmentally dependent sensitive periods for avian vocal learning. Nature: 288; 477–479, 1980.

Kuhl PK: Categorization of speech by infants. In Mehler J, Fox R (Eds), Neonate Cognition: Beyond the Blooming Buzzing Confusion. Hillsdale, NJ: Erlbaum, 1985.

Kuhl PK: The special-mechanisms debate in speech: Contributions of tests on animals (and the relations of these tests using non-speech stimuli). In Harnad S (Ed), Categorical Perception. Cambridge University Press, 1986.

Kuhl PK: Effects of linguistic experience in the first half-year of life: Implication for a theory of infant speech development. In De Boysson-Bardies D et al. (Eds), Developmental Neurocognition: Speech and Face Processing in the First Year of Life. Dordrecht: Kluwer, 1993.

Kuhl PK, Meltzoff AN: Speech as an intermodal object of perception. In Yonas A (Ed), The Minnesota Symposia on Child Psychology, Vol. 20, Perceptual Development in Infancy. Hillsdale, NJ: Erlbaum, pp. 235–266, 1988.

Kuhl PK, Williams KA, Lacerda F, Stevens KN, Lindblom B: Linguistic experiences alter phonetic perception in infants by 6 months of age. Science: 255; 606–608, 1992.

Kuhn HG, Dickinson-Anson H, Gage FH: Neurogenesis in the dentate gyrus of the adult rat: Age-related decrease of neuronal progenitor proliferation. Journal of Neuroscience: 16(6); 2027–2033, 1996.

Kutas M, Van Petten C: Psycholinguistics electrified: Event-related brain potential investigations. In Gernsbacher M (Ed), Handbook of Psycholinguistics. San Diego: Academic Press, pp. 83–143, 1994.

Lakoff G: Women, Fire and Dangerous Things: What Categories Reveal about the Mind. Chicago: University of Chicago Press, 1987.

Lalonde C, Werker J: Cognitive perceptual integration of three skills at 9 months. In Rovee-Collier C (Ed), Abstracts of the Seventh International Conference on Infant Studies, Special issue of Infant Behavior and Development 13, 464. Norwood, NJ: Ablex, 1990.

Lambrecht K: Information Structure and Sentence form: Topic, Focus, and the Mental Representations of Discourse Referents. Cambridge; New York: Cambridge University Press, 1994.

Langacker R: Foundations of Cognitive Grammar. Stanford: Stanford University Press, 1987.

Lenneberg E: Biological Foundations of Language. New York: Wiley, 1967.

Leonard LB: Children with Specific Language Impairment. Boston MA: MIT Press, 1998.

Leonard LB, Newhoff M, Mesulam L: Individual differences in early child phonology. Applied Psycholinguistics: 1; 7–30, 1980.
Leslie AM: Pretending and believing - Issues in the theory of Tomm. Cognition: 50(1–3); 211–238, 1994.
Levelt WJM: Speaking: From Intention to Articulation. Cambridge, MA: MIT Press, 1989.
Levelt WJM, Roelofs A, Meyer AS: A theory of lexical access in speech production. Behavioral and Brain Sciences: 22; 1–75, 1999.
Lidov HG, Molliver ME: Immunohistochemical study of the development of serotonergic neurons in the rat CNS. Brain Research Bulletin: 9(1–6); 559–604, 1982.
Lidow MS, Goldman-Rakic PS, Rakic P: Synchronized overproduction of neurotransmitter receptors in diverse regions of the primate cerebral cortex. Proceedings of the National Academy of Sciences USA: 88(22); 10218–10221, 1991.
Lidow MS, Rakic P: Neurotransmitter receptors in the proliferative zones of the developing primate occipital lobe. Journal of Comparative Neurology, 360(3), 393–402, 1995.
Lieberman P: Eve Spoke: Human Language and Human Evolution. New York: WW. Norton, 1998.
Lightfoot D: The child's trigger experience: Degree-0 learnability. Behavioral and Brain Sciences, 12, 321–375, 1989.
Linebarger M, Schwartz M, Saffran E: Sensitivity to grammatical structure in so-called agrammatic aphasics. Cognition: 13; 361–392, 1983.
Locke JL: Phonological Acquisition and Change. New York: Academic Press, 1983.
Locke JL: The sound shape of early lexical representations. In Smith M, Locke J (Eds), The Emergent Lexicon. New York: Academic Press, 1988.
Lu C-C, Bates E, Li P, Tzeng O, Hung D, Tsai C-H, Lee S-E, Chung Y-M: Judgements of grammaticality in aphasia: The special case of Chinese. Aphasiology: 14(10); 1021–1054, 2000.
Luskin MB: Neuroblasts of the postnatal mammalian forebrain: Their phenotype and fate. Journal of Neurobiology: 36(2); 221–233, 1998.
MacDonald MC, Pearlmutter NJ, Seidenberg MS: Lexical nature of syntactic ambiguity resolution. Psychological Review: 101(4); 676–703, 1994.
MacWhinney B: The CHILDES Project: Tools for Analyzing Talk (2nd ed). Hillsdale, NJ: Erlbaum, 1992.
MacWhinney B: Update to the CHILDES Project: Tools for Analyzing Talk (2nd ed). Hillsdale, NJ: Erlbaum, 1995.
MacWhinney B (Ed): The Emergence of Language. Mahwah, NJ: Lawrence Erlbaum, 1999.
MacWhinney B, Bates E (Eds): The Crosslinguistic Study of Sentence Processing. New York: Cambridge University Press, 1989.
MacWhinney B, Snow C: The Child Language Data Exchange System. Journal of Child Language: 17; 271–296, 1985.
MacWhinney B, Snow C: The child language data exchange system: An Update. Journal of Child Language: 12; 457–472, 1990.
Mandler J: Representation. In Damon W (Series Ed.) and Kuhn D, Siegler R (Vol. Eds), Handbook of Child Psychology: Vol. 2 Cognition, Perception and Language, 5th ed. New York: Wiley, pp. 255–308, 1998.
Marchman V, Bates E, Burkhardt A, Good A: Functional constraints on the acquisition of the passive: Toward a model of the competence to perform. First Language: 11; 65–92, 1991.
Marchman V, Miller R, Bates E: Babble and first words in children with localized brain injury. Applied Psycholinguistics: 12; 1–22, 1991.
Marcus G: The Algebraic Mind. Cambridge, MA: MIT Press, 1999.
Mareschal D, Quinn PC: Categorization in infancy. Trends in Cognitive Sciences: 4(10); 443–450, 2001.
Marslen-Wilson W (Ed): Lexical Representation and Process. Cambridge, MA: MIT Press, 1989.
Marslen-Wilson W, Tyler LK: Central processes in speech understanding. Philosophical Transactions of the Royal Society, B: 317–332, 1981.
Marslen-Wilson W, Tyler LK: Against modularity. In Garfield J (Ed), Modularity and Knowledge Representation. Cambridge, MA: MIT Press, 1987.
McCune-Nicolich L: Toward symbolic functioning: Structure of early pretend games and potential parallels with language. Child Development: 52; 785–797, 1981.
McCune-Nicolich L, Bruskin C: Combinatorial competency in play and language. In Rubin K, Pepler D (Eds), The Play of Children: Current Theory and Research. New York: Karger, 1982.
McDonough L, Choi S, Bowerman M, Mandler JM: The use of preferential looking as a measure of semantic development. In Bavin EL, Burnham D (Eds), Advances in Infancy Research. Norwood, NJ: Ablex Publishing, in press, 2002.
McRae K, Spivey-Knowlton MJ, Tanenhaus MK: Modeling the influence of thematic fit (and other constraints) in on-line sentence comprehension. Journal of Memory and Language: 38(3); 283–312, 1998.
Mehler J, Jusczyk PW, Lambertz G, Halsted N, Bertoncini J, Amiel-Tison C: A precursor of language acquisition in young infants. Cognition: 29; 143–178, 1988.
Meltzoff AN: Infant imitation and memory: Nine-month-olds in immediate and deferred tests. Child Development: 59; 217–225, 1988.
Meltzoff AN, Borton RW: Intermodal matching by human neonates. Nature: 282; 403–404, 1979.
Meltzoff AN, Moore MK: Interpreting 'imitative' responses in early infancy. Science: 205; 217–219, 1979.
Menn L: Phonological development: Learning sounds and sound patterns. In Berko Gleason J (Ed), The Development of Language. Columbus, OH: Charles E. Merrill, 1985.
Menn L, Stoel-Gammon C: Phonological development. In Fletcher P, MacWhinney B (Eds), Handbook of Child Language. Oxford: Basil Blackwell, pp. 335–359, 1995.
Milberg W, Blumstein S, Dworetzky B: Phonological processing and lexical access in aphasia. Brain and Language: 34; 279–293, 1988.
Miller B, Chou L, Finlay BL: The early development of thalam-

ocortical and corticothalamic projections. Journal of Comparative Neurology: 335(1); 16–41, 1993.

Miller JF: Assessing Language Production in Children: Experimental Procedures. Baltimore: University Park Press, 1981.

Mills DL, Coffey SA, Neville HJ: Language acquisition and cerebral specialization in 20-month-old infants. Journal of Cognitive Neuroscience: 5; 317–334, 1993.

Mills DL, Coffey-Corina SA, Neville HJ: Language comprehension and cerebral specialization from 13 to 20 months. In Thal D, Reilly J (Eds), Special issue on Origins of Communication Disorders. Developmental Neuropsychology: 13(3); 397–445, 1997.

Missler M, Eins S, Merker HJ, Rothe H, Wolff JR: Pre- and postnatal development of the primary visual cortex of the common marmoset. I. A changing space for synaptogenesis. Journal of Comparative Neurology: 333(1); 41–52, 1993.

Missler M, Wolff A, Merker HJ, Wolff JR: Pre- and postnatal development of the primary visual cortex of the common marmoset. II. Formation, remodelling, and elimination of synapses as overlapping processes. Journal of Comparative Neurology: 333(1); 53–67, 1993.

Miyake A, Carpenter PA, Just MA: A capacity approach to syntactic comprehension disorders: Making normal adults perform like aphasic patients. Cognitive Neuropsychology: 11(6); 671–717, 1994.

Molnar Z, Adams R, Blakemore C: Mechanisms underlying the early establishment of thalamocortical connections in the rat. Journal of Neuroscience: 18(15); 5723–5745, 1998.

Nass R: Plasticity: mechanisms, extents and limits. In Segalowitz SJ, Rapin I (Eds), Child Neuropsychology, Handbook of Neuropsychology, 2nd Edition, vol. 8, part I. Amsterdam: Elsevier, pp. 29–68, 2002.

Nathanielsz PW: Comparative studies on the initiation of labor. European Journal of Obstetrics, Gynecology and Reproductive Biology: 78(2); 127–132, 1998.

Nelson K: Structure and strategy in learning to talk. Monograph of the Society for Research in Child Development: 38(1 and 2, Serial #49), 1973.

Newmeyer FJ: Language Form and Language Function. Cambridge, MA: MIT Press, 1998.

Ochs E, Schieffelin B: Developmental Pragmatics. New York: Academic Press, 1979.

O'Connell B, Bretherton I: Toddler's play, alone and with mother: The role of maternal guidance. In Bretherton I (Ed), Symbolic Play: The Development of Social Understanding. New York: Academic Press, 1984.

O'Connell B, Gerard A: Scripts and scraps: The development of sequential understanding. Child Development: 56; 671–681, 1985.

Ohala JJ, Jaeger JJ (Eds): Experimental Phonology. New York: Academic Press, 1986.

O'Kusky JR: Synapse elimination in the developing visual cortex: A morphometric analysis in normal and dark-reared cats. Brain Research: 354(1); 81–91, 1985.

O'Kusky JR, Colonnier M: Postnatal changes in the number of neurons and synapses in the visual cortex (area 17) of the macaque monkey: A stereological analysis in normal and monocularly deprived animals. Journal of Comparative Neurology: 210(3); 291–306, 1982.

O'Kusky JR, Norman MG: Sudden infant death syndrome: increased synaptic density in the central reticular nucleus of the medulla. Journal of Neuropathology and Experimental Neurology: 53(3); 263–271, 1994.

O'Kusky JR, Norman MG: Sudden infant death syndrome: increased number of synapses in the hypoglossal nucleus. Journal of Neuropathology and Experimental Neurology: 54(5); 627–634, 1995.

O'Leary DD, Schlaggar BL, Tuttle R: Specification of neocortical areas and thalamocortical connections. Annual Review of Neuroscience: 17; 419–439, 1994.

Oller DK: The emergence of the sounds of speech in infancy. In Yeni-Komshian GH, Kavanaugh JF, Ferguson CA (Eds), Child Phonology: Vol. 1. Production. New York: Academic Press, 1980.

Olswang L, Bain B: Assessment information for predicting upcoming change in language production. Journal of Speech and Hearing Research: 39(2); 414–423, 1996.

O'Seaghdha P: Conjoint and dissociable effects of syntactic and semantic context. Journal of Experimental Psychology: Learning, Memory, and Cognition: 23(4); 807–828, 1997.

Osofsky JD (Ed): Handbook of Infant Development, 2nd ed. New York: Wiley, 1987.

Oyama S: The problem of change. In Johnson M (Ed), Brain Development and Cognition: A Reader. Oxford: Blackwell Publishers, pp. 19–30, 1992.

Pae Soyeong: Early vocabulary in Korean: Are nouns easier to learn than verbs? Unpublished doctoral dissertation, University of Kansas, 1993.

Parmelee AH, Sigman MD: Perinatal brain development and behavior. In Haith MM, Campos J (Eds), Infancy and the Biology of Development: Vol. 2. Handbook of child psychology. New York: Wiley, 1983.

Parnavelas JG, Kelly W, Franke E, Eckenstein F: Cholinergic neurons and fibres in the rat visual cortex. Journal of Neurocytology: 15(3); 329–336, 1986.

Parnavelas JG, Moises HC, Speciale SG: The monoaminergic innervation of the rat visual cortex. Proceedings of the Royal Society of London B: Biological Sciences: 223(1232); 319–329, 1985.

Pennington BF: The working memory function of the prefrontal cortices: Implications for developmental and individual differences in cognition. In Haith M, Benson J, Roberts R, Pennington B (Eds), The Development of Future-Oriented Processes. Chicago: The University of Chicago Press, pp. 243–289, 1994.

Perkell J, Matthies M, Lane H, Guenther F, Wilhelms-Tricarico R, Wozniak J, Guiod P: Speech motor control: Acoustic goals, saturation effects, auditory feedback and internal models. Speech Communication: 22(2–3); 227–250, 1997.

Peters A: Language-learning strategies: Does the whole equal the sum of the parts? Language: 53; 560–573, 1977.

Peters A: The Units of Language Acquisition. Cambridge: Cambridge University Press, 1983.

Petersen SE, Van Mier H, Fiez JA, Raichle ME: The effects of practice on the functional anatomy of task performance.

Proceedings of the National Academy of Sciences of the United States of America: 95(3); 853–860, 1998.
Piaget J: The Construction of Reality in the Child. New York: Ballantine, 1954.
Piaget J: Play, Dreams and Imitation. New York: Norton, 1962.
Pick A: Aphasia. (J. Brown, Ed. and Trans.) Springfield, IL: Charles C. Thomas. (Original work published 1913), 1973.
Pickett JM: The Sounds of Speech Communication: A Primer of Acoustic Phonetics and Speech Perception. Baltimore, MD: University Park Press, 1985.
Pinker S: The Language Instinct: How the Mind Creates Language. New York: William Morrow, 1994.
Pinker S: How the Mind Works. New York: Norton, 1997.
Pinker S: Words and Rules: The Ingredients of Language. New York: Basic Books, 1999.
Pinker S, Bloom P: Natural language and natural selection. Behavioral and Brain Sciences: 13; 707–784, 1990.
Plaut DC: Parallel distributed processing challenges the strong modularity hypothesis, not the locality assumption. Behavioral and Brain Sciences: 17(1); 77–78, 1994.
Prince E: Toward a taxonomy of given-new information. In Cole P (Ed), Radical Pragmatics. New York: Academic Press, 1981.
Provis JM, Penfold PL: Cell death and the elimination of retinal axons during development. Progress in Neurobiology: 31(4); 331–347, 1988.
Provis JM, Van Driel D, Billson FA, Russell P: Human fetal optic nerve: overproduction and elimination of retinal axons during development. Journal of Comparative Neurology: 238(1); 92–100, 1985.
Quartz SR, Sejnowski TJ: The neural basis of cognitive development: A constructivist manifesto. Behavioral and Brain Sciences: 20(4); 537, 1997.
Rapin I, Dunn M, Allen DA: Developmental language disorders. In Segalowitz SJ, Rapin I (Eds), Child Neuropsychology, Handbook of Neuropsychology, 2nd Edition, vol. 8, part II. Amsterdam: Elsevier, pp. 593–630, 2003.
Rakic P, Bourgeois JP, Eckenhoff MF, Zecevic N, Goldman-Rakic PS: Concurrent overproduction of synapses in diverse regions of the primate cerebral cortex. Science: 232; 232–235, 1986.
Reilly J, Bates E, Marchman V: Narrative discourse in children with early focal brain injury. In Dennis M (Ed), Special issue, Discourse in children with anomalous brain development or acquired brain injury. Brain and Language: 61(3); 335–375, 1998.
Reznick JS: Visual preference as a test of infant word comprehension. Applied Psycholinguistics: 11; 145–165, 1990.
Reznick JS, Kagan J: Category detection in infancy. In Lipsitt L (Ed), Advances in Infancy Research, 2nd ed. Norwood, NJ: Ablex, 1983.
Rice M (Ed): Toward a Genetics of Language. Mahwah, NJ: Erlbaum, 1996.
Rice M, Wexler K: Extended optional infinitive (EOI) account of specific language impairment. In MacLaughlin D, McEwen S (Eds), Proceedings of the 19th Annual Boston University Conference on Language Development, 2, 451–462. Somerville, MA: Cascadilla Press, 1995.
Rice M, Wexler K, Cleave P: Specific language impairment as a period of extended optional infinitive. Journal of Speech and Hearing Research: 38; 850–863, 1995.
Ring EN: Assessment of language comprehension and production: Child performance versus parent judgment. Unpublished master's thesis, San Diego State University, San Diego, CA, 1999.
Riva D, Cazzaniga L: Late effects of unilateral brain lesions before and after the first year of life. Neuropsychologia: 24; 423–428, 1986.
Riva D, Cazzaniga L, Pantaleoni C, Milani N, Fedrizzi E: Acute hemiplegia in childhood: The neuropsychological prognosis. Journal of Pediatric Neurosciences: 2(4); 239–250, 1986.
Rizzolatti G, Fadiga L, Gallese V, Fogassi L: Premotor cortex and the recognition of motor actions. Cognitive Brain Research: 3; 131–141, 1996.
Robertson SS, Dierker LJ, Sorokin Y, Rosen MG: Human fetal movement: spontaneous oscillations near one cycle per minute. Science: 218(4579); 1327–1330, 1982.
Rogoff B: The development of conceptual structures. In Damon W (Series Ed.) and Kuhn D, Siegler R (Vol. Eds), Handbook of Child psychology: Vol. 2. Cognition, Perception and Language, 5th ed. New York: Wiley, pp. 679–744, 1998.
Role LW, Kelly JP: The brain stem: Cranial nerve nuclei and the monoaminergic systems. In Kandel ER, Schwartz JH, Jessell TM (Eds), Principles of Neural Science, 3rd ed. Norwalk, CT: Appleton and Lange, 1991.
Ross ED: The aprosodias: Functional-anatomic organization of the affective components of of language in the right hemisphere. Archives of Neurology: 38; 561–569, 1981.
Ross ED, Mesulam MM: Archives of Neurology: 36; 144–148, 1979.
Roug L, Landberg I, Lundberg L: Phonetic development in early infancy: a study of four Swedish children during the first eighteen months of life. Journal of Child Language: 16(1); 19–40, 1989.
Rovee-Collier C: The ontogeny of learning and memory in human infancy. In Kail R, Spear N (Eds), Comparative Perspectives on the Development of Memory. Hillsdale, NJ.: Erlbaum, 1984.
Rovee-Collier C, Lipsitt L, Hayne H (Eds): Advances in Infancy Research. Norwood, NJ: Ablex, 1998.
Sacher GA: Brain maturation in the evolution of primates. In Armstrong E, Falk D (Eds), Primate Brain Evolution: Methods and Concepts. New York: Plenum Press, pp. 97–112, 1980.
Saffran EM, Aslin RN, Newport EL: Statistical learning by 8-month-old infants. Science: 274; 1926–1928, 1996.
Santelmann LM, Jusczyk PW: Sensitivity to discontinuous dependencies in language learners: Evidence for limitations in processing space. Cognition: 69; 105–134, 1998.
Savage-Rumbaugh ES: Ape Language: From Conditioned Response to Symbol. New York: Columbia University Press, 1986.
Schneider W, Bjorklund DF: Memory. In Damon W (Series Ed.) and Kuhn D, Siegler R (Vol. Eds), Handbook of Child Psychology: Vol. 2. Cognition, Perception and Language, 5th ed. New York: Wiley, pp. 467–522, 1998.

Schwartz R: Words, objects and actions in early lexical acquisition. Unpublished doctoral dissertation, Memphis State University, 1978.

Seidenberg MS: Language acquisition and use: Learning and applying probabilistic constraints. Science: 275(5306); 1599–1603, 1997.

Seidenberg MS, Petitto LA: Signing behavior in apes: A critical review. Cognition: 7; 177–215, 1979.

Shallice T: From Neuropsychology to Mental Structure. New York: Cambridge University Press, 1988.

Shatz CJ, Chun JJM, Luskin MB: The role of the subplate in the development of the mammalian telencephalon. In Peters A, Jones EG (Eds), The Cerebral Cortex (Vol. 7). New York: Plenum, 1988.

Shore C: Combinatorial play: Conceptual development and early multiword speech. Developmental Psychology: 22; 184–190, 1986.

Shore C, Bates E, Bretherton I, Beeghly M, O'Connell B: Vocal and gestural symbols: Similarities and differences from 13 to 28 months. In Volterra V, Erting C (Eds), From Gesture to Language in Hearing and Deaf Children. New York: Springer-Verlag, 1990.

Shore C, O'Connell C, Bates E: First sentences in language and symbolic play. Developmental Psychology: 20; 872–880, 1984.

Singer Harris N, Bellugi U, Bates E, Jones W, Rossen M: Contrasting profiles of language development in children with Williams and Down Syndromes. In Thal D, Reilly J (Eds), Special issue on Origins of Communication Disorders. Developmental Neuropsychology: 13(3); 345–370, 1997.

Sirevaag AM, Black JE, Shafron D, Greenough WT: Direct evidence that complex experience increases capillary branching and surface area in visual cortex of young rats. Brain Research: 471(2); 299–304, 1988.

Sirevaag AM, Greenough WT: Differential rearing effects on rat visual cortex synapses. III. Neuronal and glial nuclei, boutons, dendrites, and capillaries. Brain Research: 424(2); 320–332, 1987.

Slobin D (Ed): The Crosslinguistic Study of Language Acquisition (Vols. 1–5). Hillsdale, NJ: Erlbaum, 1985–1997.

Small S, Cottrell G, Tanenhaus M (Eds): Lexical Ambiguity Resolution: Perspectives from Artificial Intelligence, Psychology and Neurolinguistics. San Mateo: Morgan Kaufman, 1988.

Snow C, Hoefnagel-Hohle M: The critical period for language acquisition: Evidence from second language learning. Child Development: 49; 1114–1128, 1978.

Sodian B, Taylor C, Harris PL, Perner J: Early deception and the child's theory of mind: False trails and genuine markers. Child Development: 62(3); 468–483, 1991.

Spelke ES: Initial knowledge: Six suggestions. Cognition: 50; 431–445, 1994.

Spelke ES, Breinlinger K, Macomber J, Jacobson K: Origins of knowledge. Psychological Review: 99(4); 605–632, 1992.

Spelke ES, Newport EL: Nativism, empiricism, and the development of knowledge. In Damon W (Series Ed) and Lerner RM (Vol. Ed), Handbook of Child Psychology: Vol. 1. Theoretical Models of Human Development, 5th ed. New York: Wiley, pp. 275–340, 1998.

Spitz RV, Stiles J, Siegel R: Infant use of relative motion as information for form: Evidence for spatial–temporal integration of complex motion displays. Project in Cognitive and Neural Development Technical Report #89–14. La Jolla: University of California, San Diego, 1989.

Spivey-Knowlton MJ, Tanenhaus MK, Eberhard KM, Sedivy JC: Integration of visuospatial and linguistic information: Language comprehension in real time and real space. In Olivier EP, Gapp EK-P et al. (Eds), Representation and Processing of Spatial Expressions (pp. 201–214). Mahwah, NJ: Erlbaum, 1998.

Stemberger JP, Bernhardt BH: The emergence of faithfulness. In MacWhinney B (Ed), The Emergence of Language. Mahwah, NJ: Erlbaum, pp. 417–446, 1999.

Stiles J, Bates E, Thal D, Trauner D, Reilly J: Linguistic, cognitive and affective development in children with pre- and perinatal focal brain injury: A ten-year overview from the San Diego longitudinal project. In Rovee-Collier C, Lipsitt L, Hayne H (Eds), Advances in Infancy Research. Norwood, NJ: Ablex, pp. 131–163, 1998.

Stryker MP, Harris WA: Binocular impulse blockade prevents the formation of ocular dominance columns in cat visual cortex. Journal of Neuroscience: 6(8); 2117–2133, 1986.

Swinney D: Lexical access during sentence comprehension: (Re) consideration of context effects. Journal of Verbal Learning and Verbal Behavior: 18; 645–59, 1979.

Tager-Flusberg H (Ed): Constraints on Language Acquisition: Studies of Atypical Children. Hillsdale, NJ: Erlbaum, 1994.

Tager-Flusberg H (Ed): Neurodevelopmental Disorders. Cambridge, MA: MIT Press, 1999.

Tallal P, Stark R, Kallman C, Mellits D: Developmental aphasia: the relation between acoustic processing deficits and verbal processing. Neuropsychologia: 18; 273–284, 1980.

Tallal P, Stark R, Kallman C, Mellits D: A re-examination of some nonverbal perceptual abilities of language-impaired and normal children as a function of age and sensory modality. Journal of Speech and Hearing Research: 24; 351–357, 1981.

Tallal P, Stark R, Mellits D: Identification of language-impaired children on the basis of rapid perception and production skills. Brain and Language: 25; 314–322, 1985a.

Tallal P, Stark R, Mellits D: The relation between auditory temporal analysis and receptive language development: evidence from studies of developmental language disorders. Neuropsychologia: 23; 527–534, 1985b.

Tardif T: Nouns are not always learned before verbs: Evidence from Mandarin speakers' early vocabularies. Developmental Psychology: 32(3); 492–504, 1996.

Thal D: Late talkers: Are they at risk? Albert Johnson Research Award Lecture, San Diego State University, San Diego, CA, 1999, May.

Thal D, Bates E: Language and communication in early childhood. Pediatric Annals: 18(5); 299–306, 1989.

Thal D, Bates E: Continuity and variation in early language development. In Colombo J, Sagan J (Eds), Individual Differences in Infancy: Reliability, Stability, and Prediction. Hillsdale, NJ: Erlbaum, 1990.

Thal D, Bates E, Zappia M, Oroz M: Ties between lexical and grammatical development: Evidence from early talkers. Journal of Child Language: 23; 349–368, 1996.

Thal D, Katich J: Predicaments in early identification of specific language impairment: Does the early bird always catch the worm? In Cole K, Dale P, Thal D (Eds) Assessment of Communication and Language. Baltimore, MD: Brookes, 1996.

Thal D, Marchman V, Stiles J, Aram D, Trauner D, Nass R, Bates E: Early lexical development in children with focal brain injury. Brain and Language: 40; 491–527, 1991a.

Thal D, O'Hanlon L, Clemmons M, Frailin L: Validity of a parent report measure of vocabulary and syntax for preschool children with language impairment. Journal of Speech, Language and Hearing Disorders: 42; 482–496, 1999.

Thal D, Reilly J: Special issue: Origins of language disorders. Developmental Neuropsychology: 13(3); 233–238, 1997.

Thal D, Tobias S: Communicative gestures in children with delayed onset of oral expressive vocabulary. Journal of Speech and Hearing Research: 35; 1281–1289, 1992.

Thal D, Tobias S: Relationships between language and gesture in normal and late-talking toddlers. Journal of Speech and Hearing Research: 37; 157–171, 1994.

Thal D, Tobias S, Morrison D: Language and gesture in late talkers: A one-year follow-up. Journal of Speech and Hearing Disorders: 34; 604–612, 1991b.

Thelen E, Smith LB: A Dynamic Systems Approach to the Development of Cognition and Action. Cambridge, MA: MIT Press, 1994.

Thelen E, Smith LB: Dynamic systems theories. In Damon W (Series Ed) and Kuhn D, Siegler R (Vol. Eds), Handbook of child Psychology: Vol. 1. Theoretical Models of Human Development, 5th ed. New York: Wiley, pp. 563–634, 1998.

Tincoff R, Jusczyk PW: Some beginnings of word comprehension in 6-month-olds. Psychological Science: 10(2); 172–175, 1999.

Tomasello M (Ed): The New Psychology of Language: Cognitive and Functional Approaches to Language Structure. Mahwah, NJ: Lawrence Erlbaum, 1998.

Tomasello M, Call J: Primate Cognition. New York: Oxford University Press, 1997.

Tomasello M, Mervis CB: The instrument is great, but measuring comprehension is still a problem. Monographs of the Society for Research in Child Development: 59 (5, Serial No. 242); 174–179, 1994.

Turner AM, Greenough WT: Differential rearing effects on rat visual cortex synapses. I. Synaptic and neuronal density and synapses per neuron. Brain Research: 329(1–2); 195–203, 1985.

Ullman M, Corkin S, Coppola M, Hickok G, Growdon JH, Koroshetz WJ, Pinker S: A neural dissociation within language: Evidence that the mental dictionary is part of declarative memory, and that grammatical rules are processed by procedural system. Journal of Cognitive Neuroscience: 9(2); 266–276, 1997.

Van Hout A: Acquired aphasia in childhoold. In Segalowitz SJ, Rapin I (Eds), Child Neuropsychology, Handbook of Neuropsychology, 2nd Edition, vol. 8, part II. Amsterdam: Elsevier, pp. 631–658, 2003.

VanLancker D, Kempler D: Comprehension of familiar phrases by left- but not by right-hemisphere-damaged patients. Brain and Language: 32; 265–277, 1986.

Van Petten C, Coulson S, Rubin S, Plante E, Parks M: Timecourse of word identification and semantic integration in spoken language. Journal of Experimental Psychology: Learning, Memory and Cognition: 25(2); 394–417, 1999.

Vargha-Khadem F, Isaacs E, Muter V: A review of cognitive outcome after unilateral lesions sustained during childhood. Journal of Child Neurology: 9(Suppl.); 2S67–2S73, 1994.

Vargha-Khadem F, Isaacs E, Watkins K, Mishkin M: Ontogenetic specialization of hemispheric function. In Oxbury J, Polkey CE, Duchowny M (Eds), Intractable Focal Epilepsy. London: WB Saunders, 2000.

Vicari S, Albertoni A, Chilosi A, Cipriani P, Cioni G, Bates E: Plasticity and reorganization during early language learning in children with congenital brain injury. Cortex: 36; 31–46, 2000.

Vicari S, Caselli MC, Tonucci F: Asynchrony of lexical and morphosyntactic development in children with Down Syndrome. Neuropsicologia: 38; 634–644, 2000.

Vihman M: Individual differences in babbling and early speech: Predicting to age three. In Lindblom B, Zetterstrom R (Eds), Precursors of Early Speech. Basingstoke, Hampshire: MacMillan, 1985.

Vihman M, Ferguson C, Elbert M: Phonological development from babbling to speech: Common tendencies and individual differences. Applied Psycholinguistics: 7; 3–40, 1986.

Vihman M, Greenlee M: Individual differences in phonological development: Age one and age three. Journal of Speech and Hearing Research: 30; 503–528, 1987.

Volpe JJ: Neurology of the Newborn (2nd ed.). Philadelphia: Saunders, 1987.

Volterra V, Bates E: Selective impairment of Italian grammatical morphology in the congenitally deaf: A case study. Cognitive Neuropsychology: 6; 273–308, 1989.

Vu H, Kellas G, Metcalf K, Herman R: The influence of global discourse on lexical ambiguity resolution. Memory and Cognition: 28(2); 236–252, 2000.

Vu H, Kellas G, Paul ST: Sources of sentence constraint on lexical ambiguity resolution. Memory and Cognition: 26(5); 979–1001, 1998.

Weber-Fox CM, Neville HJ: Maturational constraints on functional specializations for language processsing: ERP and behavioral evidence in bilingual speakers. Journal of Cognitive Neuroscience: 8(3); 231–256, 1996.

Wells R: Language Development in the Pre-School Years. Cambridge University Press, 1985.

Werker J, Tees R: Cross-language speech perception: evidence for perceptual reorganization during the first year of life. Infant Behavior and Development: 7; 49–63, 1984.

Werner H, Kaplan B: Symbol Formation: An Organismic-Developmental Approach to the Psychology of Language. New York: Wiley, 1963.

Wexler K: The development of inflection in a biologically based theory of language acquisition. In Rice ML (Ed), Toward a Genetics of Language. Mahwah, NJ: Erlbaum, pp. 113–144, 1996.

Wong RO: Retinal waves and visual system development. Annual Review in Neuroscience: 22; 29–47, 1999.

Woo TU, Beale JM, Finlay BL: Dual fate of subplate neurons in a rodent. Cerebral Cortex: 1(5); 433–443, 1991.

Wulfeck B, Bates E: Differential sensitivity to errors of agreement and word order in Broca's aphasia. Journal of Cognitive Neuroscience: 3; 258–272, 1991.

Yakovlev P, Lecours A: The myelinogenetic cycle of regional maturation of the brain. In Minkowski A (Ed), Regional Development of the Brain in Early Life. Philadelphia: Davis Co, 1967.

Zecevic N, Bourgeois JP, Rakic P: Changes in synaptic density in motor cortex of rhesus monkey during fetal and postnatal life. Developmental Brain Research: 50(1); 11–32, 1989.

Zecevic N, Milosevic A: Initial development of gamma-aminobutyric acid immunoreactivity in the human cerebral cortex. Jouronal of Comparative Neurology: 380(4); 495–506, 1997.

Zecevic N, Rakic P: Synaptogenesis in monkey somatosensory cortex. Cerebral Cortex: 1(6); 510–523, 1991.

Zurif E, Caramazza A: Psycholinguistic structures in aphasia: Studies in syntax and semantics. In H, Whitaker HA (Eds), Studies in Neurolinguistics (Vol. I). New York: Academic Press, 1976.

Zurif E, Swinney D, Garrett M: Lexical processing and sentence comprehension in aphasia. In Caramazza A (Ed), Cognitive Neuropsychology and Neurolinguistics: Advances in Models of Cognitive Function and Impairment. Hillsdale, NJ: Erlbaum, 1990.

© 2003 Published by Elsevier Science B.V.
Handbook of Neuropsychology, 2nd Edition, Vol. 8, Part II
S.J. Segalowitz and I. Rapin (Eds)

CHAPTER 22

Developmental language disorders

Isabelle Rapin [a,b,*], Michelle Dunn [b] and Doris A. Allen [c,†]

[a] *Saul R. Korey Department of Pediatrics, Rose F. Kennedy Center for Research in Mental Retardation and Human Development, Bronx, NY 10461, USA*
[b] *Saul R. Korey Department of Neurology, Rose F. Kennedy Center for Research in Mental Retardation and Human Development, Bronx, NY 10461, USA*
[c] *Division of Child Psychiatry, Albert Einstein College of Medicine, Bronx, NY 10461, USA*

Introduction

Developmental language disorder (DLD), specific language impairment (SLI), or dysphasia (these terms are used interchangeably in this chapter) is one of the most frequent developmental disorders of higher cerebral function of early childhood. *SLI* implies that the child has no other developmental impairments, which is desirable for research purposes but is by no means always the case in the clinic. *Dysphasia* (developmental dysphasia) implies deficient acquisition of language, as opposed to acquired aphasia, the loss of previously competent language due to an acquired focal insult to the brain. Rarely, *DLD* means total lack of language; more often it means either a delay that exceeds the upper boundaries of the age for normal language acquisition, or deviance in some aspects of language development or, more typically, both.

Language is a socially-derived, rule-governed system of arbitrary signals that makes possible the interpersonal transmission of information and supports much of private thought. Speech consists of a sequence of rapid (tens of milliseconds) sound stimuli that are the vehicle for language. Language is encoded at multiple levels and its comprehension and production require a large number of sequential and parallel brain operations. Input to the common central language processing network may utilize the auditory, visual, or tactile channel, while output may be vocal or gestural (including writing). We concentrate here on the auditory/vocal channel.

The major rule-governed levels of language include pragmatics (communicative use of language), phonology (speech sounds), semantics (meaning of language), and grammar (rules for assembling words into meaningful utterances). The complexities of language call for the coordinated activation of multilevel brain networks and subroutines, any of which may be dysfunctional, resulting in a variety of language disorder subtypes. In the face of normal hearing, inadequate or deviant language acquisition implies atypical brain function, in DLD generally without clinically discernible structural brain lesion or malformation.

Diagnostic criteria

There is no biologic marker or gold standard that defines DLD which, like other developmental disorders, is a behavioral diagnosis with fuzzy borders. DLD's ill-defined borders and its overlaps with other developmental disorders are hardly surprising in view of the many factors that shape brain development (Karmiloff-Smith, 1998). The existence of several subtypes of language disorder (discussed later)

* Corresponding author. Tel.: +1-718-430-2478; Fax: +1-718-430-8786; E-mail: rapin@aecom.yu.edu
† Deceased

and the variability of their manifestations with age contribute to the fuzzy borders of DLD. The diagnosis of DLD would be straightforward if language acquisition followed a uniform time-table and if all children acquired the components of language in the same order. Because this is not the case (see chapter by Bates, Thal, Finlay and Clancy, 2003), it may be difficult to decide when a toddler's or preschooler's language skills are so delayed or deviant as to fall outside the realm of normal variation and thus justify a diagnosis of dysphasia. Also, diagnostic criteria are often a matter of one's goals. Children identified for research are selected on the basis of rigorously defined test criteria or very specific characteristics of their language. To identify children in need of remediation, the diagnosis of DLD may rest on the opinions of experienced clinicians who may use less rigorous clinical criteria.

Variability in the emergence of language is well documented (Miller, Chapman and MacKenzie, 1981). The MacArthur Communicative Development Inventories' wide ranges and substantial standard deviations index great variability in the age of acquisition of each language milestone (Fenson, Dale, Reznick et al., 1993). The Inventories were standardized on large samples of children for English and several other languages on the basis of parental reports of the receptive and expressive language of their normal children up to age 30 months. The variability in acquisition of language milestones makes it difficult to distinguish *a priori* 'late bloomers' who, on follow-up, turn out unimpaired and were genuinely 'language delayed' from 'late bloomers' who are genuinely dysphasic (Thal and Bates, 1990; Thal and Katich, 1996).

For some investigators, a diagnosis of DLD requires a language profile distinct from what one would expect of normal children at any age (see Johnston, 1988 for a review). 'Late bloomers' who turn out to have DLD on follow-up are generally those children who were not only late talkers but also late comprehenders. Although many among children with expressive and receptive language delays may speak adequately or reasonably adequately by schoolage, this does not necessarily mean that they have 'recovered' and are no longer dysphasic. Rather, the manifestations of the language disorder have changed: instead of causing overt difficulty with verbal comprehension and expression, its most salient characteristic is now likely to be inadequate acquisition of written language (dyslexia) and academic difficulty (American Academy of Child and Adolescent Psychiatry, 1998a,b).

The most frequently invoked cause for slow-to-develop language is delayed brain maturation (e.g., Locke, 1994), even though biologic evidence for immaturity of the brain is generally lacking. DLD in young children is widely referred to as 'language delay', a label that implies that the systems that underlie language are normal and that when catch up occurs the child will be asymptomatic, which is not true if the child has trouble reading and spelling at school age.

The term SLI implies that the child has no other disability to account for his or her inadequate language; it is therefore largely a diagnosis by exclusion. The most widely accepted exclusionary criteria for a diagnosis of DLD are hearing loss, a sensorimotor deficit or abnormal imaging study that denotes an overt brain lesion, anomaly, or disease, as well as autism, mental retardation, and severe social deprivation (American Psychiatric Association, 2000, pp. 58–69).

Although most of these exclusionary criteria seem straightforward and unambiguous, some are not. For example, the requirement for normal hearing seems unassailable, yet a great many infants and preschoolers suffer from repeated episodes of middle ear effusion (glue ear) and have mild or even moderate conductive hearing losses that go undetected for months. It is impractical and invalid, unless there is longitudinal documentation, to use a history of glue ear as an exclusionary criterion for DLD because its detection is so inconsistent, its duration and severity so variable. The hearing loss it causes is never severe enough to preclude the emergence of language, although more subtle influences on language and reading skills have been a matter of controversy for years (Bennett and Haggard, 1999; Klein and Rapin, 1988; Peters, Grievink, Van Bon et al., 1997). In a study conducted by the authors, there was no significant difference in the prevalence of parental reports of frequent otitis media or of middle ear effusion requiring the insertion of ventilating tubes in children with DLD compared to those with other developmental disorders (Rapin, 1996a). Even though glue ear may add another risk factor to borderline cognitive skills or an impoverished environment and slow the emergence of language in some children (Lonigan, Fischel, Whitehurst et al., 1992; Roberts and Wallace, 1997), alone it does not cause DLD (Bishop, 1997a).

The exclusion of overt brain pathology may also be ambiguous as its detection has as much to do with the power of currently available technologies as with the state of the brain. By no means do all structural insults to the developing brain give rise to overt sensorimotor deficits, to epilepsy, or to detectable abnormalities on neuroimaging tests. Even epilepsy is an ambiguous rejection criterion as the frequency and seizure-types vary so widely; some genetic epilepsies are not associated with structural brain lesions or cognitive deficits, and antiepileptic medications differ greatly in their uses and side-effects.

Mental deficiency as an exclusionary criterion for a diagnosis of DLD poses real problems when the IQ is in the borderline range. A nonverbal IQ of 80–85 is a widely accepted but arbitrary cut-off for a diagnosis of DLD rather than subnormal intelligence (Stark and Tallal, 1981), with the *caveat* that scores on performance tests may be lowered by inadequate language inasmuch as instructions for most tasks are verbal, and verbal strategies may optimize performance. The impaired verbal skills of children with DLD may result in spuriously low estimates of cognitive function based on full-scale IQ scores. Thus one needs to guard against the error of labeling young dysphasic children mentally retarded rather than language impaired. A widely used criterion is a discrepancy between verbal IQ and performance IQ, or between a test of language and nonverbal IQ, although there is no universal agreement on the size of the required cognitive/language discrepancy. One, one and half, and two standard deviations will net vastly different numbers of children (Aram, Morris and Hall, 1993; Whitehurst and Fischel, 1994). Data from monozygotic twin pairs, where one might expect very high diagnostic congruency because of shared genes and, generally, a shared environment, also cast doubt on the validity of cognitive/language discrepancy as diagnostic criterion; indeed, twin studies indicate that both twins may not have equally large verbal/nonverbal IQ discrepancies (Bishop, 1994), and that the heritability of DLD is unaffected by NVIQ (Tomblin and Buckwalter, 1998). The corollary is that it is appropriate to diagnose DLD in children with mild mental retardation based on the characteristics of their language deficits, especially as the predictive validity of the IQ in young children is limited (Krassowski and Plante, 1997).

Autistic spectrum disorders are usually considered another exclusionary criterion for DLD even though impaired communication is one of the defining deficits for a diagnosis of autism, and most preschool children on the autistic spectrum are also dysphasic (Allen and Rapin, 1992). The topic of the language disorders of children on the autistic spectrum is considered later in this chapter.

Social deprivation has to be extreme to jeopardize language development, albeit the vocabulary and complexity of the language of children growing up in impoverished environments often reflect this impoverishment (Skuse, 1988). This is not DLD, however.

Prevalence

The lack of universally accepted diagnostic criteria for DLD, the frequent lack of distinction between language disorders and speech articulation disorders, the unrepresentative samples studied, and the admixture of other causes for deficient language all contribute to wide variation in prevalence figures for DLD. Tallal (1988), among many others (see the chapter by Bellinger, Rappaport, Weiler and Beers, 2002), stresses the wide range and unreliability of prevalence estimates

Beitchman, Nair, Clegg and Patel (1986) conducted a survey in the Ottawa area and found that up to 19% of 5 year old kindergarten children scored below norms on language tests. Isolated speech impairments were found in 6.6% of boys and 6.7% of girls, speech and language impairments in 3.3% of boys and 7.1% of girls, and language impairments without speech impairments in 8.2% of boys and 8.4% of girls. The exceptionally high prevalences reported in that study are attributable to the inclusion of all possible causes of speech and language disorders, including stuttering, voice disorders, hearing loss, dysarthria, cerebral palsy, mental deficiency, and autism. The high prevalence in girls is atypical, since other studies indicate that boys are significantly more likely to be affected than girls. A more recent estimate in children of kindergarten age was 8% in boys and 6% in girls (Tomblin, Records, Buckwalter et al., 1997). Age at ascertainment must be taken into account in prevalence estimates: Whitehurst and Fischel (1994) point out that estimates range from 9–17% in 2 year olds, but drop to 3–8% at 3 years and 1–5% by age 5 years. This optimistic view does not take into account the prevalence of reading disability, much of which stems from the same phonologic deficits responsible for a sizable proportion of DLD, and is estimated to affect some 5% of the schoolage population (Lyon, 1996; Shaywitz, Shaywitz, Fletcher and Escobar, 1990). Clearly, DLD (and dyslexia, its frequent *alter ego*) are moving targets for prevalence estimates.

Causes of DLD

It is the rare child in whom DLD has a unique, medically identifiable cause. The evidence today is that genetic factors play the major causal role in the developmental disorders of brain function by jeopardizing, to a greater or lesser degree, the development of the brain networks required for mastery of complex skills like language, reading, calculation, music, and social abilities. The causal role of acquired environmentally determined insults, previously thought to be major culprits, is now considered minor. This statement does not imply, of course, that the environment in which a child develops has a trivial long term influence on cognitive potential; quite the contrary, the crucial modulatory role of enriched (and impoverished) environments on the fine structure and complexity of the developing brain has long been known in animals (Bryan and Riesen, 1989; Rosenzweig, Bennett, Diamond et al., 1969), and the beneficial effect of intensive early intervention in children at risk is clear (Brooks-Gunn, Liaw and Klebanov, 1992).

Genetics

In the San Diego longitudinal study (Tallal, 1988), 62% of children with DLD had at least one affected parent who had a history of DLD and/or learning disability, 20% had an affected sibling or more distant relative, and only 18% had no affected family member, compared to 38% of controls with an affected parent, 26% with an affected sibling or relative, and 36% with no affected relative. Concordance in monozygotic British twins was close to 100%, whereas it was 50% in same sex dizygotic twins, suggesting dominant inheritance (Bishop, North and Donlan, 1995). A very large British family with DLD was identified a decade ago (Hurst, Baraitser, Auger et al., 1990) in which dysphasia was linked to chromosome 7q31–33 (Fisher, Vargha-Khadem, Watkins et al., 1998; Lai, Fisher, Hurst et al., 2000). This trait is inherited as a dominant trait with a phenotype characterized by articulatory and grammatical deficits (Fisher et al., 1998; Gopnik and Crago, 1991). Linkage to this locus has recently also been found in autistic individuals with inadequate phonology with familial language disorders (Wassink, Piven, Vieland et al., 2001). Linkage of susceptibility to dyslexia to chromosomes 6 and 15 (Gayan, Smith, Cherny et al., 1999; Grigorenko, Wood, Meyer et al., 1997) has also been reported. Genetic heterogeneity having now been unequivocally demonstrated, what is needed are very well studied large families with some members with DLD, dyslexia, and other developmental disorders. These studies are required in order to link phenotype to genotype and, ultimately, to define root causes of the particular deficits in language development.

Syndromic conditions associated with detectable chromosome anomalies may be associated with speech and language disorders which, in some children, fulfil criteria for DLD, albeit they are generally but a facet of a wider somatic and cognitive phenotype. For example, many children with trisomy 21 (Down syndrome) have expressive disorders out of proportion with the severity of their mental deficiency (Chapman, Seung, Schwartz and Kay-Raining Bird, 1998; Laws, 1998). The expressive disorders of many Down children may be aggravated by chronic middle ear effusion which is ubiquitous if untreated. Some children with Prader-Willi syndrome, which is due to a complex molecular defect or to a deletion of a segment of the long arm of chromosome 15 also have severe expressive language deficits (Akefeldt, Akefeldt and Gillberg, 1997; Kleppe, Katayama, Shipley and Foushee, 1990). Boys who have extra X chromosomes, notably those with XXY (Klinefelter) syndrome, tend to have delayed language development, and reading and spelling deficits (Rovet, Netley, Keenan et al., 1996). Those with Fragile-X have cognitive impairments that range from severe mental deficiency to mild learning disability and, in some boys, to autism (Bailey, Hatton and Skinner, 1998).

There are a number of other genetic conditions that may affect language development. An interesting example is Williams syndrome which is associated with a small deletion of the elastin gene and other genes on the long arm of chromosome 7 (Nickerson, Greenberg, Keating et al., 1995). Children with Williams syndrome exhibit significant overall cognitive disability, typically characterized by a dissociation between adequate acquisition of oral vocabulary and syntax and musical ability in the face of deficient semantic and pragmatic skills and moderate to severe impairment in the acquisition of visual spatial skills (Bellugi, Lichtenberger, Mills et al., 1999; Volterra, Capirci, Pezzini et al., 1996).

These associations of unique genetic defects with particular subtypes of DLD must not be interpreted as evidence that there are 'language genes' — or 'syntax genes' for that matter — specific to dedicated language networks. Differences in the developmental schedules of different aspects of language (discussed later), and the dissociations of these aspects among subtypes of DLD bolster the concept of a multiplicity of genes turning on and off at various points in brain development as they influence the genesis of the networks required for the emergence of language. For example, Pinker (Pinker, 1999) conducted an exhaustive study of the acquisition of regular and irregular verbs by normal children speaking a variety of different languages. He deduced that the human brain has genetically-determined circuitry that enables children to memorize words by exposure to any spoken language, but also other circuitry that favors categorization and the learning of the rules that make possible the universal and effortless mastery of connected language. A more appealing hypothesis than the idea of language-dedicated genes is that the phenotypic expression of these genes becomes domain-specific in the course of development and that progressive modularity results from the interaction of specific genotypes with particular environmental experiences (Karmiloff-Smith, 1998). This view accounts for the fact that most developmental deficits occur as spectra rather than discrete entities, with ubiquitous overlaps among what are generally considered phenotypically distinct developmental disorders.

Atypical brain development

Because it is well established that language is strongly lateralized to the left hemisphere in virtually all right handed and in most left handed individuals, it would seem logical to suppose that left hemispheric maldevelopment or very early damage would be found in dysphasic children. No major structural lesions are detectable with brain imaging in dysphasic children, although reversal of the normal asymmetry of the *planum temporale* is demonstrable in some children with DLD or dyslexia (Habib, 2000; Semrud-Clikeman, 1997). As discussed in the Bates et al. chapter on language development and Nass' chapter on plasticity, the consequence of an early lateralized brain lesion may be delayed language acquisition but not DLD, as the requisite networks to sustain language preempt other parts of the left hemisphere or, more often, develop in the right hemisphere. This suggests that the neurologic substrate of DLD may be subtle atypical development of both hemispheres (Aram and Eisele, 1994).

There is a strong preponderance of boys over girls with DLD/dyslexia (4 : 1 is a commonly quoted figure, which at least one population study disputes (Shaywitz et al., 1990)), as well as in children with stuttering, and those with autism which also prominently affects language development. Geschwind and Galaburda (1985) hypothesized that this gender preponderance is due in part to sex-related hormonal influences on brain maturation. The existence of gender-related differences in skills is widely accepted: as a group, boys have better visuospatial (presumably right hemispheric) skills than verbal skills (left hemispheric), and better visuospatial skills than girls who tend to be superior verbally. Males of all ages are also stated to be more strongly lateralized than females (Bryden, 1988). These gender differences have been attributed to interhemispheric differences in brain maturation and organization, which remain in some dispute, however (Clarke and Zaidel,

1994; Davatzikos and Resnick, 1998). A predominant view is that the right hemisphere matures earlier than the left, although there are opposing views (see chapter by Nass, 2002, on plasticity in this volume for a discussion). Geschwind and Galaburda (1985) hypothesized that later and slower maturation of the left hemisphere during fetal life made it more vulnerable than the right to deleterious pre/perinatal exogeneous and immunological influences, especially in boys whose brains were exposed to retarding maturational effects of testosterone. The more recent evidence, that genetics rather than acquired causes are responsible for most cases of DLD suggests that this widely discussed theory needs revision.

Exogenous causes

Findings from the Collaborative Study and a more recent twin study indicate that *perinatal factors* do not cause SLI (Bishop, 1997b; Broman, Nichols, Shaughnessy and Kennedy, 1987). In 196 children with DLD studied by the present authors and others, only 2% of parents reported birth weights under 1.5 kg. and there was no difference in potentially deleterious perinatal factors reported by parents of children with DLD compared to those with autism and mental deficiency without autism (Rapin, 1996a). Thus, even when a history of prematurity or asphyxia is elicited, it is unlikely to be solely responsible for the language disorder (Aram, Hack, Hawkins et al., 1991). Although it is the case that very low birth weight infants are often quite delayed in language and motor skills as toddlers, in the vast majority of those without overt brain insults such as cerebral palsy, mental retardation, or epilepsy, language catches up during the preschool years (Klein, Hack and Breslau, 1989), even though their cognitive level may be inferior to that of their siblings. The language of even those who do have cognitive sequellae does not have the deviant characteristics of DLD.

Environmental toxins, lead in particular, have demonstrable dose-related deleterious effects on the developing brain (Needleman, 1990), although they are much more likely to lower general cognitive ability than to affect language skills selectively. In contrast to the serious cognitive consequences of moderate to high lead levels, there is no credible evidence for a specific effect of slightly elevated lead levels on language. The same can be said about intrauterine exposure to ethanol. Fetal alcohol syndrome is responsible for a sizable proportion of mild to moderate mental deficiency, often associated with attention deficit disorder, but not for pure SLI (Coles, Platzman, Raskind-Hood et al., 1997). Intrauterine exposure to cocaine and other street drugs, combined with social disadvantage, contributes significantly to the burden of developmental disorders, including language (Mentis, 1998; Msall, Bier, LaGasse et al., 1998), but again does not produce SLI.

Environmental social influences

Language is a socially dependent as well as biologically determined human characteristic. As just stated, experience interacts with genetic programs to shape the unfolding of communicative abilities. Total social and environmental deprivation precludes language acquisition, as demonstrated by isolated children like Genie, studied by Curtiss (1977). Although less extreme early deprivation often delays and impoverishes children's language (e.g., Blank and Allen, 1976; Richardson, 1981; Skuse, 1988), it rarely if ever provides a convincing cause for DLD. In the absence of genetic or congenital anomalies or gross malnutrition, delay caused by less than extreme social deprivation has a good prognosis if a more stimulating environment is provided (Skuse, 1988). Because brain plasticity decreases with age, it is widely held that adequate language acquisition is precluded by mid to late childhood, even if children are thereafter exposed to adequate language. It is true that it will not develop effortlessly and rapidly after the 'critical period' for language development is passed in early adolescence. Nonetheless the end of childhood does not totally close the door on language acquisition: a deaf adult who had no formal language — visual or auditory — and no concept of linguistic communication, with intensive education was able to discover what language was and to acquire manual language and, eventually reading (Schaller, 1991). Of course adults are able to learn new languages, but vanishingly few do so with the ease and rapidity of young children and they are unlikely to achieve fully idiomatic or phonologically unaccented speech, even in a foreign language that they have spoken fluently for years.

Bilingualism is sometimes invoked as a possible cause for inadequate acquisition of language. Normal children growing up in a bilingual (or multilingual) environment acquire both languages in the same way as they would a single language. They seem to differentiate between their languages virtually from the start even though they may use words from both languages in utterances during language acquisition (Genesee, 1988). By the same token, dysphasic bilingual children are dysphasic in both languages. Bilingualism is not a sufficient reason for dysphasia, although therapists and educators regularly recommend postponing the exposure of dysphasic children to two languages so as to decrease the demands on a partially compromised system. Hard evidence for this commonsense recommendation seems to be lacking, however.

Neurologic basis of language and dysphasia

Evidence for the neurologic basis of normal language and of dysphasia, although still largely inferential, rests on parallels between developmental and acquired disorders of language, on genetic grounds, on meager neuropathologic data, on imaging and electrophysiologic evidence, and on the presence of associated signs of brain dysfunction.

Neurologic basis of language

A much oversimplified view of the neurologic operations required for language reception include stimulation of the receptors in the ear, transmission of auditory excitation up the relays of the central auditory pathway which contribute to sharpening the auditory signal on its way to the primary and secondary auditory cortices and specialized language association areas. Phonologic, syntactic and lexical decoding entails temporary storage for processing, assisted by on-line activation of previously stored linguistic information from long term memory. The importance of the decoded verbal message is then evaluated in the light of other on-going priorities in order to select an appropriate response (or no response). Formulation and production of a verbal response involves the retrieval of needed words from the lexicon (repository of words in the brain), arranging them into a coherent grammatical utterance, programming the appropriate motor commands for speech, and, finally, execution of the planned utterance by the muscles of respiration, phonation, and articulation.

Thus language processing depends on many interconnected parallel and serial operations. Decoding is by no means an entirely sequential bottom-up process. Although the semantic interpretation of a verbal message must await a certain amount of phonologic, lexical, and grammatical decoding, top-down processing dependent on prior knowledge is activated as soon as a language input is perceived. It hastens and facilitates higher level comprehension by proceeding in parallel with lower level sequential operations. Language comprehension is the result of a widely distributed pattern of neural activation that builds up over time as potentially relevant meanings are enhanced and irrelevant meanings suppressed. Information about the structure (syntax), meaning (semantics), and intent (pragmatics) of an utterance is acquired in parallel and interacts in real time during speech comprehension. Functional MRI and PET scanning indicate that, although the conventional frontal and temporo/parietal perisylvian language cortices of the left hemisphere are activated preferentially during language processing, the language processing networks include many other areas such as the cerebellum, neostriatum, dorsolateral prefrontal cortex, anterior cingulate cortex, and others.

As comprehension and production of language require such complex and overlapping mental operations, it should come as no surprise that if one or more of these operations is defective, the constellation of spared and impaired language functions results in atypical language development compared to language acquisition in normally developing children, and in a variety of DLD subtypes.

DLD, acquired aphasias, and cerebral localization

Owing to the potential of the developing brain for reorganization following damage, children who sustain unilateral left or right brain lesions affecting the perisylvian cortex *in utero* or in early life do not have DLD (Bates, 1999; see chapter by Bates et al., 2003). Language development is somewhat delayed but competence is usually achieved before schoolage, although careful testing may show subtle lexical and syntactic deficits in children with left-sided lesions (Aram, 1988). The price for the plasticity in cerebral organization which makes it possible for anatomically aberrant circuitry for language to develop in the right hemisphere is often 'crowding out' of some visual–spatial skills that, normally, depend on that hemisphere's activity (Milner, 1974; Nass, 1997; Nass, Sadler and Sidtis, 1992; Stark and McGregor, 1997; Teuber, 1975; see chapters by Nass, 2002, and by Bates et al., 2003).

There are limits to plasticity which decreases with maturation but persists to some degree lifelong. Acquired aphasia occurring after children have mastered language produces some persistent deficits (Loonen and Van Dongen, 1990). Childhood aphasias tend to be milder than the permanent, varied, and often severe residual aphasias that follow large cortical and subcortical lesions in older children and adults whose brains have lost much of their plasticity (see chapter by Van Hout, 2003). Left anterior subcortical lesions involving the adjacent white matter are more likely to result in persistent deficits in children than cortical lesions (Aram and Eisele, 1994). The localization of lesions responsible for particular types of acquired aphasias in children parallel localization in adults (Van Hout, 2003).

With the one exception of verbal auditory agnosia (VAA), almost nothing is known about the localization of brain dysfunction in children with various DLD subtypes. This is true even though comparison of the language characteristics of clinically defined DLD syndromes with several of the acquired adult aphasias shows striking parallels (Rapin and Allen, 1988). Whether these parallels provide clues regarding localization of dysfunction in DLD remains to be determined. Tools like functional magnetic resonance imaging (fMRI) and electrophysiology may answer some of these questions, but systematic comparisons between children with well defined dysphasic syndromes and others with acquired aphasias have yet to be carried out.

Anatomic parallel between dysphasia and acquired aphasia is closest in VAA (word deafness) (Klein, Kurtzberg, Brattson et al., 1995; Klein, Tuchman and Rapin, 2000; Rapin, 1996b; Rapin, Mattis, Rowan and Golden, 1977). The adult variant results from bilateral damage to the auditory cortex in the temporal lobes. Characteristically, adult patients can speak, read, and write, but they understand little or no oral language. In some cases they have an even more pervasive deficit and cannot identify environmental sounds (auditory agnosia) or, rarely, they may be cortically deaf, especially early in the course of the disorder. In children with acquired epileptic aphasia or Landau–Kleffner syndrome (LKS) (Landau and Kleffner, 1957), the deficit too may fluctuate between cortical deafness, auditory agnosia, and VAA (Kaga, 1999). The main difference between adults and young children with developmental VAA is that, because they are in the prelinguistic stage of language acquisition, children are likely to be mute as well as unable to comprehend acoustic language. Rapid disappearance of speech is also true of preschool and young schoolage children with acquired VAA, as well as of young children with sudden cochlear deafness, for example from meningitis. In children, VAA often occurs in the context of acquired epileptic aphasia or LKS (e.g., Van Dongen, De Wijngaert and Wennekes, 1991), in which VAA is associated with either clinical seizures or an epileptiform EEG. VAA may also occur as a developmental syndrome without clinical epilepsy (Klein et al., 2000; Worster-Drought and Allen, 1930). VAA may characterize some mute severely impaired autistic children who understand little or nothing of what is said to them but who may be able to acquire some language through the visual modality (Bonvillian, Nelson and Rhyne, 1981).

Classical LKS is almost never associated with a gross brain lesion on computer tomography (CT) or MRI. The EEG abnormality is often bilateral and perisylvian (Lewine, Andrews, Chez et al., 1999), although in some children the EEG discharges are lateralized to the right or left temporo-parietal region or may fluctuate from side to side (Rapin et al., 1977). In some children these discharges have the characteristics of Rolandic epilepsy (Graf and Lischka, 1998) or of status epilepticus in slow wave sleep (Beaumanoir, Bureau, Deonna et al., 1995). Thus far, VAA is the only DLD syndrome in which there is information about localization of dysfunction and, significantly, localization conforms to what has been learned from adult aphasia and to what is known about the organization of the language networks of the brain.

Neuropathology and neuroimaging in DLD

As classic DLD is not associated with clinically detectable cerebral malformations or lesions, there are virtually no data on its neuropathology. Landau, Goldstein and Kleffner's (1960) one case would be disqualified by today's criteria as the boy's bilateral temporal porencephalies were major acquired brain lesions that would have been readily detectable by CT or MRI. Eight consecutive brains of dyslexic persons, at least four of whom were DLD children grown up, did not have the expected asymmetry between the left and right *planum temporale*, with the right being atypically large. There were also microscopic cortical scars and areas of abnormal cell migration that predominated in the dominant hemisphere of some but not all cases (Galaburda, Sherman, Rosen et al., 1985; Humphreys, Kaufmann and Galaburda, 1990). The investigators attributed these tiny scars and cortical dysgeneses to intrauterine or perinatal microvascular insults of as yet undetermined but possibly autoimmune etiology, and they speculated that the larger planum temporale on the right might reflect failure of programmed cell death or inadequate pruning of superfluous neural processes (Rosen, Galaburda and Sherman, 1990). More recent work in animals suggests that prenatal overmigration of neurons into the leptomeninges may result from abnormalities of signaling molecules under genetic control rather than from acquired intrauterine pathology (e.g., Brunstrom, Gray-Swain, Osborne and Pearlman, 1997; Sherman and Holmes, 1999).

The planum temporale, which encompasses the primary and secondary auditory cortices, is larger on the left than the right in about two thirds of normal brains (Geschwind and Levitsky, 1968), a difference already discernible in the last third of fetal life (Chi, Dooling and Gilles, 1977). Coupled with the mass of evidence for specialization of the left hemisphere for language, this asymmetry is widely considered a plausible correlate for language lateralization, with lack of asymmetry or reversed asymmetry a marker for dysphasia and dyslexia. A number of studies based on linear measurements of CT scan films report an increased prevalence of 'reversed asymmetry' in dysphasics and dyslexics, as well as a variety of other areal or volumetric changes (Habib, 2000; Plante, Swisher, Vance et al., 1991). Agreement on these findings is not universal, however, but there is preliminary evidence in normal children that the size of auditory association areas (planum temporale) may be linked to phonemic awareness and age (Leonard, Lombardino, Mercado et al., 1996). A morphometric study by Preis, Jancke, Schittler et al. (1998) describes normal left/right asymmetry in 21 children with mixed receptive/expressive DLD compared to controls, but a slightly (7%) smaller overall hemispheric size on the left. Unusual gyral morphology in the posterior perisylvian region was found in five families with an expressive dysphasia (Jackson and Plante, 1996). Thus far no pathognomonic morphometric correlate has been identified in DLD and imaging has little or nothing to offer in the clinical diagnostic evaluation of the individual child.

There is rapid progress in imaging regions of increased cerebral blood flow with fMRI or single photon emission tomography (SPECT), and imaging of enhanced oxygen or glucose utilization with positron emission tomography (PET) during the performance of various language-relevant tasks. Comparisons of activation by stimuli presented to the auditory, visual, or somatosensory modality are yielding data on the localization of activation by language or other tasks (Petersen, Fox, Posner et al., 1988). The studies show widespread focal activation of the classic language areas of the left hemisphere, even in deaf signers, but also participation of the right hemisphere, cerebellum, and other brain areas (Fiez and Petersen, 1998; Fiez, Raichle, Balota et al., 1996). The utility of these procedures in the evaluation of developmental and acquired disorders in children is reviewed in Chugani and Chugani (2003, this volume). These are exciting research techniques for elucidating the neurologic basis of language and DLD but, again, they have little or no place in the clinical evaluation of an individual child with DLD unless the child has epilepsy and its surgical treatment is being considered.

Techniques more readily applicable to infants and children are electrophysiology and magnetoencephalography (see Steinschneider and Dunn, 2002; Lee, Kuppusamy, Grueneich et al., 1999; Leppanen and Lyytinen, 1997). Electrophysiology records the sequential activation in real time of each of the relays of the auditory pathway, from the ear to the cortex.

With the use of multiple electrode arrays and appropriate mathematical methods for the localization of cortical and subcortical generators, electrophysiology provides anatomic data that can be mapped onto MRI images. Thus electrophysiology makes it possible to follow the sequential processing of the various stages and levels of language. It also makes it possible to compare language presented to the auditory channel with its presentation to the visual or tactile channel. Cochlear emissions and brain stem auditory evoked response (ABR) audiometry are the techniques of choice to rule out peripheral sensorineural loss in infants and uncooperative children as they provide hearing threshold data (Nozza, Sabo and Mandel, 1997; Stapells and Oates, 1997). Cochlear emissions probe hair cell function and the ABR provides information on auditory conduction time in the brainstem. The relevance of prolonged conduction times recorded in some children with communication disorders remains uncertain (Von Suchodoletz and Wolfram, 1996), although it might be related to the deficit in processing rapid acoustic stimuli described by Tallal (Tallal, Miller and Fitch, 1993; Tallal and Piercy, 1974).

Modern electrophysiology yields information about cortical correlates of language. Cohen and LeNormand (1998) studied the effects of focal epileptic discharges on language development. Children with focal discharges were more delayed in the development of speech production than comprehension. Event-related potentials (ERPs) are powerful tools for studying brain physiology during the performance of a variety of language tasks. For example, Neville and collaborators (Mills and Neville, 1997; Neville and Bavelier, 1998) have shown distinct correlates of the processing of small grammatical words such as articles and prepositions and of content words such as nouns, verbs, and adjectives in young children with normal or delayed language development.

Associated neurologic deficits

DLD may be associated with other signs of brain dysfunction (so-called soft signs) of insufficient severity to be exclusionary criteria for a diagnosis of DLD. Some of these signs are probably due to lack of selectivity of the pathologies responsible for the developmental disorders of higher cerebral function. Some associated deficits include mild impairment of gross and fine motor skills, visuospatial abilities, attention, memory, cognition, sociability, and, in some cases, epilepsy. Children with DLD may be clumsy, hypotonic, dyspraxic, and have oromotor deficits, with or without drooling and dysarthria (Haynes and Naidoo, 1991; Powell and Bishop, 1992; Preis, Schittler and Lenard, 1997). *Dysarthria*, a motor deficit, is quite frequent in some subtypes of DLD and may contribute to poor speech intelligibility, but it does not account for dysphasia, a language deficit, even though both may have a common underlying cause (Guerreiro, Andermann, Guerrini et al., 2000). There are occasional dysphasic children who have overt sensorimotor deficits such as spastic diplegia or congenital hemiparesis, forms of cerebral palsy not typically associated with dysphasia. As discussed earlier, if one views DLD as a specific developmental disorder and is interested in investigating its etiology, one will exclude such children because cerebral palsy signals an overt brain lesion. One could, however, argue with some justification that dysphasic children with focal brain lesions constitute a particular subgroup worthy of study among children with deficient language acquisition.

There is an increased prevalence of seizures in children with DLD (Picard, Cheliout-Héraut, Bouskraoui et al., 1998; Tuchman, Rapin and Shinnar, 1991). This is accounted for, in part but not entirely, by the syndrome of acquired epileptic aphasia or LKS, discussed earlier, which is a form of acquired aphasia rather than a dysphasia. As a group, children with all types of developmental disorders are at somewhat greater risk for epilepsy than other children, a risk that increases with the severity of the underlying pathology indexed by mental deficiency and cerebral palsy (Goulden, Shinnar, Koller et al., 1991).

Autism (pervasive developmental disorder — PDD or the autistic spectrum disorders) is virtually always associated with some form of language disorder (Allen, 1988; Dunn and Rapin, 1997). In fact, the most common presenting complaint of parents of autistic preschoolers is delayed language development or lack of speech. Communication disorder and inadequate imaginative play are the second of three behavioral domains that define the autistic spectrum (the others are impaired sociability, and behavioral rigidity, perseveration, and a narrow range of interests). This does not imply that autism is a form of DLD or a consequence of DLD, but that the brain dysfunction responsible for autism affects systems that sustain language as well as those responsible for the other manifestations of autism. In other words, autistic children are both autistic *and* dysphasic, with the notable difference that purely expressive disorders are very rare or absent in young children with autism (Allen and Rapin, 1992; Wassink et al., 2001).

There is an increased prevalence of behavior disorders among children with DLD and other developmental disorders of higher cerebral function (Beitchman, Brownlie, Inglis et al., 1996). Although some of the behavioral problems may be reactive to the social consequences of the disability, others, for example disorders of attention, are more likely a comorbid condition (Shaywitz, Fletcher and Shaywitz, 1995).

Normal versus abnormal development of the levels of language

The various levels of language do not develop in parallel or at a uniform pace. Consequently, atypical development does not affect them uniformly. This lack of uniformity contributes significantly to the various subtypes of DLD.

Pragmatics

Pragmatics is the system of rules for the communicative use of language. *Nonverbal pragmatics* includes facial expression, tone of voice, gestures and body posture, features that provide a context for the interpretation of verbal language and of the speakers's communicative intent. Pragmatics also includes rules for nonverbal indicators of comprehension and attentiveness (or boredom, impatience, etc.). *Verbal pragmatics* refers to the rules for turn-taking, initiating communication and responding, the maintenance of meaningful conversation, such as staying on topic and making one's referent clear, and for using stylistic modes of expression, such as word choices, that are appropriate to the particular social situation.

Pragmatic development starts at birth and is exemplified by the reciprocal gaze and facial expression of infants and their care takers in face-to-face interaction (Tronick, 1989; Weinberg and Tronick, 1994). At just a few months, the infant scans faces, takes turns vocalizing, and imitates and responds to the affect on the care-taker's face. This responsive looking and cooing is the start of the communicative use of language, and of the realization that language confers power over another person's behavior. The inability to develop nonverbal communicative competence must be seen as a very serious developmental failure.

Most normally developing children make communicative use of whatever language they have developed, even at the single-word stage, supplementing verbal utterances with gestures like pointing and altered tone of voice. In contrast, severe pragmatic deficits characterize individuals on the autistic spectrum, whether they are verbal or not, although some types of severely language-impaired children also exhibit pragmatic deficits (Adams and Bishop, 1989; Bishop and Adams, 1989; Rapin and Allen, 1998). Toddlers know to look up when addressed by name, and most preschoolers will have learned that one speaks to someone rather than to the wall, even though speaking aloud to no one in particular while engrossed in an activity may persist in very reduced form in some adults.

Investigation of pragmatics in children involves noting (1) what they know about engaging in interpersonal communication (e.g., initiating, responding, maintaining the topic of discourse, and observing turn-taking rules) within a specified context; (2) for what purposes they use speech (e.g., giving or requesting information or behavior from a conversational partner, requesting clarification, etc.); and (3) under what conversational circumstances they violate traditional conversation rules or make errors in comprehension, structure or semantics. In order to reduce the complexity of the analysis and to insure maximal inter-rater reliability, the number of categories to be rated should be kept to a reasonable limit (see Adams and Bishop, 1989; Bishop and Adams, 1989; Damico, 1985) for examples of this type of analysis). Bishop (1998) recently developed a checklist suitable for teachers and therapists to evaluate the pragmatic skills of schoolage children.

Phonology

Phonology is the highly encoded sound system of spoken languages. Phonemes are the basic sound units which are combined into words. In contrast to vowels, consonants are perceived categorically, that is, they have clear acoustic boundaries. Consonant and vowels are co-articulated, so that the acoustic signals for individual phonemes vary depending on the phonemes that precede and follow them. The first operation in decoding a verbal message is perception and processing of the rapid components of the acoustic signal that define its co-articulated component phonemes (Liegeois-Chauvel, De Graaf, Laguitton and Chauvel, 1999; Tallal and Piercy, 1974; Tallal et al., 1993). Prosody is the suprasegmental melody of speech that assists in conveying the intent of speakers' utterances, thus clarifying meaning.

Although the development of phonologic perception relevant to the language(s) heard starts at birth, full mastery of the production of all the phonemes of a language extends over several years. Some misarticulations may persist until the early school years, for example in English /l/, /r/ /w/ and /s/, /f/, /th/. Whether these developmental misarticulations arise from perceptual or fine motor programming deficits or delays seems to vary. For example, 6 year old children who misarticulated /r/ and /w/ were shown in one study not to perceive these speech sounds categorically like normally speaking children (Hoffman, Daniloff, Bengoa and Schuckers, 1985). Another study attributed misarticulations of lingual consonants to deficient motor control of the tongue (Gibbon, 1999). Some of the phonologic errors of normally developing young children include deletions of initial and final consonants, cluster reduction, and substitution of voiced/voiceless consonants. Many of the phonologic deficits in children with DLD are substitutions, deletions, or distortions that are not, or are rarely seen in normal children at any age, or that persist after the children become fully verbal. A good rule-of-thumb for determining whether a child has phonological *deficits,* as opposed to *developmental misarticulations,* lies in the relationship between sound production and size of vocabulary (Ingram, 1976), with normally developing children regularly 'cleaning up' their speech articulation as they become more verbal.

Semantics

Semantics refers to the meaning of individual words and the integration of these meanings in connected language. The *lexicon* is the store of the words individuals carry in their brains which are linked to complex phonologic and meaning networks. Semantics subsumes two inter-related subsystems: *lexical semantics* (vocabulary and knowledge of word classes) and *relational semantics* (more abstract meaning relations expressed through word combinations) (De Villiers and De Villiers, 1978). The study of semantic development is complicated by the fact that there is a strong relationship between the development of a lexicon and the development of cognitive concepts (e.g., temporality, causality, modality, etc.) on the one hand, and between relational semantics and both syntax and pragmatic use on the other. Both kinds of semantics have been much more widely studied in young normal children than in those with language disorders, but even in the psycholinguistic literature there is a paucity of information about normative developmental sequences in the acquisition of the semantic system.

The development of a lexicon requires the ability to recognize that words can be used to refer to such entities as people, objects, attributes, events, and locations. The ability to express relational meanings (e.g. agent, object, action) is dependent upon an awareness that the same word can stand in many different relationships to other words (e.g., the word *boy* in the sentences 'John is a boy'; 'the boy kissed the girl'; 'the boy was kissed by the girl'; 'the boy is happy'; and so on).

The two most widely used methods for assessing semantic development are the type-token-ratio (TTR, the number of different words divided by the total number of words in a language sample) (Templin, 1957) and semantic field analysis (Bloom, 1970; Brown, 1973; Greenfield and Smith, 1976; Miller, 1981; see also Bates et al., 2003). Templin reported that the TTR was approximately 0.50 across her age sample from 3.0–8.0 years.

Semantic field analysis provides a framework for determining the kinds of meaning categories that have been acquired, as well as the number of different words within categories. For example, it is well recognized that normally developing young children begin with primitive vocabulary tokens that are used generically at first (e.g., 'mommy' for all adult women; 'up' for both upward and downward directions; 'car' for all vehicles; and 'doggie' for all four-legged animals). It is quite clear that the development of such semantic fields is more than a linguistic process. Rather, the child's cognitive development interacts with vocabulary development in the formation of cognitive-linguistic categories (Bloom and Lahey, 1978).

To date, most of the semantic studies have been limited to small samples of children at the earliest stages of language development. Children with hearing losses, those with receptive language deficits, as well as those who grow up in linguistically impoverished environments are bound to have a restricted stock of words, which jeopardizes their comprehension of what is being said and their ability to express themselves, especially as word retrieval may be inefficient and grammar rudimentary. Teasing out the purely semantic deficits from deficits in the larger cognitive and linguistic networks presents a real challenge.

Grammar

Grammar refers to the rules for assigning roles to words and assembling them into complex utterances to convey the speaker's message meaningfully and unambiguously. There is considerable variability among languages regarding the relative importance of *syntax* (word order) and *morphology* (the alteration of word roots to form complex words and to indicate the role of words in sentences).

Morphology lies at the linguistic nexus of phonology, syntax and semantics. Morphemes are often referred to as the 'minimal units of meaning'. There are several types of morphemes: free and bound derivational morphemes, free and bound grammatical morphemes. Free derivational morphemes are expressed as words, whereas bound derivational morphemes are connected to a free form. Thus the word */uneasy/* is comprised of the free morpheme (easy) and the bound morpheme (un) which means 'not'. Bound grammatical morphemes may mark both grammatical and semantic meaning. In English, bound grammatical morphemes mark such various aspects of language as possessive (*boy/boy's*), past tense (*walk/walked*), plural (*boy/boys*), and third person singular (*go/goes*). There is an expected developmental order in the acquisition of free and bound morpheme production which language-impaired children may or may not follow (Brown, 1973; Miller, 1981).

There is a potentially infinite number of nouns, adjectives, verbs, and adverbs (*open class words*) in any language, and new ones are constantly being forged as the communication needs of societies change with time. Function words, on the other hand, are the *closed* (i.e., finite) *class* of free grammatical morphemes that signal relation between words in sentences or between sentences. The function words include articles (e.g., *the, a, these*), prepositions (e.g., *on, through*), conjunctions (e.g., *and, or, but, because*), personal and impersonal pronouns (e.g., *it, he, they*), and interrogative pronouns (the so-called Wh- questions words *who, what, when*, etc.).

The development of word combinations (*syntax*) in the language acquisition of normally-developing children was the primary focus of psycholinguistic research in the 1960s and 1970s (the reader is referred to Miller (1981) for results of the principal language acquisition studies). Although there has been widespread theoretical difference of opinion as to how children move from being single-word speakers to grammatically competent language users, there are some generalizations about the acquisition of English syntax in young children which have stood the test of time: (1) children regularly begin producing two-word utterances sometime between 18 and 24 months; (2) early two-word utterances are structured rather than random, but they do not resemble adult sentences that the children could have heard (this indicates that the children are learning a linguistic rule rather than parroting what they have heard) (Pinker, 1999); (3) there is a virtual explosion in the acquisition of syntactic 'rules' between the ages of 2 and 3 years; (4) early sentences are either imperatives or simple active affirmative declaratives, whereas the syntax of negation, question-formation, and passives emerges later; and (5) most children acquire all of the basic elements of language by the age of 5 years (see the chapter by Bates et al., 2003, for more detail).

The most common measure of grammatical (morphologic and syntactic) development in both normal and language impaired children is the mean length of utterance (MLU) which can be computed in terms of words or morphemes. According to Brown (1973), MLU and syntactic development are highly correlated in normal development. MLU is an indirect measure of grammar, as it also depends on the richness of the lexicon. Bishop (1989a) developed the more specific Test for the Reception of Grammar (TROG) to evaluate grammatical competence. Miller and Chapman (1981) found that between ages 1.5 and 5 years, MLU increases on average by 1.2 morphemes per year. There are some studies of language-disordered children that suggest a disconnection of MLU and syntactic development (see Johnston and Schery, 1976; Scarborough, Rescorla, Tager-Flusberg et al., 1991; Van der Lely, 1993; Van der Lely, Rosen and McClelland, 1998), particularly beyond the earliest stages of syntactic development. That is, some children with DLD produce long utterances that are missing either obligatory function words or morphologic inflections, or both. In our experience, errors of omission or substitution of grammatical morphemes are quite common in many children with expressive language disorders. According to the electrophysiologic studies of Neville and colleagues (Mills and Neville, 1997), cortical evoked responses to function words in children with DLD with deficient grammar do not have the expected left hemisphere asymmetry seen in children with normally developing language.

There is considerable controversy as to whether language-disordered children acquire grammatical morphemes and rules of syntax in the same order as normally developing children, or whether their productions differ from normals at any age. One of the reasons for disparate findings in clinical research on this topic lies in how one chooses the control group to be compared with the disordered group. Those studies that use age-matched normal controls regularly find major discrepancies between the two. Those that use younger normal children matched by MLU with the impaired group generally find that the two groups are quite similar in the order in which grammatical development proceeds, but clearly dissimilar in the rate of rule acquisition (Cromer, 1987; Johnston, 1988).

Some investigators suggest that there are children with DLD whose primary deficit is grammatical (e.g., Gopnik and Crago, 1991; Van der Lely et al., 1998), but there is contrary evidence. Detailed evaluation of the family with dominant DLD studied by Gopnick indicated that their deficits were not limited to grammar but also involved phonology, the lexicon, and verbal and nonverbal praxic deficits (Vargha-Khadem, Watkins, Alcock et al., 1995). Exciting findings in this family were linkage to chromosome 7q31 (Fisher et al., 1998; Lai et al., 2000), and cortical and subcortical frontal abnormalities on fMRI, as well as bilateral smallness of the caudate nucleus on MRI morphometry (Vargha-Khadem, Watkins, Price et al., 1998). Other evidence that brings into question the primacy of syntactic deficits in DLD is Bishop's report (Bishop, 1983, 1997a) that children with hearing losses have syntactic deficits similar to those of dysphasic children with mixed receptive–expressive deficits, suggesting that the syntactic deficits may be the consequence of inadequacy in the first step of language decoding, phonology.

Not all children with DLD have syntactic deficits. In contrast to those with mixed receptive–expressive phonologic–syntactic deficits, syntax and phonology are spared or largely spared in children with higher order processing deficits. More complex linguistic structures such as clausal embeddings, passive voice, and the like may be missing, however, even in fluent DLD children. It is important to keep in mind that syntax merely provides the frame for expressing ideas. It may very well be that some children who acquire only very simple grammars are in fact deficient in the cognitive linguistic concepts or knowledge of the semantic relations which are ordinarily expressed through more elaborate syntactic constructions.

Patterns of abnormal language functioning

Children with developmental language disorders characteristically exhibit a disturbance in the rates and sequences of acquisition of the linguistic features just described. The ways in which these disturbances manifest themselves result in different profiles of impaired and spared functions. In this section, we describe some of the deviations from expected acquisition patterns.

Dissociation of comprehension and production

In normally developing children, one ordinarily sees the onset of speech closely following the comprehension of individual words. In some DLD children, comprehension far outstrips production for an extended period of time; that is, they have a severe delay in the onset of speech despite adequate comprehension. In many of these children, language expression is poor when it finally emerges (see below). There is another, even more dramatic, dissociation between comprehension and production seen in children who can speak better than they can comprehend, a pattern that is virtually never seen in the normal population, except briefly in some toddlers who process language holistically rather than analytically. Children with better expression than comprehension are usually fluent and intelligible, but they tend to use over-learned phrases and formulaic productions which may mask considerable deficits in the comprehension of connected and abstract language. This deficit can be brought out by asking these children questions: they are likely to answer beside the point of the question, chaining to a word in the question rather than to the query. This pattern characterizes verbal children with the semantic–pragmatic language deficit syndrome (see below).

Discrepancy between lexical acquisition and intelligibility

Many language-disordered children have delayed onset of speech despite adequate comprehension. When some of these children begin to speak, their productions are sparse and effortful, with limited syntactic complexity. Their comprehension of connected speech is normal or near normal, they appear to have acquired an adequate lexicon, and they know what they want to communicate. Some of these children have a verbal dyspraxia, which may or may not be associated with oromotor dysfunction. Others are more fluent and attempt to use multi-word utterances but are largely unintelligible. Both of these patterns differ from the expected increase in intelligibility as vocabulary develops. Many children with this difficulty resort to elaborate use of gestures to make their thoughts known.

Discrepancies between language development and speech production

It is important to distinguish *dysarthria* from an expressive or mixed expressive–receptive DLD. Dysarthria is not a language disorder; it is a motor deficit involving the muscles of phonation and articulation. The hallmark of dysarthria is that it also affects swallowing and voluntary control of the tongue and lips, as well as the rhythm, fluency, volume, and clarity of articulation, and the intelligibility of speech. Dysarthria may result from impaired cerebral or cerebellar control of the orofacial muscles (*pseudobulbar palsy, oromotor dyspraxia*), for example by cerebral palsy, or be caused by pathology affecting the nerves innervating the muscles or weakness of the muscles themselves (*bulbar palsy*), for example by congenital facial palsy (Moebius syndrome). Some children with DLD are dysarthric as well as dysphasic, especially those with verbal dyspraxia, the nonfluent variant of expressive DLD (Christen, Hanefeld, Kruse et al., 2000; Ferry, Hall and Hicks, 1975; Guerreiro et al., 2000), and those with the mixed receptive–expressive deficit disorder (Stark and Blackwell, 1997).

Stuttering does not impair intelligibility but it does affect fluency and, occasionally, it may be mistaken for *spastic dysphonia*, a form of dysarthria originating from dysfunction of the basal ganglia in which children struggle to speak, but rarely if ever stutter. Stuttering is characterized by the repetition of the beginning of some words, as well as by pauses (blocks) as stutterers struggle to speak. Stuttering may be confused with the pseudo-stuttering of children with word finding problems who may repeat the first syllable of a word they are having difficulty retrieving from their lexicon (Rapin and Allen, 1983), however without the blocks of stutterers, which are often associated with facial grimacing. Some 4% of children stutter, but in the majority stuttering is transient as the prevalence of stuttering is only 1% in adults. Although the neurologic basis of stuttering is not known, it is thought to arise from competition between the two hemispheres for the control of speech production (Jones, 1966) or to be a disorder in the timing of motor control for speech (Rosenfield and Barroso, 2000). As in other developmental disorders, genetics contributes to its occurrence (Poulos and Webster, 1991).

Dissociation of vocabulary and grammatical development

Around the second birthday, most children exhibit a burst in vocabulary accompanied by the appearance of two-word utterances. The two-word stage varies in duration, but is ordinarily followed by multi-word constructions at such a rapid rate that it is difficult to determine a three-word or four-word stage. The explosive growth of the lexicon soon makes it too large to count. In some language-disordered children, vocabulary development proceeds independently of grammar, so that the size of the vocabulary is not synchronous with the MLU. That is, the children may acquire lexical forms adequately, but lack the means to express their ideas in multi-word utterances. In other children, the rules for grammatical construction may be in evidence, but the application of such rules may be faulty. For example, in describing a picture of a boy blowing out the candles on a birthday cake, one 4-year-old child said: "That boy can't blow candles at hers birthday party next week because it too hard". This child had a knowledge of negation, infinitives, plurals, gender pronouns, possession, prepositions, and temporal and causal adverbs, but clearly his acquisition of these morphological forms was not accompanied by the mastery of their grammatical use in this lengthy sentence.

Discrepancy between vocabulary size and pragmatic use

One expects young children to acquire the most primitive communicative uses of the lexicon with relative ease. That is, as vocabulary increases, most children can use their words for requesting, commenting, questioning, calling, protesting, and regulating others' behaviors. They have learned that language gives them the power to alter others' behaviors on their behalf. There are some language-disordered children who acquire impressively large and sophisticated vocabularies, but which they are able to use only for labeling purposes rather than for communicating with others. We met one such 2-year-old child who had an expressive and receptive (pointing) vocabulary of several hundred nouns (including 'artichoke' and 'Oldsmobile') but could not use even simple words to make his needs known. Another child who exhibited a dissociation between vocabulary size and communication was able to ask the question "Is this a spatula or a slotted spoon?" but was not able to answer the question "What do you do with a spoon?" This type of deficit is characteristic of young verbal children on the autistic spectrum (Dunn, Gomes and Sebastian, 1996).

Discrepancy between language ability and word retrieval

It is common for language disordered children who have acquired adequate vocabularies, grammar and pragmatic rules to have difficulty accessing their lexicons in connected speech (anomia). Their deficits may be seen in the excessive use of non-specific forms (such as 'this thing') or in circumlocutions to avoid their difficulties in lexical retrieval which in some children, as just mentioned, may result in pseudo-stuttering. Their spontaneously generated speech may be much better than language 'on demand', e.g., for labeling or answering questions; or they may be equally impaired in both situations. In either case, they have considerably more difficulty formulating coherent sentences than their overall language abilities would predict.

The dissociations and discrepancies just described and others may occur singly or in various combinations. The ways in which the areas of spared and impaired functions fall together yield different language disorder subtypes.

Classification of language disorders

Attempts to define DLD subtypes

Many investigators have attempted to define subtypes of DLD. It seemed unlikely that there would be only one type of DLD given the complexity of language and the diversity of aphasic syndromes that result from focal brain lesions in adults and in children with language competence (see chapter by Van Hout, 2003) Investigators were eager to gain an understanding of the neurologic basis of developmental dysphasias and to tailor habilitation approaches to children's individual needs.

The simplest models for the subtyping of DLD divide the dysphasias into receptive disorders, which of necessity also affect expression as impaired reception precludes language learning, and expressive disorders in which comprehension is spared or largely spared (American Psychiatric Association, 2000; Tallal, 1988; Wolfus, Moskovitch and Kinsbourne, 1980). Ajuriaguerra, De Jaeggi, Guignard et al. (1976) divided the children into fluent and nonfluent groups, and Ingram (1975) partitioned them along a severity continuum. As these simple models did not do justice to the complexity of language processing, more encompassing classifications were developed.

Aram and Nation (1975) took into account both reception, production, and repetition of language and its structural levels (phonology, syntax, and semantics). Using children's scores on formal tests of language, they divided dysphasic children into 6 subtypes and followed 30 of the original 47 children into school age to evaluate subtype stability and prognosis (Aram, Ekelman and Nation, 1984; Nation and Aram, 1990). Twenty of the children were still impaired at school age. Children with poor comprehension remained symptomatic, phonology tended to improve, and children who, at preschool, had good repetition skills did well. Bishop and Rosenbloom (1987) who also based their classification on standardized psychometric tests divided DLD children into 4 subtypes: VAA, fluent, nonfluent, and delayed. The classification of Wilson and Risucci (Wilson and Risucci, 1986) used the results of a language evaluation to guide the clustering of scores from subtests of a neuropsychologic battery. They demonstrated close correspondence of their 8 subtypes with the subtypes defined by Aram and Nation (1975) and Rapin and Allen (1983). Korkman and Hakkinen-Rihu (1994) factor analyzed scores of 6–8 year old children on a language/neuropsychologic battery and derived three main subtypes: global, dyspraxia, and impaired comprehension. They validated their classification 3 years later and found an additional, rare subtype, specific dysnomia. Coverage was 80%. They did not identify a purely expressive subtype.

The author's clinical classification of preschool DLD children's language divides them into three main groups, each with two subtypes (Table 1). The three major groups are (1) expressive deficit syndromes, in which comprehension is normal or near normal in the face of compromised expression; (2) mixed receptive/expressive deficit syndromes in which phonology, syntax and semantics are affected to a greater or lesser degree and in which comprehension may be superior to expression; and (3) higher level formulation deficit syndromes which do not primarily affect phonology or syntax but in which the deficits are at the level of the comprehension and formulation of connected discourse. Each of these three groups can be divided into two distinct subtypes, based primarily on the severity of the children's deficits. The first step in this clinical classification is to determine whether the child is verbal or nonverbal, as three subtypes — VAA (verbal auditory agnosia), the mixed phonologic–syntactic deficit and verbal dyspraxic syndromes — occur in both verbal and nonverbal children.

The authors' proposed clinical typology (Table 1); (Allen, 1989; Rapin, 1996b; Rapin and Allen, 1983) is based on the amount and character of the children's expressive language and on their ability to comprehend single words and connected language (discourse). Word finding problems (anomia) may occur in all subtypes and, therefore, are not helpful for subtyping. Anomia is particularly marked in some children with higher order formulation deficits in whom prolonged hesitations and repetitions of the first syllable of a word or word in an utterance may be mistaken for stuttering. Formulation deficits for connected discourse, for example telling a story coherently or recounting an incident, do not contribute to subtyping either as they occur in all dysphasic subtypes, including in fluent children with large expressive vocabularies. Children who speak clearly and grammatically and in whom formulation difficulties are the main language deficit often go undetected on formal tests of language, but they are identifiable when they are asked to talk about a topic of particular interest or explain how to perform a task, or to answer open-ended questions. The authors have prepared a checklist to assist nonspecialists who evaluate children with inadequate language focus on the relevant aspects of language when attempting to pigeon-hole children clinically (Table 2).

Conti-Ramsden et al. (Conti-Ramsden and Botting, 1999; Conti-Ramsden, Crutchley and Botting, 1997) evaluated with standardized language and educational tests 242 6.5–8 year old children with DLD.

TABLE 1

Preschool developmental language disorders: clinical classification [a]

A. Receptive/expressive disorders

- *Phonologic–syntactic deficit disorder*: Comprehension is equal to or better than expression. Children speak in short, ungrammatical utterances with impaired phonology and limited vocabulary. This syndrome may be associated with articulation difficulties or dysarthria of variable severity, but they are not severe enough to account for the very limited speech.
- *Verbal auditory agnosia (VAA or word deafness).* Children with this disorder have a severe deficit for phonologic decoding, so understand little or nothing of what is said. They may be nonverbal or have very limited, phonologically impaired expression.

B. Expressive disorders

- *Verbal dyspraxia.* Severely impaired, often effortful production of speech in the face of adequate or normal comprehension. Some children may be nonverbal and some have associated oromotor deficits such as drooling or inadequate imitation of oromotor movements. The deficit affects the programming of expressive language and must be distinguished from the dysarthria of bulbar or pseudo-bulbar palsy.
- Speech programming deficit disorder. Fluent or relatively fluent speech, but with very impaired phonology, limiting intelligibility. Comprehension is normal or near normal.

C. Higher order processing disorders

- *Semantic–pragmatic deficit disorder.* Children's speech is fluent and often verbose, with good phonology and syntax. Despite an often large vocabulary, children may have word-finding problems (anomia). Comprehension of discourse is often paradoxically worse than expression and comprehension of open-ended questions is limited. If children are on the autistic spectrum, they may also have perseveration on certain topics, immediate and delayed echolalia, impaired prosody, and impaired verbal and nonverbal pragmatics.
- *Lexical deficit disorder.* Children's spontaneous speech is fluent. They may speak in jargon as toddlers or preschoolers, but progress rapidly to intelligible phrases and sentences. Some have prominent word finding deficits that may result in pseudo-stuttering. Syntax is immature, better in spontaneous than elicited language. Children have difficulty formulating discourse and may be better at comprehending individual words than sentences.

[a] Adapted from Rapin and Allen, 1983 and Flax and Rapin, 1998.

Cluster analysis yielded 6 subtypes, 5 of which corresponded roughly to the Allen and Rapin lexical–syntactic deficit syndrome, verbal dyspraxia, phonologic programming deficit syndrome, phonologic–syntactic deficit syndrome, and semantic pragmatic deficit syndrome. They did not have any child with VAA, but had a small group of children whose scores were normal. They did not agree with the label verbal dyspraxia (according to them, a term that refers to children with a motor speech disorder rather than a language disorder), as the children in that cluster had global deficits except for naming. They also objected to the term 'higher order processing disorders' as the children in this broad category had a variety of deficits, with lack of phonologic deficits as the main feature they had in common. When they reevaluated the children a year later they identified the same subtypes but found that 45% of the children shifted subtype membership, mostly because of changes in phonology and vocabulary. They found no advantage to reducing the Allen and Rapin classification into three major groups (Rapin, 1996b), as opposed to six subtypes, as the three were broader and less specific. The present authors agree that, although there are prototypical children of each of their subtypes, other children are not so easily classified as they do not fall neatly into the proposed categories. Nonetheless they offer them here as they may help clinicians who are not language specialists partition children with DLD.

Language deficits in young children with autism

Studies of language in autism have focused mainly on the characteristics of verbal individuals, ignoring the large proportion of the population which is nonverbal. These studies of verbal children on the autistic spectrum report that, although expressive language is typically delayed, once it appears phonology and syntax are not affected (Tager-Flusberg, 1994). Speech onset may be very delayed, but when it emerges progress to full sentences may be atypically rapid. Salient deficits are likely to be word choices that are often pedantic, and prosody which may be sing-song, or wooden and monotonous, or have a rising intonation in assertive sentences

TABLE 2

Clinical checklist for assessing child language

Comprehension (use both verbal and nonverbal responses for evaluation!)
- does the child understand single words (pointing), simple commands (e.g., show me, give Mommy. . .), simple questions (e.g., what's that? do you want this?)?
- does the child understand discourse, multilevel commands, open-ended questions (e.g., why did you wear a coat today?)

Amount and fluency of speech
- does the child speak as much as expected for his/her age?
- how long are the child's typical spontaneous utterances? (not responses to questions!)
- is the child fluent, does the child have hesitations (pauses) or repetitions, is the child's speech effortful?

Intelligibility, grammaticality
- is the child's communicative speech easily intelligible to you, or only to parents or familiar persons?
- is much of the child's speech gibberish?
- does the child speak in full sentences that include "little words" (articles, pronouns, prepositions, conjunctions, auxiliaries, etc.)?
- does the child's sentences include markers for gender, plural, tense, etc.?
- is the word order of the child's sentences correct?

Vocabulary, word retrieval, meaningfulness of the communication
- how large and rich is the child's vocabulary?
- does the child often use vague words like "thing" as substitutes for more specific words?
- does the child have problems with word retrieval, e.g., naming?
- how meaningful are the child's utterances?

Repetition of words and sentences
- how well can the child repeat?
- how does repetition contrast with spontaneous speech in terms or amount, clarity, grammaticality?

Formulation of discourse
- can the child retell a story or recount an event coherently and intelligibly?

Communicative use of language
- does the child use all means at his/her disposal to get a point across, e.g., use gestures or mimic to supplement or replace speech?
- does the child turn/respond when addressed to look at the person speaking to him or her?
- does the child engage in reciprocal conversation, take turns as listener and speaker?
- does the child know how to start and end conversations?
- is the intonation of the child's speech appropriately modulated to assist listener's comprehension?

Abnormal features for age suggesting the possibility of an autistic spectrum disorder
- frequent failure to look up or respond when addressed (make sure the child can hear!)
- speaking fluently out loud to no one in particular, to oneself with back turned to others
- immediate echolalia, i.e., repetition of the word or sentence just heard (may indicate inadequate comprehension or formulation difficulty (this is normal in toddlers!)
- delayed echolalia, formulaic language, i.e., reciting verbatim memorized expressions or sentences in more or less appropriate context (indicates formulation difficulty)
- monotonous, stilted, singsong, high pitched speech (decreased or inappropriate affective prosody)
- intrusive, repetitious questioning after receiving the requested information
- insistence on topic maintenance, perseveration
- responding beside the point of questions, chaining to a word rather than to the gist of what was said (indicates poor comprehension of discourse)
- mutism associated with seemingly total lack of comprehension of speech (suggests verbal auditory agnosia)
- enduring mutism broken by rare, unpredictable, inconsistent production of clearly articulated words or phrases

which makes them sound like questions. Immediate echolalia and the use of memorized scripts (delayed echolalia, formulaic language) to make up for word finding deficits, poverty of ideas, or difficulty formulating discourse, and profound deficits in pragmatics have already been emphasized.

By studying the language of nonverbal or minimally verbal preschoolers with autism as well as that of verbal children on the autistic spectrum, the authors have been able to classify the language deficits of autistic preschoolers into the same proposed subtypes as those of dysphasic children, with two major differences: very few autistic children have purely expressive disorders, and their verbal and nonverbal pragmatic skills are invariably deficient (Allen, 1988; Allen and Rapin, 1992; Dunn and Rapin, 1997; Rapin and Dunn, 1997). Whereas the mixed phonologic–syntactic and lexical–syntactic (formulation) deficit syndromes occur with about equal frequency in autistic and nonautistic children, verbal auditory agnosia and the semantic–pragmatic deficit syndromes are clearly more prevalent among autistic than dysphasic children. This type of language deficit in autism has very recently been linked to gene *WNT2 on* chromosome 7q 31–33, whereas autistic children without phonologic impairment do not show this linkage (Bradford, Haines, Hutcheson et al., 2001; Wassink et al., 2001). There is a controversy about whether the semantic–pragmatic deficit syndrome is specific to autism (Boucher, 1998), which it is not in the authors' experience (Rapin and Allen, 1998), or that of Bishop (Bishop, 1998). Some professionals chose to use the term semantic–pragmatic syndrome to refer to mild autism because they consider it a less stigmatizing label than autism or Asperger syndrome (Bishop, 1989b). This practice may be confusing to parents and jeopardize children's obtaining needed intervention.

Cognitive deficits in children with DLD

Cognitive deficits reported in dysphasic children include impaired speed of auditory processing (Tallal, Miller, Bedi et al., 1996; Wright, Lombardino, King et al., 1997), auditory attention (Campbell and McNeil, 1985), processing of sequences (Tallal, Stark, Kallman and Mellits, 1981), verbal and non-verbal short-term memory (Adams and Gathercole, 2000; Fazio, 1998; Montgomery, 1995; Wyke and Asso, 1979), including short-term memory for phonological sequences (Michas and Henry, 1994; Raine, Hulme, Chadderton and Bailey, 1991), as well as deficits in hierarchic organization and planning (Cromer, 1983). More general deficits in symbolic function (Kamhi, 1981) and representation (visual imaging) (Johnston and Weismer, 1983; Savich, 1984) have been reported in other studies. Research efforts are directed toward understanding the relationships between deficits in auditory perception, deficits in higher order cognition, and linguistic processing impairments in dysphasic children.

Nonverbal intelligence is regularly higher than verbal abilities in children with SLI. Spatial abilities in many dysphasic children have been demonstrated to be just as strong or to exceed the level of their non-language impaired peers (Gillies and Light, 1997). However, there is heterogeneity even in nonverbal abilities in children with SLI. There is some evidence that children with SLI who have motor impairments demonstrate deficient performance in visual discrimination tasks that have no motor component (Powell and Bishop, 1992). Visual analogical reasoning (semantically analogous pictures, perceptually analogous geometric forms, generation of a solution to a physical problem analogous to that in an auditorally and visually presented story) does not differ in dysphasic children compared to children with typical language development when nonverbal IQ is controlled statistically (Nippold, Erskine and Freed, 1988).

Auditory perception

Tallal and colleagues have demonstrated in a series of papers (Tallal and Piercy, 1973; Tallal et al., 1993, 1996) that many language-disordered children are specifically impaired in the discrimination and sequencing of rapidly presented sensory stimuli, whether visually or acoustically presented, and that, although long tones or noises may be processed normally, there is a severe deficit in processing brief auditory stimuli. These data have been interpreted as evidence that language impairment results from specific deficits in auditory perception (Wright et al., 1997). Findings suggest that it is not only speech discrimination that is impaired in children with SLI as auditory lateralization is also affected. Cohen, Gelinas, Lassonde and Geoffroy (1991) required 7–10 year old children to discriminate consonant–vowel syllables differing in either voicing or place of articulation. The syllables were presented to each ear separately while white noise was presented to the contralateral ear. Findings indicated that dysphasic children, compared to matched normal controls, had more difficulty discriminating place of articulation only when the syllable was presented to the left ear and voicing only when the syllable was presented to the right ear.

As discussed earlier, a deficit in this earliest step in phonologically decoding acoustically presented language (speech) will jeopardize all subsequent processing and programming operations. Frumkin and Rapin (1980) found these deficits most severe in children with VAA. They found them demonstrable in children with mixed receptive/expressive deficits with impaired phonology, but not in those with adequate phonology in whom sequencing deficits suggested impaired short-term auditory memory. Not all expressively disordered children have deficient perception of phonemes they produce incorrectly (Bird and Bishop, 1992; Locke, 1975). Deficits may also lie in phonologic short term memory, or at the level of programming motor commands for speech which may overlap, but seem to be distinct from, deficient voluntary commands for the execution of nonspeech oral movements responsible for dysarthria (Stark and Blackwell, 1997). Whether deficient phonologic perception accounts for impaired phonologic memory or speech programming remains unclear. A study of cerebral palsied children with dysarthria (Bishop, Byers Brown and Robson, 1990) indicates that dysarthria itself, because of the distorted feedback it produces, may contribute to difficulty with phonologic discrimination, supporting the contention of a link between phonologic discrimination and programming in prefrontal cortex (Broca's area). In any case, phonologic perceptual deficits persist, even in SLI children who, despite them, have learned to speak adequately but may have difficulty acquiring reading skills (Bishop and Adams, 1990). They remain demonstrable by problems with phonologic awareness such as rhyming (Buonomano and Merzenich, 1998; Goswami, 1993).

Attention

Some investigators propose that impaired ability to allocate attention effectively is an underlying deficit in DLD (Campbell and McNeil, 1985). Others suggest that attention deficient disorder (ADHD) is a possible co-morbid diagnosis in children with SLI (Williams, Stott, Goodyer and Sahakian, 2000) and that the risk for a co-morbid diagnosis of ADHD is "greatest among children with general linguistic impairment" (Beitchman, Hood, Rochon and Peterson, 1989). Evidence from computerized tests of selective attention indicates that these children exhibit deficient selective auditory attention, with normal ability to allocate attention to visual stimuli. In addition, they have more difficulty with sequential auditory target tasks relative to normals. Attention deficit does not provide an adequate explanation for SLI or dyslexia, even though it may be co-morbid with both and play a contributory role (Shaywitz et al., 1995; Williams et al., 2000). Future work must address the possible relationships between deficits in selective attention and linguistic, perceptual, and memory deficits in SLI children.

Memory

In recent years there has been increasing emphasis on auditory verbal short-term memory and its possible influence on language development in children with SLI. Children with SLI have deficits in verbatim repetition of strings of digits (Graham, 1980; Wiig, Semel and Nystrom, 1982), nonsense words (Montgomery, 1995), real words (Weismer, Evans and Hesketh, 1999), and sentences (Menyuk and Looney, 1972). In a study by Montgomery (1995), children with SLI repeated fewer 3 and 4 syllable nonsense words correctly than did their normal peers. Subjects with SLI interpreted fewer redundant/longer sentences correctly than non-redundant shorter sentence and there was a positive correlation between nonsense word repetition performance and sentence comprehension. The results were interpreted as reflecting diminished phonological memory in children with SLI that interferes with sentence comprehension. Ability to repeat nonsense words was also associated with deficient production. Four year old children with poor nonsense word repetition produced shorter utterances and a more limited range of syntactic constructions than nonverbal IQ-matched peers with good nonsense word repetition. This relationship existed even when short-term memory span was assessed through non-spoken recall (suggesting that the results were not due solely to language output problems) (Gathercole and Pickering, 2000). Menyuk (1978) found that dysphasic children had more omissions than normals in sentence repetition and could not repeat syntactic structures that they produced spontaneously, whereas normals showed the opposite pattern: they could repeat more complicated structures than those they produced spontaneously. This strongly suggests that deficient short-term verbal memory (as opposed to deficient syntax) determined poor performance in the dysphasic children. Of note, even though SLI children were impaired in verbatim repetition, they retained the gist of the sentences. Memory for connected speech (in a poem) was impaired relative to nonverbal IQ/age-matched peers and language-matched normals with or without accompanying hand motions and with or without accompanying music. It is interesting, though, that long term memory for the poem two days later was significantly improved in the SLI group when taught the poem with hand movements (Fazio, 1994). Most aspects of verbal memory and learning, including rehearsal (Kirchner and Klatzky, 1985) and retrieval (Wiig et al., 1982) have been demonstrated to be deficient in children with SLI. Kirchner and Klatzky (1985) had subjects rehearse aloud after the presentation of each item in a verbal list-learning task, and observed dysphasic children to have more difficulty than normals in using rehearsal to retain the information, and to have more semantic paraphasic intrusions in their rehearsal and subsequent recall of the list. This body of work has been criticized on the grounds that the tasks were verbal, so that the so-called 'memory' deficit might be the consequence rather than the cause of deficient language (Johnston, 1988).

A few studies have examined memory for visual stimuli. Short-term memory for visual material, in children with DLD, appears to depend on the demands of the task. As task complexity (i.e., the demand for multiple mental operations) increases, working memory deficits are evident in all modalities in these children relative to age-matched controls (Gillam, Cowan and Day, 1995). Preschool children with SLI were just as strong at recognizing serial patterns of pictures of common objects and iconic images (scribble drawings and unfamiliar faces) as age and language matched controls, when the presentation rate was slow. However, under rapid presentation conditions the performance of the children with SLI was significantly below that of the controls. Fazio (Fazio, 1997) and Wyke and Asso (1979) observed 7-year-old DLD children to have more difficulty than normals in recalling the position of markers in two- or three-dimensional space compared to normals. Poor performance did not reflect perceptual deficits as the impaired children could match position. Studies of memory for visual material must be interpreted with caution because if stimuli are verbally codable it is impossible to rule out covert verbal rehearsal (Levy and Menyuk, 1977). In Wyke and Asso's study (1979) verbal coding was ruled out because verbal interference material was introduced during the delay before recall and, when asked, the children could not describe the locations verbally.

Executive functions

Six year olds with specific language impairment did not demonstrate deficient executive functions on the nonverbal subtests of the Cambridge Neuropsychological Test Automated Battery (CANTAB) (quoted in Williams et al., 2000). However, a group of children with attention deficit hyperactivity disorder (ADHD) in isolation and another with SLI with a co-morbid diagnosis of ADHD were both deficient. There were no significant interactions between SLI and ADHD on these measures (Williams et al., 2000).

There is some evidence that dysphasic children may have significant difficulty organizing isolated events into meaningful wholes (Kraemer, 1975), thereby limiting organization in service of reducing memory load, in temporally ordering ideas (Cromer, 1983), and in forming sets or expectancies for interpreting incoming information (Ceci, 1983). These deficits have direct implications for language comprehension and expression, in particular the programming of discourse, as well as for memory.

Overall cognitive abilities

As one would expect, children with DLD regularly have lower verbal than nonverbal IQ scores on intelligence batteries and their academic performance is likely to be lower as well. Despite the wide variety of cognitive deficits observed in DLD children, none of these deficits exist in all dysphasic children. The concatenation of cognitive and language deficits in dysphasia just pointed out supports the need for more detailed evaluation of individuals and more homogeneous groups than those used in many of the studies of DLD carried out to date.

Prognosis

Outcome is a function of the DLD subtype and its severity. The presence of additional developmental problems, in particular autism and cognitive impairment, worsens the outcome. In general, children with expressive subtypes do well (Whitehurst et al., 1994; Paul, 1996), with the exception of those with verbal dyspraxia. Also some children with verbal dyspraxia improve (LeNormand and Chevrie-Muller, 1991), others remain extremely dysfluent or, rarely, essentially nonverbal, despite adequate or at least reasonable comprehension which enables them to express themselves with communication boards, manual signs, or writing — by computer if manual dexterity is poor (Ferry et al., 1975; Guerreiro et al., 2000). Children with developmental VAA do even worse: because of their profound comprehension deficits they may remain unable to understand what is said to them or to develop speech. If their nonverbal intelligence is normal and provided they learn language through the visual channel and are educated accordingly, they may function essentially like deaf individuals as adults (Klein et al., 1995). Unfortunately, many remain severely and permanently impaired, especially if they are also autistic (Klein et al., 2000).

Children with less severe mixed receptive/expressive phonologic–syntactic deficits generally acquire serviceable or even reasonably normal language by schoolage, although many will require special education because of academic deficits (Shaywitz, 1998). Children with higher order processing deficits, especially those who are intelligent and are not autistic, usually do well. Adequate early intervention plays a crucial role in outcome (McLean and Cripe, 1997).

Assessment of children with DLD

The steps in the multi-disciplinary assessment of a child suspected of having DLD include: (1) determining that hearing is normal in each ear at all frequencies. Definitive testing may require physiologic tests such as otoacoustic emissions (Lichtenstein and Stapells, 1996) or brainstem auditory evoked responses (BAER); (Stapells and Oates, 1997) (2) documenting that the child in fact has a developmental language disorder; (3) characterizing the child's language comprehension, production, and use; (4) assessing the child's cognitive strengths and weaknesses in order to detect associated deficits and to plan a rational remediation program; and (5) investigating potential medical causes for the disorder and associated deficits, including dysarthria.

Screening and formal testing

Screening instruments for DLD in toddlers and preschoolers may consist of a parental checklist such as the MacArthur Communicative Development Inventories (Fenson et al., 1993), the Early Language Milestones (ELM) (Coplan, 1989), or Clinical Linguistic and Auditory Milestone Scale (CLAMS) (Capute and Accardo, 1978; Capute, Palmer and Shapiro, 1986), and, if autism as well as dysphasia is suspected, the Checklist of Autism in Toddlers (CHAT) which was standardized for infants as young as 18 months (Baird, Charman, Baron-Cohen et al., 2000; Baron-Cohen, Allen and Gillberg, 1992; Baron-Cohen, Cox, Baird et al., 1996). Table 2 provides an abbreviated checklist of language features to assist professionals who are not language experts attend to the production, comprehension, and conversational use of language. Some may want to use a somewhat more detailed checklist to document language more systematically or assist clinical evaluation (Flax and Rapin, 1998). A firm diagnosis of DLD requires confirmation by the evaluation of an experienced clinician and by testing with standardized instruments. Diagnosis may rest on discrepancies between language and chronological age or non-verbal mental age, or between verbal and performance IQ scores (Stark and Tallal, 1981), or both (Miller, 1978). The strengths and limitations of each approach have been thoughtfully considered by Lahey (1990), Aram, Morris and Hall (1992), and Bishop (1997a). Ideally, in-depth investigation of language should integrate the approaches of speech–language pathology with neuropsychology so as to maximize the complementarity of approaches and minimize redundant testing. There are a number of well standardized language batteries and specialized tests for evaluating the various aspects of language reception, processing, production and use (see Nation and Aram, 1990, and Bishop, 1997a for suggestions).

Assessing conversational language

Lahey (1990) emphasizes the need to supplement standardized tests with the sampling of language in a variety of contexts that include spontaneous interactive formats; she also recommends stressing the limits of the child's language through increasingly complex demands for both comprehension and production, as detection of some of the more subtle language impairments can only be observed in conversational use. Thus a spontaneous language sample provides a great deal of information missed by formal language tests (Miller, 1981). Having the child describe a standard videotape or retell a standard story has the advantage of uniformity of the stimulus (Dollaghan, Campbell and Tomlin, 1990). Miller (1981) recommends a 45 minute language elicitation session (15 minutes of child-directed activity with the parent, 15 minutes of the same activity with the examiner, and 15 minutes of responding to the examiner's commands and questions). It is highly desirable to audio- or video-record the conversational sample as it provides information about formulation/organization of discourse, pragmatics, and syntax in connected speech. Video rather than audio recording has the advantage of providing a richer context to evaluate the nonverbal aspects of communication which are likely to be impaired in children on the autistic spectrum. The recorded sample can be put to several uses. A pediatric speech–language pathologist or other clinician can develop a child's clinical profile by listening to (or viewing) the recording, using a check-list to score the various aspects of language as normal for age, somewhat abnormal, or very abnormal. Checklists have the advantage of providing systematic clinical data for longitudinal observation.

The major advantage of a recorded sample is formal analysis. The major drawback of formal analysis, which requires transcription of the sample, is that it is extremely labor-intensive. Transcripts are invaluable for research and provide the opportunity for more systematic in-depth clinical analysis of aspects of conversational uses of language that standardized tests of language do not capture. Phonetic transcripts are required for documenting phonologic processes in connected speech. Transcripts can be coded for computer assisted analysis. The most widely used program, which has been adapted for a number of languages besides English, is the Systematic Analysis of Language Transcripts (SALT) (Miller and Chapman, 1987). Programs of this sort have built-in systems which can automatically count and categorize specific linguistic forms and compute basic data such as mean length of utterance (MLU), construction-types, and type-token ratio (TTR). For research, transcripts can be stored in the Child Language Data Exchange System (CHILDES) (MacWhinney, 1992), an international system for exchanging transcripts of child language for cross-linguistic and other studies.

Assessing the pattern of strengths and weaknesses: the neuropsychologic evaluation

For a number of reasons, the neuropsychologic evaluation is an important part of the assessment of any child with a communication impairment. First, a single IQ score, a single language test score, or the discrepancy between them provides little information concerning the child's pattern of cognitive strengths and weaknesses. For example, a child with an IQ score of 60 who presents with an even profile of subtest scores is experiencing very different problems from a child with an IQ of 60 with very poor performance on subtests involving language and motor speed with strong performance on nonverbal problem solving. Low overall IQ indicates the presence of a problem, whereas attention to intersubtest scatter on an IQ test aids in specifying the nature of the problem. Secondly, the neuropsychologic evaluation has implications for prognosis and for planning remediation. It is important to define deficits that could interfere with remedial efforts and strengths that can be used to compensate for or remediate weaknesses. The chapters on neuropsychological assessment by O'Shea, Harel and Fein (2002) and Mattis and Luck (2002), provide lists of neuropsychological assessment instruments for evaluating preschool and schoolage children.

A thorough neuropsychologic assessment includes some or all of the following:

(a) An intelligence test, used to assess overall cognitive functioning and also as a screening instrument to provide a point of departure for testing hypotheses regarding the child's strengths and weaknesses. The IQ battery can provide information concerning fluid and crystallized intellectual abilities and concept formation. Fluid cognitive abilities are those required for solving novel problems. Crystallized abilities are cognitive skills needed to acquire and employ verbal and quantitative concepts to solve problems. They are closely associated with academic achievement.
(b) Assessment of verbal and non-verbal concept formation and problem solving.
(c) Formal and informal tests of language.
(d) Assessment of attention, short-term and long-term verbal and nonverbal memory in both auditory and visual modalities.
(e) Tests of visual perception, analysis, synthesis.
(f) Evaluation of fine motor skills (graphomotor, manual and oral praxis).
(g) Assessment of adaptive functioning (how a child uses knowledge and abilities in day to day functioning), as evaluated for example by the Vineland Adaptive Behavior Scales (Sparrow, Balla and Cicchetti, 1984) encompass communication, daily living skills, socialization, motor functioning, and maladaptive behaviors.
(h) Tests of executive functions (organizational and planning skills)
(i) Evaluation of academic skills (in school-age children).

The depth of investigation into each of these areas is driven by the referral question, and hypotheses are generated through formal quantitative results and qualitative evidence obtained throughout testing.

The behavior of the child during testing must always be considered in the interpretation of the formal results of the neuropsychological evaluation, as scores are clearly influenced by attentional and motivational factors. The goal of assessment is not only to determine the child's typical level of functioning but also to get a sense of actual ability. The 'zone of proximal development' of Vygotsky (1978) is defined as the difference between actual functional level and current potential which can only be observed if the child is given special environmental support to optimize performance. Information concerning this 'zone' is indicative of a child's ability to learn. This knowledge may also aid in determining the best style of intervention for a child at a given time.

Therefore it is important in formal testing to provide an environment which embraces the child's attention and motivation and reduces anxiety. Most often this is done by establishing good rapport with the child through social support and praise for effort. Assessment of the young severely impaired child with autism is worth special mention as normal social supports may not act to reduce anxiety or enhance motivation; in fact they may be aversive. All too frequently the child with poor social relatedness, limited turn-taking ability, impaired ability to attend to a stimulus or activity introduced by someone else, and raised anxiety in novel situations is seen in an unfamiliar room for half an hour and then declared untestable or, worse, untestable and therefore mentally retarded. Performance of such children can be optimized by allowing them to become familiar with the examiner, testing room and test materials through active independent exploration. During this period the examiner should neither intrude nor attempt to force compliance. This reduces anxiety and often makes the autistic child more amenable to testing. Adequate testing may require bringing the child back for several brief sessions. Important information is gained by helping all children to perform at their highest level.

Medical evaluation

An important role of physicians is early detection of a problem with language development as they provide 'well baby' care throughout infancy and are likely to the first professional consulted by worried parents. Table 3 provides a timetable for red flags suggesting the need to refer infants and toddlers for formal investigation. Another role of physicians is to attempt to determine whether there is a definable etiology (genetic or acquired) of the child's brain dysfunction and to make certain that there is no evidence of a progressive neurologic condition. Investigation starts with the past medical history of the

TABLE 3

When to worry about inadequate language development

- No babbling (consonant/vowel sounds) by 8 months
- No pointing by 1 year
- No words by 12–14 months
- Less than a dozen words by 18 months
- No two word phrases by 2 years
- No sentences by 3 years
- Speech unintelligible to parents at 2 years
- Speech unintelligible to strangers at 3 years
- Concern about comprehension *at any age*!
- *At any age*: lack of orienting to speech, turning to name
- Inability to use language conversationally by 2 years, 'talking to talk' rather than to communicate (request, show, etc.)
- Inability to tell a coherent story by 3 years
- Language regression *at any age*

child and a detailed family history, emphasizing not only dysphasia but learning deficits and persistently inadequate reading and spelling, as well as neurologic or psychiatric conditions, in family members.

The general physical examination is rarely informative unless it discloses unusual facial features, cutaneous abnormalities, or signs suggestive of a malformation syndrome, or a specific medical condition mandating further medical investigation. The contribution of the standard neurologic examination is to determine whether the child has associated signs of localized or, much more frequently, unlocalizable brain dysfunction, for example, motor or oromotor deficits or a disorder of attention. In order to decide whether referral to a geneticist or other professional is indicated, physicians will need to review available medical records and, in particular, the availability and results of a definitive test of hearing which is mandatory in every child who does not speak and articulate clearly. Chromosome studies are rarely indicated in children who have no dysmorphic features unless the family history suggests a condition like fragile-X syndrome.

Functional imaging, magnetic resonance imaging (MRI) morphometry, event-related potentials and other computerized electrophysiologic tests, magnetoencephalography, and genetic investigations provide crucial evidence for research and for an occasional child who may be a neurosurgical candidate because of uncontrollable epilepsy. These tests are not recommended for routine clinical purposes as their yield is vanishingly small unless there is some feature of the history of the family or child or findings on the examination that suggest a specific condition (New York State Department of Health: Early Intervention Program, 1999a; Volkmar, Cook, Pomeroy et al., 1999). MRI abnormalities were found in 70% of a sample of 35 schoolage children with DLD, compared to 22% of 27 controls (Trauner, Wulfeck, Tallal and Hesselink, 2000). However, as these were nonspecific in both groups and did not alter management, the clinical importance of the abnormalities is questioned.

The probability that neuroimaging will reveal a treatable medical condition in the absence of corroborating clinical evidence in a child with SLI is negligible, although there are rare situations where it may be justified to provide a more specific diagnosis. If diagnostic brain imaging is to be performed at all, MRI, not CT, is preferable, although it often requires anesthesia with its inherent risks. MRI may be indicated in a child with frankly dysmorphic facial features or very severe dysarthria as, in the latter case it is occasionally associated with perisylvian cortical dysgenesis (Guerreiro et al., 2000). The probability that MRI will be revealing because there is a very large discrepancy between verbal and nonverbal skills is extremely low if other abnormal neurologic findings are lacking.

In the absence of clinical seizures, the yield of abnormal EEGs is highest in children with the severe comprehension deficits and very impaired speech that suggest VAA, particularly if there is a history of language regression or marked fluctuations of language skills. The yield is also fairly high in children with clear cut autistic features, especially if they have motor deficits or are retarded (Tuchman et al., 1991; Tuchman and Rapin, 1997). The yield of abnormal EEGs is higher during sleep than awake, and is highest during all night recordings which provide an adequate sample of slow wave sleep. This can be accomplished with 24 hour ambulatory EEG recordings (provided there is an adequate number of electrodes) or by monitoring to document any suspicious events with closed circuit televising of the child and EEG in an epilepsy unit (Beaumanoir et al., 1995). Whether to prescribe medication if one detects a paroxysmal EEG in the absence of clinical seizures is controversial, as in classical VAA the seizures generally respond better than the language. There are isolated reports of amelioration of the child's language with the use of therapeutic doses of anticonvulsants, especially those indicated for the primary generalized epilepsies (valproate, ethosuccimide, clonazepam), or even steroids or ACTH (Katzman, Dagher and Patronas, 1999; Marescaux, Hirsch, Finck et al., 1990; Roulet Perez, Davidoff, Despland and Deonna, 1993). Therefore, an adequate trial of anticonvulsants may be justified in dysphasic children without clinical seizures who have a frankly paroxysmal EEG, after full disclosure to the parents of the controversial aspect of this recommendation. Subpial transection in epileptogenic cortex is said to have improved language and controlled the seizures of some children with acquired epileptic aphasia and VAA (Morrell, Whisler, Smith et al., 1995), and was said to have improved language and autistic behaviors in a child with LKS and autistic regression (Neville, Harkness, Cross et al., 1997). Nass and colleagues (Nass, Gross, Wisoff and Devinsky, 1999) reported modest improvement in a handful of autistic children with language/behavioral regression and epileptiform EEGs or seizures. At best this invasive procedure must be considered experimental until more longitudinal data on larger samples of children become available.

Remediation for children with DLD

As few well controlled research studies of remediation have been conducted, there is little empirical support for adopting one theoretically based educational approach over another. There are few well defined treatments that can be implemented easily and consistently by all therapists. The level of proficiency of the therapists, their personal style and ability to develop an alliance with the child all introduce variability into outcome data which in fact may not be accounted for by the particular technique they used. Most remediation studies employ group designs and group mean data for assessing efficacy. Frequently the groups are quite heterogeneous and subject selection criteria are not clearly specified, making interpretation of the results difficult. As a result there has been a move towards single case study designs with careful specification of the subject characteristics (e.g., Olswang, Bain, Dunn and Cooper, 1983) A further problem that plagues remediation outcome studies is the need to control for the effects of maturation.

An exhaustive review of specific interventions developed for children with DLD and their efficacies will not be attempted here (for reviews of some specific methods the reader is referred to Allen, Mendelson and Rapin, 1989; Chevrie-Muller and Narbona, 1999; Law, 1997; Monfort and Juarez Sanchez, 1996; New York State Department of Health: Early Intervention Program, 1999b; Tallal, Merzenich, Miller and Jenkins, 1998b). As no universal approach will meet every child's needs, individualized remediation plans rest on each child's pattern of linguistic and cognitive strengths and weaknesses inventoried during the comprehensive assessment which need to be shared with the teacher/therapist who is planning the intervention. This pattern should also be shared with the parents in a clear, understandable way, as this frequently helps them grasp the reason for previously inexplicable developmental problems and difficult behaviors. Parents should also be counseled as to the ways in which they can be involved in their child's treatment. This includes providing information about available programs and procedures for gaining services, and how to act as the child's advocate. In addition parents need specific recommendations for language stimulation at home and instruction in achieving behavior control, if this is needed (Allen and Mendelson, 2000).

Intervention consists of designing an individually tailored remediation program (individual educational plan — IEP), monitoring the child over time to measure progress and determine the efficacy of the recommended intervention and to detect any potential new problems. Plans for remediation bring up three questions: (1) which child requires intervention? (2) when should intervention be offered? and (3) what type of approach is likely to be most effective?

(1) In the United States, Federal guidelines (PL 94–142 and later amendments) mandate individual intervention for any child ages 0–5 years at risk for a developmental deficit. At this young age a firm diagnosis of DLD is not required. Interpretation of this guideline differs in different states. For example, in New York State the recommendation on whether to initiate speech/language therapy for

children 18–36 months depends on the severity of the disorder, and on whether there are other handicaps (New York State Department of Health: Early Intervention Program, 1999b). Any professional or the child's parents may refer the child for evaluation, which must take place within 60 days of referral and ends in a conference with the parents where recommendations for the need (if any) and type of intervention are discussed. Parents are free to accept or reject the recommendations. Those who reject the recommendation are offered the opportunity for review.

(2) As brain plasticity diminishes with maturation, the time to start intervention is when it is likely to be most efficacious, which is why the Federal guideline was promulgated. The ambiguities in deciding between language delay and DLD were discussed in an earlier section; they are the reason why a definitive diagnosis is not required with very young children before starting vigorous intervention. The older the child, the more reliable and specific the diagnosis and recommendations.

(3) The type of intervention offered depends on the nature and severity of the child's deficits, on the philosophy of the therapist/reacher, on the parents' preferences, and on availability of services in the particular community. Whitehurst and Fischel (1994) recommend that children with compromised comprehension as well as expression, or with other risk factors such as borderline cognitive skills, a deprived family environment, or other handicaps be enrolled in a specialized preschool where they can receive intensive, integrated remediation to meet all their needs. Less severely communication handicapped children may benefit from individual speech and language therapy.

The type of intervention is dictated by each child's needs. Children with minimal or no language with severe behavior disorders, especially those with autism who are unable to focus on a task introduced by someone else, may profit from a maximally structured *operant conditioning* approach (Lovaas, 1981). This so-called *Applied Behavior Analysis (ABA)* involves systematically rewarding desirable behaviors like joint attention and imitation and extinguishing undesirable behaviors by ignoring them. Operant methods are often quite effective. Once children have developed a sizable vocabulary of single words that they use for labeling and requesting, moving to an approach that takes better account of normal language developmental sequences is desirable. A more naturalistic setting helps children incorporate their language skills into their functional repertoire and generalize their use to new situations.

Some intervention strategies attack children's specific deficits directly by addressing underlying processing deficits rather than overt symptoms, the idea being to take advantage of brain plasticity to foster development along its usual paths. This approach is often advocated for young children, who are least likely to resist. The direct approach is also applicable to older children where stimuli are presented by computer in an attractive rewarding format. A recent computerized multimedia program for strengthening auditory processing and reading skills of school-age children with phonologically-based reading disabilities (Bruneau, Roux, Guérin et al., 1993; Merzenich, Jenkins, Johnston et al., 1996; Tallal, Merzenich, Miller and Jenkins, 1998a) is stated to be effective and well accepted by the children. Such programs may also be effective for some younger children with DLD able to use computers.

A second approach is to emphasize strengths and teach compensatory strategies for the weaknesses, for example presenting language to the visual modality and using contextual cues to bolster the defective auditory channel of children who understand little or no speech. Visual presentation means using gestures, pictures, or even sign language as well as speech. Teaching specific compensatory strategies is generally used with older children and adolescents, and for remediating deficits resistant to direct intervention. For example, one can teach children alternate strategies such as using semantic context to help comprehension. Rourke (1995) and others advocate interventions guided by current models of information processing. Children with word finding problems might be helped by expanding their search strategies and encouraging flexibility in their use.

Another way to compensate for deficits is to modify the environment. Stark and Bernstein (1984), influenced by the findings in Tallal's studies (Tallal et al., 1981; Tallal and Stark, 1981), recommend that the teacher modify her speech by slowing down, using short utterances and simple explanations, and then require the child to restate what was said. The teacher, by using a closed loop amplification system which requires the child to wear hearing aids, can provide signal amplification that minimizes distraction from the ambient noise of the classroom. Encouraging manual expression or the use of communication boards or computers is also appropriate for children with adequate comprehension who have little or no expressive abilities. There are now sophisticated 'talking computers' for severely affected children without speech.

Future needs

A major need of the field is to collect more detailed longitudinal data on language acquisition in both normal and language impaired children. This may assuage inadequate agreement among professionals as to whether a given child is language-disordered or simply delayed in language acquisition. Although considerable normative data have now been collected on the early stages of language acquisition and its variability, much less information is available on the normal development of language beyond the toddler years. Few studies have followed the course of language development in dysphasic children over time.

If we are to predict who, among the young dysphasic children of today, are likely to be the reading-and learning-disabled children of tomorrow, we require better information regarding which patterns of linguistic and neuropsychologic deficits are harbingers of later learning disability. We need to learn more about the cognitive processes that underlie competent and defective acquisition of language. Speculation abounds in this area while a full understanding of the facts still remains largely elusive. There is clearly a need for a wider range of standardized tests for very young children and for a more extensive series of neuropsychologic instruments for school-aged children.

Sophisticated electrophysiologic and imaging studies will no doubt add a great deal to our understanding of the neurologic basis of DLD. They may assist in deciding which children with subclinical epilepsy may benefit from medication. How much they will assist in deciding about other interventions or illuminate etiology is less clear.

We have learned that genetics probably pays a more important causative role than preventable insults to the developing brain in the developmental disorders of brain function, including dysphasia. It is unlikely that the prevention of prematurity, intrauterine exposure to substances of abuse, or better treatment of prenatal or postnatal acquired infections will prevent more than a fraction of these disorders. We do know that an impoverished environment seriously compromises the optimal cognitive and social development of all children, and especially of handicapped children. By the same token, we know that early and vigorous educational intervention has a beneficial effect in some of these children; yet resources are limited so that we cannot justify providing every possible intervention to every child. In order to determine the cost-effectiveness of various interventions, we urgently need to conduct detailed longitudinal studies of the efficacies of those interventions we currently offer to children with specific language disorder profiles and to develop novel and more effective remedial approaches.

References

Adams AM, Gathercole SE: Limitations in working memory: implications for language development. International Journal of Language and Communication Disorders: 35; 95–116, 2000.

Adams C, Bishop DVM: Conversational characteristics of children with semantic–pragmatic disorder. I: Exchange structure, translating, repairs and cohesion. British Journal of Disorders of Communication: 24; 211–239, 1989.

Ajuriaguerra J, De Jaeggi A, Guignard F, Kocher F, Maquard M, Roth S, Schmid E: The development and prognosis of dysphasia in children. In Morehead DM, Morehead AE (Eds), Normal and Deficient Child Language. Baltimore: University Park Press, pp. 345–385, 1976.

Akefeldt A, Akefeldt B, Gillberg C: Voice, speech and language characteristics of children with Prader-Willi syndrome. Journal of Intellectual Disability Research: 41(Pt 4); 302–311, 1997.

Allen DA: Autistic spectrum disorders: Clinical presentation in preschool children. Journal of Child Neurology: 3; s48–s56, 1988.

Allen DA: Developmental language disorders in preschool children: Clinical subtypes and syndromes. School Psychology Review: 18; 442–451, 1989.

Allen DA, Mendelson L: Parent–child, and professional: meeting the needs of young autistic children and their families in a multidisciplinary therapeutic nursery model. Psychoanalytic Inquiry: 20; 704–731, 2000.

Allen DA, Mendelson L, Rapin I: Syndrome specific remediation in preschool developmental dysphasia. In French JH, Harel S, Casaer P, Gottlieb MI, Rapin I, De Vivo DC (Eds), Child Neurology and Developmental Disabilities. Baltimore: Paul Brookes, pp. 233–243, 1989.

Allen DA, Rapin I: Autistic children are also dysphasic. In Naruse H, Ornitz E (Eds), Neurobiology of Infantile Autism. Amsterdam: Excerpta Medica, pp. 73–80, 1992.

American Academy of Child and Adolescent Psychiatry: Practice parameters for the assessment and treatment of children and adolescents with language and learning disorders. Journal of the American Academy of Child and Adolescent Psychiatry: 37(10 Suppl); 46S–62S, 1998a.

American Academy of Child and Adolescent Psychiatry: Summary of the practice parameters for the assessment and treatment of children and adolescents with language and learning disorders. Journal of the American Academy of Child and Adolescent Psychiatry: 37; 1117–1119, 1998b.

American Psychiatric Association: Diagnostic and Statistical Manual of Mental Disorders, 4th ed., text revision DSM-IV-TR. Washington DC: American Psychiatric Association, 2000.

Aram DM: Language sequelae of unilateral brain lesions in children. In Plum F (Ed), Language, Communication and the Brain. New York: Raven Press, pp. 171–197, 1988.

Aram DM, Eisele JA: Limits to a left hemisphere explanation for specific language impairment. Journal of Speech and Hearing Research: 37; 824–830, 1994.

Aram DM, Ekelman BL, Nation JE: Preschoolers with language disorders: 10 years later. Journal of Speech and Hearing Research: 27; 232–244, 1984.

Aram DM, Hack M, Hawkins S, Weissman BM, Borawski-Clark E: Very-low-birthweight children and speech and language development. Journal of Speech and Hearing Research: 34; 1169–1179, 1991.

Aram DM, Morris R, Hall NE: The validity of discrepancy criteria for identifying children with developmental language disorders. Journal of Learning Disabilities: 25; 549–554, 1992.

Aram DM, Morris R, Hall NE: Clinical and research congruence in identifying children with specific language impairment. Journal of Speech and Hearing Research: 36; 580–591, 1993.

Aram DM, Nation JE: Patterns of language behavior in children with developmental language disorders. Journal of Speech and Hearing Research: 18; 229–241, 1975.

Bailey DBJ, Hatton DD, Skinner M: Early developmental trajectories of males with fragile X syndrome. American Journal of Mental Retardation: 103; 29–39, 1998.

Baird R, Charman T, Baron-Cohen S, Cox A, Swettenham J, Wheelwright S, Drew A, Kemal L: A screening instrument for autism at 18 months of age: A six-year follow-up study. Journal of the American Academy of Child and Adolescent Psychiatry: 39; 694–702, 2000.

Baron-Cohen S, Allen J, Gillberg C: Can autism be detected at 18 months? The needle, the haystack, and the CHAT. British Journal of Psychiatry: 161; 839–843, 1992.

Baron-Cohen S, Cox A, Baird G, Swettenham J, Nightingale N, Morgan K, Drew A, Charman T: Psychological markers in the detection of autism in infancy in a large population. British Journal of Psychiatry: 168; 158–163, 1996.

Bates E: Plasticity, localization and language development. In Broman S, Fletcher JM (Eds), The Changing Nervous System: Neurobehavioral Consequences of Early Brain Development. New York: Oxford University Press, pp. 214–253, 1999.

Bates E, Thal D, Finlay B, Clancy B: Early language development and its neural correlates. In Segalowitz SJ, Rapin I (Eds), Child Neuropsychology, Handbook of Neuropsychology, 2nd Edition, vol. 8, part II. Amsterdam: Elsevier, pp. 525–592, 2003.

Beaumanoir A, Bureau M, Deonna T, Mira L, Tassinari CA (Eds): Continuous Spikes and Waves During Slow Sleep — Electrical Status Epilepticus During Slow Sleep — Acquired Epileptic Aphasia and Related Conditions. London: John Libbey, 1995.

Beitchman JH, Brownlie EB, Inglis A, Wild J, Ferguson B, Schachter D, Lancee W, Wilson B, Mathews R: Seven-year follow-up of speech/language impaired and control children: psychiatric outcome. Journal of Child Psychology and Psychiatry and Allied Disciplines: 37; 961–970, 1996.

Beitchman JH, Hood J, Rochon J, Peterson M: Empirical classification of speech/language impairment in children. II. Behavioral characteristics. Journal of the American Academy of Child and Adolescent Psychiatry, 28, 118–123, 1989.

Bellinger DC, Rappaport LA, Weiler MD, Beers NB: Epidemiologic perspectives on neuropsychological disorders in children. In Segalowitz SJ, Rapin I (Eds), Child Neuropsychology, Handbook of Neuropsychology, 2nd Edition, vol. 8, part I. Amsterdam: Elsevier, pp. 69–90, 2002.

Beitchman JH, Nair R, Clegg M, Patel PG: Prevalence of speech and language disorders in 5-year-old kindergarten children in the Ottawa–Carleton region. Journal of Speech and Hearing Disorders: 51; 98–110, 1986.

Bellugi U, Lichtenberger L, Mills D, Galaburda A, Korenberg JR: Bridging cognition, the brain and molecular genetics: evidence from Williams syndrome. Trends in Neurosciences: 22; 197–207, 1999.

Bennett KE, Haggard MP: Behaviour and cognitive outcomes from middle ear disease. Archives of Disease in Childhood: 80; 28–35, 1999.

Bird J, Bishop D: Perception and awareness of phonemes in phonologically impaired children. European Journal of Disorders of Communication: 27; 289–311, 1992.

Bishop DVM: Comprehension of English syntax by profoundly deaf children. Journal of Child Psychology and Psychiatry and Allied Disciplines: 24; 415–434, 1983.

Bishop DVM: Test for Reception of Grammar, 2nd ed. Manchester UK: University of Manchester Age and Cognitive Perfromance Research Centre, 1989a.

Bishop DVM, 1989b: Autism Asperger's syndrome and semantic-pragmatic disorder: Where are the boundaries? British Journal of Disorders of Communication: 24; 107–121, 1989b.

Bishop DV: Is specific language impairment a valid diagnostic category? Genetic and psycholinguistic evidence. Philosophical Transactions of the Royal Society of London – Series B: Biological Sciences: 346; 105–111, 1994.

Bishop DVM: Uncommon Understanding: Development and Disorders of Comprehension in Children. Hove East Sussex UK: Psychology Press, 1997a.

Bishop DV: Pre- and perinatal hazards and family background in children with specific language impairments: a study of twins. Brain and Language: 56; 1–26, 1997b.

Bishop DVM: Development of the Children's Communication Checklist (CCC): a method for assessing qualitative aspects of communicative impairment in children. Journal of Child Psychology and Psychiatry and Allied Disciplines: 39; 879–888, 1998.

Bishop DVM, Adams C: Conversational characteristics of children with semantic–pragmatic disorder: II. What features lead to a judgement of inappropriacy? British Journal of Disorders of Communication: 24; 241–263, 1989.

Bishop DVM, Adams C: A prospective study of the relationship between specific language impairment, phonological disorders and reading retardation. Journal of Child Psychology and Psychiatry and Allied Disciplines: 31; 1027–1050, 1990.

Bishop DVM, Byers Brown B, Robson J: The relationship between phoneme discrimination, speech production, and language comprehension in cerebral palsied individuals. Journal of Speech and Hearing Research: 33; 210–219, 1990.

Bishop DV, North T, Donlan C: Genetic basis of specific language impairment: evidence from a twin study. Developmental Medicine and Child Neurology: 37; 56–71, 1995.

Bishop DV, Rosenbloom L: Classification of childhood language disorders. In Yule W, Rutter M (Eds), Language Development and Disorders. London UK: Mac Keith Press, pp. 16–41, 1987.

Blank M, Allen DA: Understanding 'why': its significance in early intelligence. In Lewis M (Ed), Origins of Intelligence: Infancy and Early Childhood. New York: Plenum Press, pp. 266–282, 1976.

Bloom L: Language Development: Form and Function in Emerging Grammars. Cambridge MA: MIT Press, 1970.

Bloom L, Lahey M: Language Development and Language Disorders. New York: Wiley, 1978.

Bonvillian JD, Nelson KE, Rhyne JM: Sign language and autism. Journal of Autism and Developmental Disorders: 11; 125–137, 1981.

Boucher J: Clinical Forum: SPD as a distinct diagnostic entity: logical considerations and directions for future research. International Journal of Language and Communication Disorders: 33; 71–81, 1998.

Bradford Y, Haines J, Hutcheson H, Gardiner M, Braun T, Sheffield V, Cassavant T, Huang W, Wang K, Vieland V, Folstein S, Santangelo S, Piven J: Incorporating language phenotypes strengthens evidence of linkage to autism. American Journal of Medical Genetics (Neuropsychiatric Genetics): 105; 539–547, 2001.

Broman S, Nichols PL, Shaughnessy P, Kennedy W: Retardation in Young Children: A Developmental Study of Cognitive Deficit. Hillsdale NJ.: Lawrence Erlbaum Associates, 1987.

Brooks-Gunn J, Liaw FR, Klebanov PK: Effects of early intervention on cognitive function of low birth weight preterm infants. Journal of Pediatrics: 120; 350–359, 1992.

Brown R: A First Language: The Early Stages. Cambridge MA: Harvard University Press, 1973.

Bruneau N, Roux S, Guérin P, Garreau B, LeLord G: Auditory stimulus intensity responses and frontal midline theta rhythm. Electroencephalography and Clinical Neurophysiology: 86; 213–216, 1993.

Brunstrom JE, Gray-Swain MR, Osborne PA, Pearlman AL: Neuronal heterotopias in the developing cerebral cortex produced by neurotrophin-4. Neuron, 18, 505–517, 1997.

Bryan GK, Riesen AH: Deprived somatosensory–motor experience in stumptailed monkey neocortex: dendritic spine density and dendritic branching of layer IIIB pyramidal cells. Journal of Comparative Neurology: 286; 208–217, 1989.

Bryden MP: Cerebral specialization: clinical and experimental assessment. In Boller F, Grafman J (Eds), Handbook of Neuropsychology. Vol. 1. Section 1: Introduction. Amsterdam: Elsevier, pp. 143–159, 1988.

Buonomano DV, Merzenich MM: Cortical plasticity: from synapses to maps. Annual Review of Neuroscience: 21; 149–186, 1998.

Campbell TF, McNeil MR: Effects of presentation rate and divided attention on auditory comprehension in children with an acquired language disorder. Journal of Speech and Hearing Research: 28; 513–520, 1985.

Capute AJ, Accardo PJ: Linguistic and auditory milestones in the first two years of life: A language inventory for the practicing pediatrician. Clinical Pediatrics: 17; 847–853, 1978.

Capute AJ, Palmer FB, Shapiro BK: Clinical Linguistic and Auditory Milestone Scale: prediction of cognition in infancy. Developmental Medicine and Child Neurology: 28; 762–771, 1986.

Ceci S: Automatic and purposive semantic processing characteristics of normal and language/learning disabled children. Developmental Psychology: 19; 427–439, 1983.

Chapman RS, Seung HK, Schwartz SE, Kay-Raining Bird E: Language skills of children and adolescents with Down syndrome: II. Production deficits. Journal of Speech Language, and Hearing Research: 41; 861–873, 1998.

Chevrie-Muller C, Narbona J (Eds): Le language de l'enfant: aspects normaux et pathologiques, 2ème Edition. Paris: Masson, 1999.

Chi JG, Dooling EC, Gilles FH: Gyral development of the human brain. Annals of Neurology: 1; 86–93, 1977.

Christen HJ, Hanefeld F, Kruse E, Imhauser S, Ernst JP, Finkenstaedt M: Foix-Chavany-Marie (anterior operculum) syndrome in childhood: a reappraisal of Worster-Drought syndrome. Developmental Medicine and Child Neurology: 42; 122–132, 2000.

Chugani DC, Chugani HT: Positron emission tomography (PET) and single photon emission computed tomography (SPECT) in developmental disorders. In Segalowitz SJ, Rapin I (Eds), Child Neuropsychology, Handbook of Neuropsychology, 2nd Edition, vol. 8, part I. Amsterdam: Elsevier, pp. 195–215, 2002.

Clarke JM, Zaidel E: Anatomical–behavioral relationships: corpus callosum morphometry and hemispheric specialization. Behavioural Brain Research: 64; 185–202, 1994.

Cohen H, Gelinas C, Lassonde M, Geoffroy G: Auditory lateralization for speech in language-impaired children. Brain and Language: 41; 395–401, 1991.

Cohen H, LeNormand MT: Language development in children with simple-partial left-hemisphere epilepsy. Brain and Language: 64; 409–422, 1998.

Coles CD, Platzman KA, Raskind-Hood CL, Brown RT, Falek A, Smith IE: A comparison of children affected by prenatal alcohol exposure and attention deficit, hyperactivity disorder. Alcoholism: Clinical and Experimental Research: 21; 150–161, 1997.

Conti-Ramsden G, Botting N: Classification of children with specific language impairment: longitudinal considerations. Journal of Speech Language and Hearing Research: 42; 1092–1204, 1999.

Conti-Ramsden G, Crutchley A, Botting N: The extent to which psychometric tests differentiate subgroups of children with SLI. Journal of Speech Language and Hearing Research: 40; 765–777, 1997.

Coplan J: ELM Scale: The Early Language Milestone Scale (Revised). Austin TX: Pro-Ed, 1989.

Cromer R: Hierarchial planning disabilities in the drawings of a special group of severely aphasic children. Brain and Cognition: 2; 144–164, 1983.

Cromer R: Language acquisition, language disorders and cognitive development. In Yule W, Rutter M (Eds), Language Development and Disorders. London: MacKeith Press, pp. 171–188, 1987.

Curtiss S: Genie: a psycholinguistic study of a modern day 'wild child'. New York: Academic Press, 1977.

Damico JS: Clinical discourse analysis; a functional approach to language assessment. In Simon CS (Ed), Comunication Skills and Classroom Success, Assessment of Language-Learning Disabled Students, London: Taylor and Francis, 1985.

Davatzikos C, Resnick SM: Sex differences in anatomic measures of interhemispheric connectivity: correlations with cognition in women but not men. Cerebral Cortex: 8; 635–640, 1998.

De Villiers J, De Villiers P: Language Acquisition. Cambridge MA: Harvard University Press, 1978.

Dollaghan CA, Campbell TF, Tomlin R: Video narration as a language sampling context. Journal of Speech and Hearing Disorders: 55; 582–590, 1990.

Dunn M, Gomes H, Sebastian M: Prototypicality of responses in autistic language disordered and normal children in a verbal fluency task. Child Neuropsychology: 2; 99–108, 1996.

Dunn M, Rapin I: Communication in autistic children. In Accardo PJ, Shapiro BK, Capute AJ (Eds), Behavior Belongs in the Brain: Neurobehavioral Syndromes. Timonium MD: York Press, pp. 97–111, 1997.

Fazio BB: The counting abilities of children with specific language impairment: a comparison of oral and gestural tasks. Journal of Speech and Hearing Research: 37; 358–368, 1994.

Fazio BB: Learning a new poem: memory for connected speech and phonological awareness in low-income children with and without specific language impairment. Journal of Speech Language and Hearing Research: 40; 1285–1297, 1997.

Fazio BB: The effect of presentation rate on serial memory in young children with specific language impairment. Journal of Speech Language and Hearing Research: pp. 1375–1383, 1998.

Fenson L, Dale PS, Reznick JS, Thal D, Bates E, Hartung JP, Pethick S, Reilly JS: The MacArthur Communicative Development Inventories: User's guide and technical manual. San Diego CA: Singular Publishing Group, 1993.

Ferry PC, Hall SM, Hicks JL: 'Dilapidated' speech: Developmental verbal dyspraxia. Developmental Medicine and Child Neurology: 17; 749–756, 1975.

Fiez JA, Petersen SE: Neuroimaging studies of word reading. Proceedings of the National Academy of Sciences of the United States of America: 95; 914–921, 1998.

Fiez JA, Raichle ME, Balota DA, Tallal P, Petersen SE: PET activation of posterior temporal regions during auditory word presentation and verb generation. Cerebral Cortex: 6; 1–10, 1996.

Fisher SE, Vargha-Khadem F, Watkins KE, Monaco AP, Pembrey ME: Localisation of a gene implicated in a severe speech and language disorder. Nature Genetics: 18; 168–170, 1998.

Flax JF, Rapin I: Evaluating children with delayed speech and language. Contemporary Pediatrics: 15; 164–172, 1998.

Frumkin B, Rapin I: Perception of vowels and consonant-vowels of varying duration in language impaired children. Neuropsychologia: 18; 443–454, 1980.

Galaburda AM, Sherman GF, Rosen GD, Aboitiz F, Geschwind N: Developmental dyslexia: Four consecutive patients with cortical anomalies. Annals of Neurology: 18; 222–233, 1985.

Gathercole SE, Pickering SJ: Working memory deficits in children with low achievements in the national curriculum at 7 years of age. British Journal of Educational Psychology: 70; 177–194, 2000.

Gayan J, Smith SD, Cherny SS, Cardon LR, Fulker DW, Brower AM, Olson RK, Pennington BF, DeFries JC: Quantitative-trait locus for specific language and reading deficits on chromosome 6p. American Journal of Human Genetics: 64; 157–164, 1999.

Genesee F: Bilingual language development in preschool children. In Bishop D, Mogford K (Eds), Language Development in Exceptional Circumstances. London: Churchill Livingstone, pp. 62–79, 1988.

Geschwind N, Galaburda AM: Cerebral lateralization: Biological mechanisms, associations and pathology. Archives of Neurology: 42; 428–459, 521–552, 634–654, 1985.

Geschwind N, Levitsky W: Human brain: Left-right asymmetries in temporal speech region. Science: 161; 186–187, 1968.

Gibbon FE: Undifferentiated lingual gestures in children with articulation/phonological disorders. Journal of Speech Language, and Hearing Research: 42; 382–397, 1999.

Gillam RB, Cowan N, Day LS: Sequential memory in children with and without language impairment. Journal of Speech and Hearing Research: 38; 393–402, 1995.

Gillies M, Light P: Spatial cognition in language-impaired children. European Journal of Disorders of Communication: 32; 159–166, 1997.

Gopnik M, Crago MB: Familial aggregation of a developmental language disorder. Cognition: 39; 1–50, 1991.

Goswami U: Phonological skills and learning to read. Annals of the New York Academy of Sciences: 682; 296–311, 1993.

Goulden KS, Shinnar S, Koller H, Katz M, Richardson S: Epilepsy in children with mental retardation: A cohort study. Epilepsia: 32; 690–697, 1991.

Graf M, Lischka A: Topographical EEG analysis of rolandic spikes. Clinical Electroencephalography: 29; 132–137, 1998.

Graham NC: Memory Constraints in Language Deficiency. Baltimore MD: University Park Press, 1980.

Greenfield P, Smith J: The Structure of Communication in Early Language Development. New York: Academic Press, 1976.

Grigorenko EL, Wood FB, Meyer MS, Hart LA, Speed WC, Shuster A, Pauls DL: Susceptibility loci for distinct components of developmental dyslexia on chromosomes 6 and 15. American Journal of Human Genetics: 60; 27–39, 1997.

Guerreiro MM, Andermann E, Guerrini R, Dobyns WB, Kuznidecky R, Silver K, Van Bogaert P, Billain C, David P, Ambrosetto G et al.: Familial perisylvian polymicrogyria: a new familial syndrome of cortical maldevelopment. Annals of Neurology: 48; 39–48, 2000.

Habib M: The neurological basis of developmental dyslexia: an overview and working hypothesis. Brain: 123; 2373–2399, 2000.

Haynes C, Naidoo S: Children with Specific Speech and Language Impairment. London: Mac Keith Press, 1991.

Hoffman PR, Daniloff RG, Bengoa D, Schuckers GH: Misarticulating and normally articulating children's identification and discrimination of synthetic [r] and [w]. Journal of Speech and Hearing Disorders: 50; 46–53, 1985.

Humphreys P, Kaufmann WE, Galaburda AM: Developmental dyslexia in women: neuropathological findings in three patients. Annals of Neurology: 28; 727–738, 1990.

Hurst JA, Baraitser M, Auger E, Graham F, Norell S: An extended family with a dominantly inherited speech disorder. Developmental Medicine and Child Neurology: 32; 352–355, 1990.

Ingram D: Speech disorders in childhood. In Lenneberg EH, Lenneberg E (Eds), Foundations of Language Development. Volume 2. New York: Academic Press, pp. 195–261, 1975.

Ingram D: Phonological Disability in Children. London: Edward Arnold, 1976.

Jackson T, Plante E: Gyral morphology in the posterior Sylvian region in families affected by developmental language disorder. Neuropsychology Review: 6; 81–94, 1996.

Johnston JR: Specific language disorders in the child. In Lass NJ, McReynolds LV, Northern JL, Yoder DE (Eds), Handbook of Speech–Language Pathology and Audiology. Philadelphia PA: BC. Decker, pp. 685–715, 1988.

Johnston JR, Schery TK: The use of grammatical morphemes by children with communication disorders. In Morehead D, Morehead A (Eds), Normal and Deficient Child Language. Baltimore: University Park Press, pp. 239–258, 1976.

Johnston JR, Weismer SE: Mental rotation abilities in language disordered children. Journal of Speech and Hearing Research: 26; 397–403, 1983.

Jones RK: Observations on stammering after localized cerebral injury. Journal of Neurology Neurosurgery and Psychiatry: 29; 192–195, 1966.

Kaga M: Language disorders in Landau–Kleffner syndrome. Journal of Child Neurology: 14; 118–122, 1999.

Kamhi AG: Nonlinguistic symbolic and conceptual abilities of language impaired and normally developing children. Journal of Speech and Hearing Research: 24; 445–446, 1981.

Karmiloff-Smith A: Development itself is the key to understanding developmental disorders. Trends in Cognitive Sciences: 2; 389–398, 1998.

Katzman GL, Dagher AP, Patronas NJ: Incidental findings on brain magnetic resonance imaging from 1000 asymptomatic volunteers. JAMA: 282; 36–39, 1999.

Kirchner DM, Klatzky RL: Verbal rehearsal and memory in language disordered children. Journal of Speech and Hearing Research: 4; 556–565, 1985.

Klein NK, Hack M, Breslau N: Children who were very low birthweight: Development and academic achievement at 9 years of age. Developmental and Behavioral Pediatrics: 10; 32–37, 1989.

Klein SK, Rapin I: Intermittent conductive hearing loss and language development. In Bishop D, Mogford K (Eds), Language Development in Exceptional Circumstances. Edinburgh: Churchill Livingstone, pp. 96–109, 1988.

Klein SK, Kurtzberg D, Brattson A, Kreutzer JA, Stapells DR, Dunn MA, Rapin I, Vaughan HG Jr: Electrophysiologic manifestations of impaired temporal lobe auditory processing in verbal auditory agnosia. Brain and Language: 51; 383–405, 1995.

Klein SK, Tuchman RF, Rapin I: The influence of premorbid language skills and behavior on language recovery in children with verbal auditory agnosia. Journal of Child Neurology: 15; 36–43, 2000.

Kleppe SA, Katayama KM, Shipley KG, Foushee DR: The speech and language characteristics of children with Prader-Willi syndrome. Journal of Speech and Hearing Disorders: 55; 300–309, 1990.

Korkman M, Hakkinen-Rihu P: A new classification of developmental language disorders (DLD). Brain and Language: 47; 96–116, 1994.

Kraemer H: Perception of rhythmic sequences by receptive aphasic and deaf children. British Journal of Disorders of Communication: 10; 43–51, 1975.

Krassowski E, Plante E: IQ variability in children with SLI: implications for use of cognitive referencing in determining SLI. Journal of Communication Disorders: 30; 1–8, 1997.

Lahey M: Who shall be called language disordered? Some reflections and one perspective. Journal of Speech and Hearing Disorders: 4; 612–620, 1990.

Lai CS, Fisher SE, Hurst JA, Levy ER, Hodgson S, Fox M, Jeremiah S, Povey S, Jamison DC, Green ED, Vargha-Khadem F, Monaco AP: The SPCH1 region of on human chromosome 7q31: genomic characterization of the critical interval and localization of translocations associated with speech and language disorder. American Journal of Human Genetics: 67; 357–368, 2000.

Landau WM, Goldstein R, Kleffner FR: Congenital aphasia: a clinicopathological study. Neurology: 7; 523–530, 1960.

Landau WM, Kleffner FR: Syndrome of acquired aphasia with convulsive disorder in children. Neurology: 7; 523–530, 1957.

Law J: Evaluating intervention for language impaired children: a review of the literature. European Journal of Disorders of Communication: 32; 1–14, 1997.

Laws G: The use of nonword repetition as a test of phonological memory in children with Down syndrome. Journal of Child Psychology and Psychiatry and Allied Disciplines: 39; 1119–1130, 1998.

Lee BC, Kuppusamy K, Grueneich R, El-Ghazzawy O, Gordon RE, Lin W, Haacke EM: Hemispheric language dominance in children demonstrated by functional magnetic resonance imaging. Journal of Child Neurology: 14; 78–82, 1999.

LeNormand MT, Chevrie-Muller C: A follow-up case study of transitory developmental apraxia of speech; "L'enfant à voyelles". Clinical Linguistics and Phonetics: 5; 99–118, 1991.

Leppanen PH, Lyytinen H: Auditory event-related potentials in the study of developmental language-related disorders. Audiology and Neuro-Otology: 2; 308–340, 1997.

Levy C, Menyuk P: Developmental language disorders: Linguistic and nonlinguistic processing. In Burns M, Andrews J (Eds), Selected Papers in Language and Phonology. Evanston IL: Institute for Continuing Professional Education, pp. 52–62, 1977.

Lewine JD, Andrews R, Chez M, Patil AA, Devinsky O, Smith M, Kanner A, Davis JT, Funke M, Jones G, Chong B, Provencal S, Weisend M, Orrison WW Jr: Magnetoencephalographic patterns of epileptiform activity in children with regressive autism spectrum disorders. Pediatrics: 104; 405–418, 1999.

Leonard CM, Lombardino LJ, Mercado LR, Browd SR, Breier JI, Agee OF: Cerebral asymmetry and cognitive development: a magnetic resonance imaging study. Psychological Science: 7; 89–95, 1996.

Lichtenstein V, Stapells DR: Frequency-specific identification of hearing loss using transient-evoked otoacoustic emissions to clicks and tones. Hearing Research: 98; 125–136, 1996.

Liegeois-Chauvel C, De Graaf JB, Laguitton V, Chauvel P: Specialization of left auditory cortex for speech perception in man depends on temporal coding. Cerebral Cortex: 9; 484–496, 1999.

Locke JL: Memory for speech and speech for memory. Journal of Speech and Hearing Research: 18; 176–191, 1975.

Locke JL: Gradual emergence of developmental language disorders. Journal of Speech and Hearing Research: 37; 608–616, 1994.

Lonigan CJ, Fischel JE, Whitehurst GJ, Arnold DS, Valdez-Menchaca MC: The role of otitis media in the development of expressive language delay. Developmental Psychology: 28; 430–440, 1992.

Loonen MC, Van Dongen HR: Acquired childhood aphasia: outcome 1 year after onset. Archives of Neurology: 47; 1324–1328, 1990.

Lovaas OI: Teaching Developmentally Disabled Children: The Me Book. Austin TX: Pro-Ed, 1981.

Lyon GR: Learning disabilities. Future of Children: 6; 54–76, 1996.

MacWhinney B: The CHILDES Project; Tools for Analyzing Talk, 2nd ed. Hillsdale NJ: Erlbaum, 1992.

Marescaux C, Hirsch E, Finck S, Maquet P, Schlumberger E, Sellal F, Metz-Lutz MN, Alembik Y, Salmon E, Frank G: Landau–Kleffner syndrome: A pharmacologic study of five cases. Epilepsia: 31; 768–777, 1990.

Mattis S, Luck DZ: Neuropsychological assessment of school-aged children. In Segalowitz SJ, Rapin I (Eds), Child Neuropsychology, Handbook of Neuropsychology, 2nd Edition, vol. 8, part I. Amsterdam: Elsevier, pp. 281–309, 2002.

McLean LK, Cripe JW: The effectiveness of early intervention for children with communication disorders. In Guralnick MJ (Ed), The Effectiveness of Early Intervention. Baltimore MD: Paul H. Brookes, pp. 349–428, 1997.

Mentis M: In utero cocaine exposure and language development. Seminars in Speech and Language: 19; 147–164, 1998.

Menyuk P: Linguistic problems in children with developmental dysphasia. In Wyke MA (Ed), Developmental Dysphasia. London: Academic Press, pp. 135–158, 1978.

Menyuk P, Looney PL: A problem of language disorder: Length vs. structure. Journal of Speech and Hearing Research: 15; 264–279, 1972.

Merzenich MM, Jenkins WM, Johnston P, Schreiner C, Miller SL, Tallal P: Temporal processing deficits in language-learning impaired children ameliorated by training. Science: 271; 77–81, 1996.

Michas IC, Henry LA: The link between phonological memory and vocabulary acquisition. British Journal of Developmental Psychology: 12; 147–163, 1994.

Miller JF: Identifying language disorders in retarded children. School Psychology Review: 7; 27–44, 1978.

Miller JF: Assessing Language Production in Children. Austin TX: PRO-ED, 1981.

Miller JF, Chapman RS: The relation between age and mean length of utterance in morphemes. Journal of Speech and Hearing Research: 24; 154–161, 1981.

Miller JF, Chapman RS: SALT: Systematic Analysis of Language Transcripts. A computer Program Designed to Analyze Free Speech Samples. University of Wisconsin Waisman Center Language Analysis Laboratory University of Wisconsin Madison WI. (Electronic Citation), 1987.

Miller JF, Chapman RS, MacKenzie H: Individual differences in the language acquisition patterns of mentally retarded children. Proceedings of the Symposium on Research in Child Language Disorders: 2; 130–146, 1981.

Mills DL, Neville HJ: Electrophysiological studies of language and language impairment. Seminars in Pediatric Neurology: 4; 125–134, 1997.

Milner B: Visually-guided maze learning in man: Effects of bilateral hippocampal, bilateral frontal and unilateral cerebral lesions. Neuropsychologia: 3; 317–338, 1965.

Milner B: Hemispheric specialization: Scope and limits. In Schmitt FO, Worden FG (Eds), The Neurosciences. Third Study Program. Cambridge MA: MIT Press, pp. 75–89, 1974.

Monfort M, Juarez Sanchez A: L'intervention dans les troubles graves de l'acquisition du langage et les dysphasies développementales. Belgium: L'Ortho, 1996.

Montgomery JW: Sentence comprehension in children with specific language impairment: the role of phonological working memory. Journal of Speech and Hearing Research: 38; 187–199, 1995.

Morrell F, Whisler WW, Smith MC, Hoeppner TJ, De Toledo-Morrell L, Pierre-Louis SJC, Kanner AM, Buelow JM, Ristanovic R, Bergen D, Chez M, Hasegawa H: Landau–Kleffner syndrome: Treatment with subpial intracortical transection. Brain: 118; 1529–1546, 1995.

Msall ME, Bier JA, LaGasse L, Tremont M, Lester B: The vulnerable preschool child: the impact of biomedical and social risks on neurodevelopmental function. Seminars in Pediatric Neurology: 5; 52–61, 1998.

Nass R: Language development in children with congenital strokes. Seminars in Pediatric Neurology: 4; 109–116, 1997.

Nass R: Plasticity: mechanisms, extents and limits. In Segalowitz SJ, Rapin I (Eds), Child Neuropsychology, Handbook of Neuropsychology, 2nd Edition, vol. 8, part I. Amsterdam: Elsevier, pp. 29–68, 2002.

Nass R, Gross A, Wisoff J, Devinsky O: Outcome of multiple subpial transections for autistic epileptiform regression. Pediatric Neurology: 21; 464–470, 1999.

Nass RD, Sadler AE, Sidtis JJ: Differential effect of congenital versus acquired unilateral brain injury on dichotic listening performance. Evidence for sparing and asymmetric crowding. Neurology: 42; 1960–1965, 1992.

Nation JE, Aram DM: Diagnosis of Speech and Language Disorders, 3 ed. San Diego CA: Singular Press, 1990.

Needleman HL: What can the study of lead teach us about other toxicants? Environmental Health Perspectives: 86; 183–189, 1990.

Neville BG, Harkness WF, Cross JH, Cass HC, Burch VC, Lees JA, Taylor DC: Surgical treatment of severe autistic regression in childhood epilepsy. Pediatric Neurology: 16; 137–140, 1997.

Neville HJ, Bavelier D: Neural organization and plasticity of language. Current Opinion in Neurobiology: 8; 254–258, 1998.

Neville HJ, Bavelier D, Rauschecker J, Karni A, Lalwani A, Braun A, Clark V, Jezzard P, Turner R: Cerebral organization for language in deaf and hearing subjects: biological constraints and effects of experience. Proceedings of the National Academy of Sciences of the United States of America: 95; 922–929, 1998.

New York State Department of Health: Early Intervention Program: Clinical Practice Guideline for Autism/Pervasive Developmental Disorders: Assessment and Intervention for Young Children (Age 0–3 Years). Albany, NY: NYS Department of Health, 1999a.

New York State Department of Health: Early Intervention Program: Clinical Practice Guideline: Communication disorders. Assessment and intervention for young children (Age 0–3 years), 1999b.

Nickerson E, Greenberg F, Keating MT, McCaskill C, Shaffer LG: Deletions of the elastin gene at 7q11.23 occur in approximately 90% of patients with Williams syndrome. American Journal of Human Genetics: 56; 1156–1161, 1995.

Nippold MA, Erskine BJ, Freed DB: Proportional and functional analogical reasoning in normal and language-impaired children. Journal of Speech and Hearing Disorders: 53; 440–448, 1988.

Nozza RJ, Sabo DL, Mandel EM: A role for otoacoustic emissions in screening for hearing impairment and middle ear disorders in school-age children. Ear and Hearing: 18; 227–239, 1997.

Olswang L, Bain B, Dunn C, Cooper J: The effects of stimulus variations on lexical learning. Journal of Speech and Hearing Disorders: 48; 192–201, 1983.

O'Shea AG, Harel B, Fein D: Neuropsychological assessment of the preschool child. In Segalowitz SJ, Rapin I (Eds), Child Neuropsychology, Handbook of Neuropsychology, 2nd Edition, vol. 8, part I. Amsterdam: Elsevier, pp. 249–280, 2002.

Paul R: Clinical implications of the natural history of slow expressive language development. American Journal of Speech Language Pathology: 5; 5–21, 1996.

Peters SA, Grievink EH, Van Bon WH, Van den Bercken JH, Schilder AG: The contribution of risk factors to the effect of early otitis media with effusion on later language, reading, and spelling. Developmental Medicine and Child Neurology: 39; 31–39, 1997.

Petersen SE, Fox PT, Posner MI, Mintum M, Raichle ME: Positron emission tomographic studies of the cortical anatomy of single-word processing. Nature: 331; 585–589, 1988.

Picard A, Cheliout-Héraut F, Bouskraoui M, Lemoine M, Lacert P, Delattre J: Sleep EEG and developmental dysphasia. Developmental Medicine and Child Neurology: 40; 595–599, 1998.

Pinker S: Words and rules: the ingredients of language. New York: Basic Books, 1999.

Plante E, Swisher L, Vance R, Rapcsak S: MRI findings in boys with specific language impairment. Brain and Language: 41; 52–66, 1991.

Poulos MG, Webster WG: Family history as a basis for subgrouping people who stutter. Journal of Speech and Hearing Research: 34; 5–10, 1991.

Powell RP, Bishop DV: Clumsiness and perceptual problems in children with specific language impairment. Developmental Medicine and Child Neurology: 34; 755–765, 1992.

Preis S, Jancke L, Schittler P, Huang Y, Steinmetz H: Normal intrasylvian anatomical asymmetry in children with developmental language disorder. Neuropsychologia: 36; 849–855, 1998.

Preis S, Schittler P, Lenard HG: Motor performance and handedness in children with developmental language disorder. Neuropediatrics: 28; 324–327, 1997.

Raine A, Hulme C, Chadderton H, Bailey P: Verbal short-term memory span in speech-disordered children: Implications for articulatory coding in short-term memory. Child Development: 62; 415–423, 1991.

Rapin I: Historical data. In Rapin I (Ed), Preschool Children with Inadequate Communication: Developmental Language

Disorder, Autism, Low IQ. London: Mac Keith Press, pp. 58–97, 1996a.

Rapin I: Practitioner review: Developmental language disorders: A clinical update. Journal of Child Psychology and Psychiatry and Allied Disciplines: 37; 643–655, 1996b.

Rapin I, Allen DA: Developmental language disorders: Nosologic considerations. In Kirk U (Ed), Neuropsychology of Language Reading and Spelling. New York: Academic Press, pp. 155–184, 1983.

Rapin I, Allen DA: Syndromes in developmental dysphasia and adult aphasia. In Plum F (Ed), Language Communication, and the Brain. New York: Raven Press, pp. 57–75, 1988.

Rapin I, Allen DA: The semantic–pragmatic deficit disorder: classification issues. International Journal of Language and Communication Disorders: 33; 82–87, 1998.

Rapin I, Dunn M: Language disorders in children with autism. Seminars in Pediatric Neurology: 4; 86–92, 1997.

Rapin I, Mattis S, Rowan AJ, Golden GS: Verbal auditory agnosia in children. Developmental Medicine and Child Neurology: 19; 192–207, 1977.

Richardson SA: Family characteristics associated with mild mental retardation. In Begab M, Garber H (Eds), Psychosocial Influences in Retarded Performance. Volume II. Baltimore MD: University Park Press, pp. 29–43, 1981.

Roberts JE, Wallace IF: Language and otitis media. In Roberts JE, Wallace IF, Henderson FW (Eds), Otitis Media in Young Children: Medical Developmental, and Educational Considerations. Baltimore: Brookes, pp. 133–162, 1997.

Rosen GD, Galaburda AM, Sherman GF: The ontogeny of anatomic asymmetry: Constraints derived from basic mechanisms. In Scheibel AB, Wechsler AF (Eds), Neurobiology of Higher Cognitive Functions. New York NY: Guilford Press, pp. 215–238, 1990.

Rosenfield DB, Barroso AO: Difficulties with speech and swallowing. In Bradley WG, Daroff RB, Fenichel GM, Marsden CD (Eds), Neurology in Clinical Practice: Principles of Diagnosis and Management. Boston: Butterworth-Heinemann, pp. 171–185, 2000.

Rosenzweig MR, Bennett EL, Diamond MC, Wu SY, Slagle RW, Saffran E: Influences of environmental complexity and visual stimulation on development of occipital cortex in rat. Brain Research: 14; 427–445, 1969.

Roulet Perez E, Davidoff V, Despland P-A, Deonna T: Mental and behavioural deterioration of children with epilepsy and CSWS: Acquired epileptic frontal syndrome. Developmental Medicine and Child Neurology: 35; 661–674, 1993.

Rourke BP: Treatment program for the child with NLD. In Rourke BP (Ed) Syndrome of Nonverbal Learning Disabilities: Neurodevelopmental Manifestations. New York Guilford Press, pp. 497–508, 1995.

Rovet J, Netley C, Keenan M, Bailey J, Stewart D: The psychoeducational profile of boys with Klinefelter syndrome. Journal of Learning Disabilities: 29; 180–196, 1996.

Savich PA: Anticipatory imagery ability in normal and language disordered children. Journal of Speech and Hearing Research: 27; 494–501, 1984.

Scarborough HS, Rescorla L, Tager-Flusberg H, Fowler A, Sudhalter V: The relation of utterance length to grammatical complexity in normal and language-disordered groups. Applied Psycholinguistics: 12; 23–45, 1991.

Schaller S: A Man Without Words. New York: Summit Books, 1991.

Semrud-Clikeman M: Evidence from imaging on the relationship between brain structure and developmental language disorders. Seminars in Pediatric Neurology: 4; 117–124, 1997.

Shaywitz BA, Fletcher JM, Shaywitz SE: Defining and classifying learning disabilities and attention-deficit/hyperactivity disorder. Journal of Child Neurology: 10(Suppl. 1); S50–S57, 1995.

Shaywitz SE: Dyslexia. New England Journal of Medicine: 338; 307–312, 1998.

Shaywitz SE, Shaywitz BA, Fletcher JM, Escobar MD: Prevalence of reading disability in boys and girls. Results of the Connecticut Longitudinal Study. JAMA: 264; 998–1002, 1990.

Sherman GF, Holmes LB: Cerebrocortical microdysgenesis in enhanced in c57BL/6J mice exposed in utero to acetazolamide. Teratology: 60; 137–142, 1999.

Skuse DH: Extreme deprivation in early childhood. In Bishop D, Mogford K (Eds), Language Development in Exceptional Circumstances. Edinburgh: Churchill Livingstone, pp. 29–46, 1988.

Sparrow SS, Balla DA, Cicchetti DV: Vineland Adaptive Behavior Scales: A Revision of the Vineland Social Maturity Scale by Edgar Doll. Circle Pines MN: American Guidance Service, 1984.

Stapells DR, Oates P: Estimation of the pure-tone audiogram by the auditory brainstem response: a review. Audiology and Neuro-Otology: 2; 257–280, 1997.

Stark R, Bernstein L: Evaluating central auditory processing in children. Topics in Language Disorders: 4; 57–70, 1984.

Stark RE, Blackwell PB: Oral volitional movements in children with language impairments. Child Neuropsychology: 3; 81–96, 1997.

Stark RE, McGregor KK: Follow-up study of a right- and a left-hemispherectomized child: implications for localization and impairment of language in children. Brain and Language: 60; 222–242, 1997.

Stark RE, Tallal P: Selection of children with specific language deficits. Journal of Speech and Hearing Disorders: 46; 114–122, 1981.

Steinschneider M, Dunn M: Electrophysiology in developmental neuropsychology. In Segalowitz SJ, Rapin I (Eds), Child Neuropsychology, Handbook of Neuropsychology, 2nd Edition, vol. 8, part I. Amsterdam: Elsevier, pp. 91–146, 2002.

Tager-Flusberg H: Dissociations in form and function in the acquisition of language by autistic children. In Tager-Flusberg H (Ed), Constraints on Language Acquisition: Studies of Atypical Children. Hillsdale NJ: Lawrence Erlbaum, pp. 175–194, 1994.

Tallal P: Developmental language disorders. In Kavanagh JF, Truss TJ Jr (Eds), Learning Disabilities: Proceedings of the National Conference. Parkton, MD: York Press, pp. 181–272, 1988.

Tallal P, Merzenich M, Miller S, Jenkins W: Language learning impairment: integrating research and remediation. Scandinavian Journal of Psychology: 39; 197–199, 1998a.

Tallal P, Merzenich MM, Miller S, Jenkins W: Language learning impairments: integrating basic science, technology, and remediation. Experimental Brain Research: 123; 210–219, 1998b.

Tallal P, Miller S, Fitch RH: Neurobiological basis of speech: A case for the preeminence of temporal processing. In Tallal P, Galaburda AM, Llinas RR, Von Euler C (Eds), Temporal Information Processing in the Nervous System: Special Reference to Dyslexia and Dysphasia. New York: New York Academy of Sciences, pp. 27–49, 1993.

Tallal P, Miller SL, Bedi G, Byma G, Wang X, Nagarajan SS, Schreiner C, Jenkins WM, Merzenich MM: Language comprehension in language-learning impaired children improved with acoustically modified speech. Science: 271; 81–84, 1996.

Tallal P, Piercy M: Developmental dysphasia: impaired rate of nonverbal processing as a function of sensory modality. Neuropsychologia: 11; 389–398, 1973.

Tallal P, Piercy M: Defects of auditory perception in children with developmental dysphasia. Neuropsychologia: 12; 83–93, 1974.

Tallal P, Stark R: Speech acoustic cue discrimination abilities of normally developing and language impaired children. Journal of the Acoustical Society of America: 69; 568–574, 1981.

Tallal P, Stark R, Kallman C, Mellits D: A reexamination of some nonverbal perceptual abilities of language-impaired and normal children as a function of age and sensory modality. Journal of Speech and Hearing Research: 24; 351–357, 1981.

Templin MC: Certain Language Skills in Children: Their Development and Interrelationships. Minneapolis MN: University of Minnesota Press, 1957.

Teuber HL: Recovery of function after brain injury in man. Ciba Foundation Symposium: 34; 159–190, 1975.

Thal D, Bates E: Continuity and variation in early language development. In Colombo J, Sagan J (Eds), Individual Differences in Infancy: Reliability, Stability, and Prediction. Hillsdale NJ: Erlbaum, 1990.

Thal D, Katich J: Predicaments in early identification of specific language impairment. In Cole K, Dale P, Thal D (Eds), Assessment of Communication and Language. Baltimore: Brookes, pp. 1–28, 1996.

Tomblin JB, Buckwalter PR: Heritability of poor language achievement among twins. Journal of Speech Language and Hearing Research: 41; 188–199, 1998.

Tomblin JB, Records NL, Buckwalter P, Zhang X, Smith E, O'Brien M: Prevalence of specific language impairment in kindergarten children. Journal of Speech and Hearing Research: 40; 1245–1260, 1997.

Trauner D, Wulfeck B, Tallal P, Hesselink J: Neurological and MRI profiles of children with developmental language impairment. Developmental Medicine and Child Neurology: 42; 470–475, 2000.

Tronick EZ: Emotions and emotional communication in infants. American Psychologist: 44; 112–119, 1989.

Tuchman RF, Rapin I: Regression in pervasive developmental disorders: Seizures and epileptiform EEG correlates. Pediatrics: 99; 560–566, 1997.

Tuchman RF, Rapin I, Shinnar S: Autistic and dysphasic children: II. Epilepsy. Pediatrics: 88; 1219–1225, 1991.

Van der Lely HK: Specific language impairment in children: research findings and their therapeutic implications. European Journal of Disorders of Communication: 28; 247–261, 1993.

Van der Lely HK, Rosen S, McClelland A: Evidence for a grammar-specific deficit in children. Current Biology: 8; 1253–1258, 1998.

Van Dongen HR, De Wijngaert E, Wennekes MJ: The Landau–Kleffner syndrome: Diagnostic considerations. In Martins IP, Castro-Caldas A, Van Dongen HR, Van Hout A (Eds), Acquired Aphasia in Children: Acquisition and Breakdown of Language in the Developing Brain. Dordrecht: Kluwer Academic, pp. 253–261, 1991.

Van Hout A: Acquired aphasia in childhoold. In Segalowitz SJ, Rapin I (Eds), Child Neuropsychology, Handbook of Neuropsychology, 2nd Edition, vol. 8, part II. Amsterdam: Elsevier, pp. 631–658, 2003.

Vargha-Khadem F, Watkins K, Alcock K, Fletcher P, Passingham R: Praxic and nonverbal cognitive deficits in a large family with a genetically transmitted speech and language disorder. Proceedings of the National Academy of Sciences of the United States of America: 92; 930–933, 1995.

Vargha-Khadem F, Watkins KE, Price CJ, Ashburner J, Alcock KJ, Connelly A, Frackowiak RS, Friston KJ, Pembrey ME, Mishkin M, Gadian DG, Passingham RE: Neural basis of an inherited speech and language disorder. Proceedings of the National Academy of Sciences of the United States of America: 95; 12695–12700, 1998.

Volkmar F, Cook E Jr, Pomeroy J, Realmuto G, Tanguay P: Summary of the Practice Parameters for the Assessment and Treatment of Children Adolescents, and Adults with Autism and other Pervasive Developmental Disorders. American Academy of Child and Adolescent Psychiatry. Journal of the American Academy of Child and Adolescent Psychiatry: 38; 1611–1616, 1999.

Volterra V, Capirci O, Pezzini G, Sabbadini L, Vicari S: Linguistic abilities in Italian children with Williams syndrome. Cortex: 32; 663–677, 1996.

Von Suchodoletz W, Wolfram I: Early auditory evoked potentials in children with language development disorders. Klinische Pädiatrie: 208; 290–293, 1996.

Vygotsky LS: Mind in Society. Cambridge MA: Harvard University Press, 1978.

Wassink TH, Piven J, Vieland VJ, Huang J, Swiderski RE, Pietila J, Braun T, Beck G, Folstein SE, Haines JL, Sheffield VC: Evidence supporting WNT2 as an autism susceptibility gene. American Journal of Human Genetics (Neuropsychiatric Genetics): 105; 406–413, 2001.

Weinberg MK, Tronick EZ: Beyond the face: an empirical study of infant affective configurations of facial, vocal, gestural, and regulatory behaviors. Child Development: 65; 1503–1515, 1994.

Weismer SE, Evans J, Hesketh LJ: An examination of verbal working memory capacity in children with specific language impairment. Journal of Speech Language and Hearing Research: 42; 1249–1260, 1999.

Whitehurst GJ, Fischel JE: Practitioner review: Early developmental language delay — what, if anything, should the clinician do about it? Journal of Child Psychology and Psychiatry and Allied Disciplines: 4; 613–648, 1994.

Wiig EH, Semel EM, Nystrom LA: Comparison of rapid naming abilities in language-learning-disabled and academically achieving 8 year olds. Language Speech, and Hearing Services in Schools: 1; 11–23, 1982.

Williams D, Stott CM, Goodyer IM, Sahakian BJ: Specific language impairment with or without hyperactivity: neuropsychological evidence for frontostriatal dysfunction. Developmental Medicine and Child Neurology: 42; 368–375, 2000.

Wilson BC, Risucci DA: A model for clinical–quantitative classification. Generation I: Application to language-disordered preschool children. Brain and Language: 27; 281–309, 1986.

Wolfus B, Moskovitch DA, Kinsbourne M: Subgroups of developmental language impairment. Brain and Language: 10; 152–171, 1980.

Worster-Drought C, Allen IM: Congenital auditory imperception (congenital word-deafness): And its relation to idioglossia and other speech defects. Journal of Neurology and Psychopathology: 10; 193–236, 1930.

Wright BA, Lombardino LJ, King WM, Puranik CS, Leonard CM, Merzenich MM: Deficits in auditory temporal and spectral resolution in language-impaired children. Nature: 387; 176–178, 1997.

Wyke M, Asso D: Perception and memory for spatial relations in children with developmental dysphasia. Neuropsychologia: 17; 231–239, 1979.

Handbook of Neuropsychology, 2nd Edition, Vol. 8, Part II
S.J. Segalowitz and I. Rapin (Eds)

CHAPTER 23

Acquired aphasia in childhood

Anne Van Hout *

Service de Neurologie Pédiatrique, Université Catholique de Louvain, Cliniques Universitaires Saint Luc, 10 Avenue Hippocrate, 1200 Brussels, Belgium

Preliminary remarks

In adults, the foundations of neuropsychology were built on early studies of aphasia (Broca, 1861) and the discovery of its neurological basis. What these pioneering anatomic studies revealed is that a behavioral disorder was the direct consequence of an acquired focal brain lesion. The asymmetric occurrence, in favor of the left hemisphere, of the lesions responsible for aphasia, was soon apparent. It also rapidly became obvious that 'aphasia' was not a single entity but that its manifestations varied depending on the location of lesions, and that brain areas implicated in language were interconnected. Those seminal discoveries prompted the development of models to account for the interaction and dynamic architecture of brain areas concerned with language.

When it came to children, however, there were contradictory reports difficult to reconcile with concepts that arose from other fields of research. It was not until the 1980's that new data began to align childhood aphasiological data with findings from neurophysiology and neuroanatomy. As had been the case with adult aphasia, data on acquired aphasia in children served as the very foundation of childhood neuropsychology.

Childhood acquired aphasia was considered in the past to differ from adult aphasia in three major ways:

(1) The children's symptoms were said to be uniform and speech predominantly non-fluent, regardless of lesion localization;
(2) Prognosis was considered to be more favorable for children than for adults;
(3) The frequency of right hemisphere lesions was thought to be higher in aphasic children than adults.

For the most part these postulates had been formulated in the nineteenth century, when Broca (1863) and Cotard (1868) reported that language could be normal in children despite complete destruction of the language areas in their left hemispheres. No symptoms were detectable despite lesions whose localization, in adults, would have resulted in severe aphasia. It was thus believed that, in young subjects, lesions could 'spare' language, which was ascribed to immaturity in the children's brain organization. Moreover, if aphasia did occur, its manifestations were stated to be uniform in type, consisting mainly of mutism and 'expressive' symptoms. Subsequent reports of Clarus (1874), Bernhardt (1885), and Freud (1897) of a higher frequency of right-hemisphere lesions in childhood than adult aphasia were interpreted as evidence that, in young children, the right hemisphere was directly implicated in language.

Thus, the two tenets, that language could develop in the face of an extensive left-sided lesion and that a right-sided lesion could bring on an aphasia, led to the presumption that language was more diffusely represented in children than in adults. Many subsequent studies seemed to confirm these observations, which led to the hypothesis of progressive lateraliza-

* Corresponding author. Tel.: +32-202-7641925;
E-mail: dr.anne.vanhout@chello.be

tion of language to the left hemisphere during development. Two of the stronger arguments supporting this theory were the description of hemispherectomies by Basser (1962) and Lenneberg's (1967) report that aphasic symptoms paralleled biological parameters of brain development. The hypothesis of progressive lateralization of language to the left hemisphere had a strong influence on ideas regarding the neurologic basis of the considerably more prevalent language disorders of childhood, dyslexia and the developmental dysphasias. By the end of the 1970's, new neuropsychological discoveries contradicted the model of progressive lateralization of language to the left hemisphere. Kinsbourne (1976) summarized this new view as follows "Language lateralization does not develop; it is present from the start".

These challenges to the classic model of language organization in childhood began to cast doubt on the validity of the clinical data on acquired aphasia in childhood which had served as the bases for this model. The seminal article of Woods and Teuber, *Changing patterns of childhood aphasia* (1978), suggested that the reported higher prevalence of crossed (right-sided lesion) aphasias in childhood might be artefactual and raised the possibility that selection bias was responsible for the supposed uniformity of aphasic symptoms. A growing number of subsequent studies substantiated Woods and Teuber's hypotheses. The development of new testing instruments, the use of neurolinguistic and age-appropriate neuropsychological tests, and advances in radiological imagery all contributed to a better understanding of acquired childhood aphasia (ACA). The consequence was that almost every statement about ACA made before the end of the seventies was challenged.

Looking back at the early models of language organization in children, one is forced to concede that rarely in scientific history has such an important theory as that of the progressive lateralization of language been derived from such tenuous clinical facts! Contemporary findings illuminate the currently accepted theory of ACA and emphasize its enhanced compatibility with data from other fields of research in developmental neuropsychology.

At the start of 1990's, an international congress was held in Portugal (Martins, Castro-Caldas, Van Dongen and Van Hout, 1991) at which new findings gathered in the 10 years following the seminal article of Woods and Teuber were summarized. Contrary to Denckla's (1979) statement made a decade earlier: "Nothing new has occurred in this field of research", the meeting concluded that most ideas on ACA then current had been successfully challenged. One may wonder why publications in the next 10 years following the Portugal congress are so few. One reason is that despite the major conceptual importance of ACA, it is a rare condition and that the number of professionals able to study children during the acute stages of their lesions is small. Another is that because scientific publications are expected to bring out new material and ideas, most of the recent papers have focused on acquired epileptic aphasia — the Landau–Kleffner syndrome, and on explorations of other behavioral syndromes secondary to focal lesions, for instance acalculia (Martins, Pereiro and Albuquerque, 1999; Van Hout, 1998).

Delineation of the syndrome of acquired childhood aphasia

Acquired aphasia (which will be referred to here simply as aphasia) refers to a deterioration of language caused by an acquired cerebral insult. Specific tests that address the different levels of language are required in order to bring it out. In children, this definition of acquired aphasia carries with it two main implications: First, the acquired lesion must have occurred after a lesion-free period — a free interval, and thus the language disorders of aphasia differ from those of the developmental dysphasias, in which language is deviant from the start, and from insults in the perinatal period, prior to the development of language. Although modifications of babbling and early language milestones have been described in these conditions (see Bates, Vicari and Trauner, 1999), the definition of aphasic language regression relates only to alterations of a structured, syntactically formed language. Second, the child must have already developed some normal language, the accepted age-dependent boundary usually being 2 years of age, the time of the advent of the first sentences.

Nevertheless, many authors still use the term 'aphasia' for both acquired and congenital lesions

(Bates et al., 1999), and even for developmental disorders, sometimes with a connotation of severity, with 'aphasia' to denote the near absence of language and 'dysphasia' less severe impairment. We suggest, for reasons of clarity, reserving 'aphasia' for an acquired language deficit occurring after the age of 2 years and reserving the terms 'dysphasia', developmental language disability, or specific language impairment for developmental disorders. Depending on the severity and extensiveness of the underlying brain lesion, congenital disorders may give rise either to a lack of language ('congenital aphasia') or to delayed language development.

Consequently, in younger children, the main conditions to be differentiated from acquired aphasia are (1) the consequences of early lesions sustained before the age 2 years, such as the congenital aphasias secondary to extensive and bilateral perinatal lesions which frequently involve cortico-thalamic connections (Vargha-Khadem, O'Gorman and Watters, 1985). These children are generally 'non verbal', with impairment of both receptive and expressive language; (2) the delays in language development that may be seen in children with congenital hemiplegias, more often in those with a lesion of the left hemisphere (Annett, 1973); (3) and alterations of early language milestones following perinatal brain injuries (Marchman, Miller and Bates, 1991). These alterations point to involvement of either side of the brain when the lesion is frontal (babbling is transitorily affected after either right frontal or left frontal lesions), and to left sided involvement in the case of left temporal lobe damage, which results in transient deficiencies of vocabulary and grammar that resolve by age 5 years (Bates et al., 1999); (4) developmental dysphasias, in which cerebral lesions are almost never demonstrable, although brain mapping of evoked potentials may suggest their existence and Cohen, Campbell and Yagmai (1989) described minute anatomical abnormalities in language areas in one autopsied case of developmental dysphasia; (5) some investigators classify autism among the developmental dysphasias, as the children's language problems are often prominent, even when language is well developed, as in Asperger syndrome where it may take the characteristics of the semantic pragmatic subtype of dysphasia. In all of these conditions, there is no free interval of normally developing speech, although there may be exceptions, notably in those children with autism in whom language loss may be the most salient sign of regression. In older children, slowly progressive deterioration of language should suggest the so-called disintegrative disorder of the autism spectrum, incipient dementia, or schizophrenia.

The prevalence of aphasia is low in childhood compared to that of the developmental language disorders and adult aphasias. Its frequency has increased recently as a consequence of head injuries which account for nearly a third of all pediatric accidents and are thus is a major public-health concern.

Types of aphasias

The classic symptoms

Most older series regarded acquired aphasia in children as predominantly non-fluent and similar to the anterior, 'Broca-like' type of aphasia of adults (Bernhardt, 1885), particularly in children under the age of puberty (Lenneberg, 1967). However, nothing is less clearly described in the literature than the so-called 'expressive' character of symptoms. Some authors equate them with the signs observed in the expressive aphasias of adults. Others, in line with Jackson (1880) and Jakobson (1962), consider language as a hierarchical system and interpret the overall 'poverty' of clinical symptoms as a regression to an earlier stage of language acquisition.

The classic descriptions of acquired childhood aphasia include five main features: mutism, hypospontaneity of speech, dysarthria, agrammatism and negative signs, i.e., lack of the symptoms usually found in adult fluent aphasias (jargon, logorrhea, paraphasias, neologisms, long-lasting comprehension disorders).

Mutism

Earlier authors considered mutism an important symptom of acquired childhood aphasia. Differentiation from non-aphasic mutism was rarely made. We now know that non-aphasic mutism (akinetic mutism or mutism with overall reduced reactivity) can often precede aphasia or aphasic mutism, particularly in traumatic cases. Aphasic mutism seems to be both more frequent and of longer duration in children than in adults, but, as in adults, it has to be distinguished from non-aphasic mutism.

Von Cramon (1975) divided mutism into two types: (1) 'true mutism', the impossibility of uttering any sound, as a consequence of injury of the speech effectors. True mutism cannot be overcome, even with intensive sollicitation; it is produced by extensive frontal lesions or, more frequently in traumatic cases, by lesions of the midbrain, of the left basal ganglia, or by diffuse cortico-axonal shearing (Levin, Eisenberg and Miner, 1983); (2) 'word mutism' or 'aphasic mutism', which affects only verbal utterances. It often fades into hypospontaneity of speech and can be somewhat reduced by encouragement, stimulation, or emotional stress.

Hypospontaneity of speech

This refers to disinclination or, rather, unreadiness of the aphasic child to initiate speech, and, if he or she does, its sparseness. Hypospontaneilty of speech is referred to in the literature by many different terms, namely, loss of the initiation of speech, aspontaneity of speech, reduction of spontaneous speech. It is rarely seen in adult aphasia and seems to be the hallmark of acquired childhood aphasia, especially in younger children. Hypospontaneity is not always clearly distinct from mutism, and there is often a true continuity between mutism and hypospontaneity. The main differences between hypospontaneity and aphasic mutism are that hypospontaneity follows mutism, lasts longer, and is characterized by more consistent utterances. Psychological factors may contribute to hypospontaneity, as children often react to stressful situations by avoidance. When sufficiently encouraged, these children can show better language skills than one might have suspected. Yet, even in a non-threatening environment, hypospontaneity can be long lasting (Gaidolfi and Vignolo, 1980).

Hypospontaneity and reduced fluency were considered equivalent in many series and hypospontaneity was interpreted as part of the traditional expressive symptoms of acquired aphasia. More recent series indicate that it can occur in some stages of neologistic jargon, particularly in young patients (Van de Sandt-Koenderman, Smit, Van Dongen and Van Hesch, 1984; Van Hout, Evrard and Lyon, 1985). Van Hout et al. (1985) noted that many children under the age of 9, after a paraphasic stage, are reluctant to initiate speech and exhibit poverty of expression, slowness of articulation, and excessive pauses.

One is tempted to suggest that, in children, language and some non-segmental features of speech may be intimately interconnected. For this reason, Van Hout and Seron (1983) proposed that hypospontaneity of speech might be equivalent to the loss of the initiator mechanism of speech described by Steriade, Botez and Petrovici (1961) in subcortical lesions affecting the periaqueductal grey matter. Subcortical structures might play a more important role for language production in young children whose brain centers are not yet fully developed than in older children and adults. Recent studies of Martins and Ferro (1992) in children aged 2–5 with subcortical pathology, either isolated or associated with cortical lesions, do not support this hypothesis, as it was the second group which had the worst clinical picture and prognosis.

Articulation disorders

Jakobson (1962) suggested that articulation disorders observed in aphasia represent a regression to more archaic, easier to pronounce phonemes, as articulation errors follow, in reverse order, the acquisition of the phonological system by the normal child. Alajouanine and Lhermitte (1965) rejected the simple regression hypothesis and equated the articulation errors of aphasic children with the phonetic disintegration syndrome of adults with an expressive aphasia. The dystonic and paretic features of the articulation disorders may evolve either separately or in parallel. Although present with the high frequency of 80% in the series of Hécaen (1976, 1983), articulation disturbances were stated to be mild and transitory.

Assal and Campiche (1973) made a distinction between 'arthric disorders' and 'phonemic substitutions' (presumably, phonemic paraphasias), although true articulatory disorders and phonemic paraphasias can coexist (Dennis, 1980).

Syntactic disorders

Hypospontaneity of speech may play a crucial role for the occurrence of syntactic deficits. Many authors mention children's single word answers, but unfortunately they rarely provide any indication of the linguistic nature of these answers. This information would be helpful for differentiating telegraphic answers with agrammatism from a simple reduction in overall emissions. Some reports mention holophrases, again highlighting the disagreement between those who regard aphasic symptoms as a sign of a deviant system and those who view them as regression to more primitive stages of development.

A conclusion to be drawn from these early studies is the existence of a modular dissociation among the different components of language. The very authors who insisted on the similarities between the phonological problems of aphasic children and those of adult aphasics (e.g., Alajouanine and Lhermitte, 1965) considered the children's syntax to be simplified rather than erroneous. They stated that true agrammatism never occurs in children. Thus, if this was to be interpreted according to the so-called 'regression hypothesis', regressive phenomena should be much more marked for syntax, as speaking in holophrases is not unusual, than for the phonological system, in which elaborate phonological oppositions may be detected.

Assal and Campiche linked the degree of syntactic impairment to the severity of the injury. In their study too, syntactic and articulation disorders appeared to be dissociated, as articulation problems were said to be more frequent in the children with the better prognosis. In her stroke case, Dennis (1980) mentioned that agrammatism affected both expression and reception. Van Hout, Evrard and Lyon (1985) and Van de Sandt-Koenderman et al. (1984) found that severity of the aphasia and reduction in the length of utterances were often correlated, even in cases of receptive aphasias. In some recent descriptions of fluent aphasias, syntactic disorders are mentioned, but they are more often evocative of a form of paragrammatism than of agrammatism.

Naming disorders

The same disagreement between the regression and pathologic views of childhood aphasia is apparent in the labels applied to naming disorders. Either the terms naming disorders or anomia are used, evoking the well-known deficit in word retrieval common to all adult aphasics, or one finds the terms 'reduction of the lexical stock' or 'poverty of vocabulary', which imply loss or restriction of usage. Many authors have stressed the frequency of these problems in acquired childhood aphasia, but the terms used are often ambiguous.

Alajouanine and Lhermitte (1965) provided somewhat contradictory descriptions of these deficits. They stated that most children had a reduction of their lexical stock, but their description of effective facilitation procedures (syllabic cueing, automatic sentence completion) seemed to point to the existence of a real anomia. On the other hand, the statement that, upon follow-up, half of their cases had trouble describing objects suggests problems of memory or of semantic access, more in the line of an actual lexical impoverishment. Hécaen (1976) reported both a reduction of lexical stock and naming disorders as long-lasting sequellae, and their mention in school reports suggests an anomia in spontaneous speech. In recent case descriptions, the discrepancy between very low naming scores and preservation of designation or of definition is indicative of a specific anomia.

Auditory comprehension

Bernhardt (1885) was the first to mention the rarity of comprehension disorders in acquired childhood aphasia, on the basis of his description of six children with infantile hemiplegia. Most of the subsequent literature emphasized the essentially 'expressive' predominance of symptoms in children, although there were a few exceptions (Poetzl, 1926). For Hécaen (1976), auditory comprehension disorders occurred but were usually limited to the acute stages following the injury. Alajouanine and Lhermitte (1965) described comprehension deficits in one third of their cases, mostly in children above 9 years.

It is only in the Landau–Kleffner syndrome (acquired aphasia with epilepsy) that auditory comprehension disorders were described as predominant, amounting in some cases to an auditory agnosia. In this syndrome, some authors believe that receptive disorders are at first of a sensory aphasia type, then resemble auditory agnosia (Kaga, 1999). Recent studies emphasize the difficulty of isolating verbal auditory comprehension from other contextual factors. Attentional or memory factors can interfere with assessments, and, in the acute stage of a lesion, the results of such valuable tests as the Token

Test are difficult to interpret (Levin et al., 1983; Van Hout and Lyon, 1986). Impaired scores on the Token Test in fluent aphasias, even past the acute stage, reflect its lack of selectivity. Comparing the late effects of left hemispheric lesions with and without aphasia, Woods and Carey (1979) found the Token Test to not discriminate between the two groups. Noting that it is regularly impaired in the acute stage of any aphasia, Van Hout et al. (1985) suggested replacing it by more specific tests of comprehension.

Repetition disorders

Some classic series mention occasional transient echolalia (Assal and Campiche, 1973), whereas others report difficulty with repetition (Hécaen, 1976). Van Dongen, Loonen and Van Dongen (1985) state that, in their series of fluent aphasics, repetition was usually impaired, even at the level of polysyllabic words. Preserved repetition, including repetition of sentences, is an important diagnostic feature of transcortical aphasia described in some ACA series (Van Hout et al., 1985; Cranberg, Filley, Hart and Alexander, 1987). Impaired repetition with preserved comprehension, and phonemic paraphasias with self-corrections (conduite d'approche) indicate conduction aphasia (Martins and Ferro, 1987; Tanabe, Ikeda, Murasawa et al., 1989; Van Hout and Seron, 1983).

Discovering new semiologies

Most early series did not report the *clear-cut* aphasic pictures of *adults*, except in post-pubertal children. Even in older children, expressive symptoms were said to dominate the picture, with occasional descriptions of Broca-like aphasia in children aged 10 years or more (Assal and Campiche, 1973; Hécaen, 1976; Van Hout and Landrieu, 1979), and classical receptive aphasia was usually reported as non-existent. According to this earlier conception, in younger children expressive signs dominated but were not organized according to an adult typology, and in older children the full-blown expressive aphasia of adults made its appearance. All childhood aphasia was thus definitely expressive.

In their 1978 article, Woods and Teuber described what looked like a jargonaphasia in a 5-year-old child. They suggested that a bias (the criterion of hemiparesis indicative of the lesion's unilaterality) might have accounted for the supposed uniformity of aphasic symptoms in children. Following this report, increased attempts to identify more unusual signs in unselected cases of childhood aphasia resulted in the description of many symptoms previously thought never to occur in childhood aphasia (Van Dongen et al., 1985; Van Hout et al., 1985; Visch-Brink and Van de Sandt-Koederman, 1984).

In contrast to the classic negative features of childhood acquired aphasia, Van Hout et al. (1985) were among the first to describe positive symptoms in these children. These consist of verbal and literal paraphasias, perseverations, fluent speech, and long-lasting comprehension disorders. In time, these symptoms organize into differentiated clusterings. Modality-specific and category-specific aphasias were found (Van Hout et al., 1985), and many aphasiologic syndromes similar to the well delineated adult profiles were observed, even in very young children.

Anatomical correlations between symptoms and localization of lesions by EEG or neuroimaging (CT scans and MRI) are similar to those in adults. These observations indicate precocious functional specifications of left intra-hemispheric language organization. The age of 2 years seems to be the earliest at which specific aphasic symptoms are identifiable (Martins and Ferro, 1992). The youngest case in the Van Hout et al. series was 3.5 years old (Van Hout and Evrard, 1987). The investigators pointed out that in receptive aphasia the mechanism for the formation of neologisms was similar to that described in adults, but that their occurrence was lower. Nass, Leventhal, Levine et al. (1998) described a repetition disorder similar to adults' in a child aged 3 years.

These positive signs are but part of a complex symptomatology. Non-fluency still dominates the picture and represents either one of the most frequent subtypes of aphasia or occurs as a major feature in all aphasia types. Fluent aphasias, although not as rare as previously thought, occurred in only five of thirty three cases in the series of Van Dongen et al. (1985), and many children with lesions as extensive as those of these fluent cases presented with a classic expressive aphasia.

Van Hout et al. (1985) demonstrated the existence of a positive semiology in all the aphasic children they investigated, however, hypospontaneity was striking, even in children who were very fluent at times. They speculated that one explanation for the differences between the classic symptoms and the new ones they observed was the presence of hypospontaneity which may have masked some positive signs; these would have been easy to overlook if not specifically sought. Moreover, classic residual symptoms persisted in many cases even after the paraphasias had receded.

Presence of positive signs (paraphasias, perseveration, neologisms)

In most of the classic series of acquired aphasia in childhood, paraphasias (verbal or phonemic substitution of a target word), neologisms (more than half of the word replaced), verbal stereotypies (repetition of the same verbal expression), and perseveration (same answer repeated several times or given after a delay to a different question) were said to be either lacking or encountered only occasionally (Gloning and Hift, 1970). If mentioned at all, these signs were said to appear at random, without the organized clustering that occurs in adult syndromes. It was only in older children that some features resembling the adult ones were occasionally described. Alajouanine and Lhermitte (1965) stated that paraphasias were mainly literal, predominated in children over 10 years, and were 'rare'. Visch-Brink and Van de Sandt-Koederman (1984) pointed out that Alajouanine and Lhermitte (1965) did not specify whether 'rare' meant that few children made paraphasic errors or that paraphasias were rare compared to other signs, if they occurred at all.

In unselected series of childhood aphasias, Van Hout (1983) and Visch-Brink and Van de Sandt-Koederman (1984) described paraphasias, both literal and verbal, in 'fluent', 'non-fluent', or even 'mixed' forms of aphasias. Van Hout et al. (1985) also reported the frequent occurrence of perseveration and stereotypies. The presence of paraphasias has subsequently been reported in transcortical aphasias (Aram, Rose, Rekate and Whitaker, 1983; Cranberg et al., 1987) and, with marked autocorrections, in conduction aphasias (Martins and Ferro, 1987; Tanabe et al., 1989).

Visch-Brink and Van de Sandt-Koederman (1984) stressed that, contrary to the literature, paraphasias are not rare in acquired aphasia in children. They reach the frequency seen in adults with Wernicke's aphasia of more than one per minute. They also observed occasional neologisms, mostly during acute stages. As is true of paraphasias in adults, pauses that precede content words, paraphasias, and neologisms suggest an underlying anomia. Some children's speech was characterized by unsuccessful autocorrections, and the authors suggested that this post-monitoring behavior might be more marked in children than adults. Van Hout et al. (1985) described a similar tendency to self-correction at the height of neologistic jargon in a 7-year-old girl who tried to modify her errors by interrupting them in the middle, as though she were aware almost immediately of their inappropriateness. Two other children with jargon (aged 4 years and 10 years) were both fluent and unaware of the lack of meaning of their utterances (Van Hout et al., 1985). Such cases fit the diagnosis of jargonaphasia with anosognosia, so that a low post-monitoring behavior does not seem to be related to age per se.

In an unselected series of 16 aphasic children, Van Hout et al. (1985) described 11 children in whom the aphasic symptoms were unusual with regard to the prevailing views of acquired childhood aphasia. All the symptoms said to be rare or even never to appear in children were observed. Paraphasias stood out as the most frequent positive symptom, were present in all cases and persisted beyond the acute stage in half of them. The relative percentage of paraphasias was used to define subgroups in this series. The group with the highest proportion of paraphasias also had the most severe aphasiological signs, that is, a predominantly receptive aphasia with neologistic jargon. The investigators provided detailed aphasiological profiles of individual cases, a feature that is often missing even from recent series. In some children, the clinical picture was similar to classic adult aphasias, and EEG or CT scans indicated a trend toward similar anatomic correlations. These profiles consisted of anomia and tactile anomia with parietal lesions, transcortical receptive aphasia with hypoperfusion of the left hemisphere, color anomia with occipital damage, and neologistic jargon with temporal injuries. Some cases fitted the adult syndromes so closely that they bring into question theoretical positions linking localization of lesions and age-related semiology, even in adults. This question was specifically brought out in the single-case description by Van Hout and Lyon (1986) of a 10-year-old boy who presented a comprehension disorder, logorrhea, anosognosia, and neologistic jargon. Both his overall aphasiologic profile and the mode of formation of neologisms were identical to classical Wernicke's aphasia, an aphasia said to occur mainly in older adults. The severity and possibly the bilaterality of the lesion (herpes simplex encephalitis) resulting in reduction of local plasticity, might have accounted for these unusual findings in this young child. Van Dongen et al. (1985) described five cases of fluent aphasia with paraphasias and neologisms in children who were slightly older (9–11-years-old) than in the preceding series (mean age of 7). As regards anatomical correlation, involvement of the posterior part of the left temporal lobe was present on CT in three of these children.

Evolution of paraphasias

In most aphasic children, paraphasias occur in ongoing speech but are more frequent and longer lasting in confrontation naming (Van Dongen et al., 1985; Visch-Brink and Van de Sandt-Koederman, 1984). Usually, the evolution of phonemic and verbal paraphasias appears to be independent and is not correlated with fluency. Neologisms are more frequent in the acute phase, but there is no clear parallelism in the course of paraphasias and neologisms. According to Visch-Brink and Van de Sandt-Koederman (1984), the number of paraphasias continues to fluctuate after the neologisms disappear, while the word-finding difficulties persist unchanged. The disappearance of neologisms is rapid, and the authors wondered if this might be specific to children. They concluded that it might not, as they found little data on this point in the adult literature and after personally examining an elderly adult patient with jargonaphasia whose paraphasias also disappeared rapidly. Van Hout et al. (1985) reported that, in two groups of children who had few paraphasias in the early stages, phonemic paraphasias were more persistent than verbal paraphasias; in the group with receptive aphasias who had the highest number of initial paraphasias, verbal paraphasias persisted longer.

If one can draw conclusions from these small series, it appears that the more severe the aphasia the more frequent the verbal paraphasias. The child with Wernicke's aphasia described by Van Hout and Lyon (1986) presented with a large number of neologisms. Their origin could be traced to perseverations and blending mechanisms, which is consonant with the hypothesis of Buckingham, Avakian-Whitaker and Whitaker (1978) on the genesis of neologisms in the adult. This child's recovery pattern also fit the usual regression of symptoms observed in adults: decrease of neologisms that parallel an increase in the percentage of semantic paraphasias. The observation that the frequency of phonemic paraphasias remained unchanged, and generally low contradicts the conduction hypothesis of multiple phonemic substitutions (Roch-Lecours and Rouillon, 1976). Should jargon derived from phonemic substitutions, one might expect their relative percentage to be higher when neologisms are more frequent. This last finding thus provides additional support to Buckingham et al.'s (1978) perseveration hypothesis regarding the formation of neologisms. Moreover, in examining the neologisms produced by a girl aged 3.5, Van Hout and Evrard (1987) found that the mechanism of formation of the paraphasias was similar to the one described for Wernicke's aphasia in the 10-year-old boy (Van Hout and Lyon, 1986). The main difference between the two cases was a lower proportion of neologisms in the younger child.

Van Dongen and Visch-Brink (1988) attempted to relate the evolution of paraphasias and neologisms to the etiology of the aphasia by comparing the results on the Boston Naming Test in three traumatic cases with those of three non-traumatic cases. Neologisms occurred in all the traumatic cases and decreased progressively, whereas the percentage of paraphasias did not change. In the non-traumatic cases, although the aphasia was less severe there were few neologisms, and the distribution of error-types varied. Like Van Hout and Lyon, they concluded that, at least for their traumatic cases, the findings do not support the conduction theory for the production of neologisms, since there was no increase in the percentage of literal paraphasias with the decrease in neologisms.

Fluent aphasias

In adults, the schematic contrast, fluent versus nonfluent aphasia, rests on related features: non-fluency defined as a reduction of the mean length of utterances goes together with a reduction in articulatory agility, the presence of pauses, agrammatism, and dysprosody. This classic duality corresponds to the anatomic opposition of 'posterior' versus 'anterior' lesions.

Up to the present, excluding cases of Landau-Kleffner syndrome, there are only some 30 descriptions or mentions of fluent aphasia in children, the term 'fluent' usually meaning lack of articulatory disorder. The lesions were either bilateral, diffuse, or strictly left posterior. Most children also had abnormal verbal comprehension, at least on the Token Test, and often produced verbal paraphasias and neologisms in their spontaneous speech. In seven fluent cases described in detail, neologistic jargon was reported, but there was no direct correlation between the presence of neologistic jargon and fluency. In the younger children, jargon was often accompanied, even during the more acute stages, by a decrease in fluency (Van de Sandt-Koederman et al., 1984; Van Hout et al., 1985). Reduced fluency was clearly absent in the phonemic jargon of children under 8, who appeared anosognosic for their faulty speech productions (Van Dongen et al., 1985; Van Hout et al., 1985), but as clear morphemic boundaries cannot be determined in such cases, quantitative measurement criteria could not be gathered in these children.

Recent reports indicate that in young children the status of fluency differs slightly from that in adults: it is never complete and has an 'intermediate' status as paradoxically, symptoms can co-occur that pertain either to anterior aphasia types or to posterior ones in adults. In young children: neologistic jargon may coexist with well articulated sentences of reduced length. This reduction of the mean length of utterances even in sensory aphasia types might be one of the reasons why childhood aphasia was so often regarded as expressive even in cases of retrorolandic lesions. However, other expressive signs like disordered articulation do not occur in such cases, contrary to classic conceptions.

True fluent aphasias with a rapid speech tempo and long mean length of utterances do occur in children. In terms of rate of speech (number of words per minute), they can meet criteria for receptive aphasia in adults (Van Dongen et al., 1985; Van Hout and Lyon, 1986). The localizations of responsible lesions correspond to those in adults with fluent aphasias. These same localizations, however, are also found in children with non-fluent aphasias. Investigators vary in the criteria they use to define fluency. Visch-Brink and Van de Sandt-Koederman (1984) and Van Dongen et al. (1985) used the double criterion of Wagenaar, Snow and Prins (1975) which includes both mean length of utterance and speech tempo, viz., a mean length of utterance of more than four words, and for fluency a speech rate of at least 90 words per minute. Van Dongen et al. (1985) expanded the criteria, following Kerschensteiner, Poeck and Brunner (1972), to also include measures of articulatory agility. Two cases of fluent aphasia fulfilling these criteria were reported by Visch-Brink and Van de Sandt-Koederman (1984), one being a 5-year-old boy with a phonemic jargon. Van Dongen described five fluent cases in his series of 33 children. The severity of the comprehension deficit varied among the five, but all obtained severely deficient scores on the Token Test. In three of the children, CT scans showed that Wernicke's area was included in the temporal lesion. The two others had extensive destruction of the whole left hemisphere.

To assess fluency, Van Hout et al. (1985) measured mean length of utterance during a defined period of spontaneous speech in a standardized situation. Mean length of utterance was diminished in nine of their eleven cases. Two children produced a neologistic jargon, in one case with logorrhea and anosognosia. The classic literature held that this extreme form of fluency, as indexed by rapid speech tempo, did not occur in childhood aphasia in, even in cases with temporal lesions (Alajouanine and Lhermitte, 1965). As did Van Dongen et al. (1985), Van Hout et al. (1985) found that fluency varied with the time of testing and also, in the case of Wernicke's aphasia, with the nature of the task. Klein, Masur, Farber et al. (1992) conducted a detailed study over 4 years of a girl with post-traumatic fluent aphasia, aged 4.5 at the time of injury, who had not changed greatly on follow-up. She used stock phrases and made excessive pauses, with an overall profile suggesting transcortical receptive aphasia.

Broca-like semiology

Although many of the early clinical descriptions of acquired childhood aphasia referred to its expressive symptoms as Broca-like, (Bernhardt, 1885), which usually meant restricted, negative, or regressive symptoms (Jakobson hypothesis). Often, the degree of syntactic and articulatory deterioration was variable, which makes it doubtful to equate childhood aphasia with Broca's aphasia. True Broca's aphasia, with its characteristic phonologic impairment and agrammatism, is said to occur only in children above age 10 (Assal and Campiche, 1973; Hécaen, 1976; Van Hout and Landrieu, 1979).

Cranberg et al. (1987) claim to have observed Broca's aphasia of vascular etiology in younger children. Of their eight cases, five were said to have Broca's aphasia, of which three were less than 9 years old, two of them age 5, and the other three to have transcortical aphasias, one receptive and two expressive. Although the authors used standardized tests appropriate to the children's ages, one regrets their lack of precision in defining the type of aphasia; such as specifying their criteria for non-fluency or agrammatism. In some of their cases, a long-lasting comprehension disorder — at least on the Token Test, and the presence of verbal paraphasias and neologisms seem to contradict the diagnosis of a purely expressive aphasia. In many children the lesion encompassed Broca's area, although one case which appeared typical of a Broca's aphasia had a lesion which specifically spared Broca's area. One wonders whether Cranberg used the term Broca's aphasia in its broader sense of signifying expressive problems. I would recommend that the label Broca's aphasia be used only in its strict sense of phonological disturbances with agrammatism. For other cases, the term non-fluent aphasia might be more appropriate. Non-fluency may have a variety of causes, including hypospontaneity, dysarthria, reduction of sentence length, excessive pauses-both within and between words, which are often indicative of anomia, and, more rarely, of a Broca-like picture. The term expressive aphasia is appropriate if a major feature of the child's speech is represented by cortical articulatory and phoneme selection problems, together with verbs use in the infinitive.

Conclusions regarding symptomatology

Recent reports of aphasic profiles in childhood bring out the occurrence of positive signs at all ages. The concept of non-fluency as a prominent feature remains valuable, especially for very young children, but non-fluency does not necessarily correlate with other expressive signs and can also occur in receptive aphasias. Increased fluency or rate of speech is not observed in children under age 8, with the possible exception of phonemic jargon in children who seem unaware of their high pressure of speech and in whom morphemic boundaries cannot be delineated. Fluent aphasias occur even in young children as conduction aphasia, transcortical receptive aphasia, and even true Wernicke's aphasia, but fluency means lack of articulatory problems, as pauses or auto-corrections usually diminish the mean length of utterance and the rate of speech. Fluent receptive aphasias are seen mostly in children over age 8 years, and true logorrhea in children after the early teens.

In conclusion, aphasias in children appear as varied as in adults as far as their positive signs are concerned, but their fluency characteristics are more often dissociated than in adults, particularly in children under 8 in whom non fluency may coexist with jargon (Table 1).

Pathologies

A number of variables influencing symptoms and recovery need to be considered, such as age at onset, age at testing, etiology, severity and extent of the lesion, and site of injury. It is difficult to determine the contribution of all these factors because the rarity of acquired aphasia in children results in small series that preclude multivariate analyses. To dissociate these effects, examination of the characteristics of aphasias with similar etiologies would be most valuable, but this has rarely been possible.

Vascular

Vascular lesions in young children are often considered relatively benign in the traditional literature. This prevailing position may have contributed to statements regarding favorable prognosis of ACA. ACA following a stroke is rarer now than in older series of childhood aphasias, in which vascular infarcts complicating bacterial sepsis were frequent cause of ACA. Vascular thromboses are much less frequent in children than adults in whom the major etiology of aphasia is a cerebro-vascular accident,

TABLE 1

Description of aphasia in children similar to the usual adult aphasic syndromes

Type of aphasia	Fluency	Auditory comprehension	Naming	Repetition	Paraphasias in ongoing speech	Paraphasias in naming	Neologisms	Localization	Age
Fluent: Van Dongen et al., 1985	+	−	−	−	+	++	+	L T (W)	9–11
Receptive: Van Hout et al., 1985	±	−	−	−	+	++	++	L T	7
Wernicke's: Van Hout and Lyon, 1986	+++	−	−	−	+	++	+++	L T	10
Receptive: Van Hout and Evrard, 1987	±	−	−	−	+	++	+	L T	3
Conduction: Martins and Ferro, 1987	+	+	−	−	+	+	−	L (smg)	11
Conduction: Tanabe et al., 1989	+	+	−	−	+	+	−	L (smg)	10
Conduction: Nass et al., 1998	+	±	+	−	+	+	−	L (smg)	3
Transcortical receptive: Van Hout and Seron, 1983	+	−	±	+	+	+	+	L (wa)	8
Transcortical expressive: De Agostini and Kremin, 1986	−	+	±	+	+	+	+	L T	9
Transcortical receptive: Klein et al., 1992	±	−	−	+ echolalia	+	+	+	L O.T. (18, 19, 37)	4

The first column indicates the term used by the authors to specify the type of aphasia.
+ = preserved; − = impaired; ± = slightly impaired or unequally distributed over period.
Refers to the predominant areas damaged: L = left; H = hemisphere; T = temporal; G = gyrus; O.T. = occipito-temporal junction. W = Wernicke's area; Smg = supramarginal; WA = watershed areas; 18, 19, 37: specific areas in the occipital zone.

although they are not as rare as frequently supposed (Lyon and Evrard, 2000). Today, except for the probably viral acute sylvian syndrome, (Gilles Lyon, personal communication) strokes are usually are usually complication of systemic (for instance collagen/vascular diseases like Sjögren or lupus), cardio-vascular or hematological disorders (sickle cell anemia, leukemias). Bleeds from angiomas (mostly arterio-veinous malformations) may give rise to an acute aphasic disorder and, shunting of blood in arterio-veinous malformations is occasionally responsible for a progressive aphasia.

In many series of ischemic strokes in childhood, symptoms are stated to be severe and outcome unfavorable (Guttmann, 1942; Van Dongen et al., 1985). The type of aphasia, which is usually mixed receptive/expressive or global in large hemispheric ischemic or hemorrhagic strokes, may contribute to this limited recovery, as shown by Cranberg et al. (1987). In that series, mainly non-fluent aphasias had a better outcome than the mixed aphasias and than adult-type aphasias in their symptomatology and the location of underlying (both anterior and posterior) lesions. Aram et al. (1983) described an aphasiologic profile similar to that of adults in their vascular subcortical cases, except that the children made a more rapid recovery (within ten months after the lesion) than adults. Martins, Ferro and Trindale (1987) reported recovery within 6 months in their vascular cases, which were mostly prerolandic and expressive in type.

Aram, Ekelman, Rose and Whitaker, 1985 stressed the usually relatively favorable long term prognosis of ACA when the etiology was vascular, except for an unfavorable prognosis in children with combined cortical and sub-cortical lesions or bilateral insults. Compared to the long-term sequellae of lesions due to other etiologies, those following strokes consisted mainly of naming deficits, in terms of both numbers of errors and latency of retrieval, and expressive and receptive syntax (for instance on the Token test).

Tumors

In children, hemispheric neoplasms account for a comparatively small fraction of brain tumors, as the majority are located in the posterior fossa, although, in some series, half are said to be hemispheric. With the exception of acute bleeding or sudden cystic enlargement, tumors are usually slowly progressive. As a rule, aphasia develops insidiously, often as a result of mass effects on surrounding tissues, or of secondary hydrocephalus. Aphasic symptoms are usually mild and a reduction in fluency, or even mutism, are reported. Hécaen (1976) described an astrocytoma in Broca's area in a 12-year-old girl who presented only minimal and transient aphasic defects. Well-defined aphasic syndromes do occur in some children. De Agostini and Kremin (1986) described 2-year follow-up of a 9-year-old boy with transcortical expressive aphasia due to a low-grade astrocytoma in the left temporal lobe. Speech output was paraphasic and slow, with pauses preceding lexical items.

Besides the direct effects of the tumors, their treatments may be responsible for delayed language disorders (Hudson and Murdoch, 1992). In the acute stages, posterior fossa tumors are likely to cause compression of veins, the ventricles, and parenchyma. Posterior fossa tumor may give rise to mutism after their surgical removal. This absence of speech emission is now interpreted as secondary to a cerebellar surgical incision often in the inferior vermian areas (Dailey, McKahnn and Berger, 1995). This region receives inputs from the pharynx and is connected both to cortical areas implicated in speech initiation such as the supplementary motor area and to subcortical ones, i.e. the ventro-lateral thalamic nucleus. A form of oral pharyngeal apraxia may follow the initial state of mutism.

Radiotherapy and chemotherapy following surgical removal of the primary lesion may result in structural changes such as vascular necrosis and parenchymal atrophy which build up progressively and may give rise to language deficits months or even years after treatment. Hudson, Murdoch and Ozanne (1989), by using a specifically designed language battery early on, found severe language deficits in vocabulary and naming, syntax, and reading in four children out of six treated for posterior fossa tumors. On follow-up, most affected were auditory comprehension and expression, with word finding less compromised. The profiles of individual children differed markedly, for similar seeming extends and lesions locations, with expressive skills more deficient in some children and receptive skills in others.

Infections

Often complicated by vascular damage, bacterial infection was a major cause of aphasia in children in earlier series. The advent of antibiotic therapy has greatly diminished the frequency of this complication. The aphasic consequences of a left posterior cortical-subcortical abscess were extensively described by Nass et al. (1998) in a 3-year-old girl. The angular gyrus, arcuate fasciculus, and posterior corpus callosum were damaged. The girl presented symptoms of fluent though dysarthric speech with markedly impaired repetition, suggesting a conduction aphasia. Van Dongen (1989), in a long-term follow-up of acquired aphasia in childhood, found that severe lesions predominated following all kinds of infections, and that outcome was generally unfavorable.

Modern treatment has also resulted in the emergence of new syndromes, notably following herpes simplex encephalitis in which mortality has been greatly reduced by antiviral agents. Lesions are particularly severe in this form of encephalitis (Baringer, 1978), and some survivors have serious behavioral sequellae, including autism (DeLong, 1981). As herpes virus has a tropism for the temporal lobes, it has contributed to an increase in the prevalence of posterior types of aphasias. For example, Van Hout and Lyon (1986) described a 10-year-old boy with herpes simplex encephalitis who presented the classic features of Wernicke's aphasia, a type of aphasia said to occur mainly in older adults.

Epilepsy

Partial epileptic seizures can produce transient receptive or expressive aphasias. These must be differentiated from speech arrest, a simple ictal suspension of speech without aphasic manifestations. Language disturbances during a partial seizure occur more frequently during focal epilepsy, although they may not be directly correlated to the initial focus but more often to the spreading of epileptic discharges.

Ictal aphasias are amenable to anti-epileptic treatment. Ictal aphasias are usually transient as their duration is determined by the length of the seizure. If a long-lasting ictal aphasia is not directly correlated with epileptiform EEG discharges, this may suggest a lesional aphasia or a Todd's phenomenon (Efron, 1961) following a prolonged simple or partial complex seizure.

In the uncommon but much written about entity called acquired epileptic aphasia (or Landau–Kleffner syndrome), the language disturbance is of long duration (days to many months) and may fluctuate. This aphasic syndrome develops between ages 3 and 8 years in a previously normal child and may be the presenting or only clinical symptom. Clinical seizures are usually infrequent and may even be absent, but the EEG must be epileptiform to make this diagnosis, and it may consist of electrical status epilepticus in slow wave sleep (Beaumanoir, Bureau, Deonna et al., 1995). In most cases the first manifestation is a severe receptive language disorder, or even an auditory agnosia (cortical deafness) (Kaga, 1999) which may be so severe that the possibility of peripheral deafness is considered. Expressive language deterioration soon follows. The comprehension disorder often presents as a verbal auditory agnosia, which refers to the inability to decode phonology which therefore precludes all subsequent language operations, and which many authors consider to be the basis of the language disorder (Klein, Tuchman and Rapin, 2000; Rapin, Mattis, Rowan and Golden, 1977). In some children, reception is affected only during some episodes, with resultant fluctuations of speech. Rarely, expressive impairment precedes the auditory disorder (Van Dongen and Visch-Brink, 1988). A predominantly expressive aphasic pictures may occur, but only in about one case in ten is there no evidence of receptive disorder.

Aphasic symptoms vary in Landau–Kleffner syndrome, as Rapin et al. (1977) reported jargonaphasia. More frequent are mutism or syntactic deficits with preservation of naming (Metellus and Hatt, 1980; Van Dongen and Visch-Brink, 1988). Even in cases presenting with jargon, expression soon becomes limited with impaired phonology. There may be a return to babbling with perseverative utterances. As with acquired deafness in very young children, the limitation of expressive speech in auditory agnosia has been interpreted in terms of Geschwind's hypothesis (Geschwind, 1974): "Perhaps the child's

Broca's area has not adequate practice in language to run as freely as that of adults".

An alternative although not contradictory explanation can be found in an article of Van de Sandt-Koenderman et al. (1984) who observed that during the acute breakdowns of speech, when the children produced more neologisms, they were less 'inclined' to speak and had a reduced mean length of utterance, alternating with the production of 'grammatically complex' sentences. In such cases, reduction in speech utterances is part of an overall 'hypospontaneity of speech' which is common in childhood aphasia.

Non linguistic cognitive functions and emotional behavior tend to remain normal in children with the Landau–Kleffner syndrome but there are exceptions, with some children having problems with overall praxias and gnosias. Emotional symptoms are usually interpreted as secondary to the language difficulties, but in some children they precede the onset of aphasia (Petersen, Koepp, Solensen et al., 1978). Frankly autistic behavioral deterioration is much more likely to accompany language regression associated with clinical or subclinical epilepsy in toddlers than in preschool or schoolage children (Shinnar, Rapin, Arnold et al., 2001). The EEG is abnormal, usually with bilateral spikes and waves, more marked in the temporal regions. There seems to be little direct correlation between the evolution of the aphasic symptoms and seizures or the standard EEG tracings. However, the use of magnetoencephalography allowed Paeteau, Kajola and Korkman et al. (1991) to show a concentration of spikes over the temporal area, in the narrow superior bank of the auditory cortex which usually responds to auditory stimuli in normal children: left sided speech decoding could be impeded by the spikes, which also limited the amount of callosal transfer to the right hemisphere. O'Tuama, Urion, Janicek et al. (1992) confirmed this interpretation using SPECT, where hypoperfusion of the latero-superior part of the temporal lobe near the sylvian fissure was disclosed in four children, in spite of different localizations of their standard EEG spikes foci. Recently Sobel, Aung, Otsubo and Smith (2000) using magnetoencephalography were able to disclose hypoperfusion in the perisylvian areas even in children who had no spikes on standard EEG; they underline the usefulness of this technique for localizing the primary focus of epileptiform activity.

Deonna, Beaumanoir, Gaillard and Assal (1977) distinguished at least three different clinical forms of this syndrome on the basis of its temporal evolution and of the importance of associated seizures. A first type has an acute onset but rapid recovery, a second one is characterized by worsening of the aphasia with recurrent seizures, and a third by progressive worsening of aphasic symptoms despite rare seizures. Recovery occurs in at most 30% of patients on long-term follow-up. There is striking variability in the severity, outcome, and type of language deficit (Deonna et al., 1977). Recovery and age are inversely correlated, in opposition with current theories on recovery in children, with prognosis better in older children (Bishop, 1985; Toso, Moschini, Gagnin and Antonu, 1981). Besides this relationship to age, no prognostic feature has emerged, so that it is recommended that substitutive, visual, language be used as soon as possible (Deonna et al., 1977).

The most widely acknowledged pathophysiology of the language deficit in acquired epileptic aphasia is a deficit in phonological decoding. Korkman et al. (1996) for instance, analyzed the auditory perception of words, sentences, phonemes and non-verbal material in six children with Landau–Kleffner syndrome. They found that all of the children had recovered for the discrimination of non-verbal material while remaining unable to identify any verbal material, and that phonemic discrimination remained very impaired even though other speech parameters had improved. Landau–Kleffner syndrome and subclinical electrical status epilepticus induced by slow wave sleep (ESES) described by Patry, Lyagoubi and Tassinari (1971) provide a clue to the persistence and severity of the language disorder (Kellerman, 1978). He proposed that the high frequency and high speed 'bombardment' of language cortices by abnormal electrical currents during the night was responsible for their dysfunction. The theory of a causal relationship between language symptoms and continuous slow waves during sleep is supported by the observation that no sign of language recovery occurs until the disappearance of the ESES. There are clinical differences, however, between the children with ESES described by Patry et al. and children with the Landau–Kleffner syndrome. In the former children, seizures are more frequent and may give rise to diurnal status epilepticus. Those children usually have marked global intellectual deterioration as well as a language disorder, although reception tends to be less severely compromised than in children with the Landau–Kleffner syndrome. In ESES spikes usually have a more anterior location than in Landau–Kleffner syndrome; they are present predominantly during slow wave sleep, disappearing during REM sleep. In Landau–Kleffner syndrome, slow wave status sleep status has a much uneven distribution and may occur in REM sleep, sometimes exclusively, particularly when the syndrome first appears (Genton and Bureau, 1991; Genton, Maton and Ogihara, 1992; Giovardini-Rossi et al., 1988).

Maquet, Hirsch, Metz-Lutz et al. (1995) conducted a PET study to relate the localization of ictal metabolic abnormalities to the children's most salient neuropsychological deficits. In 'ESES-like syndromes' discharges were located anteriorly and neuropsychologic deficits were those attributed to frontal dysfunction. In children with Landau–Kleffner syndromes, PET abnormalities coincided with areas of maximal focal spike and wave discharges in the temporal areas of one or both hemispheres. Thus the electrical discharges in these two disorders appear to affect distinct networks mediating language and cognitive processes selectively. The distribution of glucose utilization was 'immature', which suggested the hypothesis that abnormal neuronal firings might impede the development of synaptic stabilization in the affected cortices. Potentially corroborative evidence was provided by Morrell's (1995) report that subpial transection of epileptogenic temporal cortex had a favorable effect on language in stringently selected children with Landau–Kleffner syndrome, provided those with bilateral epileptogenic foci be excluded. The goal of this neurosurgical procedure is to interrupt tangential fibers carrying epileptic currents in associative auditory cortex without causing major disruption of input/output fibers. Too few well conducted longitudinal studies of these children have been carried out to determine whether long term results are superior to the natural course of the disorder, although some anecdotal reports are encouraging.

Head trauma

Head trauma is now the main cause of acquired aphasia in children. Its prognosis was usually regarded as relatively benign. Guttmann (1942), for instance, emphasized that recovery is more complete and rapid in children with post-traumatic aphasia than in those with other causes. When comparing the outcome in children with that of adults, one must keep in mind that the traumatic lesions themselves differ in the two groups, both owing to different causative mechanism and to the structure of the brain itself. The cause of the trauma usually differs, with children often involved in accidents occurring at lower speeds than adults. The rotational acceleration forces applied to the brain are thus milder and, presumably owing to the lesser fragility of young vessels, hematomas are rarer in children. The main damage, demonstrated on MRI, is shearing of the white matter (diffuse axonal injury), therefore, after regression of brain edema and focal contusions, the long term damage is mainly subcortical.

As to the type of aphasia, even adult, trauma rarely gives rise to such clear-cut aphasic subtypes as do cerebro-vascular accidents, because it results from more diffuse lesions. Adults may present a 'subclinical' aphasia (Sarno, 1980) detectable only by testing or, more often, to an anomic aphasia. Even in the acute stage, some more defined aphasic syndromes have been described, some of which may be long-lasting. For example, Van Hout et al. (1985) described a case of jargonaphasia after head trauma in the youngest child in their series (4 years old), and Cranberg et al. (1987) described a traumatic transcortical receptive aphasia.

In children, the outcome of post-traumatic aphasia appears directly linked to the severity of the injury (Bijur, Haslum and Gloning, 1990) and the severity of the initial aphasic symptoms (Assal and Campiche, 1973). Hécaen (1976) described sixteen traumatic cases that differed from other etiologies by a higher frequency of initial mutism and by more striking naming disorders. Fletcher, Erwing-Cobbs, McLaughlin and Levin (1979), Levin et al. (1983), and Ewing-Cobbs, Levin, Eisenberg and Fletcher (1987) studied large cohorts of children and adolescents with post-traumatic aphasias which they related to the initial severity of injury. They found a positive relationship between the severity of symptoms 6 months following the injury and the extent of the lesion, with this relationship clearest for naming and writing deficits. As in adult traumatic aphasia, children presented disorders of verbal fluency and of repetition for complex verbal material, with sentence repetition more often impaired in children than in adults. Chadwick, Rutter, Shaffer and Shrout (1981) noted that, despite apparent recovery from traumatic aphasia, children's naming latencies remained prolonged for at least 2 years after the injury. Jordan and Murdoch (1990) confirmed that naming deficits resulted in increased latencies and numbers of errors; they also found that in some children deficits became more salient with age, with progressive deterioration of verbal fluency.

Thus, even if the nature of traumatic lesions differs in children and adults, symptoms are similar, anomia being the most prevailing symptom of this 'subclinical' and 'subcortical' aphasia. There is lack of evidence for a more benign course in the younger patients, as data from cohorts of very young children document that, all else being equal, the younger the child, the worse the prognosis. This also seems to be true for academic outcome as well, although one must take into account the possibility that some young, accident-prone, hyperkinetic children may have had pre-existing cognitive disorders.

Anatomic correlations in the localization of lesions

Left cortical lesions

It has been widely acknowledged that it is only after a cerebral area has acquired its anatomic specification that it can display functional competence and lesional disruption. Early studies attributed apparent predominance of expressive over receptive disorders to asynchrony of cerebral maturation, as some frontal expressive association areas were thought to differentiate earlier than posterior language ones. One needs to keep in mind, however, that the classic contrast in adults between fluent versus non-fluent aphasias and their respective posterior/anterior correlations are seen mostly in vascular lesions and that vascular lesions are rare in children. Other investigators interpreted the alleged uniformity of symptomatology in childhood aphasia to lack of functional differentiation in the immature language hemisphere. Lenneberg (1967) stated that it is only after puberty that the cortical language areas acquire their anatomic specification and, consequently, are able to display differential functional disruption. The concept of more diffuse organization of language within the language hemisphere in the immature than mature brain was bolstered by the report, in one of Hécaen's series (1983), of a higher frequency of aphasias in left-hemispheric lesions in children under ten than in adults.

Yet, even the early literature detected a trend towards some 'anterior/posterior' correlations resembling those characteristic of adults. In 1942, Guttmann observed a relation in children between comprehension disorders and left temporal lobe damage. Hécaen (1976 series) found that mutism and dysarthria were more frequent in left prerolandic lesions and receptive disorders in left temporal lobe lesions, although he stated in his 1983 series that all aphasic symptoms occurred more frequently in left frontal lobe lesions. If this finding had been confirmed, it would have constituted a strong argument in favor of the hypothesis of more advanced differentiation of the frontal areas during development, and also would have been an example in man of the phenomenon of functional reallocation with maturation described in animals by Goldman (1974a,b).

The advent of modern brain imaging techniques has made possible more precise localization of acquired lesions in recent studies and has disclosed functional/anatomic correlations similar to those in adults. These observations are at variance with Bates et al.'s (1999) view of 'constrained plasticity' in infants where even the side of the lesion does not seem to be specifically related to language impairment. It is important to stress that Bates does not always make a clear distinction between congenital injuries and lesions occurring after 2 years of age. Moreover, for the most part she relies on verbal and performance IQ discrepancies as criteria for language impairment, discrepancies that are known to be only broadly related to selective functions of the left and right hemispheres. The frequently documented impairment of visuo-spatial functions as the price to pay for recovery from aphasia further complicates interpretations. When reporting the scores from more specific language tests in an attempt to identify subtypes of aphasia, Bates doesn't take into account the interval following the injury. The studies referred to in the present review focus on children in the acute post-lesional stage of injuries acquired after age 2 years, who were examined with aphasia tests specifically designed for children; specification of the affected region of the left hemisphere with CT or MRI was based on reference to radiologic tables.

A number of these studies found correlations between neologistic jargon and left temporal lesions (Martins et al., 1987; Van Dongen et al., 1985; Van Hout et al., 1985; Visch-Brink and Van de Sandt-Koederman, 1984). Fluent aphasias were shown to occur when there was a clear involvement of Wernicke's area proper (Van Dongen et al., 1985). According to Martins et al. (1991), the size of the lesion in Wernicke's area predicts outcome: the larger the lesion, the poorer the prognosis. Cranberg et al. (1987) studied CT scans in eight children with acquired aphasias: the six with non-fluent aphasia had a Broca-like picture or a transcortical expressive aphasia; all six had prerolandic lesions, often involving Broca's area itself. These investigators attributed the non-fluent picture of two children with postrolandic lesions to the extent of the lesion rather than to lack of specificity of brain organization in children, as analogous symptoms have been reported in adults with similarly located damage.

Other aphasic syndromes with clinical features and anatomic correlates parallel to those in adults have been described in children:

- conduction aphasia with a left parietal location (Martins and Ferro, 1987; Van Hout et al., 1985) and the demonstration by MRI of involvement of the arcuate fasciculus (Nass et al., 1998; Tanabe et al., 1989);
- transcortical receptive aphasia with hypoperfusion of the left hemisphere (Van Hout et al., 1985) or with damage to the left occipito-temporal junction (Klein et al., 1992);
- color anomia with a left occipital lesion (Van Hout et al., 1985);
- fluent receptive aphasia with left temporal damage (Van Dongen et al., 1985; Van Hout and Lyon, 1986).

Subcortical lesions

Lesion of the subcortical nuclei

Extensive subcortical lesions may cause mutism, but it is usually of a non-aphasic type, akinetic mutism. Assal and Campiche (1973) reported a link between the duration of mutism and the severity of brain-stem lesions. The long term sequellae of traumatic aphasia are currently considered to represent a form of subcortical aphasia, as persistent pathology consists predominantly of white matter tears affecting frontal and callosal fibers.

At least three studies (Aram et al., 1985; Cranberg et al., 1987; Ferro, Martins, Pinto and Castro-Caldas, 1982) describe the occurrence, after subcortical lesions, of aphasic symptomatology similar to but more transient than that of adults with similar lesions. The child described by Aram et al. had a vascular lesion in the putamen, the anterior limb of the internal capsule, and the lateral aspect of the head of the caudate. The resulting aphasia was non fluent with agrammatism, verbal paraphasias, and anomia; comprehension was impaired, which the investigators attributed to destruction of the afferent auditory fibers in the internal capsule. The case of Ferro et al. (1982) was similar, but symptoms were milder. In both these cases repetition was affected, although adults with the same injury often present with a transcortical motor aphasia. The adolescent boy, thus older than the two children just discussed, included in the Cranberg et al. (1987) series, presented a traumatic transcortical receptive aphasia and, as in adult cases, his repetition was spared, even for sentences. It is usually thought that in children the thalamus may play a greater role in memory than in adults, be responsible both for deficient repetition and for a drop in learning new lexical material (Van Lieshout, Renier, Eling et al., 1990) Martins and Ferro (1992) compared outcome in two groups of five children ages 2–5 years sorted according to the severity of the initial aphasia, one group with combined subcortical and cortical lesions, the other with only subcortical pathology. What they found was that the severity of the initial aphasia and the duration of symptoms were more marked in the cases with combined subcortical and cortical lesions. The implication is that subcortical involvement in early child language does not carry a worse prognosis than in older children and adults. The descriptions of Nass, Boyce and Leventhal (2000) contradict in part those findings. Their series is composed of five children between 6 and 14 who underwent left thalamic surgery for tumors. Unexpectedly, as some language reorganization might have taken place before tumor excision, they all developed a severe aphasia after surgery (Broca's aphasia, mixed transcortical, and one conduction aphasia). Repetition problems were frequent as in reports of other children; but aphasia severity and also the extent of non-verbal cognitive problems (executive disorders, apraxia, right neglect) were more marked than in adults. They underline the role of the thalamus in childhood for verbal memory and semantic learning. However, in the acute stages of aphasias, their patients were shown to have more widespread left cortical hypoperfusion on SPECT.

Lesions of the subcortical white matter

Among those subcortical lesions, conduction aphasia is usually attributed to a disconnection of Broca's to Wernicke's areas because of disruption of the arcuate fasciculus which connects them and allows the speech input to the posterior area to be translated into articulation templates. As in the adult, conduction aphasia may be seen in the recovery phase of a receptive aphasia (Van Dongen et al., 1985), but it also arises as an independent disorder (Martins and Ferro, 1987; Nass et al., 1998; Tanabe et al., 1989; Van Hout and Lyon, 1986). MRI disclosed a lesion that affected the arcuate fasciculus in both the children described by Tanabe and by Nass. The girl in the Nass report was among the youngest children to have an ACA as she was only 3 years old; the occurrence of conduction aphasia in this child suggests that the basis of her repetition disorder was similar to the one implicated in most of the adult cases, that is, a defect in reproduction, that is a repetition disorder directly affected by an increase in the number of syllables. In this condition, a direct influence of short term verbal memory is put forward as a factor, whereas, in the other 'pure conduction' deficit, the repetition itself, non-influenced by memory factors, represents the purest but rare form of repetition disorder per se.

Damage: unilateral versus bilateral or diffuse

Hécaen (1976) described postpubertal children who recovered completely and suggested that the extent of the lesion might be more relevant to recovery than age. Van Dongen, Meulstee, Blauw-Van Mouri and Van Harskamp (1989), who used the lesion severity rating scale of Vargha-Khadem et al. (1985), concluded that it is the bilaterality of lesions, rather than their severity as assessed on CT scans, that is decisive for prognosis, as none of their seven cases with bilateral lesions recovered.

From an analysis of cases due to a single etiology, herpes encephalitis, Van Hout et al. (1985) concluded that temporal lobe involvement, if bilateral, worsened both the severity of the aphasia and the outcome. They postulated that concurrent involvement of the right brain most likely precluded interhemispheric transfer (Milner, 1974) required for the expected recovery from a left temporal lesion.

Right hemisphere lesions

Freud (1897) reported a high frequency of crossed aphasias (i.e., with right-sided pathology) in children and, in his large series of left hemispherectomies following an early lesion, Basser (1962) discovered that they did not preclude normal language development. This observation bespoke the suppletive role of the right hemisphere for language. Further, Basser's observation that a lesion of the right hemisphere gave rise to aphasia in as many as 35% of young aphasic children also suggested active participation of the right-hemisphere in language. Lenneberg's (1967) theory rested largely on Basser's report. Lenneberg suggested that, from an initial stage of hemispheric equipotentiality, lateralization of language to the left-hemisphere developed progressively until puberty. Decrease in the prevalence of crossed aphasias with age was interpreted as evidence for progressive reduction of the language capabilities of the right hemisphere.

Criticism of Lenneberg's theory bears on both the active and the vicarious roles of the right-hemisphere for language. As regards vicariance, Dennis and Kohn (1975, 1976) used elaborate language tests to assess language outcome in hemispherectomies for early lesions. Although criticized for their lack of appropriate IQ controls, their findings contradict the very notion of equipotentiality. The active role of the right hemisphere for language was strongly challenged by Woods and Teuber (1978) who found only two cases of aphasia in their series of twenty right-hemisphere lesioned children, and one of these children was left handed. They pointed out that most studies reporting a high frequency of crossed aphasias in children dated from before the 1930's. At that time, one third of childhood hemiplegias were due to complications of infectious diseases, such as cerebral hypoperfusion and electrolyte disturbances. Thus, in cases of left hemiplegia with aphasia, focal thromboses in the right hemisphere were likely to have been accompanied by diffuse lesions implicating of the language hemisphere as well, and the apparent crossed aphasia could have been artefactual. With the advent of modern treatments such as antibiotics, adequate hydration, artificial ventilation, and anticonvulsants, the incidence of aphasia in right-hemisphere lesions has dropped dramatically.

An extensive review of the literature by Dennis and Whitaker (1976) indicated that left hemisphere pathology carries greater risk for language impairment, at least after the age of 13 months (there is a 2 : 1 risk of developing language impairment after right hemiplegia before that age). The finding of a lower prevalence of crossed aphasia in children than earlier thought was subsequently confirmed by Kinsbourne and Hiscock (1977) who found not one case of aphasia in children with right hemisphere lesions. In most modern series, its prevalence is similar to that of crossed aphasia in adults, between 1% and 4% (Carter, Hohenegger and Satz, 1982).

There are, in fact, very few documented descriptions of right-hemisphere aphasias in children. One can cite the single case of crossed aphasia reported by Assal and Deonna (1977) and two cases of Ferro et al. (1982), but these latter cases were left handers. All recent studies on lesion lateralization lead to the conclusion that interhemispheric specification is defined in children from a very early age. Recent research (Locke, 1997) indicates that the early lexicon might be better developed in the right hemisphere. The suggestion of the equal participation of both hemispheres for nouns had already been put forward by Zaïdel (1977). New findings provide at least partial support for the old 'equipotentiality theory': early language development after perinatal brain lesions appears to substantiate this hypothesis, not only for the lexicon but also for syntactic development (Feldman, Holland, Kemp and Janosky, 1992).

Neuroimaging techniques in acquired childhood aphasias

The new neuroimaging techniques have been a major force in modifying current views on acquired childhood aphasia. They have provided more precise anatomical correlations between symptoms, severity, and prognosis of childhood aphasia and the location and size of lesions. Van Dongen et al. (1985) point out that the discovery of certain abnormalities in CT scans has raised the suspicion of aphasia in children who otherwise would probably not have been sent to a speech pathologist for an in-depth study. As a result, the number of identified cases of childhood aphasias has probably risen. CT scans usually provide adequate data for correlations between lesion location and aphasic symptoms, although slight differences in the plane of imaging can make it difficult to identify the sylvian fissure and determine whether the site of the lesion is anterior or posterior to it (Van Dongen et al., 1985). The atlas of Matsui and Hirano (1978) is helpful in such cases.

Van Dongen et al. (1989) used the rating scale from 1 to 5 proposed by Vargha-Khadem et al. (1985) to study the impact of severity and/or bilaterality of the lesion on the quality of outcome. They observed that, if corrections are made for these two variables, only bilaterality of the lesion is significantly predictive of a poorer outcome. Martins et al. (1989) measured the degree of involvement of Wernicke's area, using the templates of Damasio (1983), and found that the larger the destruction in this specific location, the poorer the prognosis. With reconstruction techniques described by Gado, Hanaway and Frank (1979), Klein et al. (1992) were able to define the cortical areas lesioned in their case of transcortical receptive aphasia quite precisely: they were bilateral, but the larger left lesion affected areas 18, 19 and 37 at the occipito-temporal junction. Those locations are precisely those affected in adults with the same type of aphasia. In addition, area 17 was spared, a finding usual in adults with transcortical receptive aphasia.

The new neuroimaging modalities of MRI, PET, and SPECT scans are very promising, but as yet few publications have mentioned them. It is only in cases of epileptic aphasia, and in particular the Landau–Kleffner syndrome, that application of SPECT and PET have disclosed the really new causal mechanism of impediment to synaptic stabilization (Maquet et al., 1995). MRI has brought out the importance of subcortical lesions in the case of conduction aphasia of Tanabe et al. (1989) where it disclosed involvement of the arcuate fasciculus. at the level of the left supramarginal gyrus.

The importance of subcortical tears has been increasingly invoked as an explanation for long lasting sequellae in post traumatic aphasia. Yet in children under 5 years, comparisons of the detrimental role of subcortical lesions with and without additional cortical lesions, MRI has resulted in deemphasizing the subcortical involvement per se (Martins and Ferro, 1992) and emphasizing the detrimental role of associated cortical lesions.

Language tests in aphasic children

The development of new instruments to evaluate children with ACA explains some of the differences in the symptoms described in older and more recent studies. Too many children were investigated with non-standardized tests borrowed from adult aphasiological batteries. Many studies were retrospective, because children studies were not carried out until some 3 or 6 months after onset of the aphasia. Delays of this length mean that rapidly evolving semiologies would go undetected. Often, investigators were not well acquainted with the language of young children and thus were unable to differentiate between mere developmental variations and pathological substitutions. In order to detect subtle and often transient features in childhood aphasia, one must be knowledgeable regarding both individual variations in the normal language of children and familiar with adult aphasic semiology. Testing has to be adapted to the age and psychological condition of children with brain injuries. Because these children are often reluctant to speak, an examination limited to their spontaneous speech may not reveal positive aphasiologic signs. Encouragement and an appropriate approach can overcome this frequent unwillingness to speak. Children can be discouraged and tire easily, making it impossible to administer an entire battery in a short period of time. The investigation must be extended to the more defective areas, while making sure that testing is not too demanding of the child. Rapin and Allen (1988) provided a brief checklist of aphasic symptoms suitable for repeated clinical bedside assessment of aphasia symptoms in children.

Newly developed language tests, particularly in English, now permit a more elaborate and age-adapted investigation of language symptoms. Administration of these tests to large cohorts of normal children has provided norms, with means and standard deviations. These norms make it possible to make comparisons across ages and to gather reliable estimates of recovery. Unless results are expressed in standard deviations, it may not be apparent that a 3-year-old and a 10-year-old child may be equally impaired and that they have the same type of aphasia. Availability of normed scores reduces the risk of overlooking normal individual variation due to differences in stage of language acquisition, socio-economic level, and rate of post-natal development. Yet standard deviations are inadequate for expressing qualitative differences, even among non-lesioned children. The different cognitive styles characteristic of early language development, described by Nelson (1973) as 'referential' or 'expressive', may persist in some older children. Horgan (1978) has shown that the stages of late grammatical development, with some children predominantly 'noun lovers' and others 'noun leavers', still correspond to those two major early styles. In younger children, phonology is probably the area subject to the largest developmental variations, as at age 3 years some children are still inconsistent in their pronunciation of individual sounds, even within the same word. Naming errors may also vary, some children replying more frequently to unknown items by using semantically related terms and others by using superordinates. Thus, in order to take those qualitative variations into account, one has to rely on tables, when they exist, of the acceptable variations for a given task, and also on the parents' judgment of the premorbid abilities of the child.

Although many valuable tests exist, it is important to remember that most of them are oriented toward measuring the psycholinguistic development of normal children. Simple application of age-related tests is insufficient for a diagnosis of aphasia, and it is often necessary to extract the relevant features from the test batteries or to insert additional items derived from other tests. The scores must then be recorded along dimensions pertinent to the separate functions of language, as is done for the diagnosis of adult aphasics: scores for naming, comprehension, fluency, and repetition.

Unfortunately, even recent case descriptions of childhood aphasia do not always include a whole battery of standardized tests, so that it may be difficult to get an idea of what kind of aphasia the authors are describing. Some investigators concentrated on only a few aspects of language, for example as did Van Dongen et al. (1985) whose main purpose was to demonstrate that fluent aphasias do exist in childhood, which they did very convincingly. However, they went on to make a diagnosis of conduction aphasia because repetition was significantly impaired. As pointed out by Tanabe et al. (1989), Van Dongen et al. failed to provide the reasons for failure on the repetition tests, so that this diagnosis is difficult to sustain as they reported that comprehension was impaired.

The following tests address specific aspects of childhood aphasia:

(1) Items and procedures from the Boston Diagnostic Aphasic Examination (Goodglass and Kaplan, 1972)
(2) The Boston Naming Test from the same battery, which now has normative developmental data in many languages
(3) The Gaddes and Crockett adaptations of the Spreen and Benton multilingual aphasiological battery (Gaddes and Crockett, 1975)Other, more psycho-linguistic tests have been used, such as
(4) For French speaking countries the Chevrie-Müller et al. battery (1975)
(5) A multicentric multilingual test was recently devised in the European Community, specifically aimed at analysis of ACA: ELOLA (for a French version of the test, see De Agostini, Metz-Lutz, Van Hout et al., 1998)

Fluency

At least two measures of fluency must be considered: mean length of utterance and number of words per minute (Wagenaar et al., 1975). Expanded measurements, such as those of Kerschensteiner et al. (1972) take into account four more features of expressive aspects of language: effort, articulation problems, prosody, and pauses. In adults, non-fluent aphasia often exhibits a combination of these expressive signs, together with a reduction in length of sentence and number of words used. In childhood aphasia, non-fluency can occur in the context of well-articulated speech and even of neologistic production. Therefore, to evaluate fluent speech in childhood we suggest retaining only the two criteria of number of words per minute and mean length of utterance. These extended criteria, which are valuable in adults, are non-specific in childhood and in fact serve as criteria for a diagnosis of expressive aphasia. The two classic non-fluency criteria for adults are inadequate in ACA for separating its two main causes at the word level, namely the presence of pauses within words which are due to a general slowing of articulation, and between-word slowing, when pauses are usually signs of anomia. Spectrographic measurements of speech would be useful for distinguishing between these distinct reasons for pauses. Mean length of utterance is usually linked to the syntactic complexity of the sentence although, here too, dissociations can occur. Extensive investigation of the grammatical complexity of sentences and presence of deviant syntactic structures is rarely carried out. The work of Aram et al. (1983) on the long term sequellae of left hemispheric lesions provides a model of this type of detailed investigation.

In 1994, Van Dongen, Pasquier, Raes and Creten (1994) undertook an analysis of the fluency of the spontaneous conversational speech of children with ACA, in an effort to investigate the effect of different types of linguistic parameters on fluency. They used a digital timer to measure phonation time. Their major conclusions, which confirmed their clinical impressions, were that it was possible to distinguish non-fluent aphasia from other forms of brain damage and to differentiate dysarthria from expressive aphasic deficits. This method also substantiated the existence of fluent aphasias in childhood.

Repetition

Repetition is often impaired in childhood aphasia (Van Hout et al., 1985) and has to be tested both for meaningful material and for pronounceable non-words of various lengths. It is important to remember that in order to make a diagnosis of conduction aphasia, the deficit has to be selective and comprehension must be preserved. We found that repetition is often impaired in subcortical lesions in children, whereas in adults it is usually preserved. The reason for this age difference requires investigation. In children selective preservation of repetition has been described in both expressive and receptive transcortical aphasias, with the location of the underlying lesions similar to that in adults.

Comprehension

The assessment of comprehension is difficult. In too many cases comprehension has been tested by simple commands such as "blow out your cheeks" or "stick out your tongue". Failure to respond to such commands may be confounded by an agnosia or an apraxia, or for such non-linguistic reasons as bucco-facial apraxia. Investigators often limited themselves to verbal commands in a single lexical category, and some of the commands they used were so simple that the implication of adequate comprehension because they were carried out correctly was unwarranted. More elaborate comprehension tests may require the mastery of cognitive or spatial concepts and require adequate memory and sustained attention. Even the Token Test can be criticized in this respect, and its Part V combines high syntactic loading with a large number of locative prepositions that can be misunderstood for non-linguistic reasons. Therefore it is not surprising that scores on the Token Test sometimes remain depressed over the long term, even in cases of expressive aphasias (see the series of Cranberg et al., 1987, and Cooper and Flowers, 1988) or in children who sustained a left hemispheric lesion prior the onset of language (Vargha-Khadem et al., 1985).

Examining children's replies to questions in a normal environment is not very useful either, as they may rely on contextual clues and pragmatic aspects of the examiner's communication. Multiple choice techniques (Bishop, 1988) also have their biases, such as the position of the items. Tests that have the child play with toys are probably the most reliable (Chevrie-Müller, Simon and Decante, 1975), but they are less suitable for older children for whom some tests adapted from adult batteries begin to apply. In fact, the Chevrie-Müller test, which is in French, is not intended for a particular pathology, and it is useful because it provides norms for different age ranges.

Naming

As in adult aphasia, naming disorders are frequent and may be one of the more persistent deficits in ACA. If naming deficits are severe and dominate the clinical picture, they may constitute an anomic aphasia. Specific deficits affecting a particular modality (tactile) or category (colors) have been described (Van Hout et al., 1985). Confrontation naming errors with preserved passive knowledge of words through pointing or giving a definition can help resolve the oft-debated dilemma about lack of access versus loss of lexical items. In young children, a description of their gestures or frequent pantomimes can also be used to evaluate passive knowledge. After an acute, often paraphasic stage, naming problems usually present as excessive pauses before content words and as circumlocutory descriptions. The nature of the child's errors has to be determined, as described by Van Hout and Lyon (1986), as it can provide insight into the cognitive mechanisms responsible for pathological productions like neologisms. Confrontation naming provides a convenient way to study the evolution of paraphasias over time (Van Dongen and Visch-Brink, 1988).

These are the classic measures required to diagnose the type of aphasia using age-adapted measurements. I advocate the publication of detailed single-case studies. These descriptions provide more detailed data on cognitive investigations and information on the underlying nature of the observed linguistic deficits. Only by this means does it become possible to draw meaningful parallels with the adult aphasic syndromes and to explore differences and similarities in the early and late organization of language in the brain.

Outcome

As discussed in earlier sections, relevant variables for predicting outcome include etiology, location, and extent of the lesion which interact to determine the completeness of recovery. In young children, age was said to play a favorable role for outcome. Lenneberg (1967) stated that outcome was better in children than in adults, but that it took more time, the main condition for recovery being that the lesion occur before puberty. He regarded recovery by transfer of language to the right hemisphere as the rule, a view based on the idea that the right hemisphere plays a major role for language until the emergence of left hemispheric dominance. Modern data that document incomplete recovery of language in ACA challenge the extent of right hemispheric potential for taking over language, and, consequently, the hypothesis of initial equipotentiality (Dennis, 1980; Vargha-Khadem et al., 1985; Woods and Carey, 1979), whereas Locke's (1997) demonstration of early involvement of the right hemisphere for vocabulary and naming gives partial support to early equipotentiality.

With regard to aphasic recovery based on shifting of language to the right-hemisphere, it may not be limited to children, as the studies of Kinsbourne (1971), Czopf (1972), and Yarnell, Monroe and Sorel (1976) have shown that the right hemisphere may also be the source of aphasic speech in adults. At a minimum, the universality of this recovery mechanism in children has been questioned and, as shown by Milner (1974), it appears to depend more on the location of the lesion than on age. With regard the completeness of recovery, Lenneberg (1967) observed that even after recovery of oral language, subtle deficits affecting both linguistic and non-linguistic abilities may remain as sequellae. Woods and Carey (1979) spoke of the price of recovery, a compromise of functions which depends on areas now devoted to the support of language (Teuber's crowding hypothesis). Thus, in considering outcome, one has to examine both the recession of the aphasic symptoms and the ultimate level of more subtle linguistic and non-linguistic abilities. Such deficits may lead to a failure to acquire new information and, as a result, to impaired academic performance.

Many series lack homogeneity regarding the abilities considered as recovered, and the length of follow-up. Too often, the term recovery does not differentiate between elements of prognosis whose underlying mechanisms are probably dissimilar. Some authors consider that recovery has occurred if the child regains the ability to engage in conversation; others if he can perform normally on formal testing; others still if, in addition to language recovery, school performance is appropriate for the age level.

The following table summarizes the effect of age (when available, both age at the lesioning and age at testing) on the outcome of oral language in childhood aphasia compiled from the major reported series.

Apparent contradictions among reported results may be attributable to differences in lesion characteristics, but also to differences in time of testing or to divergent assumptions regarding criteria for recovery. None the less, even in children who regained near normal oral language ability, the overall consensus is that school performance is likely to be jeopardized (Alajouanine and Lhermitte, 1965; Byers and McLean, 1962; Cooper and Flowers, 1987; Cranberg et al., 1987; Van Hout et al., 1985). The learning disabilities are often both verbal, for instance impairment of written language or auditory memory, and non-verbal. The nonverbal deficits may either be a result of compensatory mechanisms, such as the crowding effect, or be secondary to a direct effect of the insult on non linguistic cognitive abilities of the left hemisphere (Van Hout and Seron, 1983).

In short, acquired childhood aphasia does not have the uniformly good prognosis that was formerly taken for granted. Overt or subclinical language disorders may persist long term and, as a rule, there are learning disabilities. The vicarious role of the right hemisphere as a mechanism for recovery is being seriously questioned, and up to now there is no report of selective impairment in lexical acquisition in a very young child with a right hemispheric lesion (Table 2).

Conclusions

To conclude, most of what used to be thought of as specific to childhood aphasias has been challenged: symptoms are more differentiated than previously

TABLE 2

Effect of age (at lesion onset and at testing) on oral language recovery

Lenneberg (1967)	Better prognosis for lesions before puberty, but duration of recovery longer in younger children.
Alajouanine and Lhermitte (1965)	No difference in children over or under 10 years at onset (evaluated after 1 year).
Hécaen (1976)	Long-lasting language disorders (mostly naming difficulties) whatever the age onset.
Woods and Teuber (1978)	Recovery always occurs in children under 8 years, but the time necessary for recovery does not correlate with age.
Van Hout et al. (1985)	Prepubertal children do not recover more completely than older children. Language disorders persist at least for 1 year as positive signs for the more severe aphasias, and, for children under 9, also as residual negative language signs.
Van Dongen et al. (1989)	When tested at 1 year after the lesion a better prognosis is found in younger children (only for traumas).
Klein et al. (1992)	Few modifications in language of a girl aged 4 at onset, tested over a 4 year period.

thought; adult-like semiologies occur at an early age; and anatomic correlations are evocative of those observed in adults. These functional data favor early specification for language of neuronal networks in the left hemisphere whose organization is more similar to that of adults than previously thought. Analogies in symptoms, their presumed mechanisms, and localization of lesions similar to those of adults have been detected in children, at least after age 3 years (Nass et al., 1998, 2000). Data on the outcome of acquired aphasia in childhood on long-term follow-up indicate that prognosis is less optimistic than had earlier been reported, and that, besides persistent language sequellae, there are usually learning disorders.

The prevalence of aphasia in right-hemisphere lesions seems to be equal to that observed in adults, and the role of the right hemisphere for language recovery also appears quite similar to its role in adult aphasia. One hypothesis might be that this role may represent its release from an original linguistic inhibition.

As far as other unexplained and unexplored areas are concerned, investigations of aphasic symptomatology in children with developmental language disorders are beginning to be carried out. Most earlier comparisons were between the developmental dysphasias and adult aphasias (Denckla, 1979; Rapin et al., 1977; Rapin and Allen, 1988). More recently, Jordan, Ozanne and Murdoch (1988) compared the naming disorders of children recovering from traumatic aphasia with the errors made by normal children of the same age; they found that the brain lesioned children made more errors, but that there was no difference between the two groups with regard to overall rate of errors in naming. Van Hout (1993) compared the naming profiles of children with acquired anomic aphasia and children with anomic developmental dysphasia with those of two groups of controls, normal children of the same chronological age and normal children of the same naming age (thus much younger). The profiles of the two anomic groups had greater similarities than those of the two control groups. This finding suggests potential similarity of dysfunction in corresponding underlying neural networks in both developmental and acquired anomia.

ACA remains a rare condition and there is a great need for more precise descriptions, using age-appropriate measures, of the specific features of aphasic language in children. The relative contributions of plasticity and of age-dependant favorable or unfavorable neurological factors to the evolution of symptom complexes remains to be explored. New functional imaging and electrophysiologic technologies open the perspective of being able to resolve some of the enduring controversies of this field.

References

Alajouanine TH, Lhermitte F: Acquired aphasia in children. Brain: 88; 653–662, 1965.

Annett M: Laterality of childhood hemiplegia and the growth of speech and intelligence. Cortex: 9; 4–33, 1973.

Aram D, Ekelman B, Rose D, Whitaker H: Spoken syntax in children with acquired unilateral hemisphere lesion. Brain and Language: 27; 75–100, 1985.

Aram D, Rose D, Rekate H, Whitaker H: Acquired capsular striatal aphasia in childhood. Archives of Neurology: 40; 614–617, 1983.

Assal G, Campiche R: Aphasie et troubles du langage chez l'enfant après contusion cérébrale. Neurochirurgie: 19; 399–406, 1973.

Assal G, Deonna Th: Aphasie par thrombose de la carotide interne droite chez un enfant droitier. Otto-Neuro-Ophtalmologie: 49; 321–326, 1977.

Baringer JR: Herpes simplex infections of the nervous system. In Vinken D, Bruyn G (Eds): Handbook of Clinical Neurology. Amsterdam: North Holland, Elsevier, 34, pp. 145–156, 1978.

Basser LS: Hemiplegia of early onset and the faculty of speech with special reference to the effects of the hemispherectomy. Brain: 85; 427–460, 1962.

Bates E, Vicari S, Trauner D: Neural mediation of language development: perspectives from lesion studies of infants and children. In Tager-Flusberg H (Ed), Neurodevelopmental Disorders. Cambridge, MA: The MIT Press, pp. 533–582, 1999.

Beaumanoir A, Bureau M, Deonna, T, Mira L, Tassinari C: Continuous Spikes and Waves During Slow Sleep. Eastleigh, England: John Libbey, 1995.

Bernhardt M: Über die spastiche cerebral paralyse im Kindesalter (Hemiplegia spastica infantilis). Nebst einem Excurse über: Aphasia bei Kindern. Archiv für path. Anatomie und Physiologie und für Klinische Medecin: 102; 26–80, 1885.

Bijur P, Haslum M, Gloning J: Cognitive and behavioural sequelae of mild head injury in children. Pediatrics: 86; 337–344, 1990.

Bishop DV: Age of onset and outcome in acquired aphasia with convulsive disorders. Developmental Medicine and Child Neurology: 27; 705–712, 1985.

Bishop DV: Language development after focal brain damage. In Bishop D, Mogford K (Eds), Language Development in Exceptional Circumstances. London: Churchill-Livingstone, 203–219, 1988.

Broca P: Remarques sur le siège de la faculté de langage, suivies d'une observation d'aphémie. Bulletin de la Société d'Anatomie, Paris: 6; 330–357, 1861.

Broca P: Localisation des fonctions cérébrales: siège du langage articulé. Bulletin de la Société Royale d'Anthropologie 6, 463–548, 1863.

Buckingham H, Avakian-Whitaker H, Whitaker H: Alliteration and assonance in neologistic jargonaphasia. Cortex: 14; 365–380, 1978.

Byers R, McLean W: Etiology and course of certain hemiplegias with aphasia in childhood. Pediatrics: 29; 376–383, 1962.

Carter RL, Hohenegger MK, Satz P: Aphasia and speech organisation in children. Science: 218; 797–799, 1982.

Chadwick O, Rutter M, Shaffer D, Shrout PE: A prospective study of children with head injuries specific cognitive abilities. Journal of Clinical Neuropsychology: 3; 101–120, 1981.

Chevrie-Müller C, Simon AM, Decante P: Epreuves pour l'examen de langage (étalonnage chez l'enfant de 5 à 8 ans). Bayeux: Expansion Scientifique, 1975.

Clarus A: Über aphasia bei kindern. Jahresbuch für Kinder Heilkunde: 7; 360–400, 1874.

Cohen M, Campbell R, Yagmai F: Neuropathological abnormalities in developmental dysphasia. Annals of Neurology: 25; 567–570, 1989.

Collignon R, Hecaen H, Angerlergues R: A propos de douze cas d'aphasie chez l'enfant. Acta Neurologica et Psychiatrica Belgica: 68; 245–277, 1968.

Cooper JA, Flowers CR: Children with a history of acquired aphasia: residual language and academic impairment. Journal of Speech and Hearing Disorders: 52; 251–262, 1987.

Cotard J: Etude sur l'atrophie partielle du cerveau. Thèse (non publiée): Paris, 1868.

Cranberg LD, Filley CM, Hart EJ, Alexander MP: Acquired aphasia in childhood. Clinical and CT investigations, Neurology: 37; 1165–1172, 1987.

Czopf J: Role of the non dominant hemisphere in the restitution of speech. Archiv für Psychiatrie und Nervenkrankeiten: 216; 126–171, 1972.

Dailey A, McKahnn G, Berger M: Oral pharyngeal apraxia. Journal of Neurosurgery: 83; 462–475, 1995.

Damasio H: A computed tomographic guide to the identification of cerebral vascular territories. Archives of Neurology: 40; 138–142, 1983.

De Agostini M, Kremin H: Homogeneity of the syndrome of acquired aphasia in childhood revisited: case study of a child with transcortical aphasia. Journal of Neurolinguistics: 2(1); 179–187, 1986.

De Agostini M, Metz-Lutz M, Van Hout A, Chavance M, Deloche G, Pavao-Martins I, Dellatolas G: Batterie d'évaluation du langage oral de l'enfant aphasique (ELOLA): standardisation française (4–12 ans). Revue de Neuropsychologie: 3; 319–367, 1998.

DeLong G: Acquired reversible autistic syndrome in acute encephalopathic illness in children. Archives of Neurology: 38; 191–194, 1981.

Denckla MB: Childhood learning disabilities. In Heilman, K, Valentin E (Eds), Clinical Neuropsychology. New York and Oxford: Oxford University Press, pp. 535–573, 1979.

Dennis M: Stroke in childhood: communicative intent, expression and comprehension after left hemisphere arteriopathy in a right handed 9 year old. In Reiber RW (Ed), Language Development and Aphasia in Children. New York: Academic Press, 1980.

Dennis M, Kohn B: Comprehension of syntax in infantile hemiplegics after cerebral hemidecortication: left hemispheres superiority. Brain and Language: 2; 472–482, 1975.

Dennis M, Whitaker HA: Language acquisition following hemidecortication: Linguistic superiority of the left over the right hemisphere. Brain and Language: 3; 404–433, 1976.

Deonna T, Beaumanoir A, Gaillard F, Assal G: Acquired aphasia in childhood with seizure disorders: a heterogeneous syndrome. Neuropediatrie: 8; 263–273, 1977.

De Renzi E, Vignolo L: The token test: a sensitive test to detect disturbances in aphasics. Brain: 85; 665–678, 1962.

Dugas M, Grenet P, Masson M, Jaquet JP, Jaquet G: Aphasie

de l'enfant avec épilepsie. Evolution régressive sous traitement anti-épileptique. Revue neurologique: 132; 189–193, 1976.

Dugas M, Masson M, Henzey MF, Regnier N: Aphasie acquise de l'enfant avec épilepsie: douze observations personnelles. Revue neurologique: 138; 755–780, 1982.

Efron R: Post-epileptic paralysis: theoretical critique and report of a case. Brain: 381–398, 1961.

Ewing-Cobbs L, Levin H, Eisenberg H, Fletcher J: Language functions following closed head injury in children and adolescents. Journal of Clinical and Experimental Neuropsychology: 9; 575–592, 1987.

Feldman H, Holland A, Kemp S, Janosky J: Language development after unilateral brain injury. Brain and Language: 42; 89–102, 1992.

Ferro JM, Martins IP, Pinto F, Castro-Caldas A: Aphasia following right striato-insular infarction in a left-handed child: a clinico-radiological study. Developmental Medicine and Child Neurology: 24; 173–182, 1982.

Fletcher JM, Erwing-Cobbs L, McLaughlin EJ, Levin HS: Cognitive and psychological sequellae of head injury in children: implications for assessment and management. In Brooks B (Ed), The Injured Child. Austin: University of Texas press, pp. 30–39, 1979.

Freud S: Infantile Cerebral Paralysis (1897). Translated by La Russin University of Miami, Coral Gables, 1968.

Gaddes WH, Crockett DJ: The Spreen Benton aphasia tests; normative data as a measure of normal language development. Brain and Language: 2; 257–280, 1975.

Gado M, Hanaway J, Frank R: Functional anatomy of the cerebral cortex by computed tomography. Journal of Computer Assisted Tomography: 3; 1–19, 1979.

Gaidolfi E, Vignolo LA: Closed head injuries of school-aged children. Italian Journal of Neurological Sciences: 1; 65–73, 1980.

Genton P, Bureau M: Epilepsy with continuous spikes and waves discharges during slow sleep. Approches Neurologiques des Apprentissages chez l'Enfant: 3; 153–152, 1991.

Genton P, Maton B, Ogihara M: Continuous focal spikes during REM sleep in a case of acquired aphasia (Landau–Kleffner syndrome). Sleep: 15; 454–460, 1992.

Geschwind N: Disorders of higher cortical functions in children. In Cohen R, Warstofsky W (Eds), Selected Papers on Language and the Brain. Dordrecht: Reidel, 1974.

Giovardini-Rossi P, Ricciutello C, Calasso E: Afasia aquisita con anomalia convulsive: syndrome di Landa e Kleffner. In Giovardini-Rossi P (Ed), Primo corso di aggiornamento sulle epilessie dell'infanzia e dell'adolescenza. Roma: Sigma-tau, pp. 218–224, 1988.

Gloning K, Hift E: Aphasie im vorschulalter. Wiener Zeitschrift für Nervenheilkunde: 28; 20–28, 1970.

Goldman PS: Plasticity of function in the CNS. In Stein D, Rosen J, Butters N (Eds), Plasticity and Recovery of Function in the Central Nervous System. New York: Academic Press, 1974a.

Goldman PS: An alternative to developmental plasticity: heterology of CNS structures in infants and adults. In Stein D, Rosen J, Butters N (Eds), Plasticity and Recovery of Function in the Central Nervous System. New York: Academic Press, pp. 149–174, 1974b.

Goodglass PS, Kaplan E: The Assessment of Aphasia and Related Disorders. Philadelphia: Lea and Febiger, 1972.

Guttmann E: Aphasia in children. Brain: 65; 205–219, 1942.

Horgan D: Rate of language acquisition and noun emphasis. Journal of Psycholinguistic Research: 10; 629–640, 1978.

Hécaen H: Acquired aphasia in children and the ontogenesis of hemispheric functional specialisation. Brain and Language: 3; 114–134, 1976.

Hécaen H: Acquired aphasia in children revisited. Neuropsychologia: 21; 581–587, 1983.

Hudson L, Murdoch B: Chronic language deficit in children treated for posterior fossa tumour. Aphasiology: 3; 135–50, 1992.

Hudson L, Murdoch B, Ozanne A: Posterior fossa tumour in childhood: associated speech and language disorders post-surgery. Aphasiology: 3; 1–18, 1989.

Isaacson RL: The myth of recovery from early brain damage. In Ellis N (Ed), Aberrant Development in Infancy. London: Wiley, 1975.

Jackson H: On affections of speech from diseases of the brain. Brain: 2; 323–363, 1880.

Jakobson R: Langage Enfantin et Aphasie. Paris: Editions de Minuit, 1962.

Jordan F, Murdoch B: Linguistic status following closed head injury in children; a follow-up study. Brain Injury: 4; 147–54, 1990.

Jordan F, Ozanne A, Murdoch B: Performance of closed head injury children on a naming task. Brain Injury: 4; 27–32, 1988.

Kaga M: Language disorders in Landau–Kleffner syndrome. Journal of Child Neurology: 14; 118–122, 1999.

Kellerman K: Recurrent aphasia with subclinical bioelectrical status epilepticus during sleep. European Journal of Pediatrics: 128; 207–212, 1978.

Kerschensteiner M, Poeck K, Brunner E: The fluency-nonfluency dimension in the classification of aphasic speech. Cortex: 8; 233–247, 1972.

Kertesz A: Aphasia and Associated Disorders; taxonomy, localizations and recovery. New York: Grune and Stratton, 1979.

Kinsbourne M: The minor cerebral hemisphere as a source of aphasic speech. Archives of Neurology: 25; 302–306, 1971.

Kinsbourne M: The ontogeny of cerebral dominance. In Rieber RW (Ed), The Neuropsychology of Language. New York: Plenum Press, 1976.

Kinsbourne M, Hiscock M: Does cerebral dominance develop? In Segalowitz S, Gruber FA (Eds), Language Development and Neurological Theory. New York: Academic Press, 1977.

Klein S, Tuchman R, Rapin I: The influence of premorbid language skills and behavior on language recovery in children with verbal auditory agnosia. Journal of Child Neurology: 15; 36–43, 2000.

Klein SK, Masur D, Farber K, Shinnar S, Rapin I: Fluent aphasia in children: definition and natural history. Journal of Child Neurology: 7; 50–59, 1992.

Korkman M: Paper presented at the 1996 INS meeting.

Landau WM, Kleffner FR: Syndrome of acquired aphasia with convulsive disorder in children. Neurology: 7; 523–530, 1957.

Lenneberg EH: Biological Foundations of Language. Wiley, New York, 1967.

Levin HS, Eisenberg HM, Miner ME: Neuropsychologic findings in head injured children. In Shapiro K (Ed), Pediatric Head Injured Children. New York: Mount Kisco, Futura, 1983.

Locke J: A theory of neurolinguistic development. Brain and Language: 58; 265–326, 1997.

Lyon G, Evrard Ph: Neurologie Pédiatrique. Paris: Masson, 2000.

Maquet P, Hirsch E, Metz-Lutz M, Motte J, Dive D, Marescaux C, Franck G: Regional glucose metabolism in children with deterioration of one or more cognitive functions and continuous spikes and waves during sleep. Brain: 118; 1497–1520, 1995.

Marchman V, Miller R, Bates E: Babble and first words in children with focal brain injury. Applied Psycholinguistics: 12; 1–22, 1991.

Martins I, Castro-Caldas A, Van Dongen H, Van Hout A: Acquired Aphasia in Children: acquisition and breakdown of language in the developing brain. Dordrecht, Klüwer Academic, 1991.

Martins IP, Ferro JM: Acquired conduction aphasia in a child. Developmental Medicine and Child Neurology: 29; 532–536, 1987.

Martins I, Ferro JM: Acquired subcortical lesions in children. In Vallar G, Cappa S, Wallesch C (Eds), Neuropsychological Disorders Associated with Subcortical Lesions. Oxford: University Press, pp. 376–380, 1992.

Martins IP, Ferro JM, Trindale A: Crossed aphasia in a child. Developmental Medicine and Child Neurology: 29; 96–109, 1987.

Martins I, Pereiro A, Albuquerque L: Capacités de calcul chez des enfants scolarisés avec des lésions acquises. Approches Neuropsychologiques des Apprentissages de l'Enfant: 51; 6–12, 1999.

Matsui T, Hirano A: Atlas of the Human Brain for Computerized Tomography. Stuttgart: Fisher Verlag, 1978.

Messerli P, Tissot A, Rodriguez J: Recovery from aphasia. In Lebrun Y, Hoops R (Eds), Recovery in Aphasias. Amsterdam: Swets and Zeitlinger, 124–135, 1976.

Metellus J, Hatt A: Problèmes linguistiques posés par une désintégration progressive du langage chez un enfant. Grammatica: 7, Etudes Neurolinguistiques; 1, 329–351, 1980.

Milner B: Hemispheric Specialisation and Interaction. The Neurosciences: Third Study Program. Cambridge, MA: The MIT Press, 1974.

Morrell F, Whisler W, Smith M et al: Landau-Kleffner syndrome: treatment with subpial intra-cortical transection. Brain: 118; 1529–1546, 1995.

Nass R, Boyce L, Leventhal F: Acquired aphasia in children after subpial resection of left thalamic tumors. Developmental Medicine and Child Neurology: 42; 580–590, 2000.

Nass R, Leventhal F, Levine, Lebron D, Maxfield C, McCall P, George A, Allen J: Conduction aphasia in a three year old with a left posterior cortical/subcortical abscess. Brain and Language: 62; 70–88, 1998.

Nelson K: Structure and strategy in learning to talk. Monographs of the Society for Research in Child Development: 38(149); 1–118, 1973.

Nelson K: Individual difference in language development: implication for development and language. Developmental Psychology: 17; 170–187, 1981.

O'Tuama L, Urion D, Janicek M, Treeves S, Bjorston B, Moriarty J: Regional perfusion in Landau-Kleffner syndrome and related childhood aphasia. Journal of Nuclear Medicine: 33; 1758–1765, 1992.

Paeteau R, Kajola M, Korkman M, Hämäläinen M, Granstrom M, Hari R: Landau-Kleffner syndrome: epileptic activity in the auditory cortex. Neuroreport: 2; 201–204, 1991.

Patry G, Lyagoubi S, Tassinari CA: Subclinical electrical status epilepticus induced by sleep in children. A clinical and electroencephalographic study of six cases. Archives of Neurology; 24; 241–252, 1971.

Petersen U, Koepp P, Solensen M, Von Villiez M, Von Villiez H: Aphasie in Kindesalter mit EEG veränderungen. Neuropädiatrie: 9; 84–96, 1978.

Poetzl T: Über sensorische Aphasie im Kindersalter. H.N.O. Kliniek: 14; 109–118, 1926.

Rapin I, Allen D: Syndromes in developmental dysphasia and adult aphasia. In Plum F (Ed), Language, Communication and the Brain. New York: Raven, pp. 57–75, 1988.

Rapin I, Mattis S, Rowan AJ, Golden GS: Verbal auditory agnosia in children. Developmental Medicine and Child Neurology: 19; 192–207, 1977.

Shinnar S, Rapin I, Arnold S, Tuchman RF, Shulman L, Ballaban-Gil K, Maw M, Deuel RK, Volkmar FR: Language regression in childhood. Pediatric Neurology: 24; 183–189, 2001.

Sarno MT: The nature of verbal impairment after closed head injury. Journal of Nervous and Mental disorders: 168; 685–692, 1980.

Sobel D, Aung M, Otsubo H, Smith H: Magnetoencephalography in children with Landau–Kleffner syndrome. American Journal of Neuroradiology: 2; 301–307, 2000.

Spreen O, Benton AL: Neurosensory Center Comprehensive Examination for Aphasia. Neuropsychology Laboratory, University of Victoria, 1969.

Steriade M, Botez MI, Petrovici I: On certain dissociations of consciousness levels within the syndrome of akinetic mutism. Psychiatria et Neurologia, Basel: 141; 38–58, 1961.

Tanabe H, Ikeda M, Murasawa A, Yamada K, Nakagawa Y, Nishimura Y, Shiraishi J: AA case of acquired conduction aphasia in a child. Acta Neurologica Scandinavica: 80; 314–318, 1989.

Toso V, Moschini M, Gagnin G, Antonu D: Aphasie acquise de l'enfant avec épilepsie; trois observations et revue de la littérature. Revue Neurologique: 137; 425–434, 1981.

Van de Sandt-Koenderman W, Smit I, Van Dongen K, Van Hesch J: A case of acquired aphasia and convulsive disorders: some linguistics aspects of recovery and breakdown. Brain and Language: 21; 174–183, 1984.

Van Dongen H, Loonen M, Van Dongen K: Anatomical basis for

acquired fluent aphasia in children. Annals of Neurology: 17; 306–309, 1985.

Van Dongen H, Pasquier P, Raes J, Creten W: An analysis of spontaneous conversational speech fluency in children with acquired aphasia. Cortex: 30; 619–33, 1994.

Van Dongen HR: Acquired childhood aphasia, course and outcome. Paper presented at the I.N.S. Meeting, Antwerpen, 1989.

Van Dongen HR, Meulstee J, Blauw-Van Mouri, Van Harskamp F: The Landau–Kleffner syndrome, a case study with a fourteen year follow-up. European Neurology: 29; 109–114, 1989.

Van Dongen HR, Visch-Brink EG: Naming in aphasic children, analysis of paraphasic errors; Neuropsychologia: 26; 629–632, 1988.

Van Hout A: Importance of paraphasias in acquired aphasia in children. Paper presented at the meeting of the International Neuropsychological Society, Lisbon, 1983.

Van Hout A: Acquired aphasia in childhood and developmental dysphasia: are the errors similar? Analysis of errors made in confrontation naming tasks. Aphasiology: 7; 525–31, 1993.

Van Hout A: Les troubles du calcul dans les lésions cérébrales acquises chez l'enfant. In Entretiens de Bichat. Paris: Expansion Scientifique Française, pp. 168–173, 1998.

Van Hout A, Evrard Ph: Aphasie sensorielle chez un enfant de moins de quatre ans. In Narbona J, Poch-Olive M (Eds), Neuropsychologie Infantile: Données Récentes. Symposium international de Pampelune: 81, pp. 294, 1987.

Van Hout A, Evrard Ph, Lyon G: On the positive semiology of acquired aphasia in children. Developmental Medicine and Child Neurology: 27; 231–241, 1985.

Van Hout A, Landrieu P: Anterior aphasia of an unusual type in a 13 years old child. Neurosciences Letters: 1(suppl 3); 210, 1979.

Van Hout A, Lyon G: Wernicke's aphasia in a ten year old boy. Brain and Language: 29; 268–285, 1986.

Van Hout A, Seron X: L'aphasie de l'enfant. Mardaga, Bruxelles: 193 pp., 1983.

Van Lieshout P, Renier W, Eling P, de Bot K, Slis I: Bilingual language processing after a lesion in the left thalamic and temporal reegion. Brain and Language: 38; 173–180, 1990.

Vargha-Khadem F, O'Gorman AM, Watters EV: Aphasia and handedness in relation to hemispheric side, age at injury and severity of cerebral lesion during childhood. Brain: 108; 167–183, 1985.

Vihman M: Phonology and the development of the lexicon: evidence from children errors. Journal of Child Language: 8; 239–264, 1981.

Visch-Brink E, Van de Sandt-Koederman W: The importance of paraphasias in the spontaneous speech of children with an acquired aphasia. Brain and Language: 23; 258–272, 1984.

Von Cramon D: Traumatic mutism and the subsequent reorganisation of speech functions. Neuropsychologia: 19; 281–303, 1975.

Wagenaar E, Snow C, Prins RS: Spontaneous speech of aphasic patients: a psycholinguistic analysis. Brain and Language: 2; 281–303, 1975.

Woods MT, Carey S: Language deficits after apparent clinical recovery from childhood aphasia. Annals of Neurology: 6; 405–409, 1979.

Woods MT, Teuber HL: Early onset of complementary specialisation of cerebral hemispheres in man. Transactions of the American Neurological Association: 98; 113–117, 1973.

Woods MT, Teuber HL: Changing pattern of childhood aphasia. Annals of Neurology: 3; 273–280, 1978.

Yarnell P, Monroe P, Sorel L: Aphasia outcome in stroke; a clinical neurological correlation. Stroke: 7; 516–522, 1976.

Zaidel E: Auditory language comprehension in the right hemisphere following cerebral commissurotomy: a comparison with child language and aphasia. In Caramazza A, Zurif E (Eds), Language Acquisition and Language Breakdown: parallels and divergencies. Baltimore: John Hopkins University Press, 229–276, 1977.

© 2003 Published by Elsevier Science B.V.
Handbook of Neuropsychology, 2nd Edition, Vol. 8, Part II
S.J. Segalowitz and I. Rapin (Eds)

CHAPTER 24

The neuropsychology of dyslexia [1]

Sally E. Shaywitz [a,*], Bennett A. Shaywitz [a,b], Robert K. Fulbright [c], Pawel Skudlarski [c], W. Einar Mencl [a,d], R. Todd Constable [c], Kenneth R. Pugh [a,d], Jack M. Fletcher [e], G. Reid Lyon [f] and John C. Gore [c,g]

[a] *Department of Pediatrics, Yale University School of Medicine, P.O. Box 3333, New Haven, CT 06510-8064 USA*
[b] *Department of Neurology, Yale University School of Medicine, New Haven, CT, USA*
[c] *Department of Diagnostic Radiology, Yale University School of Medicine, New Haven, CT, USA*
[d] *Haskins Laboratories, Yale University School of Medicine, New Haven, CT, USA*
[e] *Department of Pediatrics, University of Texas Medical School, Houston, TX, USA*
[f] *Child Behavior and Learning Branch, National Institute of Child Health and Development, National Institutes of Health, Bethesda, MD, USA*
[g] *Department of Applied Physics, Yale University, New Haven, CT, USA*

Introduction

Dyslexia is characterized by an unexpected difficulty in reading in children and adults who otherwise possess the intelligence, motivation, and schooling considered necessary for accurate and fluent reading (Shaywitz, 1998). Recent epidemiologic data indicate that, like hypertension and obesity, dyslexia fits a dimensional model. In other words, within the population, reading ability and reading disability occur along a continuum, with reading disability representing the lower tail of a normal distribution of reading ability (Gilger, Borecki, Smith et al., 1996; Shaywitz, Escobar, Shaywitz et al., 1992).

Dyslexia is perhaps the most common neurobehavioral disorder affecting children, with prevalence rates ranging from 5 to 17.5 percent (Interagency Committee on Learning Disabilities, 1987; Shaywitz, Fletcher and Shaywitz, 1994). Previously, it was believed that dyslexia affected boys primarily (Finucci and Childs, 1981); however, more recent data indicate similar numbers of affected boys and girls (Flynn and Rahbar, 1994; Shaywitz, Shaywitz, Fletcher and Escobar, 1990; Wadsworth, DeFries, Stevenson et al., 1992). Longitudinal studies, both prospective (Francis, Shaywitz, Stuebing et al., 1996; Shaywitz, Holford, Holahan et al., 1995) and retrospective (Bruck, 1992; Felton, Naylor and Wood, 1990; Scarborough, 1984), indicate that dyslexia is a persistent, chronic condition; it does not represent a transient "developmental lag" (Fig. 1). Over time, poor readers and good readers tend to maintain their relative positions along the spectrum of reading ability (Shaywitz et al., 1995b).

Heritability

Dyslexia is both familial and heritable (Pennington and Gilger, 1996). Family history is one of the most important risk factors, with 23 percent to as much as 65 percent of children who have a parent with dyslexia reported to have the disorder (Scarborough, 1990). A rate among siblings of affected persons of approximately 40 percent and among parents ranging from 27 to 49 percent (Pennington and Gilger,

[1] Portions of this chapter appeared in and are similar to other reviews by us in: Shaywitz, 1998; Shaywitz and Shaywitz, 1999; and Shaywitz, Shaywitz, Pugh et al., 2001.

* Corresponding author. E-mail: sally.shaywitz@yale.edu

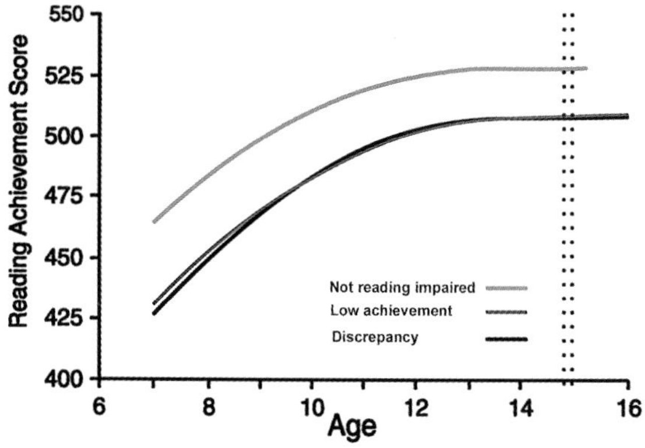

Fig. 1. Trajectory of reading skills over time in nonimpaired and dyslexic readers. Ordinate is Rasch scores (W scores) from the Woodcock–Johnson reading test (Woodcock and Johnson, 1989) and abscissa is age in years. Both dyslexic and nonimpaired readers improve their reading scores as they get older, but the gap between the dyslexic and nonimpaired readers remains. Thus dyslexia is a deficit and not a developmental lag. Figure from Francis et al. (1996).

1996) provides opportunities for early identification of affected siblings and often for delayed but helpful identification of affected adults. Replicated linkage studies of dyslexia implicate loci on chromosomes 2, 3, 6, 15 and 18 (Fisher and DeFries, 2002). Whether the differences in the genetic loci represent polygenic inheritance, different cognitive paths to the same phenotype or different types of dyslexia is not clear.

Cognitive influences

Theories of dyslexia have been proposed that are based on the visual system (Demb, Boynton and Heeger, 1998; Eden, VanMeter, Rumsey et al., 1996; Stein and Walsh, 1997), and other factors, such as temporal processing of stimuli within these systems (Talcott et al., 2000; Tallal, 2000), discussed further below. However, there is now a strong consensus among investigators in the field that the central difficulty in dyslexia reflects a deficit within the language system, although other systems and processes may also contribute to the difficulty. Investigators have long known that speech enables its users to create an indefinitely large number of words by combining and permuting a small number of phonologic segments, the consonants and vowels that serve as the natural constituents of the biologic specialization for language. An alphabetic transcription (reading) brings this same ability to readers, but only as they connect its arbitrary characters (letters) to the phonologic segments they represent. Making that connection requires an awareness that all words, in fact, can be decomposed into phonologic segments. Thus, it is this awareness that allows the reader to connect the letter strings (the orthography) to the corresponding units of speech (phonologic constituents) they represent. The awareness that all words can be decomposed into these basic elements of language (phonemes) allows the reader to decipher the reading code. In order to read, a child has to develop the insight that spoken words can be pulled apart into phonemes and that the letters in a written word represent these sounds. As numerous studies have shown, however, such awareness is largely missing in dyslexic children and adults (Bruck, 1992; Fletcher, Shaywitz, Shankweiler et al., 1994; Liberman and Shankweiler, 1991; Shankweiler, Liberman, Mark et al., 1979; Share, 1995; Shaywitz, 1998, 1996; Stanovich and Siegel, 1994; Torgesen, 1995; Wagner and Torgesen, 1987). Results from large and well-studied populations with reading disability confirm that in young school-age children (Fletcher et al., 1994; Stanovich and Siegel, 1994) as well as in adolescents (Shaywitz, Fletcher, Holahan et al., 1999) a deficit in phonology represents the most robust and specific (Morris, Stuebing, Fletcher et al., 1998) correlate of reading disability. Such findings form the basis for the most successful and evidence-based interventions designed to improve reading (Report of the National Reading Panel, 2000). While children and adults with a phonologic deficit represent the majority of cases of dyslexia, we note that other subtypes may, indeed, account for some cases of dyslexia, for example, surface dyslexia (Coltheart, Curtis, Atkins and Haller, 1993), D- and L-type dyslexia (Bakker, 1992; Bakker, Licht and Van Strien, 1991) and dyslexia resulting from deficits in naming-speed in addition to phonological deficits (double-deficit hypothesis, Wolf and Bowers, 1999).

Implications of the phonologic model of dyslexia

Basically, reading comprises two main processes — decoding and comprehension (Gough and Tunmer, 1986). In dyslexia, a deficit at the level of the phonologic module impairs the ability to segment the written word into its underlying phonologic elements. As a result, the reader experiences difficulty, first in decoding the word and then in identifying it. The phonologic deficit is domain-specific; that is, it is independent of other, nonphonologic, abilities. In particular, the higher order cognitive and linguistic functions involved in comprehension, such as general intelligence and reasoning, vocabulary (Share and Stanovich, 1995), and syntax (Shankweiler et al., 1995), are generally intact. This pattern — a deficit in phonologic analysis contrasted with intact higher-order cognitive abilities — offers an explanation for the paradox of otherwise intelligent people who experience great difficulty in reading (Shaywitz, 1996).

According to the model, a circumscribed deficit in a lower-order linguistic (phonologic) function blocks access to higher-order processes and to the ability to draw meaning from text. The problem is that the affected reader cannot use his or her higher-order linguistic skills to access the meaning until the printed word has first been decoded and identified. For example, an individual who knows the precise meaning of the spoken word 'apparition' will not be able to use his knowledge of the meaning of the word until he can decode and identify the printed word on the page and will appear not to know the word's meaning.

The phonologic deficit in adolescence and adult life

Deficits in phonological coding continue to characterize dyslexic readers even in adolescence; performance on phonological processing measures contributes most to discriminating dyslexic and average readers, and average and superior readers as well (Shaywitz et al., 1999). Children with dyslexia neither spontaneously remit nor do they demonstrate a lag mechanism for 'catching up' in the development of reading skills. That is not to say that many dyslexic readers do not become quite proficient in reading a finite domain of words that are in their area of special interest, usually words that are important for their careers. For example, an individual who is dyslexic in childhood but who, in adult life becomes interested in molecular biology and who then learns to decode words that form a minivocabulary important in molecular biology. Such an individual, while able to decode words in this domain still exhibits evidence of his early reading problems when he has to read unfamiliar words, which he then does accurately but not fluently or automatically (Ben-Dror, Pollatsek and Scarpati, 1991; Bruck, 1992, 1994; Lefly and Pennington, 1991; Shaywitz et al., 1999). In adolescents, the rate of reading as well as facility with spelling may be most useful clinically in differentiating average from poor readers. From a clinical perspective, these data indicate that as children approach adolescence, a manifestation of dyslexia may be a very slow reading rate; in fact, children may learn to read words accurately, but they will not be fluent or automatic, reflecting the lingering effects of a phonologic deficit (Lefly and Pennington, 1991). Because they are able to read words accurately (albeit very slowly) dyslexic adolescents and young adults may mistakenly be assumed to have 'outgrown' their dyslexia. Data from studies of children with dyslexia who have been followed prospectively support the notion that in adolescents, the rate of reading as well as facility with spelling may be most useful clinically in differentiating average from poor readers in students in secondary school, and college and even graduate school. It is important to remember that these older dyslexic students may be similar to their unimpaired peers on untimed measures of word recognition yet continue to suffer from the phonologic deficit that makes reading less automatic, more effortful, and slow. For these readers with dyslexia the provision of extra time is an essential accommodation; it allows them the time to decode each word and to apply their unimpaired higher-order cognitive and linguistic skills to the surrounding context to get at the meaning of words that they cannot entirely or rapidly decode. Other accommodations useful to adolescents with reading difficulties include note-takers, taping classroom lectures, using Recordings for the Blind to access texts and other books they have difficulty reading and the opportunity to take tests in alternate formats, such as short essays or even, orally (Shaywitz, 1998).

Neurobiologic studies

To a large degree these advances in understanding dyslexia have informed and facilitated studies examining the neurobiological underpinnings of reading and dyslexia. Thus, a range of neurobiologic investigations using postmortem brain specimens (Galaburda, Sherman, Rosen et al., 1985), and more recently, brain morphometry (Filipek, 1996), and diffusion tensor MRI imaging (Klingberg, Hedehus, Temple et al., 2000) suggests that there are differences in the temporo-parieto-occipital brain regions between dyslexic and nonimpaired readers.

Functional brain imaging

Rather than being limited to examining the brain in an autopsy specimen, or measuring the size of brain regions using static morphometric indices based on CT or MRI, functional imaging offers the possibility of examining brain function during performance of a cognitive task. In principle, functional brain imaging is quite simple. When an individual is asked to perform a discrete cognitive task, that task places processing demands on particular neural systems in the brain. To meet those demands requires activation of neural systems in specific brain regions and those changes in neural activity are, in turn, reflected by changes in brain metabolic activity, which in turn, are reflected, for example, by changes in cerebral blood flow and in the cerebral utilization of metabolic substrates such as glucose. The term functional imaging has also been applied to the technology of magnetic source imaging using magnetoencephalography, an electrophysiologic method with strengths in resolving the temporal sequences of cognitive processes. In this chapter we use the term functional imaging to refer to technologies that measure those changes in metabolic activity and blood flow in specific brain regions while subjects are engaged in cognitive tasks. Some of the first functional imaging studies of dyslexia used Positron Emission Tomography (PET) (Gross-Glenn, Duara, Barker et al., 1991; Hagman, Wood, Buchsbaum et al., 1992). In practice PET requires intraarterial or intravenous administration of a radioactive isotope to the subject so that cerebral blood flow or cerebral utilization of glucose can be determined while the subject is performing the task. Positron emitting isotopes of nuclei of biological interest have very short biological half-lives and are synthesized in a cyclotron immediately prior to testing, a factor that mandates that the time course of the experiment conform to the short half-life of the radioisotope.

Rumsey, Andreason, Zametkin et al. (1992) used PET and measured cerebral blood flow using ^{15}O in 14 dyslexic subjects; their task was to respond if binaurally presented real words rhymed. Dyslexics failed to activate the left parietal and left middle temporal regions. In a second report, Rumsey, Zametkin, Andreason et al. (1994) again used ^{15}O PET and studied 15 dyslexic men and 20 matched controls. Their task was a semantic judgment, that is, to listen to sentence pairs and respond if the meaning of both sentences was the same. Both normal and dyslexic readers increased cerebral blood flow in the middle temporal regions during the task, and no significant differences were observed between normal and dyslexic readers.

Paulesu, Frith, Snowling et al. (1996) used PET to compare 5 university male students with histories of reading problems but who were currently reading in the average range and 5 similarly aged subjects without a history of reading problems; one task required subjects to rhyme single letters and a companion task involved short-term memory for single letters. Dyslexics activated Broca's area during the single-letter rhyme task and Wernicke's area during the memory task, but, in contrast to controls, both language regions were not activated in concert in either task. The authors attribute the problem to a disconnection between the anterior and posterior language regions, a theory supported by their finding of underactivation in the insula in this group of compensated dyslexics.

In a later report, Rumsey, Nace, Donohue et al. (1997) used PET to study 17 dyslexic men and 14 male controls. Subjects performed two pronunciation tasks (low-frequency real words and pseudowords) and two lexical decision tasks (orthographic and phonologic). Compared to controls, dyslexic readers demonstrated reduced blood flow in temporal cortex and inferior parietal cortex, especially on the left, during both pronunciation and decision making.

Functional Magnetic Resonance Imaging (fMRI)

Functional Magnetic Resonance Imaging (fMRI) promises to supplant other methods for its ability to map the individual brain's response to specific cognitive stimuli. Since it is non-invasive and safe, it can be used repeatedly, properties which make it ideal for studying humans, especially children. In principle, the signal used to construct MRI images changes, by a small amount (typically of the order 1–5%), in regions that are activated by a stimulus or task. The increase in signal results from the combined effects of increases in the tissue blood flow, volume and oxygenation, though the precise contributions of each of these is still somewhat uncertain. MR image intensity increases when deoxygenated blood is replaced by oxygenated blood. A variety of methods can be used to record the changes that occur but one preferred approach makes use of ultrafast imaging, such as echo planar imaging (EPI), in which complete images are acquired in times substantially shorter than a second. Echo planar imaging can provide images at a rate fast enough to capture the time course of the hemodynamic response to neural activation and to permit a wide variety of imaging paradigms over large volumes of the brain. Details of fMRI are reviewed in Anderson and Gore (1997).

Recent progress using functional MRI to study reading

Functional MRI and visual processing

Eden et al. (1996) and Demb et al. (998) have used fMRI to study the role of visual processing in dyslexia. Eden et al. studied 6 dyslexic and 8 controls, a subset of men from Rumsey's subjects. Presentation of a moving stimulus activated higher order visual regions in the extrastriate cortex in controls but not in dyslexics, while presentation of a stationary visual task resulted in equivalent activations in primary visual cortex and extrastriate cortex in both dyslexic and control groups. Demb et al. studied brain activation during a visual speed discrimination task in 3 dyslexic men and 2 dyslexic women. Compared to controls, dyslexics showed reduced brain activity in primary visual cortex and several extrastriate regions. Neither of these studies used reading tasks and the implications for reading in dyslexia are uncertain. The reader is referred to a recent review (Stein and Walsh, 1997) for a more detailed discussion of how visual processing deficits might relate to dyslexia.

Functional MRI and phonological processing

A number of research groups, including ourselves, have used fMRI to examine the functional organization of the brain for reading and reading disability. Initial studies focused on the identification of those cortical sites associated with various subcomponent operations in reading in nonimpaired readers. We studied 19 neurologically normal right-handed men and 19 women (Shaywitz, Shaywitz, Pugh et al., 1995). Of particular interest were differences in brain activation patterns during phonological processing in men compared to women. This is illustrated in Fig. 2 which demonstrates that activation during phonological processing in men was more lateralized to the left inferior frontal gyrus; in contrast, activation during this same task in women resulted in a more bilateral pattern of activation of this region.

These findings provide the first clear evidence of sex differences in the functional organization of the brain for language and indicate that these differences exist primarily at the level of phonological processing. At one level, they support and extend a long held hypothesis which suggests that language functions are more likely to be highly lateralized in males but represented in both cerebral hemispheres in females (Halpern, 2000; Witelson and Kigar, 1992). It should be noted that while the basic sex difference in hemispheric activation in IFG appears statistically robust across investigations using large numbers of subjects, it is clear that there is much overlap between the distributions as well. For example, this effect has been replicated using different language processing tasks (Jaeger, Lockwood, Vanvalin et al., 1998; Kansaku, Yamaura and Kitazawa, 2000), yet other imaging experiments have not observed robust sex differences in lateralization (Price, Moore and Frackowiak, 1996). As with analogous sex differences in lateralization using visual-hemifield or binaural presentation conditions in language processing tasks, given the large overlap in distribution the basic effect may not be expected to attain significance in each

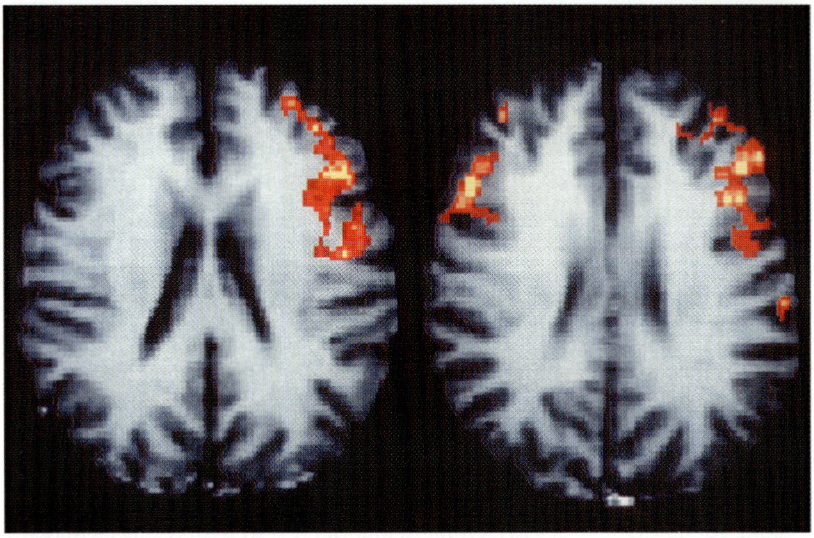

Fig. 2. Sex differences in the brain during phonological processing. Composite fMRI images showing the distribution of brain activation patterns in men (left) and women (right) during the nonword rhyming task. In men activation is lateralized to the left inferior frontal regions but in women the same region is active bilaterally. Data from Shaywitz et al. (1995a).

and every sample and for all language processing manipulations. Since our initial finding of sex differences in functional activation within IFG we have obtained three replications of the same basic sex by hemisphere pattern. In sum, the evidence from several imaging experiments seems clear — the modal pattern indicates relatively greater right hemisphere involvement for females than for males. However, laterality differences, while important with respect to sex difference research, are somewhat orthogonal to critical reading group differences that predict reading disability.

fMRI in dyslexic readers

Using tasks which tapped phonologic analysis, we compared performance and brain activation patterns (as measured by fMRI) of dyslexic (DYS) and non-impaired (NI) readers. We studied 61 right-handed subjects, 29 DYS readers (14 men, 15 women, ages 16–54 years) and 32 NI readers (16 men, 16 women, ages 18–63 years). Both groups were in the average range for IQ; DYS readers had a full scale IQ (mean $\pm$ SEM) of 91 ± 2.3 and NI readers had an IQ of 115 ± 2.2. Other than requiring that all subjects have an IQ in the average range (80 or above), we elected not to match subjects on IQ so as not to bias our sample selection in favor of less impaired readers since in adults IQ is known to be influenced by reading ability. Reading performance in the DYS subjects was significantly impaired: the mean standard score on a measure of nonword reading (Woodcock and Johnson, 1989) was 81 ± 1.9 (mean $\pm$ SEM) in DYS readers compared to 114 ± 1.5 in NI readers, with no overlap between groups.

We focused on those brain regions which previous research had implicated in reading and language (Demonet, Price, Wise and Frackowiak, 1994; Henderson, 1986; Petersen, Fox, Snyder and Raichle, 1990) and examined these for evidence of differences between the two reading groups in patterns of activation across the series of tasks. In this study we found significant differences in brain activation patterns between DYS and NI readers, differences which emerged during tasks that made progressive demands on phonologic analysis. Thus, during nonword rhyming in dyslexic readers, we found a disruption in several critical components of a posterior system involving posterior superior temporal gyrus (Wernicke's area), BA 39 (angular gyrus) and BA 17 (striate cortex) and a concomitant increase in activation in the inferior frontal gyrus anteriorly.

Most recently (Shaywitz, Shaywitz, Pugh et al., 2002), we used functional magnetic resonance imaging (fMRI) to study 144 right handed children, 70 dyslexic (DYS) readers (21 girls, 49 boys, ages 7–18 years, mean age 13.3 years) and 74 nonimpaired (NI) readers (31 girls, 43 boys, ages 7–17 years, mean age 10.9 years) as they read pseudowords and real words. We found significant differences in brain activation patterns during phonologic analysis in nonimpaired compared to dyslexic children. Specifically, nonimpaired children demonstrate significantly greater activation than do dyslexic children in left hemisphere sites including the inferior frontal, superior temporal, parieto-temporal and middle temporal–middle occipital gyri and right hemisphere sites including the inferior frontal, superior temporal, cingulate and medial orbital gyri. These data converge with reports from many investigators using functional brain imaging which show a failure of left hemisphere posterior brain systems to function properly during reading (Brunswick, McCrory, Price et al., 1999; Helenius, Tarkiainen, Cornelissen et al., 1999; Horwitz, Rumsey and Donohue, 1998; Paulesu, Demonet, Fazio et al., 2001; Rumsey et al., 1992; Rumsey et al., 1997; Salmelin et al., 1996; Seki, Koeda, Sugihara et al., 2001; Shaywitz, Shaywitz, Pugh et al., 1998; Simos, Breier, Fletcher et al., 2000; Temple, Poldrack, Protopapas et al., 2000) as well as during non-reading visual processing tasks (Demb et al., 1998; Eden et al., 1996) indicating that dysfunction in left hemisphere posterior reading circuits is already present in dyslexic children and cannot be ascribed simply to a lifetime of poor reading.

Of particular interest was the finding that there are significant correlations between performance on a reading measure out of the magnet and brain activations during fMRI tasks located in the left occipito-parietal area, suggesting that the left occipito-temporal region may be a critical component of a neural system for skilled reading.

In anterior regions NI children demonstrated greater activation during pseudoword rhyming than DYS children; this finding is consonant with two other reports in children (Corina, Richards, Serafini et al., 2001; Georgiewa, Rzanny, Hopf et al., 1999) as well as reports in adults (Gross-Glenn et al., 1991; Paulesu et al., 1996). At the same time, this finding contrasts with what we (Shaywitz et al., 1998) and others (Brunswick et al. 1999; Paulesu et al., 2001) have reported in adults, where dyslexic readers showed greater activation in the inferior frontal gyrus. Consideration of the correlation between age and brain activation provided an explanation that could resolve these differences. Specifically, we found that during the most difficult and specific phonologic task (nonword rhyming) *older* dyslexic readers engaged the left and right inferior frontal gyrus, a finding consistent with results in adult dyslexic readers which indicate an increase in activation in frontal regions (Brunswick et al., 1999; Shaywitz et al., 1998). It is reasonable to suggest that older dyslexic readers engage neural systems in frontal regions to compensate for the disruption in posterior regions. During the category task older dyslexic readers engage the right inferior frontal gyrus while older nonimpaired readers engage the left inferior frontal gyrus and right central sulcus region. The category task is considerably more complex than nonword rhyming, engaging not only phonology but lexical-semantic processes as well. The older nonimpaired readers begin to engage the left frontal systems to perform this task; in contrast, older dyslexic readers fail to engage left frontal systems but rather begin using an ancillary system, the right inferior frontal gyrus. This study was designed to minimize some of the problems encountered in previous studies, and thus we examined a large sample, particularly for a functional imaging study; we included a broad age range and studied both boys and girls. We also recognize that there are limitations of this current study, notably that inferences about development are based on the cross-sectional features of the study design. A longitudinal study of the development of reading in children with dyslexia would be of particular interest. Knowledge that dyslexic children and adults demonstrate a disruption within the neural systems engaged in accessing the sound structure of words underscores the importance of evaluating phonologic skills in the diagnosis of dyslexia and also, of focusing on these skills and their underlying neural systems as targets for informed phonologically-based interventions for children and for adults.

A neural model for reading

These data from laboratories around the world indicate that there are a number of interrelated neural

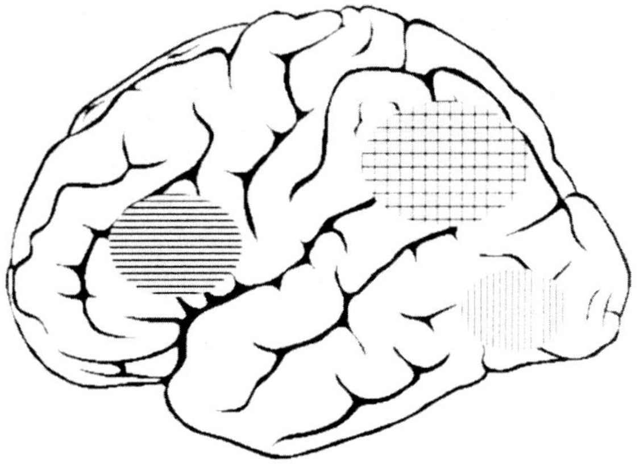

Fig. 3. Neural systems for reading. Converging evidence indicates three important systems in reading, all primarily in the left hemisphere. These include an anterior system and two posterior systems: (1) anterior system in the left inferior frontal region; (2) parieto-temporal system involving angular gyrus, supramarginal gyrus and posterior portions of the superior temporal gyrus; (3) occipito-temporal system involving portions of the middle temporal gyrus and middle occipital gyrus. For details, please see text.

systems used in reading, at least two in posterior brain regions as well as distinct and related systems in anterior regions (Fig. 3). In order to read, the beginning reader must break the reading code, that is, transform the visual features (the letters) of the word into the linguistic sounds (the phonemes) they represent and then access the meaning of the word. As early as 1891, Dejerine suggested that a portion of the posterior brain region (which includes the angular gyrus and supramarginal gyrus in the inferior parietal lobule, and the posterior aspect of the superior temporal gyrus) is critical for reading. Since that time a large literature on acquired inability to read (alexia) describes neuroanatomic lesions most prominently centered about the angular gyrus as a region considered pivotal in mapping the visual percept of the print onto the phonologic structures of the language system (Damasio and Damasio, 1983; Friedman et al., 1993; Geschwind, 1965). Thus, this temporo-parietal reading system seems to be critical for analyzing the written word, that is, transforming the orthography into the underlying linguistic structures. Another posterior brain region in the occipito-temporal area was also described by Dejerine (1892) as critical in reading.

More recently, Logan (1988, 1997) proposed two systems critical in the development of skilled, automatic processing, one involving word analysis, operating on individual units of words such as phonemes, requiring attentional resources and processing relatively slowly and the second system operating on the whole word (word form), an obligatory system that does not require attention and processes very rapidly, on the order of 150 ms after a word is read (Price et al. 1996). Converging evidence from a number of lines of investigation indicate that Logan's word analysis system is localized within the parieto-temporal region while the automatic, rapidly responding system is localized within the occipito-temporal area, functioning as a visual word form area (Cohen et al., 2000; Cohen, Lehéricy, Chochon et al., 2002; Dehaene, Le Clec'H, Poline et al., 2002; Dehaene, Naccache, Cohen et al., 2001; Moore and Price 1999). The visual word form area appears to respond preferentially to rapidly presented stimuli (Price et al., 1996) and is engaged even when the word has not been consciously perceived (Dehaene et al., 2001). Still another reading-related neural circuit involves an anterior system in the inferior frontal gyrus (Broca's area), a region that has long been associated with articulation and also serves an important function in silent reading and naming (Fiez and Peterson 1998; Frackowiak et al., 1997).

Recognition of these systems allows us to suggest an explanation for the brain activation patterns observed in dyslexic children. We suppose that rather than the smoothly functioning and integrated reading systems observed in nonimpaired children, disruption of the posterior reading systems results in dyslexic children attempting to compensate by shifting to other, ancillary systems, for example, anterior sites such as the inferior frontal gyrus and right hemisphere sites. The anterior sites, critical in articulation (Brunswick et al. 1999; Fiez and Peterson 1998; Frackowiak et al., 1997), may help the child with dyslexia develop an awareness of the sound structure of the word by forming the word with his lips, tongue and vocal apparatus and thus allow the child to read, albeit more slowly and less efficiently than if the fast occipito-temporal word identification system were functioning. The right hemisphere sites may represent the engagement of brain regions that allow the poor reader to use other perceptual processes to compensate for his or her poor phonologic skills. A number of studies of young adults with childhood histories of dyslexia indicate that although they may develop some accuracy in reading words, they remain slow, nonautomatic readers (Bruck 1992; Felton et al. 1990). These data now suggest an explanation for these observed clinical findings. In dyslexic readers disruption of both parieto-temporal and occipito-temporal left hemisphere posterior reading systems underlies the failure of skilled reading to develop, while a shift to ancillary systems in left and right anterior regions and right posterior regions supports accurate, but not automatic word reading. This notion of a shift to ancillary systems, particularly in the right hemisphere, has some similarities to the Bakker's concepts of dyslexia which emphasize the contributions of right and left hemispheres to reading (Bakker et al., 1991).

Conclusions and implications

Within the last two decades overwhelming evidence from many laboratories has converged to indicate the cognitive basis for dyslexia: dyslexia represents a disorder within the language system and more specifically within a particular subcomponent of that system, phonological processing. Recent advances in imaging technology and the development of tasks which sharply isolate the subcomponent processes of reading now allow the localization of phonological processing in brain, and, as a result, provide for the first time, the potential for elucidating a biological signature for reading and reading disability. Converging evidence from a number of laboratories using functional brain imaging indicates a disruption of left hemisphere posterior brain systems in adult dyslexic readers while performing reading tasks with an additional suggestion for an associated increased reliance on ancillary systems, for example, in the frontal lobe and right hemisphere posterior circuits. The discovery of neural systems serving reading has significant implications. At the most fundamental level, it is now possible to investigate specific hypotheses regarding the neural substrate of dyslexia, and to verify, reject or modify suggested cognitive models. From a more clinical perspective, the identification of neural systems for reading offers the promise for more precise identification and diagnosis of dyslexia in children, adolescents and adults.

Acknowledgements

The work described in this review was supported by grants from the National Institute of Child Health and Human Development (PO1 HD 21888 and P50 HD25802). We thank Carmel Lepore for her help in preparing this manuscript.

References

Anderson A, Gore J: The physical basis of neuroimaging techniques. In Lewis M, Peterson B (Eds), Child and Adolescent Psychiatric Clinics of North America. Vol. 6. Philadelphia, PA: W.B. Saunders Co., pp. 213–264, 1997.

Bakker D: Neuropsychological classification and treatment of dyslexia. Journal of Learning Disabilities: 25(2); 102–109, 1992.

Bakker D, Licht R, Van Strien J: Biopsychological validation of the L- and P-type dyslexia. In Rourke B (Ed), Neuropsychological validation of learning disability subtypes. New York, NY: Guilford Press, pp. 124–139, 1991.

Ben-Dror I, Pollatsek A, Scarpati A: Word identification in isolation and in context by college dyslexic students. Brain and Language: 40; 471–490, 1991.

Bruck M: Persistence of dyslexics' phonological awareness deficits. Developmental Psychology: 28(5); 874–886, 1992.

Bruck M: Outcomes of adults with childhood histories of dyslexia. In Joshi RM (Ed), Cognitive and linguistic bases of reading, writing, and spelling, 1994.

Brunswick N, McCrory E, Price CJ, Frith CD, Frith U: Explicit and implicit processing of words and pseudowords by adult developmental dyslexics: A search for Wernicke's Wortschatz. Brain: 122; 1901–1917, 1999.

Cohen L, Dehaene S, Naccache L, Lehericy S, Dehaene-Lambertz G, Henaff M, Michel F: The visual word form area: Spatial and temporal characterization of an initial stage of reading in normal subjects and posterior split-brain patients. Brain: 123; 291–307, 2000.

Cohen L, Lehéricy S, Chochon F, Lemer C, Rivaud S, Dehaene S: Language-specific tuning of visual cortex? Functional properties of the Visual Word Form Area. Brain: 125; 1054–1069, 2002.

Coltheart M, Curtis B, Atkins P, Haller M: Models of reading aloud: Dual-route and parallel-distributed-processing approaches. Psychological Review: 100; 589–608, 1993.

Corina D, Richards T, Serafini S, et al: fMRI auditory language differences between dyslexic and able reading children. NeuroReport: 12; 1195–1201, 2001.

Damasio AR, Damasio H: The anatomic basis of pure alexia. Neurology: 33; 1573–1583, 1983.

Dehaene S, Le Clec'H G, Poline J, Le Bihan D, Cohen L: The visual word form area: a prelexical representation of visual words in the fusiform gyrus. NeuroReport: 13; 1–5, 2002.

Dehaene S, Naccache L, Cohen L, et al: Cerebral mechanisms of word masking and unconscious repetition priming. Nature Neuroscience: 4; 752–758, 2001.

Dejerine J: Sur un cas de cécité verbale avec agraphie, suivi d'autopsie. C.R. Société du Biologie: 43; 197–201, 1891.
Dejerine J: Contribution a l'etude anatomo-pathologique et clinique des differentes varietes de cecite verbale. Memoires de la Societe de Biologie: 4; 61–90, 1892.
Demb J, Boynton G, Heeger D: Functional magnetic resonance imaging of early visual pathways in dyslexia. Journal of Neuroscience: 18; 6939–6951, 1998.
Demonet JF, Price C, Wise R, Frackowiak RSJ: A PET study of cognitive strategies in normal subjects during language tasks: Influence of phonetic ambiguity and sequence processing on phoneme monitoring. Brain: 117; 671–682, 1994.
Eden GF, VanMeter JW, Rumsey JM, Maisog JM, Woods RP, Zeffiro TA: Abnormal processing of visual motion in dyslexia revealed by functional brain imaging. Nature: 382; 66–69, 1996.
Felton RH, Naylor CE, Wood FB: Neuropsychological profile of adult dyslexics. Brain and Language: 39; 485–497, 1990.
Fiez JA, Peterson SE: Neuroimaging studies of word reading. Proceedings of the National Academy of Sciences USA: 95(3); 914–921, 1998.
Filipek P: Structural variations in measures in the developmental disorders. In Thatcher R, Lyon G, Rumsey J, Krasnegor N (Eds), Developmental Neuroimaging: Mapping the Development of Brain and Behavior. San Diego, CA: Academic Press, pp. 169–186, 1996.
Finucci JM, Childs B: Are there really more dyslexic boys than girls? In Ansara A, Geschwind N, Albert M, Gartrell N (Eds), Sex Differences in Dyslexia. Towson, MD: Orton Dyslexia Society, pp. 1–9, 1981.
Fisher S, DeFries JC: Developmental dyslexia: Genetic dissection of a complex cognitive trait. Nature Reviews Neuorscience: 3; 767–780, 2002.
Fletcher JM, Shaywitz SE, Shankweiler DP, Katz L, Liberman IY, Stuebing KK, Francis DJ, Fowler AE, Shaywitz BA: Cognitive profiles of reading disability: Comparisons of discrepancy and low achievement definitions. Journal of Educational Psychology: 86(1); 6–23, 1994.
Flynn J, Rahbar M: Prevalence of reading failure in boys compared with girls. Psychology in the Schools: 31; 66–71, 1994.
Frackowiak R, Friston K, Frith C, Dolan R, Mazziotta JC: Human Brain Function. New York: Academic Press, 1997.
Francis DJ, Shaywitz SE, Stuebing KK, Shaywitz BA, Fletcher JM: Developmental lag versus deficit models of reading disability: A longitudinal, individual growth curves analysis. Journal of Educational Psychology: 88(1); 3–17, 1996.
Galaburda AM, Sherman GF, Rosen GD, Aboitiz F, Geschwind N: Developmental dyslexia: Four consecutive patients with cortical anomalies. Annals of Neurology: 18(2); 222–233, 1985.
Georgiewa P, Rzanny R, Hopf J, et al: fMRI during word processing in dyslexic and normal reading children. NeuroReport: 10; 3459–3465, 1999.
Geschwind N: Disconnection syndromes in animals and man. Brain: 88; 237–294, 1965.
Gilger JW, Borecki IB, Smith SD, DeFries JC, Pennington BF: The etiology of extreme scores for complex phenotypes: An illustration using reading performance. In Chase CH, Rosen GD, Sherman GF (Eds), Developmental dyslexia. Neural, cognitive, and genetic mechanisms. Baltimore, MD: York Press, pp. 63–85, 1996.
Gough PB, Tunmer WE: Decoding, reading, and reading disability. Remedial and Special Education: 7; 6–10, 1986.
Gross-Glenn K, Duara R, Barker WW, Loewenstein D, Chang J-Y, Yoshii F, Apicella AM, Pascal S, Boothe T, Sevush S, Jallad BJ, Novoa L, Lubs HA: Positron emission tomographic studies during serial word-reading by normal and dyslexic adults. Journal of Clinical and Experimental Neuropsychology: 13(4); 531–544, 1991.
Hagman JO, Wood F, Buchsbaum MS, Tallal P, Flowers L, Katz W: Cerebral brain metabolism in adult dyslexic subjects assessed with positron emission tomography during performance of an auditory task. Archives of Neurology: 49; 734–739, 1992.
Halpern DF: Sex Differences in Cognitive Abilities. Third ed. Mahwah, NJ: Lawrence Erlbaum Associates, 2000.
Helenius P, Tarkiainen A, Cornelissen P, Hansen PC, Salmelin R: Dissociation of normal feature analysis and deficient processing of letter-strings in dyslexic adults. Cerebral Cortex: 4; 476–483, 1999.
Henderson VW: Anatomy of posterior pathways in reading: A reassessment. Brain and Language: 29; 119–133, 1986.
Horwitz B, Rumsey JM, Donohue BC: Functional connectivity of the angular gyrus in normal reading and dyslexia. Proceedings of the National Academy of Science USA: 95; 8939–8944, 1998.
Interagency Committee on Learning Disabilities: Learning disabilities: A report to the U.S. Congress. Washington, DC: U.S. Government Printing Office, 1987.
Jaeger J, Lockwood A, Vanvalin R, Kemmerer D, Murphy B, Wack D: Sex differences in brain regions activated by grammatical and reading tasks. Neuroreport: 9; 2803–2807, 1998.
Kansaku K, Yamaura A, Kitazawa S: Sex differences in lateralization revealed in the posterior language areas. Cerebral Cortex: 10; 866–872, 2000.
Klingberg T, Hedehus M, Temple E, Salz T, Gabrieli J, Moseley M, Poldrack R: Microstructure of temporo-parietal white matter as a basis for reading ability: Evidence from diffusion tensor magnetic resonance imaging. Neuron: 25; 493–500, 2000.
Lefly DL, Pennington BF: Spelling errors and reading fluency in compensated adult dyslexics. Annals of Dyslexia: 41; 143–162, 1991.
Liberman IY, Shankweiler D: Phonology and beginning to read: A tutorial. In Rieben L, Perfetti CA (Eds), Learning to Read: Basic Research and its Implications. Hillsdale, NJ: Lawrence Erlbaum, 1991.
Logan G: Toward an instance theory of automatization. Psychological Review: 95; 492–527, 1988.
Logan G: Automaticity and reading: perspectives from the instance theory of automatization. Reading and Writing Quarterly: Overcoming Learning Disabilities: 13; 123–146, 1997.
Moore C, Price C: Three distinct ventral occiptotemporal regions

for reading and object naming. NeuroImage: 10; 181–192, 1999.

Morris RD, Stuebing KK, Fletcher JM, Shaywitz SE, Lyon GR, Shankweiler DP, Katz L, Francis DJ, Shaywitz BA: Subtypes of reading disability: Variability around a phonological core. Journal of Educational Psychology: 90; 347–373, 1998.

Paulesu E, Demonet J-F, Fazio F, et al: Dyslexia-cultural diversity and biological unity. Science: 291; 2165–2167, 2001.

Paulesu E, Frith U, Snowling M, Gallagher A, Morton J, Frackowiak RSJ, Frith CD: Is developmental dyslexia a disconnection syndrome? Evidence from PET scanning. Brain: 119; 143–157, 1996.

Pennington BF, Gilger JW: How is dyslexia transmitted? In Chase CH, Rosen GD, Sherman GF (Eds), Developmental dyslexia. Neural, cognitive, and genetic mechanisms. Baltimore, MD: York Press, pp. 41–61, 1996.

Petersen SE, Fiez JA: The processing of single words studied with positron emission tomography. Annual Review of Neuroscience: 16; 509–530, 1993.

Price C, Moore C, Frackowiak RSJ: The effect of varying stimulus rate and duration on brain activity during reading. Neuroimage: 3(1); 40–52, 1996.

Report of the National Reading Panel: Teaching Children to Read: An Evidence-Based Assessment of the Scientific Research Literature on Reading and its Implications for Reading Instruction. Bethesda, MD: National Institute of Child Health and Human Development, National Institutes of Health, 2000.

Rumsey JM, Andreason P, Zametkin AJ, Aquino T, King C, Hamburber SD, Pikus A, Rapoport JL, Cohen RM: Failure to activate the left temporoparietal cortex in dyslexia. Archives of Neurology: 49; 527–534, 1992.

Rumsey JM, Nace K, Donohue B, Wise D, Maisog JM, Andreason P: A positron emission tomographic study of impaired word recognition and phonological processing in dyslexic men. Archives of Neurology: 54; 562–573, 1997.

Rumsey JM, Zametkin AJ, Andreason P, Hanahan AP, Hamburger SD, Aquino T, King C, Pikus A, Cohen RM: Normal activation of frontotemporal language cortex in dyslexia, as measured with oxygen 15 positron emission tomography. Archives of Neurology: 51; 27–38, 1994.

Salmelin R, Service E, Kiesila P, Uutela K, Salonen O: Impaired visual word processing in dyslexia revealed with magnetoencephalography. Annals of Neurology: 40; 157–162, 1996.

Scarborough HS: Continuity between childhood dyslexia and adult reading. British Journal of Psychology: 75; 329–348, 1984.

Scarborough HS: Very early language deficits in dyslexic children. Child Development: 61; 1728–1743, 1990.

Seki A, Koeda T, Sugihara S, et al: A functional magnetic resonance imaging study during sentence reading in Japanese dyslexic children. Brain and Development: 23; 312–316, 2001.

Shankweiler D, Crain S, Katz L, Fowler AE, Liberman AM, Brady SA, Thornton R, Lundquist E, Dreyer L, Fletcher JM, Stuebing KK, Shaywitz SE, Shaywitz BA: Cognitive profiles of reading-disabled children: Comparison of language skills in phonology, morphology, and syntax. Psychological Science: 6(3); 149–156, 1995.

Shankweiler D, Liberman IY, Mark LS, Fowler CA, Fischer FW: The speech code and learning to read. Journal of Experimental Psychology: Human Learning and Memory: 5(6); 531–545, 1979.

Share DL: Phonological recoding and self-teaching: Sine qua non of reading acquisition. Cognition: 55; 151–218, 1995.

Share DL, Stanovich KE: Cognitive processes in early reading development: Accommodating individual differences into a model of acquisition. Issues in Education: Contributions from Educational Psychology: 1(1); 1–57, 1995.

Shaywitz B, Pugh KR, Jenner A, Fulbright RK, Fletcher JM, Gore JC, Shaywitz S: The neurobiology of reading and reading disability (dyslexia). In Kamil M, Mosenthal P, Pearson P, Barr R (Eds), Handbook of Reading Research. Vol. III. Mahwah, NJ: Lawrence Erlbaum Associates, pp. 229–249, 2000.

Shaywitz B, Shaywitz S, Pugh K, Constable R, Skudlarski P, Fulbright R, Bronen R, Fletcher J, Shankweiler D, Katz L, Gore J: Sex differences in the functional organization of the brain for language. Nature: 373; 607–609, 1995a.

Shaywitz BA, Holford TR, Holahan JM, Fletcher JM, Stuebing KK, Francis DJ, Shaywitz SE: A Matthew effect for IQ but not for reading: Results from a longitudinal study. Reading Research Quarterly: 30(4); 894–906, 1995b.

Shaywitz BA, Shaywitz SE, Pugh KR, et al: Disruption of posterior brain systems for reading in children with developmental dyslexia. Biological Psychiatry: 52; 101–110, 2002.

Shaywitz S: Current Concepts: Dyslexia. The New England Journal of Medicine: 338(5); 307–312, 1998.

Shaywitz S, Shaywitz B: Dyslexia. In Swaiman K, Ashwal S (Eds), Pediatric Neurology: Principles and Practice. Third ed., Vol. 1. St. Louis, MO: Mosby, pp. 576–584, 1999.

Shaywitz S, Shaywitz B, Pugh K, Fulbright R, Mencl W, Constable R, Skudlarski P, Fletcher J, Lyon G, Gore J: The neurobiology of dyslexia. Clinical Neuroscience Research, 1, 291–299, 2001.

Shaywitz SE: Dyslexia. Scientific American: 275(5); 98–104, 1996.

Shaywitz SE, Escobar MD, Shaywitz BA, Fletcher JM, Makuch R: Evidence that dyslexia may represent the lower tail of a normal distribution of reading ability. New England Journal of Medicine: 326(3); 145–150, 1992.

Shaywitz SE, Fletcher JM, Holahan JM, Shneider AE, Marchione KE, Stuebing KK, Francis DJ, Pugh KR, Shaywitz BA: Persistence of dyslexia: The Connecticut Longitudinal Study at adolescence. Pediatrics: 104; 1351–1359, 1999.

Shaywitz SE, Fletcher JM, Shaywitz BA: Issues in the definition and classification of attention deficit disorder. Topics in Language Disorders: 14(4); 1–25, 1994.

Shaywitz SE, Shaywitz BA, Fletcher JM, Escobar MD: Prevalence of reading disability in boys and girls: Results of the Connecticut Longitudinal Study. Journal of the American Medical Association: 264(8); 998–1002, 1990.

Shaywitz SE, Shaywitz BA, Pugh KR et al: Functional disruption in the organization of the brain for reading in dyslexia. Proceedings of the National Academy of Science USA: 95; 2636–2641, 1998.

Simos P, Breier J, Fletcher J, Bergman E, Papanicolaou A: Cerebral Mechanisms Involved in Word Reading in Dyslexic Children: A Magnetic Source Imaging Approach. Cerebral Cortex: 10; 809–816, 2000.

Stanovich KE, Siegel LS: Phenotypic performance profile of children with reading disabilities: A regression-based test of the phonological-core variable-difference model. Journal of Educational Psychology: 86(1); 24–53, 1994.

Stein J, Walsh V: To see but not to read; the magnocellular theory of dyslexia. Trends in Neurosciences: 20(4); 147–152, 1997.

Talcott J, Witton C, McLean M, Hansen P, Rees A, Green G, Stein J: Dynamic sensory sensitivity and children's word decoding skills. Proceedings of the National Academy of Sciences USA: 97; 2952–2957, 2000.

Tallal P: The science of literacy: From the laboratory to the classroom. Proceedings of the National Academy of Sciences USA: 97; 2402–2404, 2000.

Temple E, Poldrack R, Protopapas A, et al: Disruption of the neural response to rapid acoustic stimuli in dyslexia: evidence from functional MRI. Proceedings of the National Academy of Science USA: 97; 13907–13912, 2000.

Torgesen JK: Phonological Awareness: A Critical Factor in Dyslexia. Orton Dyslexia Society, 1995.

Wadsworth SJ, DeFries JC, Stevenson J, Gilger JW, Pennington BF: Gender ratios among reading-disabled children and their siblings as a function of parental impairment. Journal of Child Psychology and Psychiatry: 33(7); 1229–1239:

Wagner R, Torgesen J: The nature of phonological processes and its causal role in the acquisition of reading skills. Psychological Bulletin: 101; 192–212, 1987.

Witelson SF, Kigar DL: Sylvian fissure morphology and asymmetry in men and women: Bilateral differences in relation to handedness in men. Journal of Comparative Neurology: 323; 326–340, 1992.

Wolf M: Naming speed and reading: The contribution of the cognitive neurosciences. Reading Research Quarterly: 26(2); 123–141, 1991.

Wolf M, Bowers PG: The double-deficit hypothesis for the developmental dyslexias. Journal of Educational Psychology: 91(3); 415–438, 1999.

Woodcock RW, Johnson MB: Woodcock–Johnson Psycho-Educational Battery: Revised (WJ-R). Allen, TX: Developmental Learning Materials, 1989.

Handbook of Neuropsychology, 2nd Edition, Vol. 8, Part II
S.J. Segalowitz and I. Rapin (Eds)

CHAPTER 25

Neuropsychological perspectives on reading development and developmental reading disorders

Maureen W. Lovett [a,*] and Roderick W. Barron [b]

[a] *Brain and Behaviour Program, The Hospital for Sick Children, Departments of Paediatrics and Psychology, University of Toronto, 555 University Avenue, Toronto, ON MSG 1X8, Canada*
[b] *Department of Psychology, University of Guelph, Guelph, ON N1G 2W1, Canada*

> And so to completely analyze what we do when we read would almost be the acme of a psychologist's achievements, for it would be to describe very many of the most intricate workings of the human mind, as well as to unravel the tangled story of the most remarkable specific performance that civilization has learned in all its history.
>
> *Edmund Burke Huey (1908)*

> I don't have any trouble with the sentences; it's the words that get in my way.
>
> *A 9-year-old struggling reader, 2000*

> Putting aside the intellectual excitement and cultural (and historical and evolutionary) significance inherent in understanding developmental dyslexia, the core meaning of this work is to help. . . perhaps millions of children who are struggling to master reading. Helping, however, requires understanding.
>
> *Elena L. Grigorenko, 2001*

Introduction

At the beginning of this third millennium, much has been learned about the mental processes and cognitive skills that allow humans to represent language and meaning in visible form — as print. There is greater understanding of the cognitive and biological underpinnings of this complex system of behaviors, although a great deal more remains to be discovered. As Huey marvelled in his seminal book on the psychology of reading almost a century ago, reading can be conceptualized as a skill set by which an "arbitrary conventional set of symbols is used to transfer information from one mind to another" (1908). How individuals acquire these skills and the neurobiological substrates required for their acquisition and subsequent fluent execution have been but a fraction of the central questions motivating the widespread scientific interest and activity devoted to the study of reading in past decades.

Klein and McMullen (1999) note that less than 500 years ago reading was a relatively elite and undersubscribed skill, confined to monks and a small group of scholars. Access to printed information through the invention of the printing press permitted reading to become a more universal form of information exchange. Although reading is far too recent a human achievement to be considered the product of evolution, rapid technological changes and far-reaching cultural developments have rendered the successful acquisition of reading and related literacy skills a prerequisite for individuals in any countries participating in and shaping the information age. And yet one of the most common developmental disorders of childhood involves an unexpected failure in otherwise normally developing children to learn to read.

In this chapter, we will describe this developmental neurocognitive disorder, currently labeled as developmental reading disorders. We will attempt to

* Corresponding author. E-mail: mwl@sickkids.ca

summarize what is known to date of the prevalence of these disorders and the status of current etiological speculations. Much of the chapter will focus upon identifying the core processing deficits which appear central to the signature symptom behaviors of individuals with reading disabilities. In this chapter we will ask what predicts reading acquisition success, and whether there is sufficient evidence to allow us to identify children at risk of reading disorder; in addition, we will explore the available literature on what constitutes effective early intervention. In the latter pages of this chapter, we will consider the biological foundations of the disorder, as well as the question of what constitutes effective intervention for a child with significant reading disorder and to what extent the disorder is amenable to remediation. Finally, we will suggest a set of unanswered questions relevant to diagnosis and treatment of developmental reading disorders.

Historical overview

That a small proportion of otherwise intelligent healthy children fail to recognize language in its visible form was recognized before 1900. Both Hinshelwood (1895) and Morgan (1896) discussed a syndrome they referred to as "visual word blindness". These early conceptualizations of dyslexia were shaped by what was understood of reading loss or alexia in adults with acquired brain damage (Spreen, Tupper, Risser et al., 1984), although there was early recognition of some differences between a loss of previously acquired reading skill (alexia) and a failure to ever acquire reading skills (dyslexia) (Fletcher, Foorman, Shaywitz and Shaywitz, 1999).

One of the most influential early investigators of reading disorder was the neurologist Samuel Orton (1925), who proposed that dyslexia could be attributed to incomplete or mixed cerebral dominance, suggesting that delayed development of specialization of the left hemisphere for language was potentially causal. Orton's theory has led to a number of educational interventions patterned more after the linguistic than the neurological basis of his speculations. His ideas formed the basis for a number of educational therapies for dyslexic individuals, some of which remain popular today (Ansara, 1982; Gillingham and Stillman, 1960) and are known as adaptations of the Orton–Gillingham method — a structured language program which uses multisensory feedback to reinforce the learning of letter–sound relationships for struggling readers. The approach is born of Orton's longstanding collaboration with the linguist Anne Gillingham; many other multisensory teaching programs have modified and adapted the basic theme of teaching language structure in a systematic, cumulative, and careful manner (Hall and Moats, 1999). Project Read, a recent US programming initiative for children with reading difficulties, adheres to many of the Orton–Gillingham principles. Orton's ideas have also inspired some innovative therapies purportedly designed to directly remediate incomplete cerebral dominance for language (Tomatis, 1978); controlled evaluations, however, have not demonstrated the therapeutic effectiveness of these interventions for developmental dyslexia (Kershner, Cummings, Clarke et al., 1986, 1990). Controlled evaluations of the Orton–Gillingham and related educational therapies have been limited.

Defining developmental reading disorders

In 1968, the World Federation of Neurology defined specific developmental dyslexia as "a disorder manifested by difficulty in learning to read despite conventional instruction, adequate intelligence, and sociocultural opportunity". The disorder was attributed to "fundamental cognitive disabilities which are frequently of constitutional origin" (Critchley, 1970). Dissatisfied with the exclusionary flavor and lack of etiological specificity in this definition, other authors suggested that dyslexia can be attributed "to a well-defined defect in any one of several specific higher cortical functions" (Mattis, 1978, p. 54).

Some investigators attempted greater specificity in moving towards a positive definition: Denckla (1979) described dyslexia as "usually the index symptom of a developmental language disorder too subtle to lead to a referral of the child in preschool life" (p. 550). In addition to her important early emphasis on the speech and language concomitants of dyslexia for many children, Denckla also drew attention to the plurality of the disorder, contending that there is not one dyslexia, but rather a group of dyslexias — just as in adult neurology different forms of alexia were acknowledged. In recent years, investigators from related fields have questioned the specificity of the concept of developmental dyslexia, and have demonstrated that some of the cognitive deficits considered potential precursors of the disorder may in fact be more appropriately considered as sequelae (e.g., Stanovich, 1986). Recent classification studies have confirmed the plurality of the disorder while characterizing variability around a core of more central well-defined processing deficits (Morris, Stuebing, Fletcher et al., 1998).

The concept of reading disorder as a language-based disability is still widely embraced more than 75 years after Samuel Orton's first publications on what he termed strephosymbolia. The International Dyslexia Association (previously the Orton Dyslexia Society) proposed a working definition of developmental reading disability/dyslexia in 1994. This consensus definition suggested dyslexia had to be a specific language-based disorder of constitutional origin, characterized by difficulties in single word decoding and frequently unexpected in relationship to an individual's age and other cognitive and academic abilities. According to this language-based definition, reading disability was suggested not to be the consequence of general developmental delay or specific sensory impairment, but rather to be associated with variable difficulties with different aspects of speech and language development, and often including concurrent problems with writing and spelling acquisition.

In the same year, DSM-IV, the fourth edition of the Diagnostic and Statistical Manual of Mental Disorders, published by the American Psychiatric Association, defined developmental reading disorder/dyslexia as reading achievement on individual testing found to be significantly below what would be expected on the basis of the individual's speech, intelligence, and education. To be diagnosed as having a reading disorder, the impairment could not be attributable to sensory disorder and was required to be clinically significant, interfering with academic, career, or life activities requiring literacy skills. This definition was notable for its recognition of multidimensional criteria of reading achievement; the DSM-IV suggests reading underachievement can be defined by accuracy, speed, or comprehension skill criteria on individual testing. It should be noted, however, that both definitions proposed in the mid-1990s were discrepancy-based and to some extent still diagnoses by exclusionary criteria.

Current definitional issues

Discrepancy-based definitions of reading disorder have dominated clinical practice, psychoeducational assessment, access to special education services, and a majority of clinical research studies in the field. For many decades, reading disability criteria were considered to be met only when an individual's reading achievement fell significantly below what would be predicted based on estimates of intellectual functioning. A prototypical discrepancy-based formula might place as the criterion for reading disorder reading performance on standardized assessment instruments that fell at least one and a half standard deviations below the level of achievement predicted by full-scale IQ. This formula adopts a regression-adjusted discrepancy of one-and-a-half standard errors based on a correlation between IQ and reading achievement of +0.68.

Scientifically it had long been believed that if reading disorders were defined by discrepancy-based definitions in clinical research, the investigator would be more likely to recruit samples of individuals with purer diagnostic profiles and greater specificity with respect to the core processing deficits underlying their reading disorder. Historically, it is interesting that these themes of deficit severity and intellectual context are still being discussed with regard to current classifications of reading disorder; these concepts were previewed in part in very early considerations of reading problems.

As early as 1917, Hinshelwood described the syndrome he called congenital word blindness, or "congenital dyslexia", as a disorder in which the defect in reading was very severe and related symptoms relatively pure. Hinshelwood described such children as very late to develop reading skills but responsive to remedial interventions. In contrast, Hinshelwood would diagnose the condition he called "congenital alexia" if the child experienced reading acquisition problems in the context of generally low intellectual ability. Thus Hinshelwood's diagnostic classifications for individual patients varied according to his perception of symptom severity, profile specificity, and intellectual profile.

Another approach to defining reading disorder ignores the positive correlation with IQ in classification and diagnoses individuals based upon documented underachievement relative to age and grade level expectations on standardized test instruments. The low achievement definition of reading disorder is attracting increasing support from both scientists and practitioners in the learning disabilities (Fletcher, Shaywitz, Shankweiler et al., 1994; Francis, Shaywitz, Stuebing et al., 1996; Siegel, 1992; Stanovich, 2000; Stanovich and Siegel, 1994).

An influential epidemiological study was conducted in the late 1960s and early 1970s by Rutter and Yule (1975; Rutter, 1978). These investigators collected an epidemiological sample of children on the Isle of Wight, in Wales, and in the course of their investigations of development and developmental anomalies, addressed basic concepts related to the definition and specificity of reading disability. When they studied the distribution of reading performance in their developmental sample, the distribution appeared bimodal, with what appeared as a 'hump' in the lower end of the distribution and expected patterns of normal distribution near the average. These findings led Rutter and Yule to speculate that there were indeed two different types of reading disorder in children, a disorder of "specific reading retardation" characterizing individuals with reading achievement significantly below what would be predicted based on age norms and IQ scores (i.e., discrepancy-defined cases), and a disorder they labeled "general reading backwardness" characterizing those cases with reading performance consistent with IQ expectations but significantly below age-based expectations. The latter group included children with lower IQs and poor reading achievement. These children would meet low-achievement but not IQ-discrepancy definitions of reading disability today. Thus the Isle of Wight epidemiological study was often cited to support the idea that discrepancy definitions of reading underachievement in relation to IQ were necessary to study the 'true' phenomenon of developmental dyslexia.

Although Rutter and Yule's work was a significant contribution on many developmental issues and noteworthy for its time, many methodological criticisms and interpretive reservations can now be raised particularly regarding their findings on reading disability (Fletcher, Foorman, Shaywitz and Shaywitz, 1999). In their reviews, Fletcher et al. (1999a) and Shaywitz, Fletcher and Shaywitz (1996) suggest that the bimodality results may be an artifact of a ceiling effect on the reading measures used (Van der Wissel and Zegers, 1985), skewing reading scores to the left and creating an artifactual hump in the distribution that may actually reflect not an overrepresentation of poor readers but rather an underrepresentation of good readers. The results of the Isle of Wight study can also be challenged for a failure to employ any exclusionary criteria in sample definitions (Fletcher, Francis, Shaywitz et al., 1998). The general reading backwardness group included a number of children with diagnosed CNS disorders (11.4%) and a larger subsample with suspected CNS disorders (25.3%); in contrast, the specific reading retardation group had no cases of diagnosed CNS disorders and only 18.6% with possible CNS involvement. When exclusionary criteria have been applied (typically excluding children with known causes of potential underachievement such as sensory impairment and frank neurological disorder), no evidence of bimodality or a 'hump' at the bottom of the distribution of reading scores in epidemiological samples has been replicated.

The most influential epidemiological study in this field to date is the Connecticut Longitudinal Study (CLS) in which a cohort of 445 children representative of all Connecticut children entering kindergarten in 1983 have been followed into late adolescence (Shaywitz, Fletcher, Holahan et al., 1999; Shaywitz, Shaywitz, Fletcher and Escobar, 1990). A classification study of children who met criteria for reading disorder by either discrepancy-based or low achievement criteria revealed no evidence of a bimodal distribution of reading scores. Instead the CLS data indicated that reading ability and disability fall along a normal distribution, much like blood pressure readings, and the decision of what constitutes disability in reading skill or hypertension involves selection of an arbitrary cut-off value on the distribution (Shaywitz et al., 1990; Shaywitz, Escobar, Shaywitz et al., 1992; Shaywitz et al., 1999). As Fletcher et al. (1998, 1999a) caution, the key for research purposes is to measure appropriate reading skills and to demonstrate a well-defined and replicable cut-point in dimensional classifications. As Shaywitz and her colleagues describe it, reading disorder is now recognized as the lower tail of a normal distribution: "reading difficulties, including dyslexia, occur as part of a continuum that includes normal reading ability" (Shaywitz et al., 1992, p. 145).

The CLS results also provide important insight into the nature of the processing deficits limiting reading development in children defined by IQ discrepancy vs low achievement criteria. It should be noted that 75 percent of the CLS reading disabled sample defined by IQ achievement discrepancies also meet the criterion for reading disorder by low achievement criteria (Shaywitz et al., 1996). This result parallels that obtained in the Isle of Wight study where 88% of specific reading retardation children also met criteria for general reading backwardness (Rutter, Tizard and Whitmore, 1970). When discrepancy-identified and low achievement-identified groups were compared in this CLS sample, more similarities than differences were observed, with the only meaningful differences attributable to the expected IQ disparity between the groups and inherent in their definition (Shaywitz et al., 1996).

Additional investigations of this question have confirmed that there are no meaningful differences in reading disability symptoms, long term outcomes, phenotype or genotype profiles between groups identified by these different criteria for reading disability (Fletcher et al., 1994; Francis et al., 1996; Stanovich and Siegel, 1994). There appear to be no qualitative differences in the diagnostic profiles of the two groups on reading and reading-related measures, with the most pervasive and persistent common deficit falling in the domain of phonological processing. As Stanovich and Siegel (1994, p. 48) conclude

> neither the phenotypic nor the genotypic indicators of poor reading are correlated in any reliable way with IQ discrepancy. If there is a special group of children with reading disabilities who are behaviorally, cognitively, genetically, or neurologically different, it is becoming increasingly unlikely that they can be easily identified by using IQ discrepancy as a proxy for the genetic and neurological differences themselves. Thus, the basic assumption that underlies decades of classification in research and educational practice regarding reading disabilities is becoming increasingly untenable.

While some investigators propose complete adoption of the low achievement definition in identifying disabled readers solely based on performance with respect to age level expectations (e.g., Siegel, 1988, 1989, 1992), others contend that there exist significant problems with this solution. Fletcher et al. (1998) argue that the low achievement definition alone does not address the issue of high IQ underachieving readers whose reading underachievement may not be low enough according to age norms to be detected as deficient despite being significantly below intellectual expectations. In the Fletcher et al. (1994) analyses, these children constituted less than 12% of the sample and were labelled as discrepant-only cases. Another parallel concern at the other end of the IQ distribution is the issue of where and how to distinguish learning disabilities from mental deficiency. Finally, the severity cut-off of what is significantly below age level expectations requires clarification, with obvious implications for publicly funded education systems and children's access to special educational services. Fletcher et al. (1998) recommend a move towards domain-specific assessments of achievement and related achievement-related abilities.

The prevalence of developmental reading disorders and cross-linguistic comparisons

Estimates of the prevalence of reading disorders vary considerably according to the type of definition used. When the standard IQ-achievement discrepancy definition has been used in epidemiological studies, developmental reading disability has been estimated to affect between 4% and 10% of school-age children in the U.S. (American Psychiatric Association, 1994; Shaywitz et al., 1990) and between 6 and 7% of 9 and 10-year-old children in the U.K. (Lewis, Hitch and Walker, 1994). When low achievement definitions are used, between 17% and 20% of U.S. children are considered to have reading disorders (Shaywitz et al., 1996) — one in every five children in the school system!

Prevalence estimates vary considerably around the world. A survey of data from 26 different countries was reported two decades ago by Tarnapol and Tarnapol (1981). Their review revealed the lowest prevalence of reading disorder among school-age children in Japan and China (1%), and the highest prevalence rate in Venezuela (33%). An overall median rate of 7% was reported. English-speaking countries tended to report higher prevalence rates, approximating up to 20% of the school population. In Scandinavian countries, a prevalence rate approximating 10% was reported, with a 5% rate attributed in Germany (Glezerman, 1983). The prevalence of reading disorder in Italy has been estimated to be about one half that found in the United States (Lindgren, De Renzi and Richman, 1985).

While observed differences in prevalence are undoubtedly partially attributable to differences in cultural values and educational practices around literacy instruction in different countries, there is also evidence that the relationship of orthography and phonology in different languages may play an important role in the frequency with which beginning readers encounter difficulty. Languages differ considerably in phonological characteristics (Mattingly, 1985), and in the consistency with which spelling maps onto sound in orthographic representations. In what have been called 'phonologically shallow' orthographies, letters alone or in combination are in most cases uniquely mapped to each of the speech sounds in the language; orthography represents phonology almost directly (Grigorenko, 2001; Paulesu, Démonet, Fazio et al., 2001). In 'phonologically deep' orthographies, the mapping between letters, speech sounds, and whole word pronunciations often appears highly ambiguous because restrictions on orthographic sequences are constrained not only by phonology, but also by the etymology and morphology of the language (Grigorenko, 2001; Paulesu et al., 2001).

The deepest orthographies are considered to be French, Danish, and English. Learning to read in deep orthographies like French and English is far more difficult than learning to read a language with shallow orthography like Italian (Paulesu et al., 2001). Finnish, Greek, Italian, Spanish, German, and Norwegian are considered languages with shallow orthographies. Languages such as Icelandic, Dutch, Swedish, and Portuguese are characterized as having intermediate orthographies (Grigorenko, 2001).

The enormous diversity in the regularity with which spelling maps onto sound in different languages contributes in a significant way to the difficulty of the reading acquisition process-particularly for at-risk children. At the same time, however, there is increasing consensus that phonological processes represent a universal and important foundation of reading acquisition success in all phonological writing systems. The following sections will examine prerequisite skills involved in successful reading development by normal early readers. Special attention will be paid the role of phonological awareness and phonological processing skills in early reading development and in reading acquisition failure. The core processing deficits that appear signature and potentially causal features of reading disability will be reviewed. Final sections will examine the available evidence on the neurobiology of reading disorders and the efficacy of treatment.

Phonological core processes and predictors of reading skill acquisition

Research on how reading is acquired normally provides critical foundation information for understanding developmental reading disability (Adams, 1990; Adams, Treiman and Pressley, 1998). Investigations of the cognitive and linguistic prerequisites for learning to read, particularly those dealing with the non-reading skills and knowledge that predict reading skill acquisition, have been influential in identifying the underlying deficits that characterize developmental reading disability as well as providing evidence-based rationales for prevention and remediation programs (Rayner, Foorman, Perfetti et al., 2001). Before reviewing this research on predictors of reading skill, it is important to note that obtaining meaning from print, the primary goal of learning to read, requires beginning readers to learn first how print represents their spoken language.

In order to learn to read alphabetic orthographies such as English or French or Italian, children must learn the principle that the letters of the alphabet represent the individual phonemes into which spoken words can be decomposed (Liberman, 1997, 1998, 1999). Letters themselves are not the primary problem in learning to read because they are physically discrete visual units. Phonemes are the problem.

The phonemes making up a syllable are produced by very rapid, overlapping motor gestures; this co-articulation yields a seamless representation in which the acoustic and articulatory information for the individual phonemes overlap. The result is that the phonemes are not physically discrete acoustic units; they are embedded within a syllable making it difficult for children to access them and become aware of them as separate mental objects to which graphemes (a letter or a letter cluster) can be associated (Bryne, 1998).

In practical terms, children need to know that the word *fleet*, for example, consists of the phonemes /f/, /l/, /i/, /t/. They can demonstrate this knowledge in phoneme awareness tasks that typically require listening to a word presented orally, repeating it aloud, and then matching, deleting, categorizing, identifying, counting, blending, or reordering its constituent phonemes (e.g., Stahl and Murray, 1994; Wagner and Torgesen, 1987). In phoneme elision, one of the most sensitive and widely used phoneme awareness tasks (Schatschneider, Francis, Foorman et al., 1999), a child might hear a monosyllabic word like *fleet*, repeat it, and then pronounce it after deleting the first (/f/), or second (/l/), or final phoneme (/t/). Young children (pre-schoolers) demonstrate precursors to phoneme awareness in tasks in which segmentation is required but the units are more accessible because they consist of syllables or onsets and rimes within syllables (e.g., onset = /fl/, rime = /it/) rather than individual phonemes (e.g., Bryant, Bradley, Maclean and Crossland, 1989; Lonigan, Burgess, Anthony and Barker, 1998).

Longitudinal studies indicate that individual differences in performance on phoneme awareness tasks are very stable. Wagner, Torgesen, Rashotte et al. (1997), in their seminal longitudinal study, found year-to-year correlations in phonemic awareness performance from Kindergarten through fourth grade ranging between $r = 0.83$ and 0.95; with the correlation between phoneme awareness in Kindergarten and fourth grade at $r = 0.63$. Phoneme awareness at the time of school entry (Kindergarten) accounts for unique variance in word reading skill over several subsequent grades (e.g., Wagner, Torgesen and Rashotte, 1994). Wagner et al. (1997) and Torgesen, Wagner, Rashotte et al. (1997) found that phonological awareness was a unique predictor of word reading in the first through the fifth grades even when the influence of word reading skill in prior grades (Kindergarten through the third grade) was controlled statistically. This latter finding provides crucial evidence that phonemic awareness plays a causal role in word reading acquisition because the autoregressor variable of word reading skill in the early grades is a primary predictor of word reading in the later grades and typically accounts for the majority of the word reading variance in subsequent grades.

Phonemic awareness tasks are memory-intensive, and verbal working memory is correlated with reading skill (e.g., Baddeley, 1986; Brady and Shankweiler, 1991). Measures of verbal working memory, particularly those involving oral language processing tasks such as sentence repetition and story recall, are strong predictors of reading skill (Badian, 1998). Phoneme awareness is not, however, the same thing as verbal working memory because phoneme awareness accounts for variance in reading skill even when measures of verbal working memory are controlled statistically (Cormier and Dea, 1997; Hansen and Bowey, 1994), and Wagner et al. (1997) showed that verbal working memory was not an independent, unique predictor of reading skill when compared to phonemic awareness in their longitudinal study. Finally, Bowey (1994) reported that phonemic awareness is related to reading skill even in tasks in which cognitive and memory demands are reduced through the use of matching tasks and pictures (e.g., "Which pictured item, cat or dog, begins with the same sound as cap?").

Serial, rapid automatized naming (RAN; Denckla and Rudel, 1976) tasks in which children name sequences of familiar letters, numbers, objects, and colors as rapidly as possible are also strong predictors of word reading skill (Wolf, Bally and Morris, 1986; Wolf and Bowers, 1999; Wolf, Goldberg, Gidney et al., 2002). They are statistically independent of phonological awareness in longitudinal studies (Wagner et al., 1997) and tend to be more strongly associated with measures of orthographic processing, comprehension, and fluency (Bowers, Sunseth and Golden, 1999; Manis, Seidenberg and Doi, 1999) than phoneme awareness tasks. Wagner et al. (1997; see also Manis et al., 1999) have shown that RAN is a unique predictor of word reading skill through the third grade even when the autoregressive effects of word reading skill in Kindergarten and first grade were controlled statistically. These results indicate that rapid serial naming is independent of phoneme awareness and is causally related to word reading ability but that it influences word reading over a shorter time period than phonological awareness.

There are empirical and theoretical reasons for regarding phoneme awareness and rapid serial naming as independent predictors of word reading skill, particularly with reference to subtypes of developmental reading disability and approaches to remediation which will be considered in a later section of this chapter (e.g., Lovett, Steinbach and Frijters, 2000; Wolf, 1991; Wolf and Bowers, 1999; Wolf, Bowers and Biddle, 2000; Wolf, Miller and Donnelly, 2000). Some investigators, however, regard these two skills as part of a core of phonological processing skills which involve accessing, maintaining, and using precise phonological representations of verbal information (Goswami and Bryant, 1990; Share, 1995; Stanovich, 1988, 2000; Stanovich and Siegel, 1994; Wagner et al., 1994).

Research during the past 30 years has yielded considerable agreement that word reading and nonword decoding draw heavily upon core phonological processing skills (Adams, 1990; Goswami and Bryant, 1990; Share, 1995; Stanovich, 2000). In addition to being causal predictors of reading acquisition (Bradley and Bryant, 1983; Manis et al., 1999; Wagner et al., 1997), phonological skills provide a neurocognitive signature for the phenotype of developmental reading disability when they are deficient (Bradley and Bryant, 1978; Fletcher et al., 1994, 1999a; Stanovich and Siegel, 1994). They are the primary behavioral indices used in studies of the underlying brain and genetic bases of reading skill performance and breakdown (Grigorenko, Wood, Meyer et al., 1997; Paulesu et al., 2001; Shaywitz, Shaywitz, Pugh et al., 1998; see Grigorenko, 2001; Habib, 2000; and Pennington, 1999 for reviews) as well as the primary target of efforts to improve reading skill through early intervention and later remediation (Foorman, Francis, Fletcher et al., 1998; Hatcher, Hulme and Ellis, 1994; Lovett, Steinbach and Frijters, 2000; Olson, Wise, Ring and Johnson, 1997; Pennington, 1999; Torgesen, Wagner, Rashotte et al., 1999; Vellutino, Scanlon, Sipay et al., 1996; see Lovett and Barron, 2002; Snowling, 1996; and Swanson and Hoskyn, 1998 for reviews)

Predictors of reading skill and children 'at risk' for developmental reading disorders

But reading is a very complex cognitive process. It begins with the analysis of a string of small, discrete visual patterns; integrates information from visual–spatial and auditory–temporal domains, involves rapid, precise visual–motor coordination and timing; draws upon attentional and working memory resources; utilizes syntactic and semantic as well as phonological levels of language processing; and recruits a number of different areas of the brain. In other words, there is more to reading than phonological processes and it is possible that measures other than those which index phonological processes might account for individual differences in learning to read, fluent reading performance, and reading disability. Research on the predictors of reading skill acquisition and early identification of children at risk for developmental reading disabilities is a valuable source of information on individual differences in the contribution of phonological versus non-phonological processes in the early stages of learning to read.

The skills and knowledge required to benefit from formal instruction in reading begin to be acquired during the preschool years but children arrive at school with vastly different levels of readiness and those at the lower end of the distribution may be at risk for developmental reading disability. Identifying children who are at risk is, of course, a first step toward early intervention and prevention but one major difficulty with early as opposed to later identification is that the target behavior of reading has yet to be acquired.

Scarborough (1998) conducted a comprehensive survey of concurrent and longitudinal studies of predictors of early reading skill in which the predictors were assessed one year before, at the same time, or one year after formal reading instruction began and the outcome assessment of reading was made after one to three years of instruction. Her sample was based on studies published between 1976 and 1996 and the mean correlations between representative predictors and reading outcome measures are presented in Fig. 1. The number of studies per predictor ranged from 4 to 27 and the total N per predictor ranged from 300 to over 1000.

Fig. 1 shows that print-specific predictors, such as letter identification, had the highest correlations

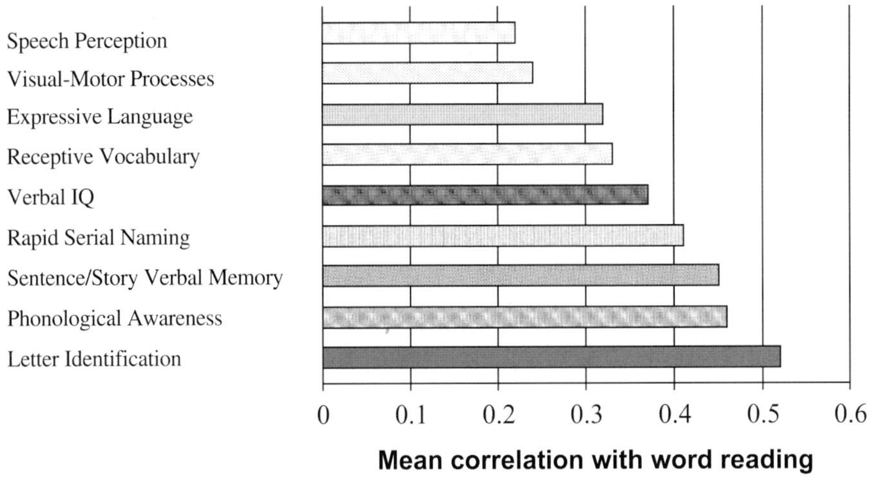

Fig. 1. Predictors of Word Reading Skill. (Adapted from Scarborough, 1998.)

with reading, while measures of language skill that involve phonological processing, such as rapid serial naming, verbal memory, and phonological awareness, have the strongest correlations among the non-print predictors. Verbal IQ, as well as measures of vocabulary, are more moderate predictors. The weakest predictors tend to involve motor skills, visual perceptual processes, and speech perception, even though the latter is often regarded as a phonologically-based language skill (e.g., McBride-Chang, 1995a,b; McBride-Chang and Manis, 1996).

Environmental influences on reading acquisition, such as the reported frequency with which parents read to their children, is also a relatively weak predictor (mean $r = 0.28$; Bus, Van Ijzendoorn and Pelligrini, 1995; Scarborough and Dobrich, 1994) although prediction is improved when a wider range of home literacy activity is measured (Frijters, Barron and Brunello, 2000). Socioeconomic status (SES) was also a relatively weak predictor (mean $r = 0.23$) when reading achievement and SES were correlated for individuals within a school. The correlation between SES and reading achievement is much higher (mean $r = 0.68$), however, when the data consist of average SES and reading achievement scores for schools and school districts rather than individuals (White, 1982).

Scarborough's (1998) survey provides further evidence that print-specific and non-print phonological processing variables are primary predictors of future reading skill. Although the list of predictors is not exhaustive, non-phonological influences such as visual, motor, socioeconomic, and home literacy variables make less of a contribution. Consistent with Torgesen et al. (1997) and Wagner et al. (1994, 1997), none of the measures was as highly correlated with word reading skill as measures of reading skill taken in prior years ($r = 0.72$). Scarborough (1998) also reported on nine studies in which multiple rather than single measures were used to predict reading skill. All of the studies contained some phonological processing measures as well as other measures and the multiple r was 0.75; these studies were fairly effective in correctly classifying children who subsequently became successful readers. Eighty-nine percent of the successful readers were initially classified as not being at risk and only four percent of the not-at-risk children subsequently developed reading problems. In contrast, seventy-eight percent of the unsuccessful readers were initially classified as being at risk and 55 percent of those initially classified as at-risk did not actually develop reading problems.

These results suggest that phonological core measures are fairly accurate in predicting who will become a successful reader but are less accurate in predicting who will become a disabled reader. This lack of accuracy may occur because there are multiple pathways to classification as developmentally reading disabled and, as a result, subtypes may exist within the phenotype. Before examining this possibility, however, we will consider the evidence that some children who receive an initial 'at risk' classification for developmental reading disability may actually be impaired by inadequate environmental experience and instruction which is mistaken for deficits in fundamental cognitive processes related to reading, particularly in the domain of core phonological skills. If this is the case, then at-risk children should vary in their response to intensive efforts at early intervention and at least some of them should end up being re-classified as normally achieving readers after a year or two of instruction.

Vellutino et al. (1996) conducted a large scale intervention study in which the initial sample included 1284 Kindergarten children. Nine percent of the sample (118 children) were identified as being at-risk for acquiring reading skill based upon their performance on phonological processing tasks, reading measures, and teacher recommendations. Beginning in first grade, 74 of these children were selected for early intervention and given one-half hour per day one-to-one tutoring by trained teachers for at least one to two semesters. The instruction consisted of 15 minutes of reading connected text and 15 minutes of word recognition training that involved word identification, decoding, phoneme awareness, and writing. Their performance was compared to 65 normal readers who were also selected from the initial sample but did not receive intervention. Overall, 67 percent of the instructed readers scored in the average range after one semester; average was defined as being above the 30th percentile or within 0.5 standard deviation of the mean on the WRMT-R Word Identification and Word Attack subtests (Woodcock, 1987). The growth functions of the 74 instructed at-risk readers were rank ordered and the top 25 percent ($N = 19$) were similar to the normal control readers at the end of the second grade in word identification and word attack (64th versus 75th percentile). The bottom 25 percent ($N = 19$), however, were not very responsive to tutoring and they were at the 14th percentile at the end of second grade. These results indicate that children identified as 'at-risk' can improve substantially with appropriate and intensive environmental input in the form of instruction that targets core phonological processing as well as reading; in fact, some may become indistinguishable from normally achieving readers.

Vellutino et al. (1996) also found that while many of the instructed children compensated for an initial 'at risk' diagnosis, their phonological processing skills were relatively weak. The group that was easy to remediate had the strongest profile of phonological skills both in Kindergarten and after one year of instruction. The group that was difficult to remediate had the most severe deficiencies in measures of phonological processing skill. These findings strongly implicate phonological processing ability as the key factor in at risk children's ability to respond positively to early intervention. The critical role of phonological processing skill is further highlighted by the finding that instructed groups did not differ in IQ among themselves or from a normal reader control group (Vellutino, Scanlon and Lyon, 2000; Vellutino et al., 1996). These groups also did not differ on semantic and syntactic measures that required minimal working memory or on measures of visual, attentional, and organizational processes. Finally, Torgesen, Wagner and Rashotte (1997) and Torgesen et al. (1999) have also reported that initial phonological processing skills of Kindergarten at-risk children predict the acquisition of word reading skills and that intensive instruction which explicitly emphasizes the phonemic structure of words is effective in moving many of them into the normal range of word recognition ability by the end of second grade.

Subtypes of developmental reading disorders

Children who are identified as having developmental reading disorder tend to be very heterogenous and, as discussed above, this heterogeneity arises from a variety of sources that involve both how reading is defined and nonreading correlates of the disorder. With respect to the issue of definition, it is important to note that developmental reading disorder is diagnosed in children and adults who experience persistent and unexpected difficulty in acquiring accurate and rapid context-free word reading skills (Shaywitz, 1998). Developmental reading disorder is persistent because it is lifelong (e.g., Bruck, 1992; Pennington, Van Orden, Smith et al., 1990); it is unexpected because it occurs despite adequate opportunity for schooling, motivation, and intelligence; and it is defined with reference to context-free word recognition because the ability to read individual words accurately and rapidly out of context is the primary skill which allows reading to proceed fluently and effortlessly (e.g., Perfetti, 1985; Stanovich, 1980, 1984). As Fletcher et al. (1999a) have pointed out, many of the inconsistent research findings in the area of developmental reading disability are associated with studies in which dyslexic readers were identified using behavioral criteria other than their ability to read aloud single, isolated words. The ability to decode nonwords is a particularly sensitive measure for identifying deficits in word reading skill in both children and adults (Rack, Snowling and Olson, 1992) and Shankweiler, Lundquist, Katz et al. (1999) have shown that nonword decoding and comprehension are highly correlated ($r = 0.79$) in a study involving a large group of children ($N = 361$), many of whom were having difficulty learning to read.

Attempts to identify subtypes of reading disabled children have involved a number of different approaches (Lovett, 1992). Some investigators have based their subtyping efforts on neurocognitive theories of dyslexia (e.g., Bakker, 1979; Castles and Coltheart, 1993; Manis, Seidenberg, Doi et al., 1996; Wolf and Bowers, 1999) while others have taken a strongly empirical perspective and used reading behavior (e.g., Boder, 1973; Doehring and Hoshko, 1977; Doehring, Trites, Patel and Fiedorowicz, 1981) or nonreading deficits (e.g, Rourke, 1985) as a basis of classification. In a landmark study, Morris et al. (1998) attempted to combine these different perspectives in a large scale study involving 232 children who varied in reading skill. They used measures derived from core phonological processing theory (phonemic awareness, verbal working memory, serial naming tasks) as well as measures of language skill (vocabulary and speech production tasks) and measures of nonverbal skill identified as being associated with reading disorders (visual–spatial, visual attention, and non-verbal memory tasks). Using multiple clustering methods, they identified 9 subtypes: two were not disabled and two were broadly deficient in language skill and yielded a uniformly low performance profile across the measures that was consistent with being "garden variety poor readers" (Stanovich, 1988). Four out of five of the remaining subtypes were all characterized by deficiency in phonological awareness with profiles of different patterns of strength and weakness in the other reading-related measures (verbal working memory and rapid serial naming) as well as language and nonverbal processing. The final subtype was characterized by relative strength in language processing but weakness in verbal and nonverbal measures of rate of processing.

The pervasive deficit in phonological awareness across eighty percent of the specific reading disability subtypes and the two garden variety subtypes is generally consistent with the core phonological deficit model (e.g., Stanovich, 1988; Stanovich and Siegel, 1994). It is noteworthy, however, that rapid serial naming was an important discriminating measure for several of the subtypes. Two of the subtypes consisted of children who were relatively deficient in both phonemic awareness *and* rapid serial naming, two others involved deficiencies just in phonemic awareness, and one involved deficiencies just in rate. This pattern of results is broadly consistent with Wolf's Double Deficit hypothesis (e.g., Wolf and Bowers, 1999) in which rapid serial naming and phonemic awareness are distinguished theoretically and empirically. Serial naming is regarded as an index of fluent reading performance and associated with measures of orthographic processing and comprehension whereas phonological awareness is associated with word, and particularly nonword, decoding skill. Wolf and Bowers (1999) have reported that children with a double deficit — impairments in both phonemic awareness and rapid serial naming — are more severely impaired than children with a single deficit (see also Lovett, Steinbach and Frijters, 2000).

One appealing feature of the double deficit perspective is that it provides a theoretical rationale for the fact that developmental reading disorders may manifest themselves as deficits in word reading fluency rather than in nonword decoding in languages such as German and Italian that have shallow orthographies (e.g., Wimmer, 1993; Wolf, Pfeil, Lotz and Biddle, 1994). This perspective also has implications for differential treatment approaches to developmental reading disorders (e.g., Lovett, Steinbach and Frijters, 2000; Wolf and Bowers, 1999).

Unlike the broad, multivariate approach of Morris et al. (1998), the Wolf and Bowers (1999) Double Deficit hypothesis is an example of a subtyping scheme that is tied to a small and theoretically-based set of measures. Another influential example of this approach to subtyping draws heavily upon research in acquired dyslexia. Castles and Coltheart (1993) extended the dual-route theoretical perspective (e.g., Coltheart, Curtis, Atkins and Haller, 1993) which had been used to identify phonological and surface dyslexic subtypes among adult readers with acquired dyslexia (e.g., Coltheart, Patterson and Marshall, 1980) to account for the reading behavior of children. Castles and Coltheart (1993) looked at the relative imbalance between nonword reading, which draws upon phonological processing skill, and exception word reading, which draws upon lexical or orthographic processing skill. Consistent with the work in acquired dyslexia, they found children who looked like surface dyslexics because they were relatively more impaired in exception word reading than nonword reading, and phonological dyslexics who were more impaired in nonword reading than exception word reading.

Subsequent research by Manis et al. (1996) and by Stanovich, Siegel and Gottardo (1997) showed that the surface dyslexia subtype was a manifestation of a developmental delay in reading acquisition and that children so classified were not distinguishable from normal younger readers who had less reading experience and therefore less opportunity to acquire the unique orthographic patterns characterizing exception words. In contrast, the phonological dyslexics emerged as a robust and stable subtype providing further evidence that children with developmental reading disorder have their primary impairment in nonword decoding (e.g., Fletcher et al., 1999a; Rack et al., 1992).

In a related line of research, Manis, McBride-Chang, Seidenberg et al. (1997) explored some of the correlates of the developmental phonological dyslexia subtype. As expected, children classified as phonological dyslexics (low nonword reading relative to exception word reading) generated a profile of impairment in core phonological processing skills similar to that shown by Morris et al. (1998) for the majority of their subtypes. Manis et al. (1996) also examined the categorical speech perception abilities of their phonological dyslexic readers on the grounds that phonological awareness skill was based on speech processing. Consistent with earlier research (e.g., McBride-Chang, 1995a,b; McBride-Chang and Manis, 1996), measures of categorical speech perception were only weakly correlated with nonword reading and phonological awareness skill. They also found, however, that some phonological dyslexics had marked deviations from the sharply rising S-shaped function associated with categorical speech perception. These children did not differ, however, in phonological awareness performance from other phonological dyslexics with normal S-shaped categorical speech perception functions. In other words, Manis et al. (1996) appeared to have identified readers with equal impairments in phonological awareness, but who differ in what is arguably the more fundamental ability of categorical speech perception.

In a subsequent study, Joanisse, Manis, Keating and Seidenberg (2000) replicated these findings and showed that the children who were impaired in both phonological awareness and speech perception were also impaired on measures of language processing, particularly those involving morphological processing. In addition to providing some additional language-based correlates of developmental reading disorder, these studies also highlight the fact that children may differ in the severity of their phonological processing deficit (see also Morris et al., 1998; Wolf et al., 2000a) and that some children who are diagnosed with developmental reading disorders may also have comorbid language disorders which may require different treatment approaches (Bishop, 1997; Bishop and Adams, 1990).

Visual and auditory temporal processing deficits

One theme cutting across the subtyping research (Morris et al., 1998) as well as surveys of research on the predictors of reading acquisition (e.g., Scarborough, 1998) is that basic visual and auditory sensory processes are not very important in identifying children with developmental reading disorders or in understanding the processes underlying the acquisition of reading skill (see also Vellutino, 1979). Furthermore, the dominant theoretical perspective in the field is that developmental reading disorders are fundamentally and irreducibly deficits in phonological processing, a central component of language skill; they cannot be further reduced to deficits in sensory processing (e.g., Liberman, 1997, 1998, 1999; Mann, 1998; Mody, Studdert-Kennedy and Brady, 1997;

Studdert-Kennedy, 2002). Nevertheless, there is continuing interest in the visual and, more recently, the auditory bases of developmental reading disorders. Research on the visual bases of reading disorders has been motivated by the obvious fact that word recognition is initially visual. Feature, letter, and letter position information involve visual pattern recognition (e.g., Massaro and Sanocki, 1993; McClelland and Rumelhart, 1981) and basic neural mechanisms of vision are engaged during the act of reading (Demb, Poldrack and Gabrieli, 1999; Joseph, Noble and Eden, 2001; Stein, 2001) as well as eye movement control systems (e.g., Rayner, 1998). Furthermore, research on the legibility of print has a substantial historical legacy in reading research (Venezky, 1993) and continues with research on the fidelity of electronically displayed printed information (e.g., Kruk, 1993). Finally, visually-based deficits tend to persist in the clinical profiles of disabled readers (Willows and Terepocki, 1993), are associated with their word reading performance (Cornelissen, Hansen, Hutton et al., 1998) and some dyslexic readers' complaints about the act of reading have a visual basis including reports that letters in words tend to exchange positions, blur, and overlap (Stein and Walsh, 1997).

Lovegrove and his colleagues (e.g., Lovegrove, Bowling, Badcock and Blackwood, 1980; Lovegrove, Garzia and Nicholson, 1990; Lovegrove, Martin and Slaghuis, 1986) were primarily responsible for initiating contemporary research on the visual basis of dyslexia with their report that dyslexic readers have impaired contrast sensitivity relative to normal reading controls in discriminating low spatial frequency grating patterns and in detecting flicker at high temporal frequencies. Dyslexic readers also have longer visible persistence than normal readers for low spatial frequency patterns. These investigators interpreted these findings in terms of the distinction between the magnocellular and parvocellular pathways in vision. There are two types of ganglion cells that are involved in relaying information from the rods and cones in the retina to the neural structures in the brain responsible for vision. The magno cells have large cell bodies with dense, heavily myelinated dendrites that ultimately project to the posterior parietal cortex. These cells have fast conduction times, short response latencies, and strong response transients; they can operate under low luminance and provide information about movement and coarse grained information about form. The parvo cells have smaller cell bodies, are tightly packed, and are much more numerous than the magno cells. They ultimately project to the inferotemporal cortex and have relatively slower conduction times, longer latencies, and weaker response transients. They provide fine grained information about form and color based on optimal responses to stimuli that are high in luminance, spatial frequency, and contrast stimuli as well as to chromatic and low temporal frequency (stationary) stimuli. Eye movement control involved in reading provides an opportunity for the two systems to interact. The parvocellular system provides high resolution information when the eye is fixated on a segment of text, but a saccadic movement to the next segment activates the magnocellular system which is hypothesized to inhibit the activity of the parvocellular system thereby preventing the new fixation from being degraded by visible persistence from the prior fixation.

Lovegrove et al. (1990) proposed that his evidence indicated that dyslexic readers have a deficient magnocellular system and one consequence of this deficiency is failure to suppress adequately the parvocellular system during saccadic eye movements. This conclusion has been controversial on several grounds. First, the findings themselves have been replicated by some investigators (e.g., Stein, 2001), but not by others (e.g., Hayduk, Bruck and Cavanagh, 1996; O'Brien, Mansfield and Legge, 2000; Skottun, 2000) with some arguing that the evidence points to suppression of the magnocellular rather than the parvocelluar system during saccadic eye movements (Skottun and Parke, 1999). Second, the theory has been challenged because it is specific to the eye movement processes and reading words in the context of connected text, and does not deal with the evidence and processes associated with deficits in context-free word identification, the primary area in which dyslexic readers experience difficulty (Hulme, 1986). Third, the characteristics of the participants in the experiments are also a source of controversy. The samples are often not well defined with respect to deficits in word recognition and core phonological processes, and the nature of pre-existing visual deficits is often not specified (Garzia, 1993) or, in some studies, they consist of a clinical population for which reports of visual problems are the primary basis for referral (Stein, Richardson and Fowler, 2000).

Eden and Zeffiro (1998) point out that magnocelluar deficits may be more general as a defining feature of developmental reading disorder than is evident from research on saccadic suppression. Eden, VanMeter, Rumsey et al., 1996 (see also Demb, Boyton and Heeger, 1997; Frith and Frith, 1996) used a motion detection task and fMRI recording to show lower levels of activation for dyslexic adults than normal reading controls in an area of the extrastriate cortex that receives substantial input from the magnocellular system (MT/V5). The two groups did not differ in activation in the V1/V2 area of the striate cortex when performing tasks involving the processing of stationary patterns. Cornelissen, Richardson, Mason et al. (1995) found that dyslexic children performed worse than normal reading controls on motion detection tasks and, in a subsequent set of studies, reported that motion detection was related to word recognition in tasks in which close attention to letter position information was required for accurate performance (Cornelissen, Hansen, Gilchrist et al., 1998; Cornelissen et al., 1998). Witton, Talcott, Hansen et al. (1998) found that motion detection performance was related to nonword reading and Cestnick and Coltheart (1999) reported an even more specific finding: motion perception was related to nonword reading but not to regular or exception word reading. These latter results concerning linkage of motion processing to nonwords appears to be contradicted by Talcott, Witton, McLean et al. (2000) who found that motion detection was more strongly correlated with exception word reading and a word (e.g., *rain*), nonword (e.g., *rane*) discrimination task than with nonword reading.

But why is a deficiency in motion detection and, by implication, a deficiency in the magnocellular system, related to single word reading at all? Drawing upon their nonword results, Cestnick and Coltheart (1999) offer one interpretation based on the greater serial, left-to-right processing requirements for reading nonwords (Rastle and Coltheart, 1998) and the possibility that letter-to-letter shifts in attention engage the magnocellular system. They suggest that the dyslexic readers' relatively poor motion detection performance is associated with their inability to engage in efficient, serial nonword decoding. Stein and Fowler, 1981 (see also Stein, 2001) offer a different interpretation. They propose that the visual world of dyslexic readers is relatively unstable, and deficiencies in the magnocellular system make them less able to compensate for unintended eye movements (retinal slips) involved in fixating small targets, such as letters (Eden, Stein, Wood and Wood, 1995). This problem is increased with binocular perception processes suggesting that dyslexic readers have a greater degree of binocular fixation instability than normal readers (Stein, 1993) and it provides a rationale for their greater tendency to produce reading errors that are orthographically inconsistent and contain sounds that are not represented in the word (e.g., *grandeen* for *garden*; Cornelissen et al., 1998). Stein et al. (2000) investigated this problem by occluding the left eye of children who were both dyslexic and had unstable binocular control. They found that stable binocular fixation was obtained by 59% of the children given the occluding patch compared to 36% for the non-occluded control after three months and that this advantage was maintained over the nine months of the study. They also reported that those readers who obtained binocular control improved their reading performance by 9.4 months compared with 3.9 months for the control group or those who were unable to achieve binocular control. Although these results appear impressive, they should be accepted with caution as the children's dyslexia may have been secondary to their visual problems; the procedures for assessing binocular instability are controversial (Bishop, 1989; Goulandris, McIntyre, Snowling et al., 1998; but see Stein, 1989); the children were classified as dyslexic based upon their performance on a single reading test; their phonological processing skills were not assessed; and direct comparisons were not made with phonologically-based procedures for improving reading skill.

Contemporary research on the possibility that deficits in auditory processing might be related to developmental dyslexia was initiated by Tallal (1980) with her report of a strong relationship (Spearman rank order correlation, $rs = 0.81$) between nonword reading errors and errors on an auditory temporal processing task. In the auditory temporal task, the children were required to make temporal order and same/different judgments of two 75 millisecond auditory stimuli that differed in fundamental frequency.

Tallal and Piercy (1973) had previously reported that children with severe specific language impairments performed poorly on this task when the interval between the two stimuli dropped below 300 milliseconds compared to younger children with normal language development. Tallal and Piercy (1974, 1975) also showed that these children had difficulty processing short duration speech and nonspeech acoustic stimuli and interpreted their results as indicating that specific language impaired children had an auditory temporal processing deficit for stimuli that were of brief duration, had brief interval between them, or were changing rapidly, such as formant transitions in consonants (see Tallal, 1978 for a review). In a subsequent series of studies, Tallal, Merzenich, and their colleagues demonstrated that the linguistic and non-linguistic temporal processing deficits in children with specific language impairments could be improved with intensive training (Merzenich, Jenkins, Johnston et al., 1996) and that their speech discrimination and language comprehension skills could be improved with computer-based algorithms that increased the duration and intensity of critical cues for speech (e.g., consonant formant transitions; Tallal, Miller, Bedi et al., 1996).

The temporal processing hypothesis continues to be very controversial with evidence that is both consistent (Habib, Espesser, Ray et al., 1999; Wright, Lombardino, King et al., 1997) and inconsistent (Bishop, Bishop, Bright et al., 1999; Bishop, Carlyon, Deeks and Bishop, 1999; Bradlow, Kraus, Nicol et al., 1999; Nittrouer, 1999; Studdert-Kennedy, 2002) in studies involving children with specific language impairments. There is also substantial debate over the definition of temporal processing in speech and non-speech modes (Farmer and Klein, 1995; Studdert-Kennedy and Mody, 1995; Tallal, 1984). Even more controversial, however, is the role the temporal processing deficit may play in accounting for developmental reading disorders. The auditory temporal processing hypothesis challenges the premise that the core processing deficits which define developmental reading disorder are based in language; instead, it encourages the view that deficits in phonological processing are surface manifestations of a fundamental auditory sensory deficit.

One central question is whether or not dyslexic readers are impaired in their ability to perceive speech categorically (a deficit specific to language) and in auditory temporal processing (a sensory deficit) or whether their impairment is confined to speech alone. This issue was addressed by Mody et al. (1997) who identified two groups of children who, though similar in age and intelligence, differed in word reading skill and in a /ba/–/da/ categorical speech perception task. The groups were compared in their ability to discriminate non-speech sine wave analogs of the second and third formants of /ba/ and /da/ presented at short and long inter-stimulus intervals. Mody et al. (1997) found that the two groups were very similar; in fact, the poor readers performed slightly better than the good readers, particularly at the short inter-stimulus intervals. Although these findings have been criticized on statistical grounds (Denenberg, 1999) and require replication, they suggest that differences between good and poor readers who differ in categorical speech perception does not extend to auditory temporal perception. As discussed above, however, the connection between basic speech perception and developmental dyslexia is not as strong as might be expected. Although dyslexic readers tend to perform more poorly than normally achieving readers, the correlations between measures of categorical speech perception and reading are in the low moderate range (McBride-Chang, 1995a,b), and Joanisse et al. (2000) report that only *some* dyslexic readers, with their characteristic profile of low phonological awareness, are also deficient in categorical speech perception. This latter group of children may have specific language impairment as well as developmental reading disorder. One implication of this conclusion is that auditory temporal processing deficits, to the extent to which they exist, may be confined to children with specific language impairment who are also having difficulty acquiring reading skill.

The possibility of a sensory basis for developmental reading disorder was approached from a different perspective by Booth, Perfetti, MacWhinney and Hunt (2000). They obtained a positive correlation between performance on a tone sequence detection task (similar to Tallal, 1980) and performance in word reading with both children and adult dyslexic readers. Witton et al. (1998) found that dyslexic adults were less sensitive than normal reading controls at detecting auditory frequency modulation (warble) compared to a pure tone and that performance in this auditory task was correlated with nonword reading performance. Stein (2001) reports similar relationships with nonword reading for amplitude modulation. Using an unselected sample of 10-year-old children, Talcott et al. (2000) found that frequency modulation was significantly correlated with a composite score consisting of nonword reading and an oral phonological processing measure involving spoonerisms, even when reading skill and intelligence were removed statistically. In contrast, both Watson and Miller (1993) and Schulte-Körne, Deimel, Bartling and Remschmidt (1999) failed to find significant relationships between measures of temporal processing and reading and spelling (see also Studdert-Kennedy, 2002). Although many of these studies indicate that performance on auditory sensory processing tasks are related to measures of literacy and phonological processing, the findings do not address directly the issue of core linguistic versus sensory bases of reading disability. Specifically, they do not directly evaluate whether or not auditory sensory task performance makes a unique contribution to word reading performance independent of variance accounted for by core phonological processes such as phonological awareness, particularly within the context of longitudinal research designs in which the autocorrelated variable of word reading performance in earlier grades can be controlled statistically (Wagner et al., 1997).

Booth et al. (2000), Talcott et al. (2000), and Witton et al. (1998) all found that measures of deficits in visual motion detection were associated with measures of orthographic processing, while measures of auditory temporal processing were associated with measures of phonological processing in the same individuals — suggesting that the two measures of sensory processes index different aspects of developmental reading disorder. These results have encouraged investigators to combine the auditory temporal processing deficit hypothesis with the visual magnocellular deficit hypothesis into a more general temporal processing deficit hypothesis (Habib, 2000; Stein, 2001; Stein and Walsh, 1997). One important basis of this proposal comes from neuroanatomical evidence for magno cells in the auditory relay nucleus of the thalamus (medial geniculate nucleus) that are responsive to changes in frequency and amplitude. Post mortem analyses indicate that these magno cells are disordered in the brains of some dyslexic individuals, particularly on the side projecting to the left hemisphere (Galaburda, Menard and Rosen, 1994). Stein (2001) speculates that both the visual and auditory magno cells are very similar and are therefore both potentially susceptible to influences that might modify their structural and functional characteristics during the course of early brain development. He has recently expanded this hypothesis to include impairments in motor development, which can accompany developmental dyslexia (e.g., Nicholson, Fawcett, Berry et al., 1999), and dysfunctions in the cerebellum, which receives substantial magnocelluar input. Along with Wolf (1991, 2001) and Tallal, Galaburda, Llinas and Von Euler (1993), Stein (2001) has suggested an even more general hypothesis: Developmental reading disorder is one manifestation of a general deficit in neuronal timing. These speculations are provocative and have the potential to move research on developmental reading disorder into the mainstream of neuroscience research and allow it to be investigated with animal as well as human models. The evidence for a fundamental, non-linguistic basis for developmental dyslexia that is defined with reference to deficits in sensory and motor processes, however, is currently fragmentary and very controversial; and even though it is possible to regard visual, auditory, and motor deficits as indexing different types of reading disorder the current state of evidence concerning dyslexic subtypes reviewed above points to deficits in linguistically-based, core phonological processes as underlying all subtypes (e.g., Morris et al., 1998).

Neurobiological substrates of reading and reading disability

While even the earliest case studies of visual word blindness included speculation on the neurobiological substrates of dyslexia, scientific interest in the neurobiology of reading and reading disability has been particularly strong in the past two decades. Several lines of investigation had been pursued to investigate brain structures and brain function involved in reading, together with a search for a neurobiological signature or profile for individuals with reading disorders. Studies of brain structure have been conducted using both autopsy and structural Magnetic Resonance Imaging (MRI) techniques. Studies of reading-related brain function have been undertaken using electrophysiological methods and recent advances in neuroimaging technology that support functional brain imaging methods (e.g., regional cerebral blood flow mapping (rCBF), positron emission tomography (PET), and functional MRI (fMRI)). This complex literature has been reviewed in detail in several recent publications and the reader is directed to these for a more complete review (c.f., Filipek, 1999; Grigorenko, 2001; Pugh, Mencl, Jenner et al., 2000).

A unique line of neuroanatomic evidence for reading disorder was provided through a series of post-mortem investigations of dyslexic brains as was reported by Albert Galaburda and his colleagues at Beth Israel Hospital. Galaburda's investigations compared at autopsy the brains of adults with and without a history of childhood dyslexia. Galaburda (1988) reported that the planum temporale (a structure believed relevant to normal language function, the posterior aspect of the superior temporal lobe) was symmetrical in all seven dyslexic brains studied; in normal readers, distinct asymmetry is typically seen with the left side greater than the right in approximately 65% of cases. Galaburda's finding could not be attributed to a smaller left planum, but reflected instead an unexpected increase in the size of the right planum in dyslexic individuals. Galaburda stated that this outcome reflected reduced cell death during fetal brain development. In five of the seven dyslexic brains analyzed, these investigators found evidence of microdysgenesis and focal dysplasia. Galaburda and Livingstone (1993) subsequently reported abnormalities in the magnocellular, but not the parvocellular, layers of five dyslexic brains.

Galaburda (1988; Galaburda and Livingstone, 1993; Galaburda, Menard and Rosen, 1994) suggested that normal asymmetry of the plana (left > right) may be a structural prerequisite for normal phonological development. The findings of these autopsy investigations have received mixed reviews and have been the subject of some controversy in the literature. Reviewers have criticized the small sample of brains studied and have noted that the nature and severity of their dyslexic symptoms represents enormous heterogeneity (Fletcher et al., 1999a). The three female brains studied (Humphreys, Kaufmann and Galaburda, 1990) were apparently those of women with comorbid attentional disorders, psychiatric problems, and head injury. That all three demonstrated highly symmetrical plana temporale cannot be taken as evidence specific to the neural substrates of developmental dyslexia, but may reflect instead a different pattern of early brain development common to multiple forms of developmental neurocognitive disorder.

Early enthusiasm for the evidence of symmetry of the plana in dyslexic brains also has been tempered by recent recognition that the planum temporale region shows significant inter-individual variability in the general population, and evidence that estimates of planum measurements tend to be imprecise (Filipek, 1995, 1999; Filipek, Kennedy and Caviness, 1992; Grigorenko, 2001; Westbury, Zatorre and Evans, 1999). Filipek concludes that direct comparisons across published studies of the plana temporale in dyslexic individuals cannot be provided currently because of the difficulty in accurately demarcating its boundaries (Filipek, 1995, 1999).

Galaburda's contribution may lie not so much in providing specific neuroanatomical profiles of dyslexic brain development but rather in the interpretation that dyslexia may be the outcome of anomalies in neural development, resulting from an event or sequence of events that occur in utero. His group has suggested that this neurocognitive disorder could stem from an interaction between the prenatal chemical environment of the fetus and differing maturation rates of different brain areas (Galaburda, 1990). Small vascular events and other sources of injury have been suggested, with later speculation that ischemic injuries may be a result of autoimmune dysfunction (Galaburda, Schrott, Sherman et al., 1996). These interactions are seen as potentially forging different paths of brain development characterized by anomalous cell migration and organization within the fetal brain (Grigorenko, 2001).

In reviewing the literature on the possible functional significance of patterns of symmetry and asymmetry in the plana temporale, Morgan and Hynd (1998) conclude that the two most consistent findings are those of symmetrical or rightward asymmetrical plana being associated with poor verbal comprehension and poor phonological processing and decoding skills. Morgan and Hynd suggest that other research on symmetry and asymmetry in posterior regions of the brain, however, suggests that atypical patterns of symmetry and asymmetry posteriorally appear generally associated with poorly developed verbal comprehension abilities. Phonological decoding deficits and perhaps automatic naming abilities and other expressive language deficits may be more uniquely associated with atypical symmetry/asymmetry of the plana specifically. These reviewers suggest the need for better controlled research, however, to determine whether there exists a relationship in nondyslexic individuals between patterns of plana symmetry/asymmetry and specific aspects of language competence.

Over the past decade, a number of structural MRI studies have compared the mapping of specific cerebral asymmetries in dyslexic and nondyslexic individuals. Deviations in the normal profile of posterior asymmetry were reported (Flowers, 1993; Hynd, Semrud-Clikeman, Lorys et al., 1990; Rumsey, 1992), with increased right measurements reported for dyslexic brains by some investigators (Duara, Kushch, Gross-Glenn et al., 1991), and decreased left measurement by other researchers (Hynd et al., 1990: Larsen, Hoien, Lundberg and Odegaard, 1990). Leonard, Voeller, Lombardion et al. (1993) reported other cerebral anomalies, including missing or duplicated gyri bilaterally in the planum and parietal operculum, suggesting these to be the consequence of genetically- or developmentally-influenced disturbances in cell migration (Grigorenko, 2001).

Quantitative MRI analyses were employed to study a large sample of dyslexic and control twins as part of the Colorado studies on brain structure and dyslexia and genetic influences on size variations in brain structure (Pennington, 1999; Pennington, Filipek, Churchwell et al., 1999). Preliminary results suggested different etiologies for individual differences in the size of cortical and subcortical brain areas. Pennington summarizes early results as supporting speculation that subcortical structures appear to be more strongly genetically influenced, while cortical structures appear to vary in size with both genetic and environmental influences. Earlier work with a cohort of monozygotic and dizygotic adolescent twin pairs with reading disability (Filipek, Pennington, Holmes et al., 1995; Pennington et al., 1999) revealed the largest operculum, temporal, and posterior-parietal/occipital regions in the subjects with reading disorder. Filipek (1999) compares these findings to similar regional brain enlargements she has reported in developmental language disorder (and autistic) cohorts (Filipek, Richelme, Kennedy et al., 1992). No differences were revealed in subcortical structure volumes (e.g., basal ganglia, thalamus). Filipek (1999) suggests that these findings are further evidence of developmental structural anomalies in RD in those brain areas thought to subserve receptive language functions (i.e., the opercular, temporal, and posterior-parietal (association) cortices). Pennington et al. (1999) also found smaller insula bilaterally and smaller frontal cortex in the adolescents with reading disability. In this study with large samples (97 twin pairs), analyses controlled for age, gender, and IQ, raising confidence in the replicability of these results.

Grigorenko (2001) concludes that while these anatomical studies provide overall support for a neurobiological model of dyslexia, there remains considerable inconsistency in the findings; she suggests that there exist few findings of brain structure differences between dyslexic and nondyslexic individuals that can be considered truly robust. Small sample sizes and variable criteria for defining subjects as dyslexic contribute to discrepant findings and a lack of consensus on the available evidence (Fletcher et al., 1999a; Pennington, 1999).

Functional neuroimaging evidence

Recent advances in neuroimaging technology that support functional brain imaging methods [e.g., regional cerebral blood flow mapping (rCBF), positron emission tomography (PET), and functional MRI (fMRI)] enable a closer examination of the neural circuitry contributing to different functions in reading and reading-related processing systems. A landmark fMRI study by Shaywitz et al. (1998) provided unique information on the different brain activation patterns of dyslexic and nondyslexic adult readers while engaged in progressively more phonologically demanding tasks. The investigation was motivated by interest in understanding the location and functional disruption of the neural systems associated with the characteristic phonological processing deficits of disabled readers.

Using a subtraction paradigm common to fMRI studies, Shaywitz et al. (1998) administered a set of hierarchically structured tasks that varied the level of linguistic coding necessary and then compared both behavioral performance and brain activation patterns of their disabled and nondisabled readers. The five tasks used in this study varied according to the processing demands made on visual–spatial processing [line orientation judgement, e.g., do (\\\/) and (\\\/) match?], orthographic processing (letter case judgement, e.g., do *bbBb* and *bbBb* match?), simple phonological analysis (single letter rhyme judgement, e.g., do *T* and *V* rhyme?), phonological assembly (nonword rhyme judgement, e.g., do *leat* and *jete* rhyme?), and lexical–semantic processing (semantic category judgement: are *corn* and *rice* in the same category?).

Systematic differences were revealed in the brain activation patterns of the two groups of subjects as task demands increased in phonological processing load. Shaywitz et al. (1998) found that the adult disabled readers failed to systematically increase activation within a large posterior cortical system as the phonological demands of print-to-sound mapping increased. In contrast, these disabled readers demonstrated patterns of relative overactivation in anterior areas on phonological tasks. The normal readers' brain activation patterns on these tasks were interpreted as providing

> functional evidence of a widely distributed computational system for reading characterized by specialization and reciprocity: within the system, task-specific responses vary from region to region.
>
> *Shaywitz et al., 1998, p. 2639*

Shaywitz and her colleagues concluded that these data revealed for dyslexic readers what appears to be a functional disruption of an extensive system of posterior cortex that encompasses both traditional visual areas and traditional language processing areas as well as an area of association cortex. The area of association cortex was noted to be of interest because it included the angular gyrus, an area speculated to be important to the cross-modality information processing functions relevant to print-to-sound mapping during reading. These investigators conclude their report with speculation that this pattern of relative *under*activation of posterior areas coupled with relative *over*activation of anterior areas may provide what may be considered "a neural signature for the phonologic difficulties characterizing dyslexia" (Shaywitz et al., 1998, p. 2640).

Further recent work from the Shaywitz and Shaywitz lab at Yale has been conducted to address the nature of the neurobiological anomalies found in dyslexic readers and their specificity to the systems subserving phonological processing (Pugh, Mencl, Shaywitz et al., 2000). This work followed up on a study by Horwitz, Rumsey and Donohue (1998) who used PET data from the Rumsey, Horwitz, Donohue et al. (1997) study to examine correlations in activation levels between the left angular gyrus and other brain sites in the superior and occipital temporal lobe during two oral reading tasks (nonword reading and exception word reading). Horwitz et al. (1998) reported strong significant correlations for able readers, but weak correlations for dyslexic readers. Pugh et al. (2000b) agree that these findings suggest a disruption of functional connectivity between the angular gyrus and related posterior cortical areas when disabled readers read exception or nonwords, but they speculate that this failure to demonstrate functional connectivity could represent a global (linguistic and nonlinguistic) deficit or a functional deficit specific to activities and processes demanding phonological assembly.

Pugh et al. (2000b) addressed this issue by assessing functional connectivity on the four tasks used in Shaywitz et al. (1998) in their fMRI study. The tasks varied in their demands on visual, orthographic, phonological, and lexical–semantic processing. Functional connectivity was operationalized as correlations between the angular gyrus and related posterior cortical areas relevant to reading (as in Horwitz et al., 1998). The results supported the specific phonological deficit rather than the global deficit hypothesis. For dyslexic readers, the functional connectivity correlations for the left hemisphere were weak on word and nonword reading tasks, but strong on the single case detection task, reaching a numerically higher R^2 than the nondyslexic readers. Pugh et al. (2000b) report that when phonological assembly is not required, even on the simple phonology task of the single letter rhyme judgements, patterns of functional connectivity between the left angular gyrus and related posterior areas for the dyslexic readers

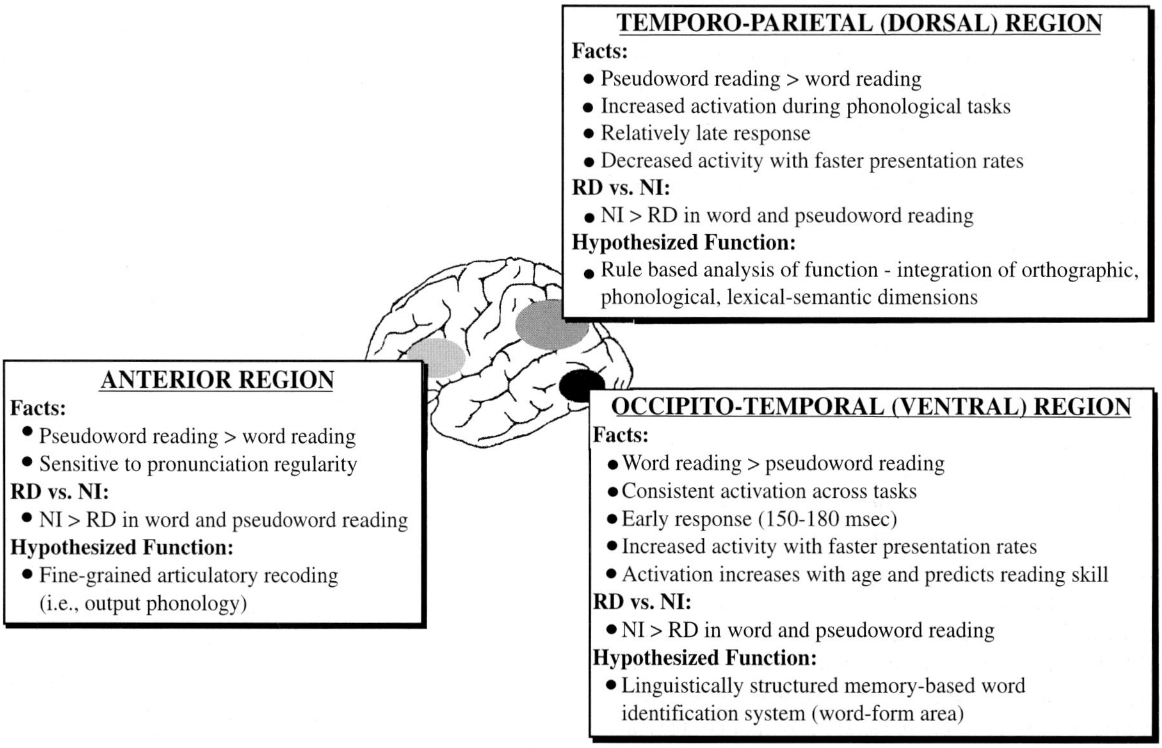

Fig. 2. A tentative model of the neural circuitry for reading. From: Pugh KR, Mencl WE Jenner AR, Katz L, Frost SJ, Lee JR, Shaywitz SE and Shaywitz BA: Neurobiological studies of reading and reading disability. Journal of Communication Disorders: 34; 479–492, 2001. Copyright 2001 by Elsevier Science Inc. Reprinted with permission.

were similar to the nondyslexic readers. The authors conclude that the disruption in functional connectivity for dyslexic individuals in the left hemisphere appears restricted to tasks with high phonological assembly demands. On print-related tasks not requiring phonological assembly, functional connectivity appeared strong for both dyslexic and nondyslexic readers. The conclusion is offered that these correlational data are consistent with a great deal of cumulative behavioral evidence that the signature neurobiological and neurocognitive deficits in dyslexia lie specifically in the phonological processing domain.

Pugh et al. (2000b) note that on those tasks where left hemisphere correlations were low for dyslexic readers, strong correlations were revealed at the corresponding right hemisphere homologues. Shaywitz et al. (1998), with the same subjects, had reported a group × hemisphere interaction at the angular gyrus, reflecting more right than left activation for dyslexic readers and more left than right activation for nondyslexic subjects. In a speculation congruent with some of those made from earlier neuroanatomical work on dyslexia (Galaburda, 1988), Pugh and his colleagues (2000b) suggest that these correlations, consistent with the earlier observation of Rumsey, Andreason, Zametkin et al. (1992) of selective rightward shifts in disabled readers on language processing tasks, may indicate some potential for compensatory overreliance on right hemisphere systems by dyslexic individuals.

In a review of functional neuroimaging studies, Pugh et al. (2000a) propose a developmental account of the neural circuitry of reading for both impaired and non-impaired readers (see Fig. 2). Pugh and his colleagues interpret converging results as suggesting that skilled reading behaviors, such as fluent word recognition, depend upon the functional integrity of two consolidated posterior systems in the left hemisphere. These authors contend that a dorsal (temporal–parietal) and a ventral (occipital–temporal) left hemisphere system serve different functions in the normally developing reader's brain and subserve different phases of successful reading acquisition. Both of these posterior systems and their functional connectivity appear deviant in the brains of reading disabled individuals and two patterns of compensatory activity have been shown related to this left hemisphere posterior anomaly. Impaired readers demonstrate increased reliance on the inferior frontal gyrus during reading; Pugh et al. (2000a) suggest that such a reliance may support articulatory or covert speech recoding as an attempt to cope with phonological processing demands. Impaired readers also demonstrate increased activation in the right hemisphere homologues of the disrupted left hemisphere posterior systems. It is suggested that this right hemisphere shift may represent development of compensatory non-phonological, visual–semantic pattern recognition processes to support word identification learning.

Pugh and his collaborators propose that in normal reading acquisition the successful development of LH posterior reading systems, especially the ventral occipital–temporal circuit, depends upon finely organized integration of phonological and lexical–semantic information about words represented within overlapping neural circuits. It is proposed that this integration of information and representations depend upon intact and functional processing in the temporal–parietal systems which support initial learning. Deficits within this dorsal LH learning system preclude subsequent development of the rapid ventral word identification circuit. For the reading disabled child with phonological processing deficits, the signature temporo-parietal problems disrupt the developmental course which integrates these two posterior reading circuits during the reading acquisition of non-impaired children.

This account of the neurobiological course of successful reading development provides an important first model for the development of both reading skill and reading disorder. The developmental model of a poorly articulated occipital–temporal system, resulting from an initial disruption of normal temporo-parietal functioning, provides a credible framework for understanding both the phonological decoding failures of struggling readers and their characteristic ensuing course of dysfluent and poorly automated word identification learning. As Pugh et al. (2000a, p. 207) suggest in summary,

> We propose a neurobiological account suggesting that for normally developing readers the dorsal circuit predominates at first, and is associated with analytic processing necessary for learning to integrate orthographic features with phonological and lexical–semantic features of printed words. The ventral circuit constitutes a fast, late-developing word identification system which underlies fluent word recognition in skilled readers.

A subsequent report by Paulesu et al. (2001) compared neurocognitive and neuroimaging data on dyslexic and nonimpaired adult readers from three countries with languages varying in the depth/shallowness of their orthographies. Impaired Italian readers were relatively better performers on literacy tasks than their French and English dyslexic peers, a behavioral difference attributed to their more shallow orthographic system. In Italian, print maps more uniquely onto speech sounds than in deeper more complex orthographies like French and English; shallow orthographies pose fewer difficulties during reading acquisition particularly if the beginning reader has phonological processing problems. When PET data from scans conducted during explicit and implicit reading activities were analyzed, impaired adult readers from all three countries demonstrated a common profile of reduced activation in the left middle, inferior, and superior temporal cortex and in the middle occipital gyrus. Significantly greater activation was demonstrated through this large region of left cortex by the nonimpaired control readers in each country. These investigators conclude that reading disability or dyslexia is characterized by a universal neurocognitive profile in the brain regardless of the depth or shallowness of the orthography, and is associated with the characteristic deficit in phonological processing. The depth/shallowness of the orthography impacts upon the extent to which the phonological deficits will impede reading acquisition and limit reading behavior, but the brain activation differences during reading appear universal regardless of orthographic depth.

The genetics of reading ability and reading disability

It had long been known that reading disabilities appeared to run in families, with family history one of the most important risk factors for the disorder. Pennington and Smith (1988) summarized the results of investigations of familial risk for dyslexia: 40% of boys and 18% of girls with an affected parent were estimated to exhibit RD profiles. Rumsey (1992) suggests this risk to approximate a seven-fold increase for boys and a 12-fold increase for girls over the estimated risk for the general population. A prospective study of the offspring of one or two dyslexic parents revealed that approximately 31% of these children were school-identified as impaired readers by the end of second grade. The prevalence of reading impairment was doubled (62%) when this prospective sample was assessed on objective test instruments (Finucci, Gottfredson and Childs, 1985; Grigorenko, 2001; Wood and Grigorenko, 2001). As Wood and Grigorenko (2001) make explicit, however, in their methodological review, a higher familial aggregation of reading disorders in the families of reading disabled individuals is "a necessary but not sufficient observation" for inferring genetic etiology. Families also share common environments, and these authors contend that these environments may also influence adult levels of reading achievement attained by both impaired and non-impaired readers.

Scientific interest in whether or not reading disorders are hereditary dates back to the late 1950s. In the first twin study of dyslexia, Hermann (1959) reported that 10 out of 10 monozygotic (MZ) twin pairs (100%) were concordant for reading disorders while only 11 of 33 dizygotic pairs (33%) he studied exhibited such concordance. Later twin studies varied in their reported concordance rates (100% MZ, 35% DZ: Zerbin-Rüdin, 1967; 84% MZ, 20% DZ: Bakwin, 1973: 85% MZ, 55% DZ: Decker and Vandenberg, 1985), although all were consistent in reporting high MZ concordance rates and DZ concordance rates of just under 50 percent on average.

Methodological concerns that a possible referral bias in RD twin sample ascertainment and a higher tendency to report concordant rather than discordant results may have exaggerated these findings (Grigorenko, 2001; Harris, 1986; Wood and Grigorenko, 2001) led a group of Colorado researchers to readdress this issue with ascertainment of a large sample of reading disabled twins from school performance records and detailed follow-up testing in a laboratory situation. With these precautions, DeFries and Alarcón (1996) reported an unbiased concordance rate of reading disorder for MZ twins of 68% and for DZ twins of 38%. As Grigorenko (2001) concludes, even if early RD twin samples had been biased, the concordance rates they reported for MZ and DZ pairs were quite accurate by today's standards. These concordance studies were powerful evidence that reading disorders likely are subject to significant genetic etiological influences, but they did not allow estimates of the relative magnitude of genetic vs. environmental influences, nor did they reveal possible mechanisms of genetic transmission across families.

Twin studies of reading disorder in the late 1980s and 1990s were influenced by growing recognition that dyslexia exists on a continuum with normal reading skill rather than as a discrete diagnostic entity (Fletcher et al., 1999a; Francis et al., 1996; Shaywitz, 1996; Shaywitz et al., 1990; Van der Wissel and Zegers, 1985). This evidence required behavioral geneticists to develop new statistical methodologies appropriate for evaluating etiology for sample membership on the tails of normal distributions for different skills (Grigorenko, 2001; Wood and Grigorenko, 2001). The DeFries–Fulker regression method was specifically developed for such investigations (DeFries and Fulker, 1985).

DeFries, Fulker and LaBuda (1987) were the first to apply the new regression methodology to twin analyses of specific reading disability. With relatively modest but carefully defined samples of 64 MZ and 55 DZ twin pairs, these investigators estimated group heritability to be a statistically significant but relatively modest 0.29. When analyses were redone with an enlarged sample of twins defined as having the same phenotype, a substantially higher estimate of group heritability at 58% was reported (Wadsworth, Olson, Pennington and DeFries, 2000). DeFries and Alarcón (1996; Alarcón and DeFries, 1997) went on to investigate the heritability of reading performance in both reading disabled and normal reading samples of Colorado's twins. The estimated proportion of genetic influence on the groups' composite reading scores (PIAT word recognition, reading comprehension, spelling recognition) had been reported at 56%. This second study found reading performance to be highly heritable in both disabled (0.82) *and* normal reader (0.66) groups. Estimates of shared environmental influences appeared extremely low (RD 0.01, control 0.18) by comparison.

With this new regression methodology and increased understanding of the multidimensional nature of the reading process and its component skills, investigators attempted to estimate the heritability of different reading-related skills. Olson, Wise, Conners et al. (1989) reported heritable group deficits for phoneme awareness, phonological decoding, and word identification, but not for orthographic coding measures. Later multivariate analyses revealed higher genetic covariance estimates for word recognition and phonological decoding than for word recognition and orthographic decoding (DeFries, Olson, Pennington and Smith, 1991).

Subsequent investigators have challenged the negative finding of Olson et al. (1989) regarding the heritability of orthographic coding. Hohnen and Stevenson (1995) reported strong heritability results for both phonological and orthographic reading-related measures. Recent results from Gayán and Olson (1999) on greater numbers of twin pairs confirmed substantial heritability for *all* component reading-related processes examined. Shared environmental influences were also identified for all measures.

Grigorenko, 1996 (as cited in Grigorenko, 2001) assessed genetic and environmental correlations for different reading-related processes in analyses of large extended families. Her results were suggestive of common genetic influences for phonemic awareness and decoding (0.77; sd = 0.15), for phonemic awareness and rapid naming (0.77; sd = 0.13), and for decoding and rapid naming (0.92; sd = 0.06). Common environmental influences were suggested for phonological decoding and rapid naming (0.57; sd = 0.09).

As evidence on phenotypic correlations has emerged, investigators have sought to estimate shared vs. independent genetic influences among related cognitive and achievement measures. Light, DeFries and Olson (1998), for example, sought to understand the etiology of phenotypic correlations between reading and math performance scores in two samples of normal and disabled readers. They compared two statistical models in an effort to understand the potential basis of these observed relationships. One model included indicators of verbal ability and phonological coding with word recognition and math achievement composite scores; the other model included a short-term memory measure with the math and reading scores. In the first case, when the variation in verbal intelligence and phonological decoding ability was controlled, the observed correlation between reading and math achievement scores decreased approximately three-fold. These investigators reported that approximately 80% of the genetic correlations between reading and math achievement scores were accounted for by genetic factors common to these underlying abilities, mainly verbal aptitude and phonological decoding ability. In contrast, when short-term memory was substituted in the reading and mathematics achievement model, only about 20% of the genetic correlations between reading and math achievement could be accounted for by genetic factors common to these abilities and short-term memory.

The specificity and complexity of the interrelationships among key reading-related processing measures render the study of genetic and environmental influences particularly challenging in reading disability research. Growing recognition of these issues underlies recent calls for greater precision in phenotype measurement, increased awareness of the multidimensional nature of complex reading behaviors and their developmental course, and awareness of common methodological hurdles encountered in this area of behavioral genetics (Grigorenko, 2001; Wood and Grigorenko, 2001).

Chromosomal linkage findings: recent advances in the genetics of reading and reading disability

As the science of behavioral genetics has become more sophisticated both with respect to phenotype and genotype characterization, a number of reports have been published linking reading ability/disability to specific parts of the human genome. Linkage analysis assesses "whether heritable variations at two (genetic) loci. . . are transmitted together in relatives at a rate that is greater than would be expected by chance" (Smith, Kelley, Askew et al., 2001, p. 513). Significant linkage is interpreted as evidence that the two loci are located close together on the same chromosome. Different chromosomal linkage findings, from current molecular techniques of genetic linkage analysis, suggest the possibility of at least six different genes contributing to reading disability and two contributing to language impairment (Barr, 2002, personal communication). More will undoubtedly be found within the next decade.

The first report of genetic linkage to reading disability was published in 1983 by Smith, Kimberling, Pennington and Lubs. In an influential paper in *Science*, they reported a study using nine multigenerational families and finding linkage to chromosome 15 in a subset of these families. The finding was not replicated in other families (Bisgaard, Eiberg, Moller et al., 1987; Cardon, Smith, Fulker et al., 1994; Lubs, Duara, Levin et al., 1991). This discrepancy was interpreted as evidence of locus heterogeneity: that different chromosomal regions were involved in the etiology of reading disability in different families. Recent evidence, however, has been reported linking spelling disability to the chromosome 15 locus in six extended families (Schulte-Körne, Brimm, Nöthen et al., 1997); and Morris, Robinson, Turic et al. (2000) have reported linkage between reading disability and the long arm of chromosome 15q. There has been some continuing replication, therefore, for genetic linkage between reading disability and chromosome 15.

In 1994, an important finding was reported by Cardon and colleagues, identifying a quantitative trait locus (QTL) for reading disability on chromosome 6 within what is known as the human leukocyte antigen (HLA) region. This quantitative trait locus was derived from interval mapping of genetic data from two independent samples of sibling pairs. This region of chromosome 6 was specifically searched because of an association that had been observed previously between reading disorder and immune disorders, most notably by Norman Geschwind (Galaburda, Sherman, Rosen et al., 1985), and existing evidence that specific fragments of chromosome 6 contain genes contributing to disorders like hay fever, migraine headaches, asthma, thyroid disease, and allergies (Grigorenko, 2001; Lazarus and Owen, 1994). In 1987, Pennington and his colleagues had advanced the case for exploring this region on chromosome 6 for dyslexia susceptibility loci (Pennington, Smith, Kimberling et al., 1987). Although subsequent research has not confirmed the association between dyslexia and autoimmune disorders, pursuit of the HLA region of the short arm of chromosome 6 has proven productive.

Further interest in the behavioral genetics of reading disability was fuelled by a finding in 1997 by Elena Grigorenko and her colleagues, suggesting susceptibility loci for different components of reading disorder on chromosomes 6 and 15. These investigators found a phenotype related to single word reading difficulties that linked to a marker on chromosome 15, and a phenotype implicating phonological awareness difficulties linking to markers on the short arm of chromosome 6. These findings appeared to be different linkage results for correlated phenotypes of developmental reading disorder. Initially, the evidence was enthusiastically interpreted by some to suggest cognitively dissociable components of reading that might be linked to different genes.

Bruce Pennington urged caution to such interpretations and to enthusiasm for the belief that science may be close to mapping genes to specific cognitive functions, at least in 1997. In an editorial that accompanied the Grigorenko et al. report in the *American Journal of Human Genetics*, Pennington (1997) suggested that one should not consider the QTLs affecting reading disorder that appeared to be localized to regions on chromosomes 6 and 15 to be genes for reading ability or reading disability. Rather Pennington cautioned that these were more likely genes that somehow lead to disruption in epigenesis and brain development, and that this disruption eventually alters the developmental process of reading acquisition and visible language learning.

For more than a decade, Plomin (1990; Plomin and Crabbe, 2000; Plomin, DeFries, McClearin and Rutter, 1997) has warned of oversimplification in studying the role of inheritance in behavior and cognition. Plomin argued that applications of molecular biological techniques to the study of cognition and behavior may prove unproductive if we embrace simplistic assumptions that one or two major genes will prove largely responsible for genetic variation. More than a decade ago, Plomin (1990) recommended an alternative approach, recognizing the identification of multiple genes, each accounting for a relatively small amount of variance; with this perspective, both genetic and nongenetic sources of variance may be equally significant in accounting for observed variations in behavior and cognitive performance.

The Grigorenko et al. (1997) study included multiple measures of reading and reading-related processes and attempted to use components of reading ability as behavioral phenotypes for linkage. Six extended families were classified on measures of phonological awareness, phonological decoding, rapid naming, and word identification. Although the report provided evidence of significant linkage between phoneme awareness and chromosome 6 and word identification and chromosome 15, a significant difference between the results for each measure in each genetic location was not observed. This is undoubtedly because single word identification is not cognitively separate from phonemic awareness and therefore overlap in genetic linkage would be expected. A later study by this group included two new families and found word identification was significantly linked more to chromosome 6 markers (Grigorenko, Wood, Meyer and Pauls, 2000).

The linkage findings implicating chromosome 6 and chromosome 15 in reading disability have been replicated (Table 1). In particular, the chromosome 6 finding has strong and consistent replication from a number of groups. Fisher and colleagues (1999) have provided empirical support for the locus influencing reading ability at chromosome 6p. Fisher, Marlow, Lamb et al. (1999) tested 181 sibling pairs from 82 nuclear families on multiple measures of word identification skill. These investigators assessed word identification, exception word reading, and nonword decoding and concluded that the linkage finding related to both phonological and orthographic skills and was not specific to phonemic awareness as originally suggested in Grigorenko's 1997 paper.

TABLE 1

The genetics of reading disability: two strong linkage findings replicated for chromosomes 6 and 15

Chromosome 6 (6p just distal to the HLA)	Chromosome 15
Smith, Kimberling and Pennington, 1991	Smith et al., 1983
Fisher et al., 1999	Schulte-Körne et al., 1999
Cardon et al., 1994	Grigorenko et al., 1997
Gayán et al., 1999	
Grigorenko et al., 1997	
Grigorenko et al., 2000	

Locus heterogeneity exists (different chromosomal regions in different families).
Both appear to be dominant transmission.

Gayán, Smith, Cherny et al. (1999) also provided additional support for the locus influencing reading ability at chromosome 6p. These investigators assessed a new sample of 126 sib pairs, measuring performance on multiple tests of word recognition, orthographic coding, phonological decoding, and phoneme awareness. Evidence for linkage varied among different defined phenotypes, which may suggest that this locus may influence measures of reading and language performance differentially (Barr, 2002, personal communication).

A complete genome scan for reading disorders has recently been published by Fisher, Francks, Marlow et al. (2002). Two sets of reading disabled families were used in this study, one from the United Kingdom and one from the United States; and both families had previously been reported to exhibit genetic linkage to chromosome 6p. Fisher et al. reported the most significant single point finding to be for markers on chromosome 18p for a measure of single word identification ability. Performance measures of orthographic and phonological processing skill also exhibited evidence of linkage to this locus. Barr, Wigg, Feng et al. (2001) suggest that this locus may influence a number of reading-related processes and constitute a more general risk factor for reading disability influencing several reading-related skills. Wood and Grigorenko (2001) contend that the chromosome 6 genotype may have a cognitive impact that is not specifically restricted to reading acquisition processes per se.

Additional loci for reading disability have been reported in individual investigations. A region on chromosome 2 was identified during a genome scan of a large Norwegian family in which dyslexia had been identified as an autosomal dominant trait (Fagerheim, Raeymaekers, Tonnessen et al., 1999). Additional evidence supporting this locus was reported from a sample of Canadian families (Petryshen, Kaplan, Hughes et al., 2002). Evidence for linkage to chromosome 1 has also been provided in individual reports but is not yet well replicated (Grigorenko et al., 2000; Rabin, Wen, Hepburn and Lubs, 1993).

While these linkage findings are extremely promising and represent substantial progress in the genetics of reading and its disorders, it should be recognized that to date no single genes have been implicated. A recent effort to assess the MOG gene on chromosome 6p21.3 as a candidate gene for reading disability yielded negative results (Smith et al., 2001). Different linkage findings suggest a minimum of six different genes potentially influencing reading disability, with the likelihood that more will be identified. Recognition of the heterogeneity of both genetic and environmental contributions to the development of reading disorders has provided a more realistic and a more sophisticated perspective on this complex developmental disorder.

A important degree of replication in the recent literature bodes well for what may be learned in the next five years about the genetic substrates of neurocognitive development and of reading disability and related neurocognitive disorders. There is already some evidence emerging of overlapping genetic influences with other developmental learning disorders frequently comorbid with developmental reading disorders, such as Attention Deficit Hyperactivity Disorder (ADHD) (Willcutt and Pennington, 2000; Willcutt, Pennington and DeFries, 2000; Wood and Flowers, 1999), specific language impairment (SLI Consortium, 2002), and mathematical learning disorders (Light and DeFries, 1995), although not all these associations are well understood or well replicated at the present time.

Long-term outcomes for children with reading disorders

Research on adolescent and adult outcomes of children with developmental reading disorders indicates that reading ability *does* improve with age and intervention for most reading disabled children. At the same time, core signature deficits of reading disorder clearly persist into adulthood, particularly in more severe cases. Phonological deficits persist, even in cases with good literacy outcomes (Bruck, 1992, 1998; Scarborough, 1984; Shaywitz et al., 1999). Problems persist with spelling accuracy, word recognition speed, and in reading rate, particularly in the reading of more technical expository text.

Prospective longitudinal data from the Connecticut Longitudinal Study reveal that the natural course of reading disorder follows a deficit rather than the developmental lag model over time (Francis et al., 1996; Shaywitz et al., 1999). When children who met criteria for persistent reading disability in Grades 2 through 6 were compared with normally developing children with average and superior reading skills in those grades, the persistently poor readers continued to exhibit deficits in phonological coding in adolescence and to demonstrate continuing problems in reading, spelling, and reading rate (Shaywitz et al., 1999).

The children who were classified as reading disabled early in their elementary school careers remained inferior readers relative to other students in the CLS longitudinal sample in high school. Shaywitz and her colleagues (1998, 1999) considered these results “sobering”, particularly since children in the persistent poor reader group all had received special education services. There was no evidence that children in the persistent RD group had caught up in their reading skills by high school. When nonacademic outcomes were considered, no differences were found between good and poor readers in 12th grade on student and teacher reports of the prevalence of legal problems, or of alcohol or tobacco use. Similarly, there was no evidence from these student and teacher reports of any differences between the groups in the prevalence of conduct or attention problems.

This result is contrary to findings from another longitudinal sample suggesting that adolescent learning disorders were associated with a three-fold increase in the risk for substance abuse problems after the contribution of concurrent behavior problems and family structure had been controlled (Beitchman, Wilson, Douglas et al., 2001). Beitchman and his colleagues concluded that persistent learning disorders in adolescence (at ages 12 and 19) were associated with a generally elevated risk for adverse outcomes in young adulthood, including lower family SES status, lower IQ scores, and lower educational and occupational attainments at age 19. This sample included a range of learning disorders, however, including reading and/or spelling and/or math disorders. Earlier follow-up studies of reading disabled children had reported negative findings (Bruck, 1985; Spreen, 1987), similar to the Shaywitz et al. (1999) results, although neither study had the prospective longitudinal design and methodological strengths of the CLS (Shaywitz et al., 1990) or the Ottawa Language Study (Beitchman, Nair, Clegg et al., 1986; Beitchman, Wilson, Douglas et al., 2001).

Considerable variability exists in the standard of literacy attained by adults with childhood diagnoses of reading disability. Data published by Bruck (1985, 1989, 1998) suggest that although many of her subjects had been educationally successful, and as adults had significantly increased their level of reading skill, the core dyslexic processing deficits had endured. In a series of studies examining patterns of word recognition processing in adolescents and adults with childhood diagnoses of dyslexia, and age- and reading-age matched control subjects, Bruck found that the pattern of deficits characterizing dyslexic children were the very same patterns of deficits that continued to characterize adults with childhood histories of developmental dyslexia. Although standards of literacy were significantly improved in many subjects, the mechanisms of word recognition processing did not appear to change or mature with time and learning. The highest word identification scores were attained by dyslexics who had pursued college education (Bruck, 1989); but the average word recognition score for these dyslexics was placed only at the 32nd percentile (Bruck, 1998). Scores on standardized reading comprehension tests tended to be reliably higher than those on standardized word identification tests, again confirming the most severe deficits for these individuals to reside at lexical and sublexical levels of processing.

Another sample of university-enrolled dyslexics, with mean standardized reading, word attack (nonword reading), and reading comprehension scores within the average range, were compared with controls at the same campus; the controls scored more than one standard deviation above average on word identification and word attack tests and were consistently superior to the "compensated" dyslexics on a range of phonological processing tasks (Wilson and Lesaux, 2001). These data attest to the range of literacy outcomes that have been observed in adult follow-ups of students earlier diagnosed with dyslexia or reading disability. Despite the strong converging evidence of the persistence of core phonological processing deficits into adulthood, there appears to be no scientific evidence on the efficacy of phonologically-oriented or other remedial training for adults with dyslexia who want to improve their basic literacy skills.

Treatment outcome research on developmental reading disorders

Although the phenomenon of developmental reading disorders has been recognized for well over a century, and many approaches to treating reading disorders had been advocated and attempted, it was only in the mid- to late-1980s that any reliable or credible evidence from well controlled studies of the efficacy of different interventions have been reported. This dearth of scientific evidence over so many decades led to inevitable questions about the amenability of the disorder to treatment (Lovett, 1997, 1999; Lovett and Barron, 2002).

Longitudinal evidence documenting the depth and longevity of core phonological processing deficits for individuals with reading disorders (Bruck, 1992; Felton and Brown, 1990) had led to understandable concerns about their amenability to remediation (e.g., Wagner et al., 1994). With an ambitious research funding program announced by the National Institute of Child Health and Human Development in the US in the 1990s, clear incentives to conduct rigorous research on remedial interventions for phonologically-based reading disabilities became available (Lyon, 1995; Lyon and Moats, 1997; Moats and Foorman, 1997); large-scale scientific research on what constitutes effective remediation for developmental reading disorders started in earnest. Advances in our understanding of the neurobiological and genetic substrates of reading disability and other developmental neurocognitive disorders in the mid-1990s (Filipek, 1995, 1999; Grigorenko et al., 1997; Pennington, 1997; Shaywitz et al., 1998) served to focus increased research attention on the nature and underlying causes of these learning disabilities and the extent to which the core cognitive processing deficits could be ameliorated with effective intervention methods.

Within the last several years, a relatively large number of controlled and comparative research studies have been reported assessing the efficacy of different instructional approaches to the remediation of reading acquisition problems in the early elementary grades (Foorman, Francis, Winikates et al., 1997;

Foorman et al., 1998; Scanlon and Vellutino, 1997; Torgesen et al., 1997; Torgesen, Wagner, Rashotte et al., 1999; Vellutino et al., 1996, 2000). Positive results from controlled intervention studies focussing on the core phonological and word identification deficits of reading disabled children in later grades have also been reported (Lovett and Steinbach, 1997; Lovett, Steinbach and Frijters, 2000; Olson et al., 1997; Torgesen, Alexander, Wagner et al., 2001; Wise and Olson, 1995; Wise, Ring and Olson, 1999; Wise, Ring, Sessions and Olson, 1997). Converging evidence has been reported indicating that significant improvement can be attained on speech-based and phonological reading measures for both disabled readers and young children at risk for reading disability (Foorman et al., 1998; Olson et al., 1997; Torgesen et al., 1997, 1999; Vellutino et al., 1996), confirming the contention that phonologically-based decoding and early reading skills are "teachable aspects of reading for most children" (Moats and Foorman, 1997, p.188). Additional evidence from controlled intervention studies on reading disorder reveals that, with intensive systematic intervention focussed on remediation of core deficits, measurable progress in phonological reading skills *can* be achieved throughout the elementary school years even with the most severely impaired readers of a clinical sample (Lovett and Steinbach, 1997; Lovett, Steinbach and Frijters, 2000).

Despite the improvements observed in children's phonologically-based word attack and decoding skills, many of the above investigators have found that remedial gains do not reliably generalize to other aspects of reading acquisition. Children who, after intervention, could 'sound out' new words or nonwords were not always improved relative to comparison groups in their word recognition, text reading, or reading comprehension skills. In fact, generalization of remedial gains has proven a formidable hurdle for many intervention methods evaluated in the literature (Olson et al., 1997; Torgesen et al., 1997) and for those which we have assessed in early remediation studies at The Hospital for Sick Children in Toronto (Lovett, Ransby and Barron, 1988; Lovett, Ransby, Hardwick et al., 1989; Lovett, Warren-Chaplin, Ransby and Borden, 1990). As Moats and Foorman noted in their summary of a set of intervention studies, "generalization and transfer of decoding proficiency to fluent word recognition and better reading comprehension was not automatic and constitutes a . . . phase of remediation that needs . . . additional study" (1997, p. 188).

Generalization in disabled readers' response to treatment: components of effective instruction for reading disabilities

Torgesen et al. (1997) have suggested that the generalization problem in these treatment studies may reflect in part the complexity of the processing impairments seen in more severely disabled readers. In fact, it is now recognized that the core processing deficits of many disabled readers extend beyond the realm of phonological awareness to other domains of function. Wolf and Bowers have identified the deficit in naming speed as potentially causal to developmental reading disability (Bowers and Wolf, 1993; Wolf, 1991; Wolf and Bowers, 1999, 2000). Both phonological awareness and naming speed deficits interfere with reading acquisition at the lexical level and the existence of both deficits in combination are known to constitute a risk factor for more severe forms of reading disability than demonstration of either deficit separately (Lovett, Steinbach and Frijters, 2000; Wolf et al., 2000a).

Many of the generalization failures observed in disabled readers' response to instruction could also be attributed to a more general difficulty with acquiring effective, flexible word identification strategies and with monitoring the effectiveness of their strategic efforts. Problems in specific aspects of executive functioning and strategy learning appear to exist in learning disabled readers independent of their phonological processing difficulties (Levin, 1990; Swanson, 1999; Swanson and Alexander, 1997). Recent research has also confirmed the specificity of the transfer-of-learning deficit, however: Transfer-of-learning difficulties for disabled readers appear specific to printed language learning and are not evident on other learning tasks with similar cognitive demands but no phonological processing requirements (Benson, 2000; Benson, Lovett and Kroeber, 1997).

Our clinical research program at The Hospital for Sick Children in Toronto has maintained a long history of interest in generalization and transfer-of-learning issues. Difficulties in achieving generalization of remedial gains has motivated some of our most recent research with severely reading disabled children referred to our laboratory classrooms. We have described research in which children were randomly assigned to one of two remedial reading programs or to an active control treatment that worked on helping them acquire better study, organizational, and problem solving skills (Lovett et al., 1994; Lovett and Steinbach, 1997; Lovett, Steinbach and Frijters, 2000). Both of the reading programs targeted the problem of generalization of treatment gains in word identification learning, but they addressed this problem with quite different instructional approaches and at different levels of print-to-sound segmentation.

The PHAB/DI (Phonological Analysis and Blending/Direct Instruction) Program consists of lessons from the direct instructional programs developed by Engelmann and his colleagues at the University of Oregon and trains phonological analysis, phonological blending, and letter–sound association skills in the context of word recognition and decoding instruction (see Reading Mastery I/II Fast Cycle, and Corrective Reading Programs: Engelmann and Bruner, 1988; Engelmann, Carnine and Johnson, 1988; Engelmann, Johnson, Carnine et al., 1988). The second remedial reading program is called WIST for Word Identification Strategy Training. WIST has a strong metacognitive focus and teaches the children how to use and monitor the application of four metacognitive decoding strategies. The WIST Program was developed in our laboratory classrooms at The Hospital for Sick Children, and is based in part on the original Benchmark School Word Identification/Vocabulary Development Program developed by Irene Gaskins and her colleagues (Gaskins, Downer and Gaskins, 1986). WIST adapts the Benchmark Program's dialogue structure for strategy instruction, their keywords, and their compare/contrast strategy (a strategy of word identification by analogy). WIST differs from the Benchmark Program in its inclusion of three additional word identification strategies, its direct training focus on the subskills necessary for strategy implementation, and its provision of a metacognitive 'Game Plan' to train flexibility in strategy choice and evaluation of the success of those choices.

PHAB/DI and WIST work on subsyllabic segmentation using subword units of different size: PHAB/DI focuses on the smallest spelling-to-sound units (letter–sound) and WIST trains recognition of larger subsyllabic units, particularly the rime. Both programs attempt to promote generalization of word identification learning in different ways — PHAB/DI by intensive systematic remediation of core sound analysis and blending deficits, WIST by teaching a set of flexible word identification strategies and the specific skills and content required to implement them successfully. Every lesson of PHAB/DI and WIST includes practice applying new word identification skills in context — by reading connected text with controlled vocabulary and at carefully selected levels of difficulty.

In controlled research, both PHAB/DI and WIST proved far more effective than previous interventions from the perspective of achieving generalization of remedial gains (Lovett et al., 1988, 1989, 1990): PHAB/DI- and WIST-trained children were found to be significantly improved on several standardized and experimental measures and achieved generalization on a set of word reading measures including transfer probes varying in their distance from instructed target words used in the PHAB/DI and WIST lessons. While both approaches were associated with large positive effects, different patterns of transfer were observed following the two programs, confirming the existence of some treatment-specific effects. The phonological program, PHAB/DI, resulted in broader-based and deeper generalization within the phonological skill domain (speech- and print-based), and WIST, with its strategy training focus, resulted in broader-based generalization for real English words (i.e., regular *and* exception words).

Three findings from this research were particularly encouraging: (i) the achievement of generalization within the word identification domain; and (ii) the demonstration that the phonological skills and letter–sound learning of severely disabled readers could be improved with focussed intensive remediation of this type, and (iii) effects were achieved even with later (e.g., Grades 5/6) intervention (Lovett and Steinbach, 1997) and even for the most disabled children (Lovett, Steinbach and Frijters, 2000). The phonological processing and reading deficits of these children were not ameliorated after short-term in-

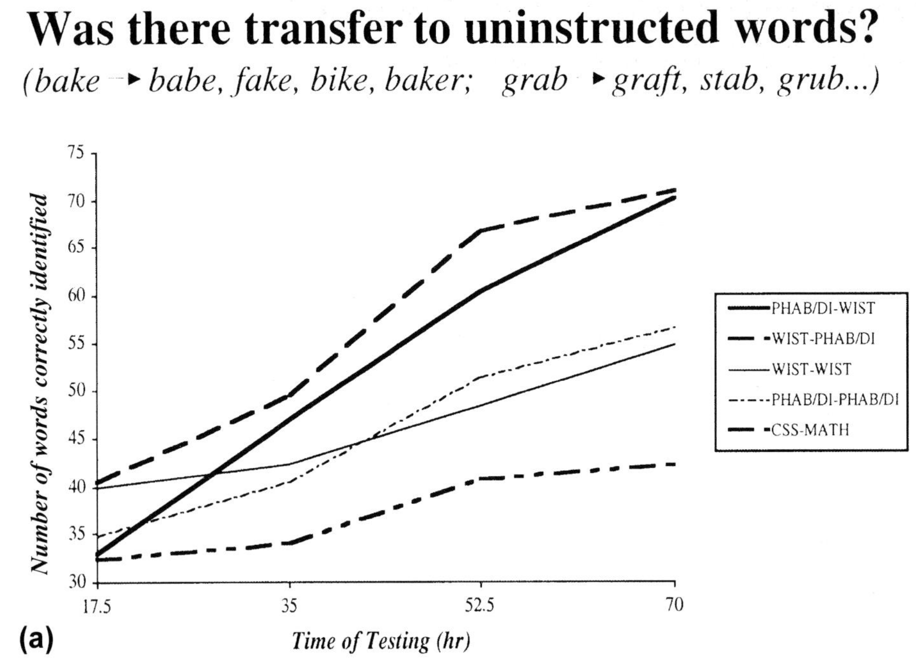

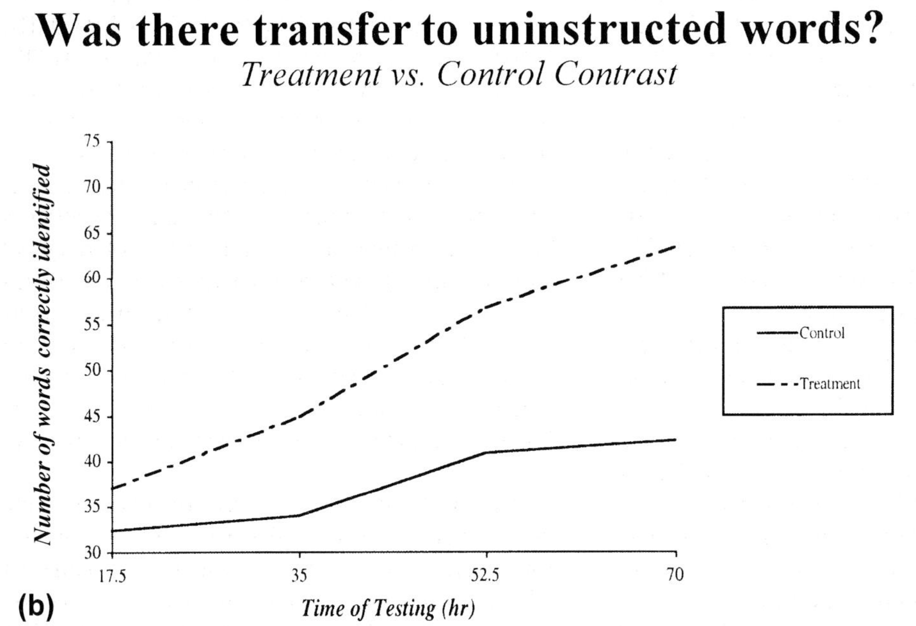

Fig. 3. (a–c) Learning curves for disabled readers receiving a sequential combination of phonological and strategy-based instruction (PHAB/DI → WIST; WIST → PHAB/DI); phonological (PHAB/DI) or strategy-based instruction alone (WIST); or a control treatment program (CSS → MATH). From: Lovett MW, Lacerenza L, Borden SL, Frijters JC, Steinbach KA, De Palma M: Components of effective remediation for developmental reading disabilities: Combining phonological and strategy-based instruction to improve outcomes. Journal of Educational Psychology: 92(2); 263–283, 2000. Copyright 2000 by the American Psychological Association. Reprinted and adapted with permission.

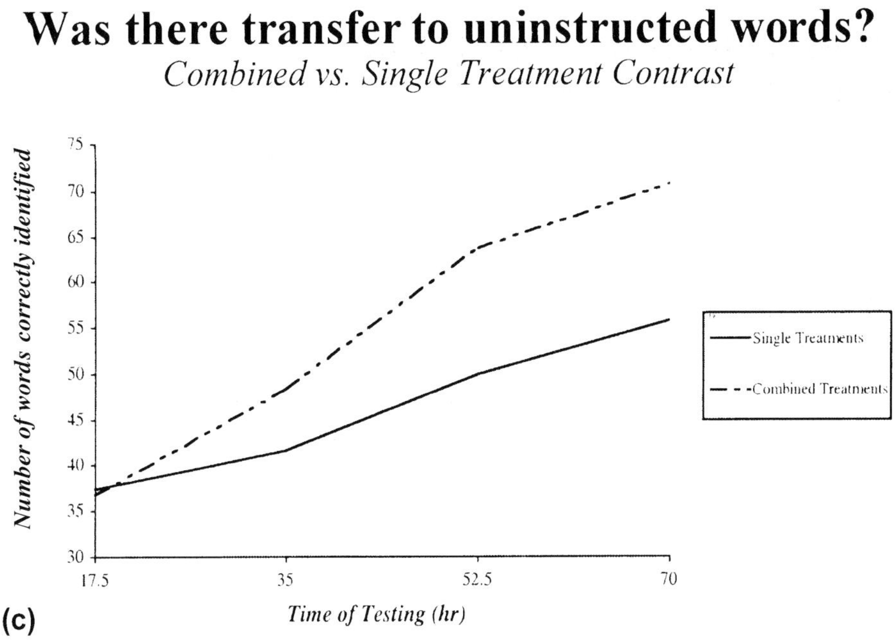

(c)

Fig. 3 (continued).

tervention, but both print- and speech-based phonological skills were significantly improved and closer to age-appropriate levels. After 35 hours of instruction, PHAB/DI and WIST graduates typically were not reading at grade level; however, they demonstrated markedly improved letter–sound knowledge, better decoding abilities, and better word identification skills. Before their remedial interventions, these severely disabled readers were incorrectly identifying one-syllable words like *way*, *left*, and *put*: After PHAB/DI or WIST lessons, many of these children were able to decode accurately (although often very slowly) difficult multisyllabic words like *unintelligible*, *mistakenly*, and *disengaged*.

In a recent sequential crossover design, we addressed the question of whether phonologically-based remediation is sufficient to achieve the best remedial outcomes for children with severe reading disabilities, or whether a combination of phonological and strategy training approaches produces superior outcomes (Lovett, Lacerenza, Borden et al., 2000). The efficacy of a combination of these two approaches was compared to that of longer-term intervention with each approach separately. Eighty-five severely reading disabled children, 7–13 years of age, were randomly assigned to 70 hours of remedial instruction in one of five program sequences: PHAB/DI $\rightarrow$ WIST; WIST $\rightarrow$ PHAB/DI; PHAB/DI $\times$ 2; WIST $\times$ 2; or CSS $\rightarrow$ MATH (Classroom Survival Skills $\rightarrow$ Mathematics, a control treatment offering study skills and then math instruction). Each child's performance was assessed at five time points: before, at three points during, and following 70 hours of intervention to allow a closer examination of the time course of remedial gains and their generalization within the different instructional conditions. Generalized treatment effects were achieved on standardized measures of word identification, passage comprehension, and nonword reading, confirming the effectiveness of the present instructional programs on multiple indices of reading skill.

The most critical results were the demonstration of superior outcomes and steeper learning curves for children who received a sequential combination of the phonological and strategy-based instruction (Fig. 3). A combination of PHAB/DI and WIST proved superior to either intervention alone on measures of phonological reading skill (nonword reading), measures of letter–sound and keyword knowledge, and three word identification measures (two of near and far transfer words and the third of uninstructed multisyllabic challenge words). These results provide evidence of the separate instructional contributions of both the phonological and the strategy-based methods and demonstrate that generalization from nonword decoding to other reading measures can be best achieved with a *combination* of effective remedial components.

The findings of this intervention research suggest that phonologically-based approaches alone are *not* sufficient for achieving optimal remedial outcomes with reading disabled individuals. While phonologically-based and deficit-directed interventions appear necessary to achieve gains, generalization of gains is more probable if a multidimensional approach to core reading-related deficits is implemented. Our findings indicate that faster learning and better outcomes are achieved when a broader-based approach is used — particularly one combining direct and dialogue-based instructional methods, teaching children different levels of subsyllabic segmentation, and training them in the acquisition and effective use of multiple decoding strategies. The critical importance of strategy instruction and the promotion of a flexible approach to word identification and text reading tasks cannot be overemphasized.

This conclusion is compatible with recent findings from a meta-analysis of the treatment outcome literature on learning disabilities: Swanson and Hoskyn (1998) reviewed 180 intervention studies and concluded that the optimal approach in instructing children with learning disabilities was a combined intervention model that included both direct instruction and strategy instruction methods. Additional work by Swanson (1999) focussed specifically on meta-analytic analyses of remedial reading interventions and demonstrated that a combined direct/strategy training approach is particularly important when outcomes in the domain of reading comprehension and text reading are considered.

A recent development in our laboratory classrooms at The Hospital for Sick Children has been to integrate these approaches into a single intervention program. Called the PHAST Track Reading Program (PHAST for Phonological *and* Strategy Training), this program begins with PHAB/DI's program of phonological remediation and uses it as a framework on which each of the four WIST strategies are introduced and scaffolded (Fig. 4). A detailed description of the instructional design of the PHAST Track Reading Program, of its component instructional parts (PHAB/DI and WIST), of the dialogue structure acquired for the learning of each word identification strategy, and of sample instructional materials developed for each program section has been published (Lovett, Lacerenza and Borden, 2000). PHAST attempts to build context-free word identification skills and strategies and facilitate their immediate application to the desired goal — reading connected text for meaning. The daily PHAST lessons include many opportunities for the children to practice applying a metacognitive Game Plan (Table 2) in daily story reading and in various Challenge Word Games. Pyramid Challenge, for example, provides a gameboard on which readers navigate a pyramid's levels and tunnels by accurately decoding difficult challenge words. The challenge games present the struggling readers — now armed with a treasure chest of multiple effective decoding strategies — a playing field on which to expedite various decoding plans and hone their skills and strategies.

The PHAST Track Reading Program is intended to be situated in a linguistically-enriched and literature-based balanced literacy program. PHAST is an intensive program to develop word identification and word attack skills and to facilitate the development of the basic skills necessary to allow independent decoding and reading for meaning. The metacognitive instructional focus and dialogue structure of the PHAST Program is compatible with dialogue-based approaches to text comprehension and writing training. Ideally, full implementation of the PHAST Program in a classroom setting would place it as part of an integrated approach to reading, spelling, and writing instruction to allow intense instruction in spelling-to-sound and sound-to-spelling analysis at the subsyllabic, lexical, and connected text levels. The goal is to foster the development of reading, spelling, comprehension, and literacy skills that would equip the child for a world where the demands for fluent, effective, multifaceted literacy skills are ever increasing. The PHAST Track Reading Program was developed for the struggling readers in our laboratory classrooms, but it is adaptable to the needs of precocious and average readers in the early elementary years. Future developments and refinements to the PHAST Program are under way

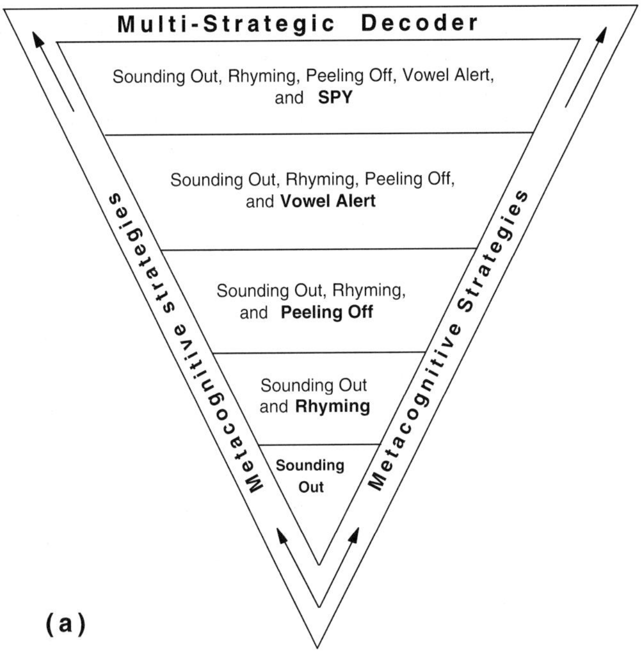

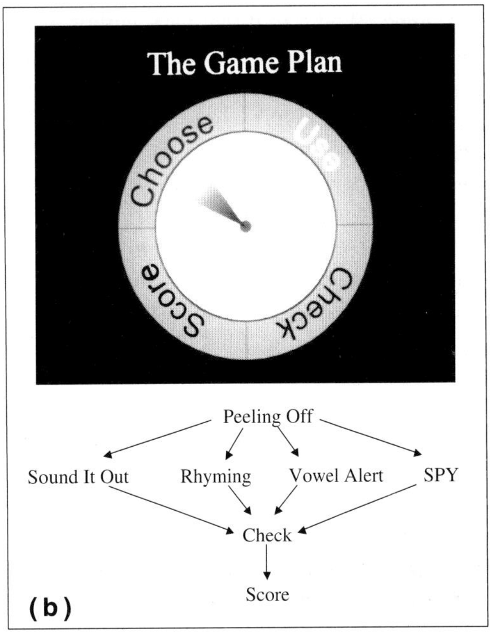

Fig. 4. (a) The PHAST Track: The acquisition of multiple word identification strategies and the sequence of their introduction in the PHAST Track Reading Program. (b) The Game Plan: A formula for strategy selection, application, monitoring, and evaluation. From: Lovett MW, Lacerenza L, Borden SL: Putting struggling readers on the PHAST track: A program to integrate phonological and strategy-based remedial reading instruction and maximize outcomes. Journal of Learning Disabilities: 33(5); 458–476, 2000. Copyright 2000 by PRO-ED, Inc. Reprinted with permission.

TABLE 2

A sample of strategy execution using the metacognitive dialogue "GAME Plan" from the PHAST Track Reading Program

The following is an example of the prompts and the dialogue of Game Plan as it is used to decode the word *unstacking*:

Step 1. CHOOSE:
"My Game Plan is to first use Peeling Off. Then I am going to use the Rhyming Strategy and look for spelling patterns I know."

Step 2. USE:
"I am Peeling Off *un* and *ing*. My next Game Plan is Rhyming. I see the spelling pattern *a-c-k*. The key word is *pack*. If I know *pack*, then I know *stack*"

Step 3. CHECK:
"I have to *stop and think* about whether I'm using the strategy(ies) properly. Is it working? Yes, I'll keep on going. I will put all the parts together — *un-stack-ing*."

Step 4. SCORE/RE-CHOOSE:
"The word is *unstacking*. I scored! I used Peeling Off and Rhyming to help me figure out this word and they worked." (If the strategy did not result in a real word, the child begins again at Step 1, and *chooses* another strategy to try.)

From: Lovett MW, Lacerenza L, Borden SL: Putting struggling readers on the PHAST track: A program to integrate phonological and strategy-based remedial reading instruction and maximize outcomes. Journal of Learning Disabilities: 33(5); 458–476, 2000. Copyright 2000 by PRO-ED, Inc. Reprinted with permission.

to develop an extended reading comprehension track and to develop an adaptation of PHAST for older individuals with reading disorders.

The PHAST Track Reading Program is being evaluated in a large multi-site intervention study funded by NICHD: In this project, Robin Morris,

Maryanne Wolf, and the first author are assessing the effectiveness of two different dual-focus, deficit-directed intervention programs for young disabled readers [PHAST (Lovett, Lacerenza and Borden, 2000) and PHAB/DI + RAVE-O (Wolf et al., 2000b; see below)] against both an alternative treatment control program (Classroom Survival Skills + Math, see Lovett, Steinbach and Frijters, 2000) and a phonological treatment control program (PHAB/DI + CSS). The reader is referred to the published papers for a more detailed description of the interventions described in these pages.

Beyond the acquisition of basic reading skills: the attainment of reading fluency in individuals with developmental reading disorders

In a recent study comparing two intensive individualized remediation programs for 8–10-year-old disabled readers, Torgesen and his colleagues (Torgesen et al., 2001) found significant improvement in generalized reading skills that were sustained over a two year follow-up period, but little impact in terms of disabled readers' continued impairment in reading speed. Although extended individual instruction in both programs (each 67.5 hours and differing in the pedagogical focus of the phonological training) was associated with rapid growth in these children's reading skills, and graduates of the two programs scored on average within the age-appropriate range of reading achievement two years after intervention, these improvements were demonstrated for measures of word identification and passage comprehension only. The children remained two standard deviations below age norms on measures of reading rate at follow-up despite an overall increase in the number of words per minute read over this time and documented improvement in basic reading skills. Torgesen and his colleagues speculate that to "close the gap" for older disabled readers, they would have to add sight words (words that can be recognized immediately, without phonologically mediated decoding) to their lexicons at a rate in excess of that of their non-disabled age-mates. In addition they acknowledge that some of the disabled readers may have constraints upon levels of processing speed as indexed for example by the naming speed deficits on rapid automatized naming tasks (Wolf et al., 1986; Wolf and Bowers, 1999).

There has been growing recognition that different models of remedial intervention will need to be developed if disabled readers are to make gains in phonological processing skills, word identification and text reading accuracy *and* in word identification speed and text reading fluency with intervention. In fact, there remains little consensus in definitions of reading fluency (Meyer and Felton, 1999; Wolf and Katzir-Cohen, 2001). Meyer and Felton defined fluency as "the ability to read connected text rapidly, smoothly, effortlessly, and automatically with little conscious attention to the mechanics of reading such as decoding" (1999, p. 284), similar to the early model of LaBerge and Samuels (1974) of reading fluency as resulting from the automatization of component processes thus allowing attentional resources to be reallocated to other levels of processing. Berninger, Abbott, Billingsley and Nagy (2001) advocate a "systems" conceptualization of reading fluency, based upon their body of research examining components of reading, spelling, and written language development. Berninger et al. suggest that fluency is dependent upon three main sources of influence: characteristics of the stimulus input (visual or speech), the efficiency and automaticity of component language processing systems, and management and coordination by an executive function system.

Wolf and Katzir-Cohen (2001) propose a developmental and component-based framework for understanding and facilitating the acquisition of reading fluency. They define reading fluency as

> the product of the initial development of accuracy and the subsequent development of automaticity in underlying sublexical processes, lexical processes, and their integration in single-word reading and connected text. These include perceptual, phonological, orthographic, and morphological processes at the letter, letter-pattern, and word level, as well as semantic and syntactic processes at the word level and connected text level. After it is fully developed, reading fluency refers to a level of accuracy and rate where decoding is relatively effortless; where oral reading is smooth and accurate with correct prosody; and where attention can be allocated to comprehension.
>
> *Wolf and Katzir-Cohen, 2001, p. 219*

It should be noted, however, that much remains unknown about the nature and reciprocity of the relationships between reading fluency and text comprehension. Although it has long been assumed that increased efficiency and automatization of word identification and decoding processes will result in a freeing of attentional resources for comprehension processing, the question of whether there exist direct reciprocal relationships between fluency and comprehension is not established (Meyer and Felton, 1999; Wolf and Katzir-Cohen, 2001).

Following this developmental model of reading fluency, Wolf and her colleagues at Tufts University have developed an experimental reading intervention program called RAVE-O to facilitate its development (Wolf et al., 2000b). RAVE-O is only to be taught in combination with a systematic phonologically-based intervention program that teaches letter–sound knowledge, decoding, and word identification skills while remediating the speech-based phonological processes of disabled readers. In combination with this decoding program, RAVE-O (for Retrieval, Automaticity, Vocabulary Elaboration, Engagement, and Orthography) seeks (i) to facilitate accuracy and automaticity in reading subskills and component processes; (ii) to develop fluency in word identification, word attack, and text reading and comprehension processes; and (iii) to retrain the attitudes and affect of disabled readers in their approach to words and written language. RAVE-O helps the children learn to play with their language through animated computer games (Wolf and Goodman, 1996), building of imaginative word webs, the teaching of systematic yet playful word retrieval strategies, and the reading of minute mystery stories.

As with the PHAST Track Reading Program described above, the RAVE-O program in conjunction with the previously described PHAB/DI Program (Engelmann and Bruner, 1988; Lovett et al., 1994) is being evaluated in the large multi-site intervention study funded by NICHD in which Robin Morris, Maryanne Wolf and the first author are assessing the effectiveness of two different dual-focus, deficit-directed intervention programs for young disabled readers [PHAB/DI + RAVE-O; and PHAB/DI + WIST - i.e., PHAST (Lovett, Lacerenza and Borden, 2000)] against both an alternative treatment control program (Classroom Survival Skills + Math, see Lovett, Steinbach and Frijters, 2000) and a phonological treatment control program (PHAB/DI + CSS). Again, the reader is referred to the published papers for a more detailed description of the interventions described in these pages.

Findings of the National Reading Panel and questions for further intervention research

Within the past decade, substantial evidence has been amassed that significantly increases our understanding of what constitutes effective intervention for individuals with developmental reading disorder, and what components of instruction are critical for young children at risk of reading acquisition failure. As more large-scale controlled research studies are reported, the next years should herald a better integrated, methodologically more sophisticated, research literature about developmental reading disorders, their characterization and etiologies, and optimal methods of intervention.

The recent Report of the Subgroups from the National Reading Panel (2000) in the United States reviewed the available scientifically credible literature on intervention, and made clear recommendations about how to develop phonological awareness, decoding, and word identification skills in struggling readers. Even the NRP Report, however, notes that despite substantial advances in our understanding of the importance of phonologically-based instruction in remediating developmental reading disorders, there remain important but neglected questions requiring future research. Among their recommendations are research into the "active ingredients" in effective systematic phonics-based reading programs, study of the influence of motivational factors in learners *and* in teachers, and the importance of using decodable text in phonologically-based programs.

There were, in addition, areas of instruction where evidence was too sparse for the NRP to make recommendations for practice. The Panel was reluctant to suggest a particular method of vocabulary instruction, for example, because of the paucity of replicated research studies on different methods. The NRP found a more extensive body of studies on guided oral reading procedures (designed to facilitate the development of reading fluency), and suggested that these procedures tended to result in improved word recognition, fluency, and comprehension with most groups. Their analysis of the effectiveness of other programs to encourage fluency and foster more reading experience revealed equivocal results and inadequate evidence to sustain many claims.

Although many methodological and measurement limitations were noted to characterize reading comprehension studies, the best available evidence supported the superiority of comprehension instruction that involved the training of multiple comprehension strategies and a metacognitive approach that emphasizes flexibility in strategy application. The NRP concluded that the teaching of a variety of reading comprehension strategies was associated with increased learning of the strategies, better transfer of learning, better retention and comprehension of new texts, and occasionally with generalized improvement in reading comprehension skill. More research was suggested as to how to effectively prepare teachers for the instruction of multiple flexible strategies. Metacognitive methods, scaffolding, socratic questioning, and cognitive strategy instruction require considerable teacher expertise — and access to sufficient mentoring while these skills are being developed.

Final comments: asking neurobiological questions about treatment response

The neuropsychological and neurobiological literatures reviewed in earlier pages have yielded a better integrated, more focused, and enriched knowledge base about developmental reading disorders, their neurobiological substrates, their developmental precursors, and the interaction of genetic predisposition and environmental experience that may influence the emergence of reading disorders. Substantial increases in evidence-based treatment approaches now allow the posing of more refined research questions about the combination of treatment components that are most effective, characteristics of optimal treatment delivery, and moderators and mediators of long-term treatment outcome.

As advances have been made in our understanding of the core processing deficits on a behavioral and cognitive level, key issues with respect to definition, and phenotypic and genotypic clarifications of what constitutes reading disorder, there have emerged new questions regarding potential neurobiological correlates of performance gains with effective intervention. Specifically, many investigators have questioned whether it is possible that the neurobiological substrates for reading behavior can change with behavioral evidence of improvements in reading skill. And if change can be observed at a neurobiological level, are there limits to plasticity in these brain regions with respect to establishing more effective functional circuitry to subserve newly developing literacy skills? Is there a developmental window beyond which literacy cannot be attained?

Recent findings by Simos, Fletcher, Bergman et al. (2002) offer some empirical support for these speculations. These investigators obtained Magnetic Source Imaging (MSI) scans on eight dyslexic readers and eight normal readers while subjects decoded nonwords (i.e., completed a visual pseudoword rhyme detection task, e.g., *yoat* and *wote*). The dyslexic children received 80 hours of intense, individualized, phonologically-based remediation and were scanned before and after the intervention. The normal readers were scanned on two separate occasions two months apart, and no significant changes were observed as a function of time in their activation profiles. Before remediation, dyslexic subjects demonstrated limited activation of the superior temporal gyrus, the signature profile of impaired readers in this area of the brain involved with phonological processing. Similar to imaging studies reviewed earlier, the dyslexic subjects also showed increased activation in corresponding right hemisphere areas. After effective remediation, associated with normalization of phonological decoding scores for these dyslexic individuals, their MSI activation profiles during nonword decoding were observed to change "by several orders of magnitude": the investigators report "normalization of the brain activation profiles in *all* children" (Simos et al., 2002), with the most marked intervention-related changes in activation in the posterior portion of the left superior temporal gyrus. In the majority of dyslexic subjects, changes in degree of activation in these regions yielded post-intervention activation profiles that were described as "virtually indistinguishable" from those of the age-matched normal readers. If replicated with larger samples, these findings offer encouraging evidence that the atypical functional organization of the brain in disabled readers can be altered with intervention techniques that are effective and sufficiently intense to move their decoding and word identification skills into the age-appropriate range. This provides an optimistic perspective on the amenability of the disorder to intervention, and insight into the neurobiological and functional changes that remain possible even into adolescence. (Subjects in the study ranged from 7 to 17 years of age, with a mean of 11.4 years.)

Research findings such as these, when translated into practice, should impact upon the lives of reading disabled individuals, particularly children, and greatly enhance their chances to access effective literacy instruction and become fully involved in their world as literate individuals, participating in and shaping the information age. It is the hope of many involved in the scientific investigation of normal and atypical reading development, its cognitive, neurobiological, and genetic substrates, that our increased understanding will translate into productive literacy initiatives so that we no longer share the shame that half of our world's population remains illiterate.

Acknowledgements

Preparation of this chapter was supported by a National Institute of Child Health and Human Development Grant (HD30970–01A1) to Georgia State University, Tufts University, and The Hospital For Sick Children/University of Toronto. The remediation research reported here was supported, in addition, by operating grants to the authors from the Ontario Mental Health Foundation, the Velleman Foundation, and the Social Sciences and Humanities Research Council of Canada.

We gratefully acknowledge the conceptual contributions of our collaborators and colleagues over the years, particularly those of Robin Morris and Maryanne Wolf. We also gratefully acknowledge the intellectual contributions of senior members of the Learning Disabilities Research Program at The Hospital For Sick Children — Nancy J. Benson, Karen A. Steinbach, Maria De Palma, Jan C. Frijters, Lea Lacerenza and the whole LDRP staff who have contributed so much to past and current intervention studies.

References

Adams MJ: Beginning to Read: Thinking and Learning About Print. Cambridge, MA: The MIT Press, 1990.

Adams MJ, Treiman R, Pressley M: Reading, writing, and literacy. In Sigel IE, Renninger KA (Vol. Eds), Damon W (Ed), Handbook of Child Psychology, Vol. 4 (5th ed.). New York, NY: Wiley, pp. 275–355, 1998.

Alarcón M, DeFries JC: Reading performance and general cognitive ability in twins with reading difficulties and control pairs. Personality and Individual Differences: 22; 793–803, 1997.

American Psychiatric Association: Diagnostic and Statistical Manual of Mental Disorders (4th ed.). Washington, DC: American Psychiatric Association, 1994.

Ansara A: The Orton-Gillingham approach to remediation. In Malatesha RN, Aaron PG (Eds), Reading Disorders: Varieties and Treatment. New York: Academic Press, pp. 409–433, 1982.

Baddeley AD: Working Memory. Oxford: Oxford University Press, 1986.

Badian NA: A validation of the role of preschool phonological and orthographic skills in the prediction of reading. Journal of Learning Disabilities: 31; 472–481, 1998.

Bakker DJ: Hemispheric differences and reading strategies: Two dyslexias? Bulletin of the Orton Society: 29; 84–100, 1979.

Bakwin H: Reading disability in twins. Developmental Medicine and Child Neurology: 15; 184–187, 1973.

Barr CL, Wigg K, Feng Y, Hayes C, Azeke O, Ickowicz A, Schachar R, Tannock R, Roberts W, Malone M, Kennedy JL, Anderson B, Lovett M, Young A, Humphries T: Linkage study of reading disabilities and attention-deficit hyperactivity disorder in the chromosome 6p region. The American Society of Human Genetics 51st Annual Meeting. San Diego, CA. American Journal of Human Genetics: 69(4: 2129); 544, 2001.

Benson NJ: Analysis of specific deficits: Evidence of transfer in disabled and normal readers following oral–motor awareness training. Journal of Educational Psychology: 92(4); 646–658, 2000.

Benson NJ, Lovett MW, Kroeber CL: Training and transfer-of-learning effects in disabled and normal readers: Evidence of specific deficits. Journal of Experimental Child Psychology: 64(3); 343–366, 1997.

Beitchman JH, Nair R, Clegg M, Ferguson B, Patel PG: Prevalence of psychiatric disorders in children with speech and language disorders. American Academy of Child Psychiatry: 25; 528–535, 1986.

Beitchman JH, Wilson B, Douglas L, Young A, Adlaf E: Substance use disorders in young adults with and without LD: Predictive and concurrent relationships. Journal of Learning Disabilities: 34(4); 317–332, 2001.

Beitchman JH, Wilson B, Johnson CJ, Atkinson L, Young A, Adlaf E, Escobar M, Douglas L: Fourteen-year follow-up of speech/language-impaired and control children: Psychiatric outcome. Journal of the American Academy of Child and Adolescent Psychiatry: 40(1); 75–82, 2001.

Berninger VW, Abbott RD, Billingsley F, Nagy W: Processes underlying timing and fluency of reading: Efficiency, automaticity, coordination, and morphological awareness. In Wolf M (Ed), Dyslexia, Fluency, and the Brain. York Press, 2001.

Bisgaard ML, Eiberg H, Moller N, Niebuhr E, Mohr J: Dyslexia and chomosome 15 heteromorphism: Negative lod score in a Danish material. Clinical Genetics: 32; 118–119, 1987.

Bishop DVM: Unfixed reference, monocular occlusion, and developmental dyslexia — a critique. British Journal of Ophthalmology: 73; 209–215, 1989.

Bishop DVM: Uncommon Understanding: Development and Disorders of Language Comprehension in Children. Hove, East Sussex, UK: Psychology Press, 1997.

Bishop DVM, Adams C: A prospective study of the relationship between specific language impairment, phonological disorders and reading retardation. Journal of Child Psychology and Psychiatry: 31(7); 1027–1050, 1990.

Bishop DVM, Bishop SJ, Bright P, James C, Delaney T, Tallal P: Different origin of auditory and phonological processing problems in children with language impairment: Evidence from a twin study. Journal of Speech, Language, and Hearing Research: 42; 155–168, 1999.

Bishop DVM, Carlyon RP, Deeks JM, Bishop SJ: Auditory temporal processing impairment: Neither necessary nor sufficient for causing language impairment in children. Journal of Speech, Language, and Hearing Research: 42; 1295–1310, 1999.

Boder E: Developmental dyslexia: A diagnostic approach based on three atypical reading-spelling patterns. Developmental Medicine and Child Neurology: 15; 663–687, 1973.

Booth JR, Perfetti CA, MacWhinney B, Hunt SB: The association of rapid temporal perception with orthographic and phonological processing in children and adults with reading impairment. Scientific Studies of Reading: 4; 101–132, 2000.

Bowers PG, Sunseth K, Golden J: The route between rapid naming and reading progress. Scientific Studies of Reading: 3; 31–53, 1999.

Bowers PG, Wolf M: Theoretical links between naming speed, precise mechanisms, and orthographic skill in dyslexia. Reading and Writing: An Interdisciplinary Journal: 5; 69–85, 1993.

Bowey JA: Phonological sensitivity in readers and nonreaders. Journal of Experimental Psychology: 58; 134–159, 1994.

Bradley L, Bryant PE: Difficulties in auditory organization as a possible cause of reading backwardness. Nature: 271(5647); 746–747, 1978.

Bradley L, Bryant PE: Categorizing sounds and learning to read: a causal connection. Nature: 301; 419–421, 1983.

Bradlow AR, Kraus N, Nicol T, McGee TJ, Cunningham J, Zecker SG, Carrell TD: Effects of lengthened format transitions duration on discrimination and neural representation of synthetic CV syllables by normal and learning disabled children. Journal of the Acoustical Society of America: 106; 2086–2096, 1999.

Brady SA, Shankweiler D: Phonological processes in literacy: A tribute to Isabelle Y. Liberman. Hillsdale, NJ: Lawrence Erlbaum Associates, Inc., 1991.

Bruck M: The adult functioning of children with specific learning disabilities: A follow-up study. In Siegel IE (Ed), Advances in Applied Developmental Psychology. Vol. 1. Norwood, NJ: Ablex, pp. 91–129, 1985.

Bruck M: Prevalence and ethiology of adjustment problems of children with learning disabilities. In Dumont JJ, Nakken H (Eds), Learning Disabilities: Cognitive, Social and Remedial Aspects. Amsterdam: Swets and Zeitlinger, pp. 73–86, 1989.

Bruck M: Persistence of dyslexics' phonological awareness deficits. Developmental Psychology: 28; 874–886, 1992.

Bruck M: Outcomes of adults with childhood histories of dyslexia. In Hulme C, Joshi RM (Eds), Reading and Spelling: Development and Disorders. Mahwah, NJ: Lawrence Erlbaum Associates Inc., pp. 179–200, 1998.

Bryant PE, Bradley L, Maclean M, Crossland J: Nursery rhymes, phonological skills and reading. Journal of Child Language: 16(2); 407–428, 1989.

Bryne B: Foundations of Literacy: The Child's Acquisition of the Alphabetic Principle. Hove, East Sussex, UK: Psychology Press, 1998.

Bus AG, Van Ijzendoorn MH, Pelligrini AD: Joint book reading makes for success in learning to read: A meta-analysis on intergenerational transmission of literacy. Review of Educational Research: 65; 1–21, 1995.

Cardon LR, Smith SD, Fulker FW, Kimberling WJ, Pennington BF, DeFries JC: Quantitative trait locus for reading disability on chromosome 6. Science: 266; 276–279, 1994.

Castles A, Coltheart M: Varieties of developmental dyslexia. Cognition: 47; 149–180, 1993.

Cestnick L, Coltheart M: The relationship between language-processing and visual-processing deficits in developmental dyslexia. Cognition: 71; 231–255, 1999.

Coltheart M, Curtis B, Atkins P, Haller M: Models of reading aloud: Dual-route and parallel-distributed-processing approaches. Psychological Review: 100(4); 589–608, 1993.

Coltheart M, Patterson KE, Marshall JC (Eds): Deep dyslexia. Hillsdale, NJ: Lawrence Erlbaum Associates, 1980.

Cormier P, Dea S: Distinctive patterns of relationship of phonological awareness and working memory with reading development. Reading and Writing: An Interdisciplinary Journal: 9; 193–206, 1997.

Cornelissen PL, Hansen PC, Gilchrist I, Cormack F, Essex J, Frankish C: Coherent motion detection and letter position encoding. Vision Research: 38; 2181–2191, 1998.

Cornelissen PL, Hansen PC, Hutton JL, Evangelinou V, Stein JF: Magnocellular visual function and children's single word reading. Vision research: 38; 471–482, 1998.

Cornelissen PL, Richardson AJ, Mason AJ, Fowler S, Stein JF: Contrast sensitivity and coherent motion detection measured at photopic luminance levels in dyslexics and controls. Vision Research: 35; 1483–1494, 1995.

Critchley M: The Dyslexic Child. Springfield, IL: Charles C. Thomas, 1970.

Decker SN, Vandenberg SG: Colorado twin study of reading disability. In Gray D, Kavanaugh J (Eds), Biobehavioral Measures of Dyslexia. Baltimore, MD: York Press, pp. 123–135, 1985.

DeFries JC, Alarcón M: Genetics of specific reading disability. Mental Retardation and Developmental Disabilities Research Reviews: 2; 39–47, 1996.

DeFries JC, Fulker DW: Multiple regression analysis of twin data. Behavior Genetics: 15; 467–478, 1985.

DeFries JC, Fulker DW, LaBuda MC: Reading disability in

twins: Evidence for a genetic etiology. Nature: 329; 537–539, 1987.

DeFries JC, Olson RK, Pennington RF, Smith SD: Colorado reading project: An update. In Duane D, Gray DB (Eds), The Reading Brain: The Biological Basis of Dyslexia. Parkton, MD: York Press, Inc., pp. 53–87, 1991.

Demb JB, Boyton GM, Heeger DJ: Brain activity in the visual cortex predicts individual differences in reading performance. Proceedings of the National Academy of Sciences USA: 94; 13363–13366, 1997.

Demb JB, Poldrack RA, Gabrieli JDE: Functional neuroimaging of word processing in normal and dyslexic readers. In Klein RM, McMullen PM (Eds), Converging method for understanding reading and dyslexia. Cambridge, MA: MIT Press, pp. 245–304, 1999.

Denckla MB: Childhood learning disabilities. In Heilman KM, Valenstein E (Eds), Clinical Neuropsychology. New York: Oxford University Press, 1979.

Denckla MB, Rudel RG: Rapid 'automatized' naming (RAN): Dyslexia differentiated from other learning disabilities. Neuropsychologia: 14; 471–479, 1976.

Denenberg VL: A critique of Mody, Studdert-Kennedy and Brady's 'Speech perception deficits in poor readers: auditory processing or phonological coding?' Journal of Learning Disabilities: 32; 379–383, 1999.

Doehring DG, Hoshko IM: Classification of reading problems by the Q-technique of factor analysis. Cortex: 13; 284–294, 1977.

Doehring DG, Trites RL, Patel PG, Fiedorowicz CAM: Reading Disabilities: The Interaction of Reading, Language, and Neuropsychological Deficits. New York: Academic Press, 1981.

Duara R, Kushch A, Gross-Glenn K, Barker WW, Jallad B, Pascal S, Loewenstein DA, Sheldon J, Rabin M, Levin B: Neuroanatomic differences between dyslexic and normal readers on magnetic resonance imaging scans. Archives of Neurology: 48; 410–416, 1991.

Eden GF, Stein JF, Wood HM, Wood FB: Differences in eye movements and reading problems in dyslexic and normal children. Vision Research: 34; 1345–1358, 1995.

Eden GF, VanMeter JW, Rumsey JM, Maisog JM, Woods RP, Zeffiro TA: Abnormal processing of visual motion in dyslexia revealed by functional brain imaging. Nature: 382(6586); 66–69, 1996.

Eden GF, Zeffiro TA: Neural systems affected in developmental dyslexia revealed by functional neuroimaging. Neuron: 21; 279–282, 1998.

Engelmann S, Bruner EC: Reading Mastery I/II Fast Cycle: Teacher's Guide. Chicago: Science Research Associates, Inc., 1988.

Engelmann S, Carnine L, Johnson G: Corrective Reading: Word Attack Basics, Decoding A. Chicago: Science Research Associates, Inc., 1988a.

Engelmann S, Johnson G, Carnine L, Meyer L, Becker W, Eisele J: Corrective Reading: Decoding Strategies, Decoding B1. Chicago: Science Research Associates, Inc., 1988b.

Fagerheim T, Raeymaekers P, Tonnessen FE, Pedersen M, Tranebjaerg L, Lubs HA: A new gene (DYX3) for dyslexia is located on chromosome 2. Journal of Medical Genetics: 36; 664–669, 1999.

Farmer ME, Klein RM: Evidence for a temporal processing deficit linked to dyslexia: a review. Psychonomic Bulletin and Review: 2; 460–493, 1995.

Felton RH, Brown IS: Phonological processes as predictors of specific reading skills in children at risk for reading failure. Reading and Writing: An Interdisciplinary Journal: 2; 39–59, 1990.

Filipek PA: Neurobiological correlates of developmental dyslexia: What do we know of how dyslexics' brains differ from those of normal readers? Journal of Child Neurology: 10(supplemental); S62–S69, 1995.

Filipek PA: Neuroimaging in the developmental disorders: The state of the science. Journal of Child Psychology and Psychiatry: 40(1); 113–128, 1999.

Filipek PA, Kennedy DN, Caviness VSJ: Neuroimaging in child neuropsychology. In Rapin I, Segalowitz SJ (Eds), Handbook of Neuropsychology. Vol. 6. New York, NY: Elsevier Science, pp. 301–329, 1992.

Filipek PA, Pennington BF, Holmes JF, Lefly D, Kennedy DN, Meyers JM, Lang JE, Gayán J, Galaburda AM, Simon JM, Filley CM, Caniness VS, DeFries JC: Developmental dyslexia: Cortical and subcortical anomalies by MRI-based morphometry (Abstract). Annals of Neurology: 38; 509, 1995.

Filipek PA, Richelme C, Kennedy DN, Rademacher J, Pitcher DA, Zidel SY, Caviness VS: Morphometric analysis of the brain in developmental language disorders and autism (Abstract). Annals of Neurology: 32; 475, 1992.

Finucci JM, Gottfredson L, Childs B: A follow-up study of dyslexic boys. Annals of Dyslexia: 35; 117–136, 1985.

Fisher SE, Francks C, Marlow AJ, MacPhie IL, Newbury DF, Cardon LR, Ishikawa-Brush Y, Richardson AJ, Talcott JB, Gayán J, Olson RK, Pennington BF, Smith SD, DeFries JC, Stein JF, Monaco AP: Independent genome-wide scans identify a chromosome 18 quantitative-trait locus influencing dyslexia. Nature Genetics: 30(1); 86–91, 2002.

Fisher SE, Marlow AJ, Lamb J, Maestrini E, Williams DF, Richardson AJ, Weeks DE, Stein JF, Monaco AP: A quantitative-trait locus on chromosome 6p influences different aspects of developmental dyslexia. American Journal of Human Genetics: 64; 146–156, 1999.

Fletcher JM, Foorman BR, Shaywitz SE, Shaywitz BA: Conceptual and methodological issues in dyslexia research: A lesson for developmental disorders. In Tager-Flusberg H (Ed), Neurodevelopmental Disorders. Cambridge, MA: MIT Press, pp. 271–305, 1999a.

Fletcher JM, Francis DJ, Shaywitz SE, Lyon GR, Foorman BR, Stuebing KK, Shaywitz BA: Intelligent testing and the discrepancy model for children with learning disabilities. Learning Disabilities Research and Practice: 13(4); 186–203, 1998.

Fletcher JM, Shaywitz SE, Shankweiler DP, Katz L, Liberman IY, Stuebing KK, Francis DJ, Fowler AE, Shaywitz BA: Cognitive profiles of reading disability: Comparisons of discrepancy and low achievement definitions. Journal of Educational Psychology: 86(1); 6–23, 1994.

Fletcher JM, Shaywitz SE, Shaywitz BA: Comorbidity of learning and attention disorders: Separate but equal. Pediatric Clinics of North America: 46(5); 885–897, 1999b.

Flowers DL: Brain basis for dyslexia: A summary of work in progress. Journal of Learning Disabilities: 26; 575–582, 1993.

Foorman BR, Francis DJ, Fletcher JM, Schatschneider C, Mehta P: The role of instruction in learning to read: Preventing reading failure in at-risk children. Journal of Educational Psychology: 90(1); 37–55, 1998.

Foorman BR, Francis DJ, Winikates D, Mehta P, Schatschneider C, Fletcher JM: Early interventions for children with reading disabilities. Scientific Studies of Reading: 1(3); 255–276, 1997.

Francis DJ, Shaywitz SE, Stuebing KK, Shaywitz BA, Fletcher JM: Developmental lag versus deficit models of reading disability: A longitudinal, individual growth curves analysis. Journal of Educational Psychology: 88(1); 3–17, 1996.

Frijters JC, Barron RW, Brunello M: Direct and mediated influences of home literacy and literacy interest on prereaders' oral vocabulary and early written language skill. Journal of Educational Psychology: 92; 466–477, 2000.

Frith C, Frith U: A biological marker for dyslexia. Nature: 382; 19, 20, 1996.

Galaburda AM: The pathogenesis of childhood dyslexia. Research in Nervous Mental Disorders: 66; 127–138, 1988.

Galaburda AM: Address to the 16th Annual Rodin Remediation Society Meeting. Boulder, CO, 1990.

Galaburda AM, Livingstone M: Evidence for a magnocellular defect in developmental dyslexia. Annals of the New York Academy of Sciences: 68(Temporal Information Processing in the Nervous System); 70–82, 1993.

Galaburda AM, Menard MT, Rosen GD: Evidence for aberrant auditory anatomy in developmental dyslexia. Proceedings of the National Academy of Sciences of the United States of America: 91; 8010–8013, 1994.

Galaburda AM, Schrott LM, Sherman GF, Rosen GD, Denenberg VH: Animal models of developmental dyslexia. In Chase CH, Rosen GD, Sherman GF (Eds), Developmental Dyslexia. Baltimore, MD: York Press, pp. 3–14, 1996.

Galaburda AM, Sherman GF, Rosen GD, Aboitiz F, Geschwind N: Developmental dyslexia: Four consecutive patients with cortical anomalies. Annals of Neurology: 18; 222–233, 1985.

Garzia RP: Optometric factors in reading disability. In Willows DM, Kruk RS, Corcos E (Eds), Visual processes in reading and reading disabilities. Hillsdale, NJ: Lawrence Erlbaum Associates, pp. 419–434, 1993.

Gaskins IW, Downer MA, Gaskins RW: Introduction to the Benchmark School Word Identification/Vocabulary Development Program. Media, PA: Benchmark School, 1986.

Gayán J, Olson RK: Reading disability: Evidence for a genetic etiology. European Child and Adolescent Psychiatry: 8(Suppl. 3); 52–55, 1999.

Gayán J, Smith SD, Cherny SS, Cardon LR, Fulker DW, Brower AM, Olson RK, Pennington BF, DeFries JC: Quantitative-trait locus for specific language and reading deficits on chromosome 6p. American Journal of Human Genetics: 64; 157–164, 1999.

Gillingham A, Stillman BW: Remedial Training for Children with Specific Disability in Reading, Spelling, and Penmanship (7th ed.). Cambridge, MA: Educators Publishing Service, 1960.

Glezerman TB: Mozgovye disfunktsii u detei (Minimal brain dysfunctions in children). Moscow: Nauka, 1983.

Goswami U, Bryant PE: Phonological Skills and Learning to Read. Hove, East Sussex: Lawrence Erlbaum Associates, 1990.

Goulandris N, McIntyre A, Snowling M, Bethel JM, Lee JP: A comparison of dyslexic and normal readers using orthoptic assessment procedures. Dyslexia: 4; 30–48, 1998.

Grigorenko EL: A family study of dyslexia. Unpublished dissertation, 1996.

Grigorenko EL: Developmental dyslexia: An update on genes, brains, and environments. Journal of Child Psychology and Psychiatry: 42(1); 91–125, 2001.

Grigorenko EL, Wood FB, Meyer MS, Hart LA, Speed WC, Shuster A, Pauls DL: Susceptibility loci for distinct components of developmental dyslexia on chromosomes 6 and 15. The American Journal of Human Genetics: 60; 27–39, 1997.

Grigorenko EL, Wood FB, Meyers MS, Pauls DL: Chromosome 6p influences different dyslexia-related cognitive processes: Further confirmation. American Journal of Human Genetics: 66; 715–723, 2000.

Habib M: The neurological basis of developmental dyslexia: An overview and working hypothesis. Brain: 123; 2373–2399, 2000.

Habib M, Espesser R, Ray V, Giraud K, Bruas P, Gress C: Training dyslexics with acoustically modified speech: Evidence of improved phonological performance. Brain and Cognition: 40; 143–146, 1999.

Hall SL, Moats LC: Straight Talk About Reading: How Parents Can Make a Difference During the Early Years. Chicago, IL: Contemporary Books, 1999.

Hansen J, Bowey JA: Phonological analysis skills, verbal working memory, and reading ability in second grade children. Child Development: 65; 938–950, 1994.

Harris EK: The contribution of twin research to the study of the etiology of reading disability. In Smith SD (Ed), Genetics and Learning Disabilities. San Diego, CA: College Hill Press, pp. 3–19, 1986.

Hatcher PJ, Hulme C, Ellis AW: Ameliorating early reading failure by integrating the teaching of reading and phonological skills: The phonological linkage hypothesis. Child Development: 65; 41–57, 1994.

Hayduk S, Bruck M, Cavanagh P: Low-level visual processing skills of adults and children with dyslexia. Cognitive Neuropsychology: 13; 975–1016, 1996.

Hermann K: Reading Disability: A Medical Study of Word Blindness and Related Handicaps. Springfield, IL: Charles C. Thomas, 1959.

Hinshelwood J: Word blindness and visual memories. Lancet: 2; 1566–1570, 1895.

Hinshelwood J: Congenital Word Blindness. London: HK Lewis, 1917.

Hohnen B, Stevenson J: Genetic effects in orthographic ability: A second look. Behavior Genetics: 25; 271, 1995.

Horwitz B, Rumsey JM, Donohue BC: Functional connectivity of the angular gyrus in normal reading and dyslexia. Proceedings of the National Academy of Sciences of the United States of America: 95; 8939–8944, 1998.

Huey EB: The Psychology and Pedagogy. New York, NY: MacMillan, 1908.

Hulme C: The implausibility of low-level visual deficits as a cause of children's reading difficulties. Cognitive Neuropsychology: 5; 369–374, 1986.

Humphreys P, Kaufmann WE, Galaburda AM: Developmental dyslexia in women: Neuropathological findings in three cases. Annals of Neurology: 28; 727–738, 1990.

Hynd GW, Semrud-Clikeman M, Lorys AR, Novey ES, Eliopulos D: Brain morphology in developmental dyslexia and attention deficit disorder/hyperactivity. Archives of Neurology: 47; 919–926, 1990.

Joanisse MF, Manis FR, Keating P, Seidenberg MS: Language deficits in dyslexic children: Speech perception, phonology, and morphology. Journal of Experimental Child Psychology: 77(1); 30–60, 2000.

Joseph J, Noble K, Eden G: The neurobiological basis of reading. Journal of Learning Disabilities: 34; 566–579, 2001.

Kershner JR, Cummings RL, Clarke KA, Hadfield AJ, Kershner BA: Evaluation of the Tomatis Listening Training Program with learning disabled children. Canadian Journal of Special Education: 2(1); 1–32, 1986.

Kershner JR, Cummings RL, Clarke KA, Hadfield AJ, Kershner BA: Two-year evaluation of the Tomatis Listening Training Program with learning disabled children. Learning Disability Quarterly: 13; 43–53, 1990.

Klein RM, McMullen PA: Introduction: The reading brain. In Klein RM, McMullen PA (Eds), Converging Methods for Understanding Reading and Dyslexia. Cambridge, MA: The MIT Press, pp. 1–22, 1999.

Kruk RS: Processing text on monitors. In Willows DM, Kruk RS, Corcos E (Eds), Visual processes in reading and reading disabilities. Hillsdale, NJ: Lawrence Erlbaum Associates, pp. 457–472, 1993.

LaBerge D, Samuels SJ: Toward a theory of automatic information processing in reading. Cognitive Psychology: 6; 293–323, 1974.

Larsen JP, Hoien T, Lundberg I, Odegaard H: MRI evaluation of the size and symmetry of the planum temporale in adolescents with developmental dyslexia. Brain and Language: 39; 289–301, 1990.

Lazarus JM, Owen WF: Role of bioincompatibility in dialysis morbidity and mortality. American Journal of Kidney Diseases: 24; 1019–1032, 1994.

Leonard CM, Voeller KKS, Lombardion LJ, Morris MK, Hynd GW, Alexander AW, Andersen HG, Garofalakis M, Honeyman JC, Mao J, Agee OF, Staab EV: Anomalous cerebral structure in dyslexia revealed with magnetic resonance imaging. Archives of Neurology: 50; 461–469, 1993.

Levin BE: Organizational deficits in dyslexia: Possible frontal lobe dysfunction. Developmental Neuropsychology: 6; 95–110, 1990.

Lewis C, Hitch GJ, Walker P: The prevalence of specific arithmetic difficulties and specific reading difficulties in 9- to 10-year old boys and girls. Journal of Child Psychology and Psychiatry and Allied Disciplines: 35(2); 283–292, 1994.

Liberman AM: How theories of speech affect research on reading and writing. In Blachman B (Ed), Foundations of Reading Acquisition and Dyslexia. Mahwah, NJ: Lawrence Erlbaum Associates, pp. 3–19, 1997.

Liberman AM: Why is speech so much easier than reading? In Hulme C, Joshi RM (Eds), Reading and Spelling: Development and Disorders. Mahwah, NJ: Lawrence Erlbaum Associates, Inc., pp. 5–17, 1998.

Liberman AM: The reading researcher and the reading teacher need the right theory of speech. Scientific Studies of Reading: 3; 95–111, 1999.

Light JG, DeFries JC: Comorbidity of reading and mathematics disabilities: Genetic and environmental etiologies. Journal of Learning Disabilities: 28; 96–106, 1995.

Light JG, DeFries JC, Olson RK: Multivariate behavioral genetic analysis of achievement and cognitive measures in reading-disabled and control twin pairs. Human Biology: 70; 215–237, 1998.

Lindgren SD, De Renzi E, Richman LC: Cross-national comparisons of developmental dyslexia in Italy and the United States. Child Development: 56(6); 1404–1417, 1985.

Lonigan CJ, Burgess SR, Anthony JL, Barker TA: Development of phonological sensitivity in 2- to 5-year-old children. Journal of Educational Psychology: 90(2); 294–311, 1998.

Lovegrove WJ, Bowling A, Badcock D, Blackwood M: Specific reading disability: Differences in contrast sensitivity as a function of spatial frequency. Science: 210; 439–440, 1980.

Lovegrove WJ, Garzia RP, Nicholson SB: Experimental evidence for a transient system deficit in specific reading disability. Journal of the American Optometric Association: 61; 137–146, 1990.

Lovegrove WJ, Martin F, Slaghuis W: A theoretical and experimental case for a visual deficit in specific reading disability. Cognitive Neuropsychology: 3; 225–267, 1986.

Lovett MW: Developmental dyslexia. In Rapin I, Segalowitz SJ (Eds), Handbook of Neuropsychology. Vol. 7. Child Neuropsychology. Amsterdam: Elsevier Science, pp. 163–185, 1992.

Lovett MW: Developmental reading disorders. In Feinberg TE, Farah MJ (Eds), Behavioral Neurology and Neuropsychology. New York: McGraw-Hill, pp. 773–787, 1997.

Lovett MW: Defining and remediating the core deficits of developmental dyslexia: Lessons from remedial outcome research with reading disabled children. In Klein R, McMullen P (Eds), Converging Methods for Understanding Reading and Dyslexia. Language, Speech, and Communication. Cambridge, MA: MIT Press, pp. 111–132, 1999.

Lovett MW, Barron RW: The search for individual and subtype differences in reading disabled children's response to remediation. In Molfese DL, Molfese VJ (Eds), Developmental Variations in Learning: Applications to Social, Executive Function, Language, and Reading Skills. Mahwah, NJ: Lawrence Erlbaum Associates, Inc., pp. 309–337, 2002.

Lovett MW, Borden SL, DeLuca T, Lacerenza L, Benson NJ, Brackstone D: Treating the core deficits of developmental dyslexia: Evidence of transfer-of-learning following phonologically- and strategy-based reading training programs. Developmental Psychology: 30(6); 805–822, 1994.

Lovett MW, Lacerenza L, Borden SL: Putting struggling readers on the PHAST track: A program to integrate phonological and strategy-based remedial reading instruction and maximize outcomes. Journal of Learning Disabilities: 33(5); 458–476, 2000a.

Lovett MW, Lacerenza L, Borden SL, Frijters JC, Steinbach KA, De Palma M: Components of effective remediation for developmental reading disabilities: Combining phonological and strategy-based instruction to improve outcomes. Journal of Educational Psychology: 92(2); 263–283, 2000b.

Lovett MW, Ransby MJ, Barron RW: Treatment, subtype, and word type effects in dyslexic children's response to remediation. Brain and Language: 34; 328–349, 1988.

Lovett MW, Ransby MJ, Hardwick N, Johns MS, Donaldson SA: Can dyslexia be treated? Treatment-specific and generalized treatment effects in dyslexic children's response to remediation. Brain and Language: 37; 90–121, 1989.

Lovett MW, Steinbach KA: The effectiveness of remedial programs for reading disabled children of different ages: Is there decreased benefit for older children? Learning Disability Quarterly: 20(3); 189–210, 1997.

Lovett MW, Steinbach KA, Frijters JC: Remediating the core deficits of developmental reading disability: A double deficit perspective. Journal of Learning Disabilities: 33(4); 334–358, 2000.

Lovett MW, Warren-Chaplin PM, Ransby MJ, Borden SL: Training the word recognition skills of reading disabled children: Treatment and transfer effects. Journal of Educational Psychology: 82; 769–780, 1990.

Lubs HA, Duara R, Levin B, Jallad B, Lubs M-L, Rabin M, Kushch A, Gross-Glenn K: Dyslexia subtypes: Genetics, behavior, and brain imaging. In Duane DD, Gray DB (Eds), The Reading Brain: The Biological Basis of Dyslexia. Parkton, MD: York Press, pp. 89–118, 1991.

Lyon GR: Research initiatives in learning disabilities: Contributions from scientists supported by the National Institute of Child Health and Human Development. Journal of Child Neurology: 10(1); S120–S126, 1995.

Lyon GR, Moats LC: Critical conceptual and methodological considerations in reading intervention research. Journal of Learning Disabilities: 30(6); 578–588, 1997.

Mann V: Language problems: A key to early reading problems. In Wong B (Ed), Learning About Learning Disabilities (2nd Ed.). San Diego, CA: Academic Press, pp. 163–201, 1998.

Manis FR, McBride-Chang C, Seidenberg MS, Keating P, Doi LM, Peterson A: Are speech perception deficits associated with developmental dyslexia? Journal of Experimental Child Psychology: 66(2); 211–235, 1997.

Manis FR, Seidenberg MS, Doi L: See Dick RAN: Rapid naming and the longitudinal prediction of reading subskills in first and second graders. Scientific Studies of Reading: 3; 129–157, 1999.

Manis FR, Seidenberg MS, Doi LM, McBride-Chang C, Peterson A: On the basis of two subtypes of developmental dyslexia. Cognition: 58; 157–195, 1996.

Massaro DW, Sanocki T: Visual information processes in reading. In Willows DM, Kruk RS, Corcos E (Eds), Visual processes in reading and reading disabilities. Hillsdale, NJ: Lawrence Erlbaum Associates, pp. 139–162, 1993.

Mattingly IG: Did orthographies evolve? Special Issue: Phonology and the problems of learning to read and write. RASE: Remedial and Special Education: 6; 18–23, 1985.

Mattis S: Dyslexia syndromes: A working hypothesis that works. In Benton AL, Pearl D (Eds), Dyslexia: An Appraisal of Current Knowledge. New York: Oxford University Press, 1978.

McBride-Chang C: Phonological processing, speech perception, and reading disability: An integrative review. Educational Psychologist: 30; 109–121, 1995a.

McBride-Chang C: What is phonological awareness? Journal of Educational Psychology: 87(2); 179–192, 1995b.

McBride-Chang C, Manis FR: Structural invariance in the associations of naming speed, phonological awareness, and verbal reasoning in good and poor readers: A test of the double deficit hypothesis. Reading and Writing: An Interdisciplinary Journal: 8; 323–339, 1996.

McClelland JL, Rumelhart DE: An interactive activation model of context effects in letter perception: Part 1. An account of basic findings. Psychological Review: 88; 375–407, 1981.

Merzenich MM, Jenkins WM, Johnston P, Schreiner C, Miller SL, Tallal P: Temporal processing deficits of language-learning impaired children ameliorated by training. Science: 271; 77–81, 1996.

Meyer MM, Felton RH: Repeated reading to enhance fluency: Old approaches and new direction. Annals of Dyslexia: 49; 283–306, 1999.

Moats LC, Foorman BR: Introduction to special issue of SSR: Components of effective reading instruction. Scientific Studies of Reading: 1(3); 187–189, 1997.

Mody M, Studdert-Kennedy M, Brady S: Speech perception deficits in poor readers: Auditory processing or phonological coding? Journal of Experimental Child Psychology: 64; 199–231, 1997.

Morgan WP: A case of congenital word-blindness. British Medical Journal: 2; 1378, 1896.

Morgan AE, Hynd GW: Dyslexia, neurolinguistic ability, and anatomical variation of the planum temporale. Neuropsychology Review: 8(2); 79–93, 1998.

Morris DW, Robinson L, Turic D, Duke M, Webb V, Milham C, Hopkin E, Pound K, Fernando S, Easton M, Hamshere M, Williams N, McGuffin P, Owen MJ, O'Donovan MC, Williams J: Family-based association mapping provides evidence for reading disability on chromosome 15q. Human Molecular Genetics: 9; 843–848, 2000.

Morris RD, Stuebing KK, Fletcher JM, Shaywitz SE, Lyon GR, Shankweiler DP, Katz L, Francis DJ, Shaywitz BA: Subtypes of reading disability: Variability around a phonological core. Journal of Educational Psychology: 90(3); 1–27, 1998.

National Reading Panel: Teaching children to read: An evidence-based assessment of the scientific research literature on reading and its implications for reading instruction. Report of the

Subgroups of the National Reading Panel. Washington, DC: National Institute of Child Health and Human Development, 2000.

Nicholson RI, Fawcett AJ, Berry EL, Jenkins IH, Dean P, Brooks DJ: Motor learning difficulties and abnormal cerebellar activation in dyslexic children. Lancet: 353; 43–47, 1999.

Nittrouer S: Do temporal processing deficits cause phonological processing problems? Journal of Speech, Language, and Hearing Research: 42; 925–942, 1999.

O'Brien BA, Mansfield JS, Legge GE: The effect of contrast on reading speed in dyslexia. Vision Research: 40; 1921–1935, 2000.

Olson RK, Wise B, Conners F, Rack M, Fulker D: Specific deficits in component reading and language skills: Genetic and environmental influences. Journal of Learning Disabilities: 22; 339–348, 1989.

Olson RK, Wise B, Ring J, Johnson M: Computer-based remedial training in phoneme awareness and phonological decoding: Effects on the posttraining development of word recognition. Scientific Studies of Reading: 1(3); 235–254, 1997.

Orton ST: 'Word-blindness' in school children. Archives of Neurology and Psychiatry: 14; 581–615, 1925.

Paulesu E, Démonet J-F, Fazio F, McCrory E, Chanoine V, Brunswick N, Cappa SF, Cossu G, Habib M, Frith CD, Frith U: Dyslexia: Cultural diversity and biological unity. Science: 291; 2165–2167, 2001.

Pennington BF: Using genetics to dissect cognition. The American Journal of Human Genetics: 60; 13–16, 1997.

Pennington BF: Dyslexia as a neurodevelopmental disorder. In Tager-Flusberg H (Ed), Neurodevelopmental Disorders. Cambridge, MA: MIT Press, pp. 307–330, 1999.

Pennington BF, Filipek PA, Churchwell J, Kennedy DN, Lefly D, Simon JH, Filley CM, Galaburda A, Alarcón M, DeFries JC: Brain morphometry in reading-disabled twins. Neurology: 53; 723–729, 1999.

Pennington BF, Smith SR, Kimberling WJ, Green PA, Haith MM: Left-handedness and immune disorders in familial dyslexics. Archives of Neurology: 44; 634–639, 1987.

Pennington BF, Smith SR: Genetic influences on learning disabilities: an update. Journal of Consulting and Clinical Psychology: 56; 817–823, 1988.

Pennington BF, Van Orden GC, Smith SD, Green PA, Haith MM: Phonological processing skills and deficits in adult dyslexics. Child Development: 61; 1753–1778, 1990.

Perfetti CA: Reading Ability. New York: Oxford University Press, 1985.

Petryshen TL, Kaplan BJ, Hughes ML, Tzenova J, Field LL: Supportive evidence for the DYX3 dyslexia susceptibility gene in Canadian families. Journal of Medical Genetics: 39(2); 125–126, 2002.

Plomin R: The role of inheritance in behavior. Science: 248; 183–188, 1990.

Plomin R, Crabbe J: DNA. Psychological Bulletin: 126(6); 806–828, 2000.

Plomin R, DeFries JC, McClearin GE, Rutter M: Behavioral Genetics (3rd Ed.). New York, NY: Freeman, 1997.

Pugh KR, Mencl WE, Jenner AJ, Katz L, Lee JR, Shaywitz SE, Shaywitz BA: Functional neuroimaging studies of reading and reading disability (developmental dyslexia). Mental Retardation and Developmental Disabilities Review: 6; 207–213, 2000a.

Pugh KR, Mencl WE, Shaywitz BA, Shaywitz SE, Fulbright RK, Constable RT, Skudlarski P, Marchione KE, Jenner AR, Fletcher JM, Liberman AM, Shankweiler DP, Katz L, Lacadie C, Gore JC: The angular gyrus in developmental dyslexia: Task-specific differences in functional connectivity within posterior cortex. Psychological Science: 11(1); 51–59, 2000b.

Rabin M, Wen XL, Hepburn M, Lubs HA: Suggestive linkage of developmental dyslexia to chromosome lp34–36. Lancet: 342; 178–179, 1993.

Rack JP, Snowling M, Olson RK: The nonword reading deficit in developmental dyslexia: A review. Reading Research Quarterly: 27(1); 28–53, 1992.

Rastle K, Coltheart M: Whammy and double whammy: Length effects in nonword naming. Psychonomic Bulletin and Reviews: 5; 277–282, 1998.

Rayner K: Eye movements in reading and information processing: 20 years of research. Psychological Bulletin: 124(3); 372–422, 1998.

Rayner K, Foorman BA, Perfetti CA, Pesetsky D, Seidenberg MS: How psychological science informs the teaching of reading. Psychology in the Public Interest: 2; 31–74, 2001.

Rourke BP: Neuropsychology of Learning Disabilities: Essentials of Subtype Analysis. New York: Guilford Press, 1985.

Rumsey JM: The biology of developmental dyslexia. Journal of the American Medical Association: 19; 912–915, 1992.

Rumsey JM, Andreason P, Zametkin AJ, Aquino T, King AC, Hamburger SD, Pikus S, Rapoport JL, Cohen RM: Failure to activate the left temporoparietal cortex in dyslexia. An oxygen 15 positron emission tomographic study. Archives of Neurology: 49; 527–534, 1992.

Rumsey JM, Horwitz B, Donohue BC, Nace K, Maisog JM, Andreason P: Phonological and orthographic components of word recognition: A PET-rCBF study. Brain: 1997(120); 739–759, 1997.

Rutter M: Prevalence and types of dyslexia. In Benton A, Pearl D (Eds), Dyslexia: An Appraisal of Current Knowledge. New York: Oxford University Press, 1978.

Rutter M, Tizard J, Whitmore K: Education, Health, and Behavior. New York: Krieger, 1970.

Rutter M, Yule W: The concept of specific reading retardation. Journal of Child Psychiatry: 16; 181–197, 1975.

Scanlon DM, Vellutino FR: A comparison of the instructional backgrounds and cognitive profiles of poor, average, and good readers who were initially identified as at risk for reading failure. Scientific Studies of Reading: 1(3); 191–216, 1997.

Scarborough HS: Continuity between childhood dyslexia and adult reading. British Journal of Psychology: 75(3); 329–348:

Scarborough HS: Early identification of children at risk for reading disabilities. In Shapiro BK, Accardo PJ, Capute AJ (Eds), Specific Reading Disability: A View of the Spectrum. Timonium, MD: York Press, pp. 75–119, 1998.

Scarborough HS, Dobrich W: On the efficacy of reading to preschoolers. Developmental Review: 14(3); 245–302, 1994.

Schatschneider C, Francis DJ, Foorman BR, Fletcher JM, Mehta P: The dimensionality of phonological awareness: An application of item response theory. Journal of Educational Psychology: 91(3); 439–449, 1999.

Schulte-Körne G, Brimm T, Nöthen MM, Müller-Myhsok B, Propping P, Remschmidt H: Evidence for linkage of spelling disability to chromosome 15. American Journal of Medical Genetics. Neuropsychological Genetics: 74; 661, 1997.

Schulte-Körne G, Deimel W, Bartling J, Remschmidt H: The role of phonological awareness, speech perception, and auditory temporal processing for dyslexia. European Child and Adolescent Psychiatry: 8; 28–34, 1999.

Shankweiler D, Lundquist E, Katz L, Stuebing KK, Fletcher JM, Brady S, Fowler A, Dreyer LG, Marchione KE, Shaywitz SE, Shaywitz BA: Comprehension and decoding: Patterns of association in children with reading difficulties. Scientific Studies of Reading: 3(1); 69–94, 1999.

Share DL: Phonological recoding and self-teaching. Sine qua non of reading acquisition. Cognition: 55; 151–218, 1995.

Shaywitz SE: Dyslexia. Scientific American: November; 98–104, 1996.

Shaywitz SE: Dyslexia. The New England Journal of Medicine: 338(5); 307–312, 1998.

Shaywitz SE, Escobar MD, Shaywitz BA, Fletcher JM, Makuch R: Evidence that dyslexia may represent the lower tail of a normal distribution of reading ability. The New England Journal of Medicine: 326(3); 145–150, 1992.

Shaywitz SE, Fletcher JM, Holahan JM, Shneider AE, Marchione KE, Stuebing KK, Francis DJ, Pugh KR, Shaywitz BA: Persistence of dyslexia: The Connecticut longitudinal study at adolescence. Pediatrics: 104(6); 1351–1359, 1999.

Shaywitz SE, Fletcher JM, Shaywitz BA: A conceptual model and definition of dyslexia: Findings emerging from the Connecticut Longitudinal Study. In Beitchman JH, Cohen NJ, Konstantareas MM, Tannock R (Eds), Language, Learning, and Behavior Disorders. New York, NY: Cambridge University Press, pp. 199–223, 1996.

Shaywitz SE, Shaywitz BA, Fletcher JM, Escobar MD: Prevalence of reading disability in boys and girls: Results of the Connecticut Longitudinal Study. Journal of the American Medical Association: 264(8); 998–1002, 1990.

Shaywitz SE, Shaywitz BA, Pugh KR, Fulbright RK, Constable RT, Mencl WE, Shankweiler DP, Liberman AM, Skudlarski P, Fletcher JM, Katz L, Marchione KE, Lacadie C, Gatenby C, Gore JC: Functional disruption in the organization of the brain for reading in dyslexia. Proceedings of the National Academy of Sciences of the United States of America: 95(March); 2636–2641, 1998.

Siegel LS: Definitional and theoretical issues and research on learning disabilities. Journal of Learning Disabilities: 21(5); 264–266, 1988.

Siegel LS: IQ is irrelevant to the definition of learning disabilities. Journal of Learning Disabilities: 22; 469–478, 1989.

Siegel LS: An evaluation of the discrepancy definition of dyslexia. Journal of Learning Disabilities: 25(10); 618–629, 1992.

Simos PG, Fletcher JM, Bergman E, Breier JI, Foorman BR, Castillo EM, Davis RN, Fitzgerald M, Papanicolaou AC: Dyslexia-specific brain activation profile becomes normal following successful remedial training. Neurology: 1–10; 2002.

Skottun BC: The magnocellular deficit theory of dyslexia: the evidence from contrast sensitivity. Vision Research: 40; 111–127, 2000.

Skottun BC, Parke LA: The possible relationship between visual deficits and dyslexia: Examination of a critical assumption. Journal of Learning Disabilities: 32; 2–5, 1999.

SLI Consortium: A genomewide scan identifies two novel loci involved in specific language impairment. American Journal of Human Genetics: 70(2); 384–398, 2002.

Smith SD, Kelley PM, Askew JW, Hoover DM, Deffenbacher KE, Gayán J, Brower AM, Olson RK: Reading disability and chromosome 6p21.3: Evaluation of MOG as a candidate gene. Journal of Learning Disabilities: 34(6); 512–519, 2001.

Smith SD, Kimberling WJ, Pennington BF: Screening for multiple genes influencing dyslexia. Reading and Writing: An Interdisciplinary Journal: 3; 285–298, 1991.

Smith SD, Kimberling WJ, Pennington BF, Lubs HA: Specific reading disability: Identification of an inherited form through linkage analysis. Science: 219; 1345–1347, 1983.

Snowling MJ: Contemporary approaches to the teaching of reading. Journal of Child Psychology and Psychiatry: 37; 139–148, 1996.

Spreen O: Learning disabled children growing up: A follow-up into adulthood. Lisse, The Netherlands: Swets and Zeitlinger, 1987.

Spreen O, Tupper D, Risser A, Tuokko H, Edgell D: Human Developmental Neuropsychology. New York: Oxford University Press, 1984.

Stahl SA, Murray BA: Defining phonological awareness and its relationship to early reading. Journal of Educational Psychology: 86; 221–234, 1994.

Stanovich KE: Toward an interactive-compensatory model of individual differences in the development of reading fluency. Reading Research Quarterly: 16; 32–71, 1980.

Stanovich KE: The interactive-compensatory model of reading: A confluence of developmental, experimental, and educational psychology. RASE: Remedial and Special Education: 5(3); 11–19, 1984.

Stanovich KE: Matthew effects in reading: Some consequences of individual differences in the acquisition of literacy. Reading Research Quarterly: 21; 360–407, 1986.

Stanovich KE: Explaining the differences between the dyslexic and the garden-variety poor reader: The phonological-core variable-difference model. Journal of Learning Disabilities: 21; 590–604, 1988.

Stanovich KE: Early acquisition and the causes of reading difficulty: The contributions to research on phonological processing. In Stanovich KE (Ed), Progress in Understanding Reading: Scientific Foundations and New Frontiers. New York, NY: Guilford Press, pp. 57–79, 2000.

Stanovich KE, Siegel LS: Phenotypic performance profile of children with reading disabilities: A regression-based test of the phonological-core variable-difference model. Journal of Educational Psychology: 86(1); 24–53, 1994.

Stanovich KE, Siegel LS, Gottardo A: Converging evidence for phonological and surface subtypes of reading disability. Journal of Educational Psychology: 89(1); 114–127, 1997.

Stein JF: Unfixed reference, monocular occlusion, and developmental dyslexia: a critique. British Journal of Ophthalmology: 73; 319–320, 1989.

Stein JF: Visuospatial perception in disabled readers. In Willows DM, Kruk RS, Corcos E (Eds), Visual Processes in Reading and Reading Disabilities. Hillsdale, NJ: Lawrence Erlbaum Associates, pp. 331–346, 1993.

Stein JF: The neurobiology of reading difficulties. In Wolf M (Ed), Dyslexia, Fluency, and the Brain. Baltimore, MD: York Press, 2001.

Stein JF, Fowler S: Visual dyslexia. Trends in Neuroscience: 4; 77–80, 1981.

Stein JF, Richardson AJ, Fowler MS: Monocular occlusion can improve binocular control and reading in dyslexics. Brain: 123; 164–170, 2000.

Stein JF, Walsh V: To see but not to read; the magnocellular theory of dyslexia. Trends in Neuroscience: 20; 147–152, 1997.

Studdert-Kennedy M: Deficits in phoneme awareness do not arise from failures in rapid auditory processing. Reading and Writing: An Interdisciplinary Journal: 15; 5–14, 2002.

Studdert-Kennedy M, Mody M: Auditory temporal deficits in the reading impaired: A critical review of the evidence. Psychonomic Bulletin and Review: 2; 508–514, 1995.

Swanson HL: Reading comprehension and working memory in learning-disabled readers: Is the phonological loop more important than the executive system? Journal of Experimental Child Psychology: 72; 1–31, 1999.

Swanson HL, Alexander JE: Cognitive processes as predictors of word recognition and reading comprehension in learning-disabled and skilled readers: Revisiting the specificity hypothesis. Journal of Educational Psychology: 89(1); 128–158, 1997.

Swanson HL, Hoskyn M: Experimental intervention research on students with learning disabilities: A meta-analysis of treatment outcomes. Review of Educational Research: 68(3); 277–321, 1998.

Talcott JB, Witton C, McLean MF, Hansen PC, Rees A, Green GGR, Stein JF: Dynamic sensory sensitivity and children's word decoding skills. Proceedings of the National academy of Sciences USA: 97; 2952–2957, 2000.

Tallal P: An experimental investigation of the role of auditory temporal processing in normal and disordered language development. In Caramazza A, Zurif EB (Eds), Language acquisition and language breakdown. Baltimore, MD: Johns Hopkins University Press, pp. 25–61, 1978.

Tallal P: Auditory temporal perception, phonics and reading disabilities in children. Brain and Language: 9; 182–198, 1980.

Tallal P: Temporal or phonetic processing deficit in dyslexia? That is the question. Applied Psycholinguistics: 5; 13–24, 1984.

Tallal P, Galaburda AM, Llinas RR, Von Euler C (Eds): Temporal information processing in the nervous system: Special reference to dyslexia and dysphasia. Annals of the New York Academy of Sciences: 682; 1–441, 1993.

Tallal P, Miller SL, Bedi G, Byma G, Wang X, Nagarajan SS, Schreiner C, Jenkins WM, Merzenich MM: Language comprehension in language-learning impaired children improved with acoustically modified speech. Science: 271; 81–84, 1996.

Tallal P, Piercy M: Developmental aphasia: Impaired rate of nonverbal processing as function of sensory modality. Neuropsychologia: 11; 389–398, 1973.

Tallal P, Piercy M: Developmental aphasia: Rate of auditory processing and selective impairment of consonant perception. Neuropsychologia: 12; 83–93, 1974.

Tallal P, Piercy M: Developmental aphasia: The perception of brief vowels and extended stop consonants. Neuropsychologia: 13; 69–74, 1975.

Tarnapol L, Tarnapol M: Comparative Reading and Learning Difficulties. Lexington: Lexington Books, 1981.

Tomatis A: Education and Dyslexia. France-Quebec: Les Editions, 1978.

Torgesen JK, Alexander AW, Wagner RK, Rashotte CA, Voeller KKS, Conway T: Intensive remedial instruction for children with severe reading disabilities: Immediate and long-term outcomes from two instructional approaches. Journal of Learning Disabilities: 34(1); 33–58, 2001.

Torgesen JK, Wagner RK, Rashotte CA: Approaches to the prevention and remediation of phonologically-based reading disabilities. In Blachman BA (Ed), Foundations of Reading Acquisition and Dyslexia: Implications for Early Intervention. Mahwah, NJ: Lawrence Erlbaum Associates, Inc., pp. 287–304, 1997.

Torgesen JK, Wagner RK, Rashotte CA, Burgess S, Hecht S: Contributions of phonological awareness and rapid automatic naming ability to the growth of word-reading skills in second- to fifth-grade children. Scientific Studies of Reading: 1(2); 161–185, 1997.

Torgesen JK, Wagner RK, Rashotte CA, Lindamood P, Rose E, Conway T, Garvan C: Preventing reading failure in young children with phonological processing disabilities: Group and individual responses to instruction. Journal of Educational Psychology: 91(4); 579–593, 1999.

Van der Wissel A, Zegers FE: Reading retardation revisited. British Journal of Developmental Psychology: 3; 3–9, 1985.

Vellutino FR: Dyslexia: Theory and Research. Cambridge, MA: MIT Press, 1979.

Vellutino FR, Scanlon DM, Lyon R: IQ scores do not differentiate between difficult to remediate and readily remediated poor readers: More evidence against the IQ achievement discrepancy definition of reading disability. Journal of Learning Disabilities: 33; 223–238, 2000.

Vellutino FR, Scanlon DM, Sipay ER, Small SG, Pratt A, Chen R, Denckla MB: Cognitive profiles of difficult-to-remediate and readily remediated poor readers: Early intervention as a vehicle for distinguishing between cognitive and experiential deficits as basic causes of specific reading disability. Journal of Educational Psychology: 88(4); 601–638, 1996.

Venezky RL: History of interest in the visual component of reading. In Willows DM, Kruk RS, Corcos E (Eds), Visual

Processes in Reading and Reading Disabilities. Hillsdale, NJ: Lawrence Erlbaum Associates, pp. 1–30, 1993.

Wadsworth SJ, Olson RK, Pennington BF, DeFries JC: Differential genetic ediology of reading disability as a function of IQ. Journal of Learning Disabilities: 33; 192–199, 2000.

Wagner RK, Torgesen JK: The nature of phonological processing and its causal role in the acquisition of reading skills. Psychological Bulletin: 101; 192–212, 1987.

Wagner RK, Torgesen JK, Rashotte CA: Development of reading-related phonological processing abilities: New evidence of bidirectional causality from a latent variable longitudinal study. Developmental Psychology: 30(1); 73–87, 1994.

Wagner RK, Torgesen JK, Rashotte CA, Hecht SA, Barker TA, Burgess SR, Donahue J, Garon T: Changing relations between phonological processing abilities and word-level reading as children develop from beginning to skilled readers: A five year longitudinal study. Developmental Psychology: 33(3); 468–479, 1997.

Watson BU, Miller TK: Auditory perception, phonological processing and reading ability/disability. Journal of Speech and Hearing Research: 36; 850–863, 1993.

Westbury CF, Zatorre RJ, Evans AC: Quantifying variability in the palnum temporale: A probability map. Cerebral Cortex: 9; 382–405, 1999.

White KR: The relation between socioeconomic status and academic achievement. Psychological Bulletin: 91; 461–481, 1982.

Willcutt EG, Pennington BF: Comorbidity of reading disability and attention-deficit/hyperactivity disorder: Differences by gender and subtype. Journal of Learning Disabilities: 33(2); 179–191, 2000.

Willcutt EG, Pennington BF, DeFries JC: Etiology of inattention and hyperactivity/impulsivity in a community sample of twins with learning difficulties. Journal of Abnormal Child Psychology: 28(2); 149–159, 2000.

Willows DM, Terepocki M: The relation of reversal errors to reading disabilities. In Willows DM, Kruk RS, Corcos E (Eds), Visual Processes in Reading and Reading Disabilities. Hillsdale, NJ: Lawrence Erlbaum Associates, pp. 31–56, 1993.

Wilson AM, Lesaux NK: Persistence of phonological processing deficits in college students with dyslexia who have age-appropriate reading skills. Journal of Learning Disabilities: 34(5); 394–400, 2001.

Wimmer H: Characteristics of developmental dyslexia in a regular writing system. Applied Psycholinguistics: 14; 1–33, 1993.

Wise BW, Olson RK: Computer-based phonological awareness and reading instruction. Annals of Dyslexia: 45; 99–122, 1995.

Wise BW, Ring J, Olson RK: Training phonological awareness with and without explicit attention to articulation. Journal of Experimental Child Psychology: 72; 271–304, 1999.

Wise BW, Ring J, Sessions L, Olson RK: Phonological awareness with and without articulation: A preliminary study. Learning Disability Quarterly: 20(3); 211–225, 1997.

Witton C, Talcott JB, Hansen PC, Richardson AJ, Griffiths TD, Rees A, Stein JF, Green GGR: Sensitivity to dynamic auditory and visual stimuli predicts nonword reading ability in both dyslexic and normal readers. Current Biology: 8; 791–797, 1998.

Wolf M: Naming speed and reading: The contribution of the cognitive neurosciences. Reading Research Quarterly: 26; 123–141, 1991.

Wolf M (Ed): Dyslexia, Fluency, and the Brain. Baltimore, MD: York Press, 2001.

Wolf M, Bally H, Morris R: Automaticity, retrieval processes, and reading: A longitudinal study in average and impaired readers. Child Development: 57(4); 988–1000, 1986.

Wolf M, Bowers PG: The double-deficit hypothesis for the developmental dyslexias. Journal of Educational Psychology: 91(3); 415–438, 1999.

Wolf M, Bowers PG: Naming-speed processes and developmental reading disabilities: An introduction to the special issue on the double-deficit hypothesis. Journal of Learning Disabilities: 33(4); 322–324, 2000.

Wolf M, Bowers PG, Biddle K: Naming-speed processes, timing, and reading: A conceptual review. Journal of Learning Disabilities: 33(4); 387–407, 2000a.

Wolf M, Goldberg A, Gidney C, Lovett MW, Cirino P, Morris RD: The second deficit: An investigation of the independence of phonological and naming-speed deficits in developmental dyslexia. Reading and Writing: An Interdisciplinary Journal: 15(1/2); 43–72, 2002.

Wolf M, Goodman G: Speed wizards [Computerized reading program]. Tufts University, Boston and Rochester Institute of Technology, Rochester, NY, 1996.

Wolf M, Katzir-Cohen T: Reading fluency and its intervention. Scientific Studies of Reading: 5(3); 211–239, 2001.

Wolf M, Miller L, Donnelly K: Retrieval, automaticity, vocabulary elaboration, orthography (RAVE-O): A comprehensive, fluency-based reading intervention progam. Journal of Learning Disabilities: 33(4); 375–386, 2000b.

Wolf M, Pfeil C, Lotz R, Biddle K: Towards a more universal understanding of the developmental dyslexias: The contribution of orthographic factors. In Berninger VW (Ed), The Varieties of Orthographic Knowledge, I. Dordrecht: Kluwer Academic Press, pp. 137–171, 1994.

Wood FB, Flowers DL: Functional neuroanatomy of dyslexic subtypes: A survey of 43 candidate regions with a factor analytic validation across 100 cases. In Duane DD (Ed), Reading and Attention Disorders: Neurobiological Correlates. Baltimore, MD: York Press, pp. 129–159, 1999.

Wood FB, Grigorenko EL: Emerging issues in the genetics of dyslexia: A methodological review. Journal of Learning Disabilities: 34; 503–511, 2001.

Woodcock RW: Woodcock Reading Mastery Tests-Revised. Circle Pines, MN: American Guidance Service, 1987.

Wright BA, Lombardino LJ, King WM, Puranik CS, Leonard CM, Merzenich MM: Deficits in auditory temporal and spectral resolution in language-impaired children. Nature: 387; 176–178, 1997.

Zerbin-Rüden E: Cogential word-blindness. Bulletin of the Orton Society: 17; 47–54, 1967.

© 2003 Published by Elsevier Science B.V.
Handbook of Neuropsychology, 2nd Edition, Vol. 8, Part II
S.J. Segalowitz and I. Rapin (Eds)

CHAPTER 26

Developmental dyscalculia

Ruth S. Shalev *

Neuropediatric Unit, Shaare Zedek Medical Center, P.O. Box 3235, Jerusalem 91031, Israel

Introduction

Children have a biologically-based propensity to acquire arithmetic skills (Ginsburg, 1997). Unlike reading, which needs to be taught, certain numerical skills develop naturally without formal schooling. Children growing up in cultures where formal schooling is not available learn how to count, add, compare and understand quantities (Ginsburg, 1997). This numerical capacity is thought to be an inherent trait, present as early as infancy as babies are able to discriminate between small numbers and engage in numerical computation (Wynn, 1998). Piaget's studies of the development of number concepts led him to conclude that younger children count largely by rote and by and large do not possess a conceptual understanding of number related activities until they are older (Piaget, 1965). However, preschool toddlers understand simple mathematical relations and can correctly calculate exercises in addition and subtraction for numbers up to 3 (Bryant, 1995). Developmental studies in children for whom formal schooling is the norm have shown that they are able to count 3–4 items and comprehend the concept the number represents at age 3–4 years. By age 8 years, children recognize arithmetic symbols and do elementary exercises in addition and subtraction. Further proficiency in addition, subtraction, multiplication and division is acquired between ages 9–12 years of age (Dehaene, 1997, pp. 118–143; Shalev, Manor, Amir et al., 1993).

Within the normal population, there is a subgroup of children who do not acquire arithmetic skills in this fashion. Some of them have trouble learning the arithmetic tables, others never comprehend algorithms of addition, subtraction, multiplication and division, while others have problems understanding the concept of numbers or cannot write, read or identify the correct word to the numeral. These children have developmental dyscalculia (DC) and are the focus of this chapter.

Definition

Until some decades ago, poor performance in arithmetic had been perceived as yet another nonspecific cognitive symptom in mentally retarded children (Guttmann, 1937). In 1974, Kosc redefined DC as a specific, genetically determined learning disability in a child with normal intelligence (Kosc, 1974). This definition is consistent with the current concept of learning disabilities, in the sense that they are brain-based disorders, governed by genetic influences which occur in children of normal intelligence (Geary, 1993; Hammill, 1990). A more recent definition as per the Diagnostic and Statistical Manual of Mental Disorders 4th edition (DSM-IV) (American Psychiatric Association, 1994, pp. 50–51), defines DC as a learning disability in mathematics, the diagnosis of which is established when the performance in arithmetic is substantially below that expected for age, intelligence and education. Alternative operative definitions of DC, like for other

* Corresponding author. Tel.: +972-2-6555345; Fax: +972-2-6422481; E-mail: odeds@cc.huji.ac.il

learning disabilities, rely on the discrepancy between intellectual potential and achievement, or a discrepancy of at least 2 years between the chronological grade and the level of achievement (Reynolds, 1984; Semrud-Clikeman, Biederman, Sprich-Buckminster et al., 1992). The latter definition has limited usefulness for both younger children and older individuals since a 2 year discrepancy in these age groups is not meaningful. The former definition will also identify gifted children whose achievement in a particular learning domain is within the normal range albeit significantly less than expected for the child's intellectual potential. Specific learning disabilities are not the only reason why a gifted child may not perform according to aptitude, so the clinician will ultimately have to determine which child in this category has a bona fide learning disability meriting interventions (Brody and Mills, 1997). Since we do not have a biological marker for learning disabilities, there is still no correct definition or one single way to classify a child. Thus, the choice of definition often rests upon social policy, clinical or research needs. The definition chosen may also arbitrarily determine which child will benefit from educational interventions offered by school or government bodies (Hammill, 1990). For example, children classified as learning disabled according to the achievement-potential discrepancy criterion may qualify for help even though their learning skills are in the normal range. Conversely, other children who are significantly impaired but do not fit the discrepancy criterion may find themselves ineligible for aid.

Clinical description

The manifestations of DC are age and grade related. First graders present with impaired counting skills, for example failing to detect when an object is counted more than once or out of order. They perform poorly both on tasks requiring memory retrieval for basic arithmetic facts and on computing arithmetic exercises, which are thought to reflect their immature counting skills (Geary, 1994). The clinical picture of DC in older elementary school children, i.e. third grade and above, is characterized by deficits in retrieval of presumably overlearned information. The solutions to number facts such as $17 - 9$ or 6×7 are not readily available to these children who will then use immature and inefficient strategies in attempts to solve the problems (Fig. 1a). They are also impaired in completing the arithmetic procedures necessary to solve more complex arithmetic problems in addition, subtraction, multiplication and division. They commit errors resulting from incomplete mastery of the principles and procedures necessary to finish the exercise, i.e., errors of inattention to the arithmetic sign, usage of the wrong sign, forgetting to carry over, misplacement of digits, rotations and undertaking the arithmetic exercise in the wrong direction (Fig. 1b) (Gross-Tsur, Manor and Shalev, 1996; Shalev, Manor and Gross-Tsur, 1997). Unlike the younger children however, they have succeeded by this time in mastering counting skills and are able to match written arabic numerals to quantities, understand concepts such as more, less and equivalence, recognize the numerical values of numerals, are able to determine which of a pair of numerals is the greater or smaller and correctly arrange numbers in serial order both from lowest to highest and highest to lowest. They also are able to write numbers both to dictation and copy.

There are rare case reports of children in whom the developmental arithmetic problem is characterized by a dissociation between arithmetic fact abilities and procedural skills (Temple, 1994). For example, a child will have mastered number facts but doesn't know which steps are needed to solve the entire problem. In one case study, the problem was attributed not to lack of procedural knowledge but to an inability to monitor the sequence of operations required by the arithmetic exercise (Semenza, Miceli and Girelli, 1997).

In spite of the cognitive difficulties that children with DC display, they are able, for the most part, to cope with the everyday demands of arithmetic such as dealing with money and calendrical information (unpublished data). We have encountered only a handful of adolescents and young adults with DC whose problem was so dense that they could not handle change, write checks, or understand the dynamics of dates and years.

It appears therefore that the deficits in numerical competence have a developmental pattern and are apt to change with increasing age. Thus, children at kindergarten age and early elementary school,

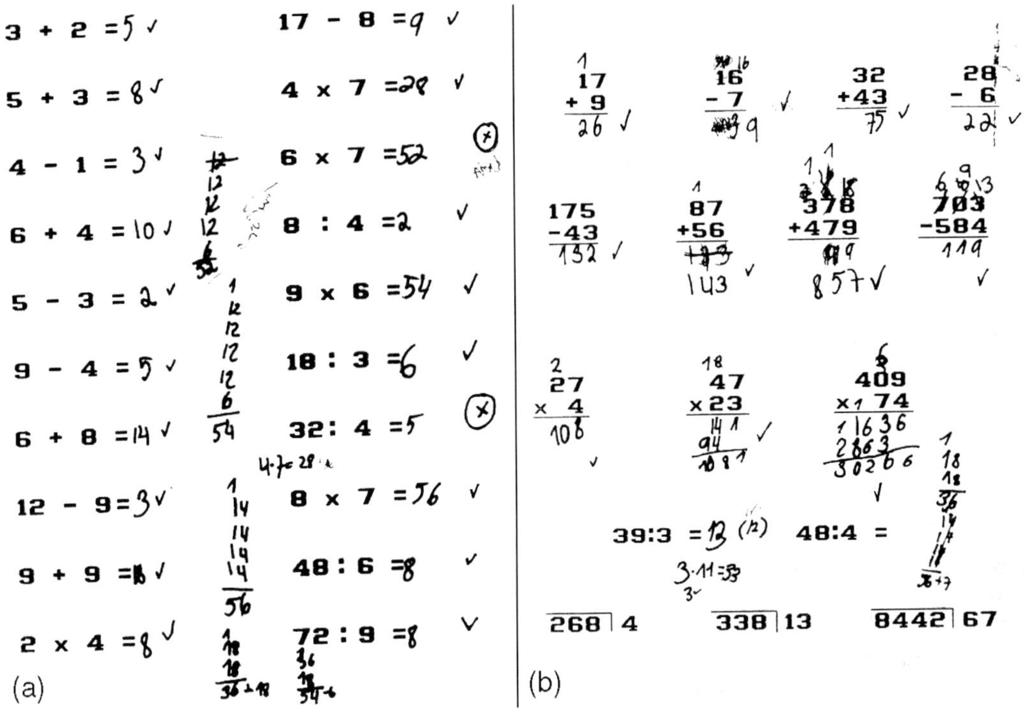

Fig. 1. Arithmetic work-sheets of a 14-year-old-boy with an IQ of 136 and developmental dyscalculia. Note the immature strategies used for multiplication facts in (a). Although the correct answers were ultimately achieved, the numerous errors and corrections seen in (b) indicate that the rules of arithmetic have not been adequately learned for addition, subtraction and multiplication. Division exercises were not attempted.

present with deficits in number concepts and use of immature counting strategies, while in older children the major deficit is recalling overlearned number facts and executing the procedural aspects of complex addition, subtraction, multiplication and division exercises.

Prevalence

The prevalence of DC in the normal population ranges from 3–6%. This figure has been found in population studies carried out in the United States (Badian, 1983), England (Lewis, Hitch and Walker, 1994), Germany (Hein, Bzufka and Neumärker, 2000; Von Aster, 1994) and Israel (Gross-Tsur et al., 1996). Although the DSM-IV (American Psychiatric Association, 1994, pp. 50–51) still states that DC is a rare learning disability with a prevalence of 1%, a more realistic estimate is 5%, which is similar to that of developmental dyslexia and attention deficit hyperactivity disorder (ADHD).

In the Israel prevalence study of DC, we found an estimated prevalence of 6.5% among elementary school children. The population studied included all 10–11-year-old children attending 4th grade in municipally run schools. Using an initial screening procedure for arithmetic skills followed by an individually administered arithmetic test, a cohort of 140 children with DC was identified. The cohort was characterized by a slightly higher prevalence of girls than boys (1.1 : 1.0), an unexpected finding considering that learning disabilities in general are at least 3-fold more prevalent in boys than girls (American Psychiatric Association, 1994). Furthermore, the majority of children had DC as an isolated learning disability with only 17% also having dyslexia and 26% ADHD. It is noteworthy, however, that children with the dual diagnosis of DC and dyslexia were more profoundly impaired on arithmetic skills and had overall poorer performance on neuropsychologic tests than children with DC alone or DC and ADHD (Shalev et al., 1997).

Comorbid conditions and developmental dyscalculia

DC is a common manifestation in many neurological disorders, and in some it is the most frequently encountered learning disability (Gross-Tsur, Manor and Shalev, 1993). Epilepsy, for example, carries an undue risk of DC. Among the learning problems these children have, the academic skill most likely to be impaired is arithmetic (Seidenberg, Beck, Geisser et al., 1986). The cognitive profile for chromosomal disorders such as Turner's syndrome (Temple and Carney, 1993) and girls with Fragile X syndrome includes dyscalculia (Hagerman, Jackson, Amiri et al., 1992). DC is also common in children with phenylketonuria who have been appropriately treated by diet (Pennington, 1991). Twenty percent of boys with ADHD have DC (Faraone, Biederman, Lehman et al., 1993) and it is one of the major criteria of the developmental right hemisphere syndrome (Gross-Tsur, Shalev, Wertman-Elad et al., 1995).

DC is a frequently encountered learning problem in children with delayed language development. Kindergarten children with developmental language disorder perform less well on arithmetic than controls even when there is no difference in their level of intelligence (Manor, Shalev, Joseph and Gross-Tsur, 2001). The frequency of DC in elementary school children who had been diagnosed in kindergarten as suffering from developmental language delay is 55%, a figure 10-fold greater than the 5–6% in the normal population. Although as many as 25% of these children have ADHD, this percentage is still less than the 55% with DC (Shalev, 1998). In this study, no relationship between particular aspects of arithmetic and language impairment could be discerned. In contrast, Fazio (1994) showed that such children were impaired in the sequential aspect of learning number words, counting, reciting numerals backwards and simple addition facts. She ascribed this arithmetic problem to a malfunctioning of the storage and retrieval of rote sequential material (Fazio, 1994, 1996).

The interrelationship between DC and developmental language disorders may be rooted in the impaired linguistic skills, which might be responsible for both the language disorder and the arithmetic dysfunction. Alternatively, both disabilities may reflect a single brain disorder with abnormalities affecting contiguous cortical networks involved in both language and arithmetic processing.

Prognosis

Longitudinal studies of learning disabilities indicate that for many children the problem may be long-lasting. Although Shaywitz, Escobar, Shaywitz et al. (1992) found that 80% of children diagnosed with dyslexia in the first grades of elementary school had a good outcome, this prognosis may not be pertinent when the diagnosis is made at an older age. In the Isle of Wight study of dyslexia that involved 9-year-old boys, more than half of the boys continued to be dyslexic five years later (Rutter, Tizard, Yule et al., 1976). As far as ADHD is concerned, 85% of boys with this disorder still meet research criteria for this condition 4 years later (Biederman, Faraone, Milberger et al., 1996).

Experience indicates that DC has a similar natural history. Between first and second grade, there is considerable improvement in counting procedures (Geary, 1994, p. 164). However, when 10–11-year-old boys and girls with DC were prospectively followed and reexamined at age 13–14 years, the arithmetic achievement in 95% of them fell in the lowest quartile of their school class and almost half continued to meet research criteria for DC (Shalev, Manor, Auerbach et al., 1998). Factors associated with persistence of DC were severity of the arithmetic disorder at the time of the original diagnosis, and the presence of arithmetic problems in siblings of the proband. Factors which were not associated with persistence were socio-economic status, gender, the co-occurrence of another learning disability and the extent or types of educational interventions received by these children (Shalev et al., 1998).

Etiology

Not all researchers agree that DC is a biologically-based brain disorder. Poor teaching, environmental deprivation, low intelligence, and 'mathematical anxiety' have all been implicated as possible causes or contributing factors for developmental arithmetic disabilities (Broman, Bien and Shaughness, 1985; Ashcraft and Faust, 1994; Miller and Mercer, 1997).

Poor teaching may be one of the reasons why children don't learn arithmetic. Most arithmetic curricula have not been field-tested so that teaching programs are chosen by educators without prior knowledge of the effectiveness of a particular text. Furthermore, arithmetic texts commonly used in the school systems are predicated on the 'basal' approach, in which numerous simple arithmetic skills are introduced rapidly to be re-taught at a more complex level in subsequent grades. Experience, however, has shown that this is not the case: the initial learning is superficial and the second, re-teaching phase, does not materialize (Miller and Mercer, 1997). Other drawbacks are overcrowded classrooms and the diversity of the student body (Ginsburg, 1997). Thus, students who haven't mastered a basic arithmetic skill will be handicapped as the teachers proceed with the curriculum. Furthermore, the trend towards mainstreaming means that children with difficulties will be receiving much of their instruction in general classrooms and not in resource rooms geared to better address their special needs (Miller and Mercer, 1997).

Another issue that may masquerade or exacerbate dyscalculia is mathematical anxiety, sufferers of which are perceived as less competent in arithmetic. Mathematics anxiety correlates with lower aptitude for arithmetic and underachievement and avoidance of mathematics courses. Highly anxious subjects are willing to sacrifice accuracy for speed and report more extraneous thoughts during an arithmetic task (Ashcraft, 1995). A lower performance is seen even on overlearned first and second grade addition problems. Mathematical anxiety is apparently due to a decrease in working memory capacity and not to lower competence in arithmetic (Faust, Ashcraft and Fleck, 1996). Competence scores improve significantly after therapeutic intervention for mathematical anxiety.

Light and Defries (1995) provide evidence for the role of genetics in children with the dual diagnosis of dyscalculia and dyslexia. They used a twin study paradigm and found that genetic factors contribute to the observed comorbidity between reading and arithmetic disabilities. In a study of twins with DC, Alarcon, Defries, Gillis Light and Pennington (1997) found that 58% of monozygotic co-twins and 39% of dizygotic co-twins of DC probands also have DC. The concordance rates were 0.73 and 0.56, respectively, further supporting a genetic etiology. The impact of familiality for DC was documented by Shalev, Manor, Kerem et al. (2001) who, using a family study paradigm, demonstrated that approximately half of all siblings and parents of children with DC also have DC. The risk was 5–10 times greater than that of the general population and the intraclass correlation between parents and siblings was 0.2. Taken together, these results highlight the role of heredity in the etiopathogenesis of DC as Kosc (1974) had hypothesized 25 years earlier.

Neurological substrate

Studies in adult patients have demonstrated that lesions in either hemisphere of the brain can cause acquired dyscalculia although injury to the left posterior quadrant appears to result in the most profound and pervasive arithmetic deficits (Grafman, Passafiume, Faglioni and Boller, 1982). This information led Grafman (1988) to speculate that both number processing and the ability to calculate are localized to the left temporal–parietal area. However, lesions leading to dyscalculia are not exclusive to the cortical regions of the brain. Structural abnormalities in subcortical areas have also been documented. For example, severe dyscalculia has been reported in patients with a basal ganglia lesions (Corbet, McCusker and Davidson, 1986; Hittmair-Delazer, Semenza and Denes, 1994) and electrical stimulation of the thalamus was found to disrupt arithmetic processing (Ojemann, 1974). Thus, involvement of cortical and subcortical structures in arithmetic alludes to the existence of a neural network, embedded within cortico-thalamo-striatal circuits.

Whalen, McCloskey, Lesser and Gordon (1997) demonstrated that selective electrical stimulation to the left anterior parietal area transiently impairs arithmetic fact retrieval, particularly for multiplication, thereby correlating between a specific arithmetic function and a particular brain region. Functional–neuroanatomical correlations were also reported by Kiefer and Dehaene (1997) who utilized event-related potentials to investigate localization of simple and complex multiplications. They found that simple multiplication exercises are processed by the left parietal cortex, whereas complex exercises generated activity in both centro-parietal areas, albeit slightly greater on the left. Neuroimaging studies support these electrophysiological findings. Functional MRI (fMRI) of normal individuals engaged in arithmetic shows bilateral activation of prefrontal and inferior parietal cortices (Rueckert, Lange, Partiot et al., 1996). Functional MRI was exploited by Dehaene and colleagues (1999) to delineate the neuroanatomy of specific arithmetic tasks in normal individuals. The authors were able to show that execution of language-dependent exact calculations activated a large area in the left inferior frontal lobe. Performing tasks of number approximation, on the other hand, activated both parietal lobes. Event related potentials bolstered the fMRI data: for exact arithmetic exercises, electrical activation appeared over the left frontal lobe while for calculation tasks requiring an approximate response, activation was greatest in the parietal lobes.

Functional MRI has also been used in the study of an adolescent with dyscalculia who endured a right temporal lobe hemorrhage in infancy. The activation pattern differed from the normal pattern in that it was primarily unilateral, localized to the frontal and parietal regions of the intact left hemisphere (Levin, Scheller, Rickard et al., 1996). In another report, magnetic resonance spectroscopy demonstrated a wedge shaped defect in the left parieto-temporal area in a young adult with developmental dyscalculia who had no known structural abnormalities (Levy, Reis and Grafman, 1999). Both studies highlight the importance of the left hemisphere, particularly the parieto-temporal areas, in the evolution of dyscalculia.

A testimony to the pivotal role of the parietal lobes in mathematics can be deduced from the brain of the legendary Albert Einstein. Although the gross anatomy of his brain was surprisingly unremarkable, the parietal lobes were distinguished by their absolute size as well as by their unique morphological (Witelson, Kigar and Harvey, 1999) and histological features (Diamond, Scheibel, Murphy and Harvey, 1985).

Classification

In an attempt to understand the neuropsychologic and clinical features of DC, children with this disorder have been classified in different ways. Badian (1983) categorized DC according to coexisting neuropsychological characteristics: aphasia, visuo-spatial dysfunction, attention problems, anarithmetia and combinations of these categories. This classification was derived from that of Hecaen, Angelergues and Houillier (1961) used for adults with acquired dyscalculia. In Badian's sample of children with DC, the category of attention problems comprised the largest number of children suggesting a close association between arithmetic and attention skills. Geary categorized DC into three types: fact-retrieval deficit, procedural deficits and deficits in the ability to spatially represent numerical information (Geary, 1994, pp. 170–175). Rourke (1993) used the absence, presence and severity of an associated reading disorder to distinguish between different types of DC. Children with an isolated arithmetic disorder had the most profound arithmetic inadequacy and a particular neurobehavioral profile. The characteristics of this profile were normal psycholinguistic skills but impaired tactile–perceptual and visuo-perceptual functions, profound difficulties on nonverbal problem-solving tasks and in adapting to novel problem-solving situations. On the other hand, the neurobehavioral profile of children with DC and dyslexia was characterized by deficits in sequential processing.

The usefulness of the classification of Rourke (1993) and Badian (1983) was reevaluated in both a population-based cohort of children with DC (Shalev et al., 1997) and in a referred group (Shalev, Manor, Amir et al., 1995). In the former (Shalev et al., 1997), dyslexia, ADHD and neuropsychological functions were studied in a group of 140 children. In contrast to what might have been expected from the evidence provided by Rourke (1993), children with both DC and dyslexia had the most profound arithmetic problem involving multiple domains of arithmetic function (Shalev et al., 1997). Visuo-spatial dysfunction, contrary to what would have been predicted by Geary (1994, pp. 170–175), did not impact on arithmetic performance of these children with DC (Shalev et al., 1997). Furthermore, attention problems, which comprised the largest subgroup of children according to Badian (1983), were found in only a quarter of the children with DC. The co-occurrence of attention problems in children with DC did not alter their neuropsychological profile nor affected the severity of the arithmetic disorder. The second study of referred children with DC was composed of children with associated language problems, presumably reflecting left hemispheric dysfunction, and children with visuo-spatial dysfunction, allegedly reflecting right hemisphere dysfunction. Neither the domains of impaired arithmetic nor their severity differentiated between these groups. Furthermore, errors in arithmetic performance attributable to visuo-spatial performance were not confined to children with DC and right hemisphere dysfunction. Thus, the results of these two studies do not support the specific subtypes of DC delineated by Badian (1983) or by Rourke (1993).

Kosc (1974) divided DC into 6 subgroups each of which could occur as an isolated deficit: (1) verbal dyscalculia — a disturbed ability to verbally name mathematical terms and relations; (2) practognostic dyscalculia — an inability to execute mathematical computations or estimate magnitude with concrete objects; (3) lexical dyscalculia — an impairment in reading mathematical symbols (digits, numbers, operational signs); (4) graphical dyscalculia — a disability in writing numerals, multidigit numbers and symbols; (5) ideognostical dyscalculia — a lack of understanding of arithmetic procedures an example of which is that 9 is 1 less than 10 or equal to 3×3; (6) operational dyscalculia — an inability to carry out mathematical operations, also termed anarithmetia by Hecaen et al. (1961) and Badian (1983). This classification of DC has both theoretical and practical implications. It incorporates many of the components of the neurocognitive models of normal arithmetic functioning (Dehaene and Cohen, 1995; McCloskey, Caramazza and Basili, 1985) that can be selectively impaired. It is also a clinically oriented classification, the potential usefulness of which is rooted in specific error-types that can be readily identified.

Another type of DC appears within the context of the developmental Gerstmann's syndrome, the symptom complex consisting of: dysgraphia, dyscalculia, finger agnosia and right–left disorientation. Although the existence of this entity has been questioned (Benton, 1961), Gerstmann's syndrome is still recognized by its classical tetrad of symptoms and cases with this syndrome continue to be of scientific interest (Cipolotti, Butterworth and Denes, 1991; PeBenito, Fisch and Fisch, 1988; Suresh and Sebastian, 2000). A developmental version of the Gerstmann's syndrome is also characterized by impaired spatial tasks and figure-ground discrimination, reading and writing retardation and a relatively low performance IQ (Kinsbourne and Warrington, 1963; Spellacy and Peter, 1978). Benson and Geschwind (1970) hypothesized that an underlying disorder of spatial orientation may account for the arithmetic problem. Kinsbourne and Warrington (1963) felt that the multiplicity of symptoms in this group of children resulted from a problem of ordering which in and of itself was sufficient to disrupt the various cognitive processes affected. Implicit in their conception of the neuropsychological basis of the developmental Gerstmann's syndrome was that the symptomatology could not be explained by damage to contiguous cortical areas. Even though all these hypotheses are theoretically based, we have not been able to subdivide DC in children, including those with the Gerstmann's syndrome, according to any particular neuropsychological feature (Shalev et al., 1997).

The anatomical substrate in adults with Gerstmann's syndrome is the dominant parietal lobe, particularly the angular, supramarginal and inferior parietal gyri or, in the right parietal lobe when the syndrome occurs in left handed patients with reversed dominance (Moore, Saver, Johnson and Romero, 1991). The anatomical correlate for children with the developmental Gerstmann's syndrome is unknown. Miller, Benson and Wolff (1984) felt that an injury in the dominant parietal lobe in the developing brain could also result in Gerstmann's syndrome although Kinsbourne and Warrington speculated that areas other than the dominant parietal lobe play a role in the developmental syndrome. Rourke and Conway (1997) thought that the right hemisphere is involved since the symptomatology of the developmental Gerstmann's syndrome shares features with the syndrome of nonverbal learning disabilities, a disorder hypothesized to result from right hemisphere dysfunction. Another possibility is that both parietal lobes are involved in this syndrome. This hypothesis is consistent with the fMRI activation pattern seen in normal individuals undertaking calculation Dehaene et al., 1999). Support for this supposition, albeit indirect, comes from Butterworth (1999) who theorized that the neurological basis of digital representation of numbers is localized to the parietal lobes and dependent upon finger knowledge, a major criterion of the Gerstmann's syndrome. For those children with the developmental Gerstmann's syndrome who also have developmental dyslexia, the left parietal lobe may be more extensively affected while those with non-verbal learning disabilities, and/or interpersonal problems, may have more severe dysfunction of the right lobe.

Cognitive models

The clinical classifications of DC, which emerged from an interest in comprehending the symptomatology of arithmetic dysfunction, predate the elaboration of neurocognitive models of arithmetic. These models were developed to understand how arithmetic is processed in the normal brain. Their validity was tested on individuals who had had no previous problem in arithmetic, but in the wake of brain damage, exhibited dyscalculia. The model proposed by McCloskey et al. (1985) divides arithmetic skills into three main groups: comprehension of number concepts, production of numbers and calculation. This model has proved valid for adults with acquired dyscalculia in whom an isolated deficit in a specific area of arithmetic has been identified while other facets of arithmetic function — as defined by the model — remain intact. The model has also been useful in understanding the selective arithmetic deficits which may occur in DC. Temple (1989) provided a detailed description of a boy with DC who had an isolated deficit in lexical number processing rendering him unable to attribute the precise word value to a digit. The boy made errors when reading arabic numbers aloud even though he encountered no difficulty in reading simple or unfamiliar words. His errors followed a consistent pattern; he would identify the numerical relationship between the numerals in the number involved, misread the number but correctly identified the syntactical position (i.e. whether they were units, tens, hundreds, etc.) of the numeral within the word. The example cited for this child is his performance in the number 9172 which he read as "six thousand, six hundred and seventy-two". The magnitude of the number was correctly identified although individual numerals were misread. Temple (1994) also identified other specific arithmetic deficits in children, including problems in the acquisition of arithmetic tables and in the execution of arithmetic laws in complex number procedures.

Another model, coined the 'triple-code model', has been proposed by Dehaene and Cohen (1995). The three elements of this model are a verbal system, a visual numeral form and magnitude representation. Mental arithmetic operations are linked to the verbal system residing in the left hemisphere, whereas more complex arithmetic procedures which require magnitude estimation and visual representations are bilaterally localized. This model is supported by case reports of patients with brain lesions as well as from studies on healthy subjects with normal arithmetic function. For example, a patient with a left hemisphere lesion exhibited dissociation of rote, overlearned arithmetic facts and knowledge of number magnitude; the patient was unable to recall arithmetic facts but retained an intact ability to estimate number magnitude. A reverse pattern was described in a strongly left handed patient (with presumed right hemisphere dominance for language) who had a right parietal lesion; the patient lost the sense of number magnitude while retaining the knowledge of arithmetic facts (Dehaene and Cohen, 1997). Evidence from split-brain patients who can neither compute simple arithmetic operations nor name digits with their right hemisphere also fits the predictions of this model (Sperry, Gazzaniga and Bogen, 1969; Teng and Sperry, 1973). Normal individuals performing overlearned arithmetic exercises which are presumably language dependent exhibit an fMRI activation pattern localized to the left frontal lobe. When the calculations are more complex, requiring combined visual and numerical magnitude representations, both parietal lobes are activated (Dehaene, Spelke, Pinel et al., 1999). Based on these data, Dehaene et al. (1999) have proposed two distinct neural circuits for arithmetic processing, both necessary for complex arithmetic calculations. One is a visuo-spatial based circuit harboring representations of approximate quantities. The second is a linguistic based circuit, containing representations of exact, rote arithmetic facts. The triple-code model is attractive since inherent within it are both the neuropsychological mechanisms necessary for arithmetic processing as well as its neuroanatomical substrate.

DC as a primary or secondary neuropsychological deficit

An alternative approach to the neuropsychological basis of DC is to determine whether this learning disability derives from a primary cognitive deficit. Evidence for a primary deficit is predicated on data from infants who are able to identify numerosities of up to four elements (Antell and Keating, 1983), reason about numbers and objects and distinguish between larger and smaller numerosities (Wynn, 1998). Auxiliary evidence for a primary deficit comes from studies on genetic disorders of the X chromosome, i.e. Turner's syndrome (Temple and Carney, 1993) and females with the Fragile X syndrome (Hagerman et al., 1992). In spite of normal intelligence, subjects with these disorders demonstrate a specific learning disability in the domain of arithmetic (Shalev, 1998). Furthermore, DC can appear as an isolated learning disability in an otherwise healthy child with normal or above normal intelligence (Gross-Tsur et al., 1996). Indeed, Ta'ir, Brezner and Ariel (1997) described such a case: an 11-year-old boy of normal intelligence and intact neuropsychological status but with profound DC. A detailed examination of the child's numerical skills revealed that his arithmetic disability resulted from a discrete deficit in the concept of quantity and seriation, sparing other domains of number logic. The authors proposed that the deficit in quantity and seriation affected other arithmetic skills such as perceiving and conserving quantities, maintaining one-to-one correlation and comprehending mathematical relations. This phenomenon, which the authors chose to coin "cardinal/ordinal skills acquisition device", resulted in the patients profound dyscalculia.

The notion that dyscalculia is secondary to a more general neuropsychological dysfunction rather than one specific to arithmetic must also be addressed. Rourke (1993) has suggested that the underpinnings of DC can be secondary either to visuo-spatial dysfunction or to verbal and auditory–perceptual dysfunction, both of which can result in multiple cognitive manifestations, only one of which is dyscalculia. Koontz and Berch (1996) have proposed that DC results from a relatively poor working memory resources for information in general.

Perhaps it is more appropriate to speak about DC in terms of a neural network rather than of a particular neuropsychological function. Neural networks have been demonstrated for both attention (Posner and Raichle, 1994) and language processing (Posner, Petersen, Fox and Raichle, 1988) and may also be relevant for arithmetic processing. Evidence for a network stems from fMRI studies which have delineated activity in multiple areas of the brain, primarily bifrontal and biparietal, in individuals executing mental arithmetic (Dehaene, 1997; Dehaene et al., 1999; Rueckert et al., 1996). Thus, different patterns of arithmetic dysfunction might result from the extent and localization of damage to the arithmetic neural network.

Arithmetic assessment batteries

Several standardized arithmetic tests, covering a broad range of ages, are available to assess arithmetic skills in children. The arithmetic subtests of the WRAT-R (Jastak and Wilkinson, 1984) and the Young's Group Mathematics Test (Young, 1971) are among tests that have been used to classify children with DC (Faraone et al., 1993; Lewis et al., 1994). These are timed tests that emphasize arithmetic achievement, which for elementary school children is manifested by competence in arithmetic facts and procedural problems. Von Aster (2001) developed a battery of arithmetic tests called Neuropsychological Test Battery for Number Processing and Calculation in Children (NUCALC). The test battery, which was validated for grades 2–4 in Switzerland and France, was designed to assess number concepts, number facts and arithmetic procedures (Deloche, Von Aster, Dellatolas et al., 1995; Von Aster, Deloche, Dellatolas and Meier, 1997). Shalev et al. (1993, 1998) have validated an arithmetic battery in Israel for grades 3–8 and 10th. The test assesses arithmetic skills, number comprehension, number production and calculation, based on the cognitive model as articulated by McCloskey et al. (1985).

Educational interventions

Effective educational techniques for children with arithmetic disabilities are those which incorporate modeling and feedback procedures, reinforcement of previously acquired arithmetic skills, a concrete-to-abstract teaching sequence, verbalization while solving problems, creative strategies for problem solving, frequent monitoring of student's progress and teaching skills to mastery (Miller and Mercer, 1997; Naglieri and Gottling, 1997).

Circumventing the impaired neuropsychological functions while basing the teaching on those which are intact has also been suggested (Rourke, 1993; Temple, 1990). For example, children for whom the presumed underpinnings of dyscalculia are perceptual and visual–spatial or verbal and auditory–perceptual, would be likely to benefit from interventions tailored to the underlying problem (Rourke and Conway, 1997). Ginsburg (1997) has suggested that memorization should be avoided if the pitfall is in learning number facts, allowing for use of pocket calculators. Impediments in understanding the concepts underlying addition/subtraction/multiplication and division require creative solutions. For some children it is useful to take a 'time-out' period until some developmental change occurs. Clearly, it is imperative to ascertain that children with DC become familiar with arithmetic concepts needed for daily life, e.g. understanding street addresses, handling money, reading calendars and writing checks.

The teacher has to be careful not to project subliminal messages. Children with learning disabilities are often perceived by their teachers as having 'a sickness' so that the teachers' approach may be edged with pity, and acceptance of academic failure to a degree that wouldn't occur for their nondisabled peers. This approach, instead of helping children, may impact negatively on an already precarious self esteem (Clark, 1997).

In summary

Developmental dyscalculia (DC) is a specific learning disability affecting the acquisition of arithmetic skills in an otherwise normal child. Although poor teaching, environmental deprivation and low intelligence have been implicated in the etiology of DC, the consensus is that this learning disability is a brain-based disorder with a familial–genetic predisposition in which the parietal lobes play a pivotal role. The prevalence of DC in the school population is about 5–6%, a frequency similar to that of developmental dyslexia and attention deficit hyperactivity disorder (ADHD). Unlike the latter two disorders, DC is as common in girls as in boys. DC is frequently encountered in diverse neurological disorders, examples of which include ADHD, developmental language disorder, epilepsy, treated phenylketonuria and Fragile X syndrome. Although the long term prognosis of DC is as yet unknown, current data indicate that DC is a stable learning disability persisting, at least for the short term, in about half of affected children. The consequences of DC and its impact on education, employment and psychological well-being have yet to be determined.

Acknowledgements

I would like to thank Drs. V. Gross-Tsur, I. Rapin, J. Auerbach and S. Segalowitz for their comments and suggestions and to acknowledge the support of the Mirsky Foundation and the Office of the Chief Scientist, Israel Ministry of Health.

References

Alarcon M, Defries JC, Gillis Light J, Pennington BF: A twin study of mathematics disability. Journal of Learning Disability: 30; 617–623, 1997.

American Psychiatric Association: Diagnostic and Statistical Manual of Mental Disorders, Fourth edition. Washington DC, pp. 48–55, 83–84, 1994.

Antell S, Keating DP: Perception of numerical invariance in neonates. Child Development: 54; 695–701, 1983.

Ashcraft MH: Cognitive psychology and simple arithmetic: A review and summary of new directions. Mathematical Cognition: 1; 3–34, 1995.

Ashcraft MH, Faust MW: Mathematical anxiety and mental arithmetic performance: An exploratory investigation. Cognition and Emotion: 8; 97–125, 1994.

Badian NA: Arithmetic and nonverbal learning. In Myklebust HR (Ed), Progress in Learning Disabilities, Vol. 5. New York: Grune and Stratton, pp. 235–264, 1983.

Benson DF, Geschwind N: Developmental Gerstmann syndrome. Neurology: 20; 293–298, 1970.

Benton A: The fiction of the Gerstmann syndrome. Journal of Neurology, Neurosurgery and Psychiatry: 24; 176–181, 1961.

Biederman J, Faraone S, Milberger S, Curtis S, Chen L, Marrs A, Ouellete C, Moore P, Spencer T: Predictors of persistence and remission of ADHD into adolescence: Results from a four-year prospective follow-up study. Journal of American Academy of Child and Adolescent Psychiatry: 35; 343–351, 1996.

Brody LE, Mills CF: Gifted children with learning disabilities: A review of the issues. Journal of Learning Disabilities: 30; 282–296, 1997.

Broman S, Bien E, Shaughness P: Low Achieving Children: The first seven years. Hillsdale: Erlbaum, p. ix, 1985.

Bryant P: Children and arithmetic. Journal of Child Psychology and Psychiatry: 36; 3–32, 1995.

Butterworth B: A head for numbers. Science: 284; 928–929, 1999.

Clark MD: Teacher response to learning disability: A test of attributional principles. Journal of Learning Disabilities: 30; 69–79, 1997.

Cipolotti L, Butterworth B, Denes G: A specific deficit for numbers in a case of dense acalculia. Brain: 114; 2619–2637, 1991.

Corbet AJ, McCusker EA, Davidson OR: Acalculia following a dominant-hemisphere subcortical infarct. Archives of Neurology: 43; 964–966, 1986.

Dehaene S: The Number Sense. Oxford: Oxford University Press, pp. 118–143; 207–230, 1997.

Dehaene S, Cohen L: Towards an anatomical and functional model of number processing. Mathematical Cognition: 1; 83–120, 1995.

Dehaene S, Cohen L: Cerebral pathways for calculation: double dissociation between rote verbal and quantitative knowledge of arithmetic. Cortex: 33; 219–250, 1997.

Dehaene S, Spelke E, Pinel P, Stanescu R, Tsivkin S: Sources of mathematical thinking: Behavioral and brain-imaging evidence. Science: 284; 970–974, 1999.

Deloche G, Von Aster MG, Dellatolas G, Gaillard F, Tieche C, Azema D: Traitement des nombres et calcul en CE1 et CE2, quelques donnees et principes d'elaboration d'une batterie. Approche Neuropsychologique des Apprentissages chez l'Enfant (A.N.E.A.): Hors serie 42–51, 1995.

Diamond MC, Scheibel AB, Murphy GM Jr, Harvey T: On the brain of a scientist: Albert Einstein. Experimental Neurology: 88; 198–204, 1985.

Faraone SV, Biederman J, Lehman BK, Spencer T, Norman D, Seidman LJ, Kraus I, Perrin J, Chen WJ, Tsuang MT: Intellectual performance and school failure in children with attention deficit hyperactivity disorder and in their siblings. Journal of Abnormal Psychology: 102; 616–623, 1993.

Faust MW, Ashcraft MH, Fleck DE: Mathematics anxiety effects in simple and complex addition. Mathematical Cognition: 2; 25–62, 1996.

Fazio BB: The counting abilities of children with specific language impairment: a comparison of oral and gestural tasks. Journal of Speech and Hearing Research: 37; 358–368, 1994.

Fazio BB: Mathematical abilities of children with specific language impairment: a 2-year follow-up. Journal of Speech and Hearing Research: 39; 839–849, 1996.

Geary DC: Mathematical disabilities: Cognitive, neuropsychological, and genetic components. Psychological Bulletin: 114; 345–362, 1993.

Geary DC: Mathematical Disabilities In: Children's Mathematical Development. Washington, DC: American Psychological Association, pp. 155–187, 1994.

Ginsburg HP: Mathematics learning disabilities: A view from developmental psychology. Journal of Learning Disabilities: 30; 20–33, 1997.

Grafman J: Acalculia. In Boller F, Grafman J (Eds), Handbook of Neuropsychology, Vol. 1. Amsterdam: Elsevier, pp. 415–431, 1988.

Grafman J, Passafiume D, Faglioni P, Boller F: Calculation disturbances in adults with focal hemispheric damage. Cortex: 18; 37–50, 1982.

Gross-Tsur V, Manor O, Shalev RS: Developmental dyscalculia, gender and the brain. Archives of Disease in Childhood: 68; 510–512, 1993.

Gross-Tsur V, Manor O, Shalev RS: Developmental dyscalculia: prevalence and demographic features. Developmental Medicine and Child Neurology: 38; 25–33, 1996.

Gross-Tsur V, Shalev RS, Manor O, Amir N: Developmental right hemisphere syndrome: the clinical spectrum of the nonverbal learning disability. Journal of Learning Disabilities: 38; 80–86, 1995.

Guttmann E: Congenital arithmetic disability and aculculia (Henschen). British Journal of Medical Psychology: 16; 16–35, 1937.

Hagerman RJ, Jackson C, Amiri K, Cronister Silverman A, O'Connor R, Sobesky W: Girls with fragile X syndrome: physical and neurocognitive status and outcome. Pediatrics: 89; 395–400, 1992.

Hammill DD: On defining learning disabilities: an emerging consensus. Journal of Learning Disabilities: 23; 76–84, 1990.

Hecaen H, Angelergues R, Houillier S: Les varietes clinicques des acalculies au cours des lesions retro-rolandiques: Approche statistique du probleme. Revue Neurologique: 105; 85–103, 1961.

Hein J, Bzufka MW, Neumärker KJ: The specific disorder of arithmetic skills. Prevalence studies in a rural and an urban population sample and their clinico-neuropsychological validation. European Journal of Child Adolescent Psychiatry: 9(Suppl 2); 87-101, 2000.

Hittmair-Delazer M, Semenza C, Denes G: Concepts and facts in calculation. Brain: 117; 715–728, 1994.

Jastak S, Wilkinson GS: Wide Range Achievement Test Revised: Administration Manual. Wilmington, DE: Jastak Associates, 1984.

Kiefer M, Dehaene S: The time course of parietal activation in single-digit multiplication: evidence from event-related potentials. Mathematical Cognition: 3; 11–30, 1997.

Kinsbourne M, Warrington EK: The developmental Gerstmann Syndrome. Archives of Neurology: 8; 490–510, 1963.

Kosc L: Developmental dyscalculia. Journal of Learning Disabilities: 7; 46–59, 1974.

Koontz KL, Berch DB: Identifying simple numerical stimuli: Processing inefficiencies exhibited by arithmetic learning disabled children. Mathematical Cognition: 2; 1–23, 1996.

Levin HS, Scheller J, Rickard T, Grafman J, Martinkowski K, Winslow M, Mirvis S: Dyscalculia and dyslexia after right hemisphere injury in infancy. Archives of Neurology: 53; 88–96, 1996.

Levy LM, Reis IL, Grafman J: Metabolic abnormalities detected by ^{1}H-MRS in dyscalculia and dysgraphia. Neurology: 53; 639–641, 1999.

Lewis C, Hitch GJ, Walker P: The prevalence of specific arithmetic difficulties and specific reading difficulties in 9 to 10 year old boys and girls. Journal of Child Psychology and Psychiatry: 35; 283–292, 1994.

Light JG, Defries JC: Comorbidity of reading and mathematics disabilities: Genetic and environmental etiologies. Journal of Learning Disabilities: 28; 96–106, 1995.

Manor O, Shalev RS, Joseph A, Gross-Tsur V: Arithmetic skills in kindergarten children with developmental language disorders. European Journal of Paediatric Neurology: 5(2); 71–87, 2001.

McCloskey M, Caramazza A, Basili A: Cognitive mechanisms in number processing and calculation: evidence from dyscalculia. Brain and Cognition: 4; 171–196, 1985.

Miller BL, Benson DF, Wolff D: Developmental syndrome of the angular gyrus. Bulletin of Clinical Neurosciences: 49; 4–7, 1984.

Miller SP, Mercer CD: Educational aspects of mathematics disabilities. Journal of Learning Disabilities: 30; 47–56, 1997.

Moore MR, Saver JL, Johnson KA, Romero JA: Right parietal stroke with Gerstmann's syndrome. Archives of Neurology: 48; 432–435, 1991.

Naglieri JA, Gottling SH: Mathematics instruction and PASS cognitive processes: An intervention study. Journal of Learning Disabilities: 30; 513–520, 1997.

Ojemann G: Mental arithmetic during human thalamic stimulation. Neuropsychologia: 12; 1–10, 1974.

PeBenito R, Fisch CB, Fisch ML: Developmental Gerstmann's syndrome. Archives of Neurology: 45; 977–982, 1988.

Pennington BF: Genetics of learning disabilities. Seminars in Neurology: 11; 28–34, 1991.

Piaget J: The Child's Perception of Number. New York: Norton, pp. 41–95, 1965.

Posner MI, Petersen SE, Fox P, Raichle ME: Localization of cognitive operations in the human brain. Science: 240; 1627–1631, 1988.

Posner MI, Raichle ME: Images of Mind. New York: WH Freeman and Company, pp. 145–178, 1994.

Reynolds CR: Critical measurement issues in learning disabilities. Journal of Special Education: 18; 451–476, 1984.

Rourke BP: Arithmetic disabilities, specific and otherwise: A neuropsychological perspective. Journal of Learning Disabilities: 26; 214–226, 1993.

Rourke BP, Conway JA: Disabilities of arithmetic and mathematical reasoning: Perspectives from neurology and neuropsychology. Journal of Learning Disabilities: 30; 34–46, 1997.

Rueckert L, Lange N, Partiot A, Appollonio I, Litvar I, Le Bihan D, Grafman J: Visualizing cortical activation during mental calculation with function MRI. NeuroImage: 3; 97–103, 1996.

Rutter M, Tizard J, Yule W, Graham P, Whitmore K: Research report: Isle of Wight studies 1964–1974. Psychological Medicine: 6; 313–332, 1976.

Seidenberg M, Beck N, Geisser M, Giordani B, Sackellares JC, Berent S, Dreifuss FE, Boll TJ: Academic achievement of children with epilepsy. Epilepsia: 27; 753–759, 1986.

Semenza C, Miceli L, Girelli L: A deficit for arithmetical procedures: Lack of knowledge or lack of monitoring? Cortex: 33; 483–498, 1997.

Semrud-Clikeman M, Biederman J, Sprich-Buckminster S, Krifcher Lehman B, Faraone SV, Norman D: Comorbidity between ADDH and learning disability: a review and report in a clinically referred sample. Journal of American Academy of Child and Adolescent Psychiatry: 31; 439–448, 1992.

Shalev R: Developmental dyscalculia. In Perat MJ (Ed), New Developments in Child Neurology. Bologna: Monduzzi Editore, pp. 635–641, 1998.

Shalev RS, Manor O, Amir N, Gross-Tsur V: Acquisition of arithmetic in normal children: assessment by a cognitive model of dyscalculia. Developmental Medicine and Child Neurology: 35; 593–601, 1993.

Shalev RS, Manor O, Amir N, Wertman-Elad R, Gross-Tsur V: Developmental dyscalculia and brain laterality. Cortex: 31; 357–365, 1995.

Shalev RS, Manor O, Auerbach J, Gross-Tsur V: Persistence of developmental dyscalculia: what counts? Results from a three year prospective follow-up study. Journal of Pediatrics: 133; 358–362, 1998.

Shalev RS, Manor O, Gross-Tsur V: Neuropsychological aspects of developmental dyscalculia. Mathematical Cognition: 33; 105–120, 1997.

Shalev RS, Manor O, Kerem B, Ayali M, Badichi N, Friedlander Y, Gross-Tsur V: Familial–genetic facets of developmental dyscalculia. Journal of Learning Disabilities: 34; 59–65, 2001.

Shaywitz SE, Escobar MD, Shaywitz BA, Fletcher JM, Mackuck R: Evidence that dyslexia may represent the lower tail of a normal distribution of reading ability. New England Journal of Medicine: 324; 145–150, 1992.

Spellacy F, Peter B: Dyscalculia and elements of the developmental Gerstmann syndrome in school children. Cortex: 14; 197–206, 1978.

Sperry RW, Gazzaniga MS, Bogen JE: Interhemispheric relationships: the neocortical commissures: syndromes of hemisphere disconnection. In Vinken PJ, Bruyn HW (Eds), Handbook of Clinical Neurology, Vol. 4. Amsterdam: North-Holland Publishing company, pp. 273–290, 1969.

Suresh PA, Sebastian S: Developmental Gerstmann's syndrome: A distinct clinical entity of learning disabilities. Pediatric Neurology: 22; 267–278, 2000.

Ta'ir J, Brezner A, Ariel R: Profound developmental dyscalculia: Evidence for a cardinal/ordinal skills acquisition device. Brain Cognition: 35; 184–206, 1997.

Temple CM: Digit dyslexia: a category-specific disorder in developmental dyscalculia. Cognitive Neuropsychology: 6; 93–116, 1989.

Temple CM: Developmental dyscalculia. In Segalowitz SJ, Rapin I (Vol. Eds) — Boller F, Grafman J (Eds), Handbook of Neuropsychology, Vol. 7. Amsterdam: Elsevier, pp. 211–222, 1990.

Temple CM: The cognitive neuropsychology of the developmental dyscalculias. Current Psychology of Cognition: 13; 351–370, 1994.

Temple CM, Carney RA: Intellectual functioning of children

with Turner syndrome: A comparison of behavioral phenotypes. Developmental Medicine and Child Neurology: 35; 361–369, 1993.

Teng EL, Sperry RW: Interhemispheric interaction during simultaneous bilateral presentation of letters and digits in commissurotomized patients. Neuropsychologia: 11; 131–140, 1973.

Von Aster MG: Developmental dyscalculia in children: Review of the literature and clinical validation. Acta Paedopsychiatrica: 56; 169–178, 1994.

Von Aster MG: ZAKERI: Neuropsychologische Testbatterie fur Zahlenvararbeitung und Rechen bei Kindern. Lisse: Swets Test Services, 2001.

Von Aster MG, Deloche G, Dellatolas G, Meier M: Zahlenverarbeitung und Rechnen bei Schulkindern der 2. und 3. Klassenstufe: Eine vergleichende Studie franzosischsprachiger und deutschsprachiger Kinder. Zeitschrift fur Entwicklungspsychologie und Padagogische Psychologie: 29; 151–166, 1997.

Whalen J, McCloskey M, Lesser RP, Gordon B: Localizing arithmetic processes in the brain: Evidence from a transient deficit during cortical stimulation. Journal of Cognitive Neuroscience: 9; 409–417, 1997.

Witelson SF, Kigar DL, Harvey T: The exceptional brain of Albert Einstein. The Lancet: 353; 2149–2153, 1999.

Wynn K: Psychological foundations of number: numerical competence in human infants. Trends in Cognitive Sciences: 2; 296–303, 1998.

Young D: Group Mathematics Test. Sevenoaks: Hodder and Stoughton, 1971.

Handbook of Neuropsychology, 2nd Edition, Vol. 8, Part II
S.J. Segalowitz and I. Rapin (Eds)

CHAPTER 27

Disorders of memory in childhood with a focus on temporal lobe disease and autism

G. Robert DeLong *

Department of Pediatrics (Neurology), Duke University Medical Center, Durham, NC 27710, USA

Introduction

Childhood memory and its pathologic correlate, childhood amnesia, historically have attracted little attention. Before 1997, very few cases of childhood amnesia were to be found in the literature (Ostergaard, 1987; Vargha-Khadem, Isaacs and Mishkin, 1994; Wood, Brown and Felton, 1989). Nor were the consequences of medial temporal lobe damage in early life known. Geschwind (1972) suggested that early-life medial temporal lobe lesions would preclude cognitive development and result in mental retardation, but had no patient material. Learning, which assuredly implies memory, has been much more emphasized by observers of childhood for obvious reasons: Learning and its disorders constitute a major field of childhood studies, and conversely, specific examples of amnesia appear rarely in children. In this chapter I will not attempt to encompass the intricacies of learning, nor even the various types of memory fundamental to learning. Rather, my focus is on clinical aspects of memory disturbances, and the principles underlying them, as far as those have been elucidated by clinical neurological evaluation of children.

One might be tempted to say that amnesia in childhood is no different from that in adulthood, and therefore has no special interest. In one respect, however, there is an inescapable difference: the adult who suffers an anmestic insult has already acquired, by learning/memory, a great body of knowledge which largely remains even though new learning is impaired. A young child who suffers an insult impairing memory, and therefore learning, presumably would not be able to acquire a body of learned knowledge and thus would appear profoundly mentally barren. However, some have speculated that plasticity of the infant brain is such that no abnormality would ensue after early-life bilateral damage to the hippocampal system.

Here, and throughout this chapter, I refer to cognitive learning, which may be equated with declarative memory (memories of which the subject is conscious, meaning that the subject can declare the context of the memories explicitly [Gloor, 1997]). Aspects of motor and habitual learning persist in the face of profound deficits of cognitive learning; these disparate forms of learning, including habits, skills, and simple Pavlovian and emotional conditioning are termed procedural memory. They do not depend on integrity of the hippocampal system, but are impaired variably by lesions of the striatum (for certain skills and habit formation), association cortex (for priming [priming is the use of partial or fragmented stimuli to trigger recognition of the original stimulus]), and amygdala (for emotional conditioning [conditioning emotional responses to perceptual stimuli]) (Gloor, 1997). I will not attempt to discuss these. In the paragraph above I refer to a 'body' of knowledge; it is more accurate to speak of a 'structure' of knowledge. At the risk of being simplistic, what

* E-mail: delon006@mc.duke.edu

is remembered from the perception of experience over time is a highly complex structure of knowledge that approximates the interrelation between the remembering individual and external reality; this is called semantic knowledge and the process that produces it, semantic memory. The word semantics refers to meaning: semantic knowledge is knowledge that provides meaning to the individual about his experience of the world (and in this context, the world includes the individual's own internal feeling states). Semantic memory is usually contrasted to episodic memory, which is the conscious memory of particular events or episodes. It should also be distinguished from rote memory, which is an item-wise, specific, concrete, unanalyzed record of perception of external experience. Is rote memory different from episodic memory? Yes, in that episodic memory can be incorporated — in part at least — into semantic memory, while rote memory as used here implies a pathological failure to be incorporated into the semantic structure. Cognition as used here refers to the acquisition and use of episodic and semantic memory. Finally, I will discuss 'savant' phenomena (meaning specific cognitive skills or abilities which are highly-developed, precocious, out of proportion to overall intelligence, and not explainable by special training) in which prodigies of memory play a large part.

Information flow in the brain

To study memory disorders in children, one must have in mind the basic structure of learning and memory in the brain. Of course, learning takes place at individual synapses, which grow and become strengthened or weakened according to the activity impinging on them. But our interest is in the way synapses, neurons, and neural tissue are organized to learn and remember complex information. It is useful and justifiable to think of a flow of information through the brain: sensory information from vision, hearing, olfaction, taste, and somesthesis (touch) is processed to extract significant patterns and features. This occurs in the primary and association cortex related to the specific sensory modality. For example, visual information is processed in the visual cortex by two systems, one yielding information about the visual object seen (dog) which is then forwarded to the temporal lobe, and the second yielding information about the location of the object in visual space (nearby on the left) which is forwarded to the parietal lobe (see Gilmore's chapter, 2003, this volume). This information then passes to higher-level association cortex that combines, for example, visual and auditory information (picture of the nearby dog and his bark). This combined information then flows to the temporal lobe, specifically the neocortex of the lateral temporal lobe, where entire immediate experiences are believed to be assembled (for example, a dog barking while you pet it, in the backyard of your house, on a beautiful spring day with the fragrance of blossoms in the air). This kind of complete memories of a past experience can be elicited by electrical stimulation of the temporal lobe (lateral cortex and amygdala), as pioneered by Penfield (Penfield and Jasper, 1954).

The next level of information processing has two components: (1) the experience becomes related to an emotional or affective quality, that is, it is recognized as pleasant or frightening, or whatever. This probably involves the amygdala, a structure in the medial temporal lobe. (The emotional coloration may come through another pathway, much more primitive, arising from the brainstem, hypothalamus, and related structures.) (2) The experience becomes related to previous experiences: this implies that it must be compared to the memory of previous experiences, so that novel aspects of the new experience become registered as a new memory, modifying the structure of pre-existing memory. This comparison with previous remembered experience appears to be a function of the hippocampal system of the medial temporal lobe (Fig. 1). This system includes the parahippocampal gyrus as well as the hippocampus proper; the hippocampal system may be compared to the neck of a funnel, or the central exchange of a telephone system, in which there is a serial and increasing convergence of current experiential information. There is reason to believe this convergence represents the site of highest integration of immediate cognitive experiential information. Two important terms are commonly used to characterize the work of the hippocampus: it receives and deals with *configural* patterns of information; and it is concerned with *contextual* relations. By *configural* is meant that the hippocampus registers a configuration

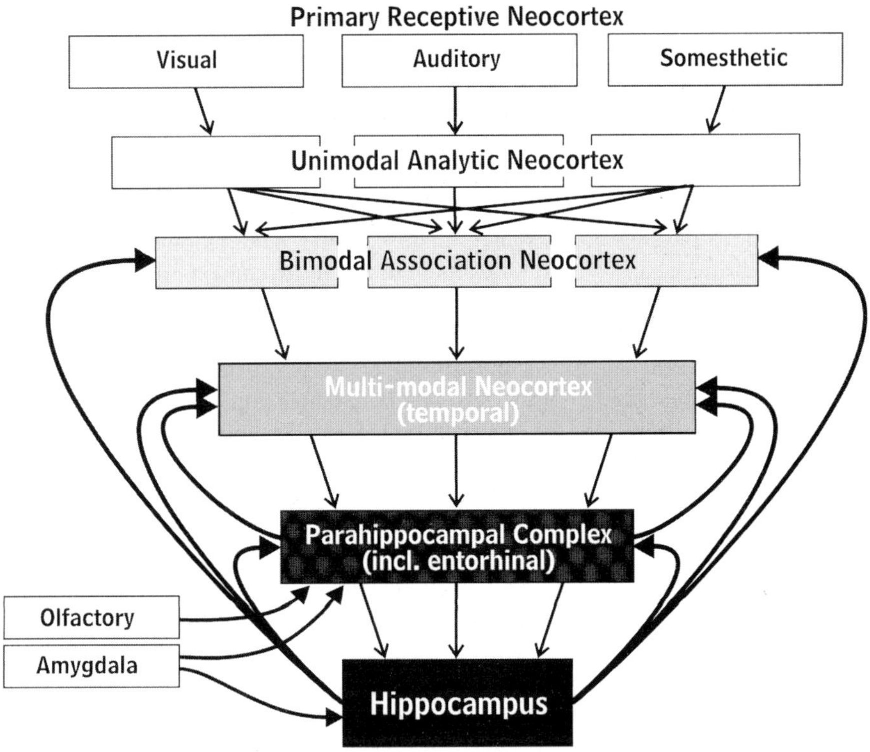

Fig. 1. Diagram characterizing information flow to and from the hippocampus. Information from primary sensory neocortex (visual, auditory, somesthetic) is successively analyzed, then combines with information from other modalities in association cortex. There is successive convergence in temporal neocortex, then into the parahippocampal structures (including entorhinal cortex), and finally at the highest level of convergence into the hippocampus. It is thought that the hippocampus may be an equipotential field, on which experience is 'configured' and also bound together (thus the 'binding' function) with past experience and motivational cues to represent a complete experience or event. (Or think of it as a staging area where all the pieces of a structure are brought together to be assembled.) The information thus configured in the hippocampus then feeds back (curved arrows) to association cortex, where it presumably modifies previously stored information in light of the new experience; thus the association cortex becomes the site of long-term memory storage.

of experiential information; this configuration is new and unique, and temporary. The hippocampus seems to be uniquely structured as an equipotential, multi-dimensional field — in a real sense a matrix capable of encompassing all possible experiences — which can transiently register the configuration of information in a present experience (Hampson, Simeral and Deadwyler, 1999). A homely but reasonable analogy is the old telephone plug-in switchboard, whose two-dimensional array of plug-in sites represented all possible combinations (configurations) of connections. The word *contextual* describing hippocampal function refers to the fact that the hippocampus deals with information not only in the present configuration of experience, but correlates this experience more widely, that is to the context of past experience (this is properly the cognitive memory function) and to the significance of the present experience for the organism (for example, relating the present experience to appetites and motivations). The term *episodic memory* refers to the more or less intact conscious memory of a specific incident of experience.

Long-term memories are not stored in the hippocampus, as shown by the fact that damage to the hippocampus which prevents the formation of new cognitive memories does not destroy many old memories. There appears to be a period of consolidation of memories, lasting several hours to several weeks or longer, during which hippocampal function is necessary for those memories to become permanent. This is demonstrated by the phenomenon of retrograde amnesia after hippocampal injury, in which memories incurred during a period of time before the injury was sustained are irretrievably lost. If memory is not permanently stored in the hippocampus, where then is it stored? Apparently in the neocortex for the most part, and probably other areas of brain also. The hippocampal system not only has a massive convergent system for information inflow, as described above, but it also has an equally massive outflow to neocortical areas, including those from which information originally passed to the hippocampal system. Thus information from transient configural patterns in the hippocampus flows back to cortical areas to stabilize information and make it permanent. It is thought that the hippocampus maintains what amounts to an address of these patterns of neocortical information storage, so that it can retrieve the data for future use for comparison with new episodic experiences. Again the new resultant pattern of information returns to neocortex to be stored, only to be shuttled back to hippocampus again as needed. And so the shuttle weaves.

This is not the complete story of information flow through the brain, of course. Information from hippocampal systems also goes to executive systems of the brain, primarily in the frontal lobes, where decisions for action are made and elaborated. And in the case of repeated, familiar experiences where there is no mismatch between experience and expectation, no new memory is necessary and the hippocampal system appears to be inactive. There are massive systems of fibers sending information directly from the posterior sensory association areas to the frontal executive association areas, bypassing the hippocampal system completely. These presumably handle the mass of routine information flow by which sensory perceptions inform decisions about action. (However, very new data from magnetoencephalography has identified hippocampal activation related to the interactive processing of sensory input and motor output, indicating the hippocampus may be more closely involved with small-scale sensorimotor integration than previously recognized [Tesche and Karhu, 1999].) In addition, there are known to be important systems for working memory involving the prefrontal lobes, which retain information temporarily in a 'scratch-pad' memory during the execution of a task (Baddeley, 1992; Goldman-Rakic, 1990). Also, there are other forms of memory, involving different systems not so tied to the hippocampus, that are beyond our scope: for example, the motoric memory of how to ride a bicycle or write in cursive; simple stimulus-response and associational memories resulting from a summation of repeated experiences; and others (McDonald and White, 1993; Squire, 1992). The astounding human ability to consciously retain complex patterns of experience and to relate them to the entire context of previous experience — to build from them a coherent integrated structure of meaning — depends on the hippocampal system. The hippocampal system is able to do this because of its remarkable capacity for convergence of information, presentation of that information transiently and configurally in a multi-dimensional array, and dispersal of information to neocortex for storage, with the address retained for future recall.

The studies of language and memory have traditionally been rather separate. That is beginning to change, and one of the purposes of this chapter is to examine the interrelations between the two, especially in development. Some authors (see MacKay, Stewart and Burke, 1998, discussed later) are beginning to argue that there is no dividing line between language and memory for verbal materials. They introduce the concept, familiar from the above discussion, that the hippocampus is responsible for 'binding'; that is, new experiences are comprehended by binding with old data, to form new memories. ('Binding' also has a broader signification, that of the convergence of all different elements of experience to guarantee the unity of consciousness.) MacKay et al. find that this binding is also impaired in the language of adult patients with bilateral hippocampal lesions, as evidenced by incapacity in comprehension and in semantic-level language production. According to this conception, every new sentence of language that an individual generates and every new sentence understood involves the semantic memory system and requires hippocampal system function. This idea about hippocampal activation in language is reminiscent of the finding of hippocampal activation in sensorimotor integration mentioned above (Tesche and Karhu, 1999); that is, it begins to describe a finer grain of hippocampal activity than previously known.

In this chapter we will consider: (1) memory impairment occurring *before* versus that occurring *after* the child's early period of formative learning (including particularly acquisition of language, social interaction, and complex purposive activities); (2) impairment affecting episodic memory versus that affecting semantic memory; and (3) impairment affecting normal flexible semantic versus rote memory. Current advances in understanding these subjects have depended on new functional imaging techniques, but also on new intellectual formulations. The disease processes contributory to this work include abnormalities of the temporal lobes, particularly medial temporal lobes, and autism.

Bilateral complete medial temporal lesion in early life: severe failure of all cognitive memory in infancy and early childhood

Bilateral medial temporal lobe damage in adults is associated with severe retrograde and anterograde amnesia, but with preservation of language and of intelligence as measured by standard IQ tests, as exemplified by the classic case of HM who underwent bilateral medial temporal ablations for treatment of epilepsy (Corkin, 1984; Scoville and Milner, 1957).

We have studied four children who sustained bilateral hippocampal sclerosis as a result of status epilepticus within ages 6–30 months of life (that is, before or during the period of initial language learning). Bilateral hippocampal sclerosis was diagnosed by magnetic resonance scans, including oblique coronal fast spin echo images of the temporal lobes, and appeared to involve the entire hippocampus including the subiculum bilaterally, but not parahippocampal structures nor other parts of the brain, in each case (DeLong and Heinz, 1997; see Fig. 2). ^{18}FDG PET (18-fluorodeoxyglucose positron emission tomography, showing local glucose [energy] metabolism in brain) scans, done in two children, showed isolated bilateral anterior temporal lobe hypometabolism including neocortex. Despite adequate motor and sensory functions all four children failed to develop language (or lost attained language), social skills, and complex purposive or adaptive activity, even after epilepsy was controlled. We concluded that bilateral hippocampal destruction in early life appeared to be associated with a profound failure of cognitive capacities, including language learning and learning of complex social and adaptive skills in general. The deficits correspond to the cognitive deficits of severe infantile autism. (Autism is characterized by three basic features in the young child: failure to develop normal communicative language; failure to develop normal interpersonal interactions; and failure to develop normal patterns of organized adaptive activity, with a consequent limitation to a narrow range of repetitive stereotyped activity patterns.) The children appear autistic, and are routinely so diagnosed by experienced clinicians. Hippocampal function, or more generally medial temporal lobe function, appears necessary for language learning in the infant, as well as for complex social and adaptive learning. This may be likened to complete anterograde amnesia, operative from the beginning of cognitive development, which prevents any accumulation of memory stores or semantic content. It is a dramatic and distinctive form of severe mental retardation in children who otherwise appear normal and have normal motor and sensory function. We recognize it in perhaps one out of two hundred retarded children in our pediatric neurology clinic.

More widespread bilateral temporal lobe disease has often been described as the neuropathological substrate for autism, including herpes simplex encephalitis (DeLong, Bean and Brown, 1981), West syndrome with infantile spasms (Chugani, Da Silva and Chugani, 1996), tuberous sclerosis with bilateral temporal location of tubers (Bolton and Griffiths, 1997), and bilateral dysgenesis of temporal cortex (Lee, Radtke, Gray et al., 1994). On ^{18}FDG PET scanning (Lee et al., 1994) these entities as well as the bilateral hippocampal sclerosis cases in the preceding paragraph have shown hypometabolism throughout the anterior temporal lobe, including temporal neocortex. This could be explained by direct damage to the temporal neocortex; alternatively, it is possible that damage to any part of the information-transfer pathway within the temporal lobe causes dysfunction (diaschisis) in other areas joined by major connecting pathways. Such pathways between temporal neocortex and medial temporal lobe structures characterize temporal lobe connections and information transfer.

The temporal lobe was compared above to a funnel, in which information coming to temporal association neocortex from other parts of the hemisphere is then transmitted to the entorhinal and parahip-

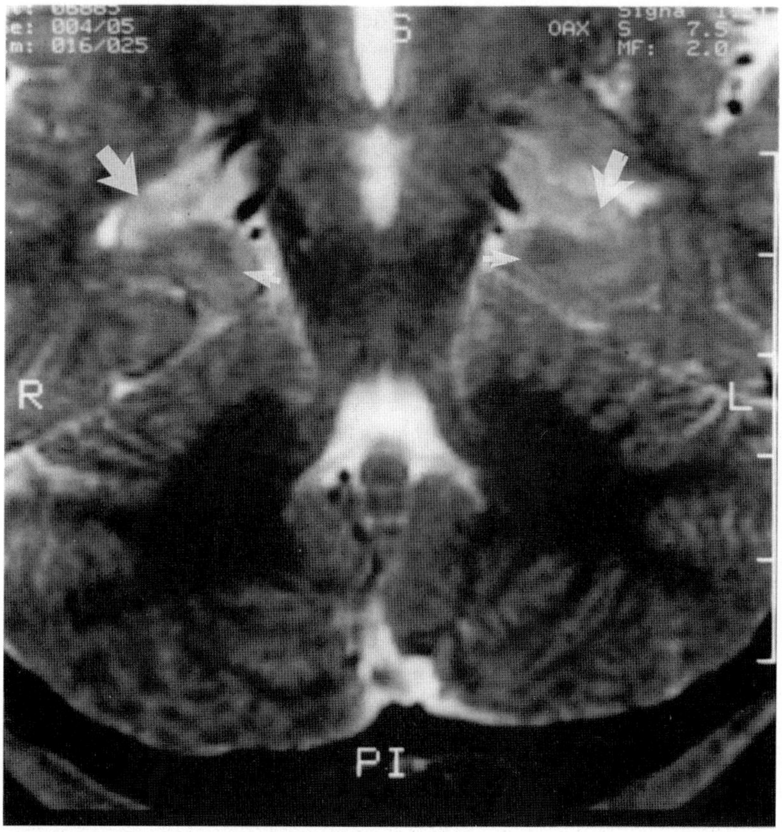

Fig. 2. MRI of coronal section of brain showing complete sclerosis (atrophy and increased signal) of both hippocampi [large arrows]. The sclerotic area does not appear to extend beyond the hippocampus proper, but increased signal in entorhinal cortex [small arrows] cannot be excluded. 18-Fluorodeoxyglucose positron-emission tomography (PET) showed hypometabolism in the temporal lobes bilaterally. This girl did not develop language or cognitive skills after severe status epilepticus occurring at age 2 years.

pocampal areas (the "gateways" [Gloor, 1997] to the hippocampus), and then to the hippocampus proper, which represents the apex of the information-flow pathway (Fig. 3). The intensity of information integration increases at each step of this path, culminating in the hippocampus. From the hippocampus, the bulk of information relays feed back into the parahippocampal structures and thence back to neocortex generally. It is clear from extensive anatomical, neurophysiological and behavioral data that the medial temporal structures (or hippocampal system, comprising the hippocampus, parahippocampal, perirhinal, and entorhinal cortices) function not simply as memory repositories. Rather, they integrate and bind together novel perceptions with motivational signals and past experience to produce new memories (or semantic constructs) which are then stored and utilized by the neocortex generally. The hippocampus might be expected to mediate the most flexible, widespread, and highest-dimensional associations among various items, thus performing the most extensive 'binding' as well as discrimination function for memory and learning. All information about its anatomic structure and connections and experimental analysis of its function suggest this is so.

A recent study of neonatal lesions of the medial temporal lobes in monkeys made the surprising observation that this lesion disrupted the normal regulation of striatal dopamine activity by the dorsolateral prefrontal cortex during adulthood (Saunders, Kolachana, Bachevalier and Weinberger, 1998). These monkeys showed increased locomotor stereotypies, especially in stressful situations such as social interactions (Malkova, Mishkin, Suomi and Bachevalier,

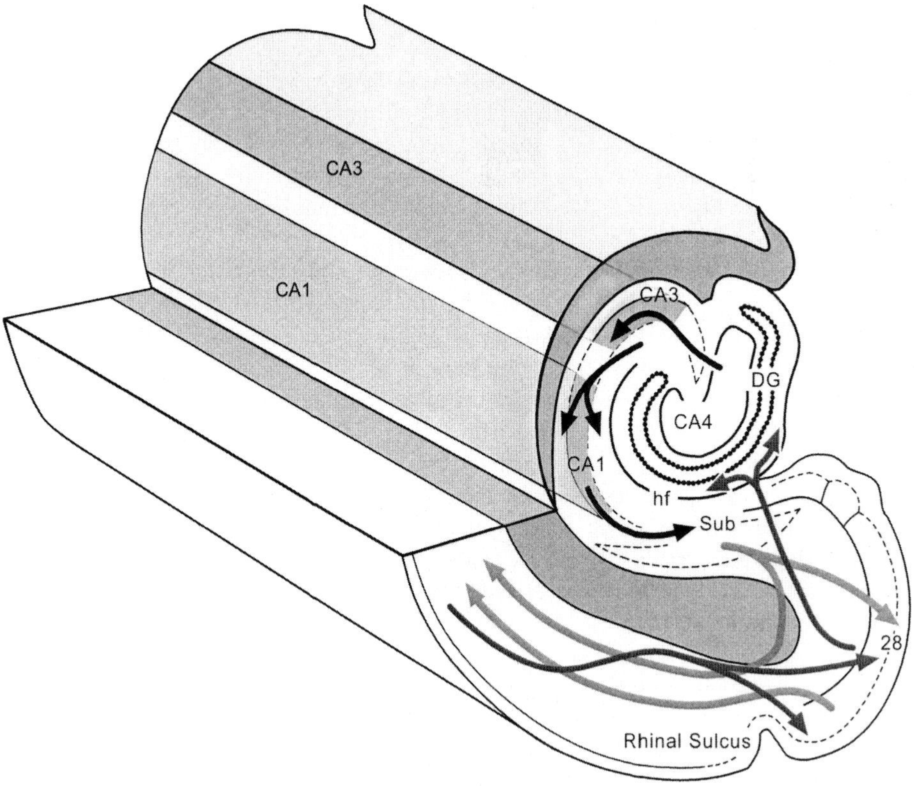

Fig. 3. Cartoon of information flow in the hippocampus. Information [dark gray arrows] from temporal neocortex funnels to entorhinal cortex (area 28) and subiculum (Sub); from these areas further pathways project into the hippocampus to synapse with dendrites of the dentate gyrus (DG). Information from dentate gyrus neurons then passes to CA3, shown here as a field of cortex, and then to CA1, another cortical field, both extended along the length of the hippocampus. Both fields are equipotential areas of hippocampal cortex with afferent fibers arranged laterally [black arrows] and longitudinally [not shown]. Patterns of information can be arrayed on these fields (as firing patterns of the cortical neurons). The patterns of neuronal activity on these cortical fields can represent spatial information, but can also represent fundamental non-spatial information about a task or situation. Thus the CA3 and CA1 fields act very much like a stage where new relationships between various aspects of a task or situation are joined together (Hampson et al., 1999). Outflow information passes to the subiculum, then [light gray arrows] back to the entorhinal cortex, then further back to temporal neocortex and throughout the cerebral hemispheres.

1997). Similar bilateral medial temporal lesions made in adulthood did not disrupt the normal patterns of regulation nor locomotor behavior. These findings after neonatal lesions enhance the parallels with autism, and also serve as reminders of the immense complexity of brain structure and function, especially when the developmental dimension is included.

Bilateral partial medial temporal lesion in early life: typical amnestic syndrome in young children

Vargha-Khadem, Gadian, Watkins et al. (1997) presented three children with early bilateral hippocampal pathology showing a different pattern of involvement from that just described. Their cases each showed a typical amnestic syndrome with severe loss of episodic memory but with relatively intact general cognitive development, based mainly on preserved semantic memory. The authors thus demonstrate clearly that episodic memory can be impaired with preservation of semantic memory. They argue that bilateral lesions of hippocampus alone produce this episodic memory loss without loss of semantic memory.

Certainly none of the children was autistic in the least. Two of them had onset of memory impairment following acute illness, one at age 4 and the other at age 9 years (status epilepticus and seizures with respiratory arrest, respectively). Since these insults occurred after the completion of the bulk of language learning, the children's clinical pictures might be expected to differ little from adult amnestic patients. The third child, however, is particularly instructive. She was born after a difficult delivery, sustained an hypoxic–ischemic insult at birth, and had generalized seizures sporadically for 2 to 3 days. Apart from persistent brachial plexus palsy, no neurological problems were evident until age 5 when memory difficulties were first noted on her entrance into a mainstream school. On neuropsychological testing (at age 12 : 10) she scored VIQ (verbal IQ) 82, PIQ (performance IQ) 61, and MQ (memory quotient) 83 (standard scores) although digit span was a normal 6 forward, 5 backward. The authors tested 6 normal children with similar VIQ, and found that their MQs were on average 20 points higher; thus they suggest that Beth, the patient, has a memory deficit as well as mildly impaired verbal intellectual development (and more serious retardation of performance intelligence). She scored extremely low on delayed testing of recall of stories and reproduction of designs, although immediate memory for a word list, digit span, and a spatial analogue of digit span, were all normal. She (and the others as well) had difficulty in daily life in (1) finding their way in familiar surroundings, and remembering where objects are usually located, or where they might have been placed; (2) orientation in space and time, being aware of regularly scheduled classes or activities; (3) giving a reliable account of episodic events such as the day's activities, or remembering telephone conversations, messages, visitors, holidays, and so on. Despite these difficulties, Beth fared well in mainstream education. She learned to read, write, and spell at a level commensurate with her IQ.

Magnetic resonance imaging of the brain showed that the hippocampi were abnormally small bilaterally, with volumes 43% of the mean value of normals; hippocampal water T2 values were elevated bilaterally (117–119 versus 108 normal, indicative of tissue damage with replacement gliosis). Other temporal lobe regions, examined by a different technique (^{1}H magnetic resonance spectroscopy, measuring the concentration of several brain chemicals) appeared normal, although low in the normal range (−1 SD on one side, −2 SD on the other); the authors note the possibility that the pathology extended into the underlying perirhinal and entorhinal cortices. Additionally, Beth had an increase in T2-weighted signal intensity in the periventricular and particularly peritrigonal white matter, accompanied by a marked loss of white matter bulk and thinning of the corpus callosum; the authors noted this could well be the cause of her impaired intellectual development. Hippocampal cross-sectional areas were very small bilaterally in the anterior half of the hippocampi, but only about 2 SD below the normal mean at the level of slices 9 and 10 (representing about one-eighth of the length of the hippocampus). The latter point suggests some functioning hippocampus may remain bilaterally in Beth. Some evidence exists that the hippocampus is an equipotential field, thus any remaining portion of it might carry out the function of the whole, albeit less efficiently (Rolls, 1996). The possibility remains that this remnant accounts for the semantic memory function that Beth retains.

For other reasons, Beth is difficult to evaluate. The three anmestic subjects as a group performed normally on a series of two-choice recognition tasks not sensitive to hippocampal lesions; but since only grouped data are presented, it is not clear whether she performed normally on these tasks. As noted earlier, her measured memory quotient did not differ from her VIQ; only by indirect comparison with other children with marginal VIQs (75–84) was it concluded that her memory quotient was lower than expected. In the face of these various uncertainties, it is difficult to use the case of Beth to conclude that early-life (pre-language) hippocampal damage affects only episodic, but not semantic, memory. The conclusion is tenable only by grouping Beth with the other two, who had a very different history in that their lesion and amnesia occurred much later. It is not possible to speculate further about the other two subjects from the data available, but the onset of their amnesia after the bulk of language learning was complete may make these cases fundamentally different from Beth. Clearly, however, both continued to show semantic learning after the onset of amnesia. In two cases of childhood amnesia found in the literature, semantic learning continued, albeit slowly (Ostergaard and Squire, 1990; Wood et al.,

1989). In another recently-reported case (Broman, Rose, Hotson et al., 1997) — the only other one I have found — a boy had amnesia following respiratory arrest at 8 years of age and was followed for 19 years. Anatomical lesions were restricted to the hippocampal formation bilaterally. Comparison of IQ and academic scores with earlier scores revealed that his literacy skills, certain basic language functions and vocabulary development were arrested by his memory disorder. In contrast, development of mathematical skill was less curtailed, and verbal and nonverbal logical abilities developed to adult levels. Neuropsychological examination at the age of 27 years elicited a pattern of memory deficits similar to those found in HM (Corkin, 1984), who underwent bilateral mesial temporal lobe ablation in adulthood. The authors note that the limitations to intellectual development imposed by severe amnesia in childhood are not pervasive, but rather are limited to specific types of abilities, namely those of language. This is further examined below.

It may be useful to compare and contrast Vargha-Khadem et al.'s cases with our four cases of bilateral hippocampal sclerosis and severe failure of cognitive development. Ours all had onset before 30 months with immediate or early loss of cognitive progress (and retrogression of previously-attained skills), while amnesia was delayed in two of Vargha-Khadem et al.'s three patients. The two of our patients having ^{18}FDG PET scans had extensive hypometabolism in the entire anterior temporal lobes, thought to be due to diaschisis (suppression of function in an area because of decreased input from a connecting damaged area); PET data were not available for their patients. The T2 water values (a measure of gliosis) in magnetic resonance images were slightly elevated in their patients, and markedly elevated in ours. This suggests more severe damage in our cases, but it must be taken into account that their patients were several years older when studied, so that early hyper-intensity might have subsided (our children were all imaged before age 5 years; Beth was imaged at age 12 years). We have reviewed the MRIs in our cases, and find the visually detectable lesions to be limited to the hippocampus proper (not extending beyond the subiculum).

We have seen two further children whose stories may be contributory. A boy, age 6, came to attention because of poor memory, which mother and teachers had noted only in the preceding year. Cognitive development was otherwise normal. There had been a period of high fever and poor responsiveness at age 6 months; past history was otherwise normal. MRI with special hippocampal views was normal; two small areas of increased T2 signal were seen subjacent to the anterior–inferior insular cortex bilaterally, of uncertain significance (such changes sometimes accompany hippocampal sclerosis, which was not visible). ^{18}FDG scan was normal. The degree of memory difficulty increased somewhat during the next two years of observation, but remains unexplained. The second boy, now 15 years old, had normal language development, assiduously documented by his father (a professor of English) until age 36 months, when he suffered a bout of status epilepticus which left him without speech. He made essentially no further language or cognitive development thereafter, and was diagnosed as autistic. At age 15, he has essentially no language, although if sufficiently excited he may utter a phrase such as "Later, alligator." His MRI shows severe complete bilateral hippocampal atrophy, without apparent involvement beyond the hippocampus proper. We suppose that his residual language reflects the language attainments preceding the hippocampal injury.

Thus, a complete bilateral early-life (pre-language) lesion of the hippocampi may produce an essentially complete failure of cognitive development. Conceivably this result may require more widespread injury of parahippocampal structures, but this seems unlikely, since such structures appear intact by MRI examination. (Recall, however, that the two patients so studied, the entire anterior temporal lobes showed hypofunction on ^{18}FDG PET imaging.) Certainly, as shown by Vargha-Khadem et al., a hippocampal lesion can produce amnesia affecting episodic memory while sparing semantic memory.

Vargha-Khadem et al. raise the question whether semantic memory is truly spared out of proportion to episodic memory; if so, this suggests that semantic memories can be stored partly independently of episodic memory. They suggest a way this could be achieved: they administered a series of two-choice, recognition memory tasks to the three anmestic patients and normal controls; the only ones that yielded group differences were voice–face and object–place associations. These findings in the anmestic patients are similar to those in monkeys with hippocampal lesions, who are severely impaired in learning object–place associations and yet are unimpaired on other two-choice (non-spatial) recognition tasks. These latter tasks, however, are severely disrupted by ablation of the perirhinal and entorhinal cortices adjacent to the hippocampus. The authors conclude that the basic sensory memory functions of the cortex subjacent to the hippocampus are substantially spared in the anmestic patients just as they are in hippocampectomized monkeys. They suggest that the basic sensory memory functions of the perirhinal and entorhinal cortices may be sufficient to support the formation of semantic memories but not of episodic memories, which must therefore require the additional processing provided by the hippocampal circuitry. They note that anatomically the higher order cortical sensory areas and the hippocampus communicate with each other only indirectly through the perirhinal and entorhinal cortices. Because of this hierarchical arrangement, the latter cortices are in a position to mediate the acquisition of some forms of memory independent of the hippocampus. (Evidence from studies in mice indicate that the parahippocampal region mediates the encoding of specific memory cues, maintains stimulus representations, and supports recognition memory) (Young, Otto, Fox and Eichenbaum, 1997).

On reflection, the primary acquisition of language, social skills, and organized patterns of activity during the second and third year of life may well occur without episodic memory; we have no direct evidence, to my knowledge, of episodic memories at this age. The first verifiable specific (episodic) childhood memory usually occurs after age 3 years (Fitzgerald, 1991). This suggests the possibility of a developmental approach to the question of semantic versus episodic memory; it appears that semantic memory (in the form of language learning) is well advanced before age 3 years, while episodic memory only occurs after age 3 years. May this mean that parahippocampal function is active before 3 years, while the hippocampus itself only matures to full function at the onset of episodic memory? The question has at least the virtue of being potentially answerable.

The episodic–semantic distinction is subject to further interpretation, however, as described by Eichenbaum (1997) in commenting on the Vargha-Khadem thesis. Functional magnetic resonance imaging has provided further clues about the distinct memory functions of the hippocampus and parahippocampal region. A part of the hippocampus was maximally activated when human subjects indirectly accessed the memory of a word cued by a picture of the corresponding object, whereas the parahippocampal region was maximally activated during simple differentiation and encoding of novel pictures for later recognition (Gabrieli, Brewer, Desmond and Glover, 1997). Similarly, single-cell recordings in both monkeys and rats have shown that parahippocampal cortex, like other cortices, encodes specific memory cues and can sustain and regenerate these item-specific representations. By contrast, the activity of hippocampal neurons reflects myriad combinations of items or abstract relations between stimuli (Young et al., 1997). Thus the hippocampus is suited to promote more flexible associations by recognizing transient (episodic) relations among items, thus permitting encoding of each unique episode; it may also serve to relate this episodic pattern into semantic knowledge. Finally, current data from animals with amnesia, as well as computational modeling, indicate that the hippocampus may interleave patterns with the memory network so as to provide access to the whole knowledge structure from any point. Eichenbaum (1997) suggests that these amnesiacs' memory failure for unique episodes, as well as their forgetting of a story or drawing, can be attributed to a partially compromised memory capacity doing poorly on any type of complex material experienced only once. He notes that rigidity of access and sensitivity to interference are hallmarks of human amnesiacs' difficulty in conscious recollection, suggesting that hippocampal function is necessary for flexibility of memory expression. In a later paper, Mishkin, Vargha-Khadem and Gadian (1998) concede that given the system's hierarchical form of organization, the dissociation of episodic and semantic deficits is difficult to prove, because a quantitatively limited deficit in a non-dissociable single system will nearly always be a viable alternative explanation. There is independent evidence from anmestic adults of some preservation of semantic learning in the face of a total lack of episodic learning (Kitchener, Hodges and McCarthy, 1998; Tulving, Hayman and Macdonald,

1991). Thus a final choice between these alternative views must await further data.

So far we have not solved the problem of our children with extensive, virtually total early-life hippocampal sclerosis who fail to develop language or other high-level cognitive function. There would be no problem with our model if we assume they have extensive parahippocampal deficits. Bilateral early-life parahippocampal damage — not only destroying parahippocampal function but interrupting information flow between hippocampi and the rest of the cortex — clearly is sufficient to cause failure of cognitive development. Whether complete bilateral early-life destruction of the hippocampi proper alone is sufficient to preclude cognitive development must remain unsettled at present. Our cases suggest it may be sufficient; but Vargha-Khadem's case Beth would indicate otherwise. The completeness of hippocampal damage in Beth, and the limitation of damage to the hippocampi solely in our cases, remain the crucial questions. In a subsequent paper Vargha-Khadem et al. (Maguire, Vargha-Khadem and Mishkin, 2001) report on functional MRI studies during successful retrieval of real-world memories in one of their children with selective bilateral hippocampal pathology resulting from perinatal hypoxia. In spite of 50% volume loss bilaterally in his hippocampi, retrieval was associated with increased activation of the hippocampi. He activated the same network of brain regions (albeit bilaterally) as did normal controls, and with the same pattern of response in the hippocampus. In light of these results, we can say that Vargha-Khadem's hypothesis that complete hippocampal damage results only in defects of episodic memory is not established. Their children with episodic memory deficits but relatively preserved semantic memory may have only partial hippocampal damage, as in the case just described. Our patients, with complete loss of semantic as well as episodic memory, appear to have complete hippocampal loss bilaterally, with preservation of parahippocampal structures (although the volume of the latter is reduced about 40% (unpublished observations)). Thus it is a viable hypothesis that hippocampus proper is necessary for both episodic and semantic memory, and that complete destruction of the hippocampi bilaterally in early life precludes both semantic and episodic learning.

The relation of amnesia and autism

It is impossible to separate the study of memory from that of autism in children. We have seen the typically anmestic cases of Vargha-Khadem et al., which are definitely not autistic; and the cases of early-life complete bilateral hippocampal formation sclerosis of DeLong and Heinz, who are clearly autistic with severe failure of cognitive development. In an earlier paper, the interrelationship of autism and amnesia was explored in detail (DeLong, 1992). That discussion will be summarized here briefly as a prelude to discussing recent observations, particularly the distinction between left and right hemisphere memory and its relation to autism. The three cardinal features of autism were listed above, but it may be useful here to describe autism in somewhat greater detail; in particular, to note that the three cardinal features all show a wide range of severity. Thus, a child with high-functioning autism may have a great deal of language, but it may be rote, echolalic, repetitive (sometimes consisting of repetitions of commercial slogans or video dialogue) but little useful for communication with other persons. Likewise, the child may manifest interpersonal interactions, but they are stiff, uneasy, and fragmentary. All patterns of activity, even those at a high level, tend to be obsessive, narrow, and repetitive.

A second important aspect of autism — particularly high-functioning autism — is the difference between the very defective language function, poor abstraction and generalization and poor sequential function suggestive of left hemispheral deficits; and normal visual–spatial skills, ability to solve visual puzzles, excellent topographic ability, musical sense, and other skills associated with right hemisphere function. Children with relatively high-functioning autism often have disproportionately low verbal IQ scores, and normal performance IQ (Minshew, Goldstein and Siegel, 1997). The reverse situation is also seen (so-called Asperger's syndrome) in which verbal skills are typically high, but non-verbal, social, and visual–spatial skills are deficient; it is generally considered a variant of autism (Ehlers, Nyden, Gillberg et al., 1997).

The symptoms of autism can be seen from another point of view, as well. Autistic children often show features of affective disorder, including extreme anxiety, obsessive and compulsive behaviors, anhedonia (lack of "joie de vivre" [Rapin, 1997]), social withdrawal, constriction of interest, irritability and temper outbursts, and mood swings. All these will be recognized as symptoms of major affective disorders. Indeed, there is strong reason to believe that a large portion of children with idiopathic autism (i.e., autism with no known neurological etiology) in fact suffer from an early-onset major affective disorder. The evidence for this assertion comes from several sources, apart from the prominence of affective symptoms as just described. Such children have a high incidence of major affective disorder in family members; they respond in part to pharmacological agents used in treatment of major affective disorders (for example, SSRIs [selective serotonin reuptake inhibitors], mood-stabilizing agents, and atypical antipsychotics); they have disturbances of brain serotonin metabolism (Chugani, Musik, Rothermel et al., 1997; Chugani, Muzik, Behen et al., 1999) as posited in major affective disorder (Grahame-Smith, 1992); and finally, genetic studies now suggest, but do not yet confirm, a correspondence between genes implicated in autism and those implicated in familial bipolar disorder (reviewed in DeLong, 1999). About 60% of such children responded to treatment with fluoxetine (an SSRI, making more serotonin available in the brain) with improvement in mood, social interaction, and breadth of attention; decrease in obsessive behaviors; and most strikingly by a spurt in language usage and competence (DeLong, Teague and Kamran, 1998).

Boucher and Warrington (1976) investigated memory function in autistic children, demonstrating that their memory functions are in some respects qualitatively similar to those of anmestic adults; retention tested by recall and recognition can be impaired, whereas cued recall is consistently normal. In one task the data from autistic children conflicted with that from anmestic adults: autistic children showed normal learning of unrelated word pairs. (Interestingly, anmestic adults differ from hippocampectomized monkeys in that the latter were able to learn a 20-object pair concurrent-discrimination, as shown by Squire, Zola-Morgan and Chen, 1988.)

The question of parallels between autism and amnesia is being clarified by the evolution of concepts of amnesia. Amnesia is not simply a deficit of memory, but of a fundamental central cognitive processor that permits flexible multidimensional association of perceptual stimuli, stored information, and motivational states (Bunsey and Eichenbaum, 1996; DeLong, 1992). It is recognized that anmestic individuals are capable of some limited kinds of new learning; it is also possible to demonstrate retrieval of stored material by means of cueing. When learning can be demonstrated in anmestic humans it tends to be rigid, hyperspecific, pairwise, and rote. Schacter (1985) states that anmestic patients "may be limited to the acquisition of rigid pairwise associations that represent linkages between preexisting unitized structures, and *they may be unable to acquire flexible new configurations in which multiple relations are formed among constituent units*" (emphasis added). Failure of this process results in rigid, invariant and rote behavior, thought and language — at least as far as new information is concerned. The parallel with autism is obvious.

Classic studies of cognitive function in autism are those of Hermelin and O'Connor (1970). Clinically they recognized the autistic child's "generally very restricted and repetitive behavior repertoire." They remarked on the limited ability to process verbal sequences. Most strikingly, they found that autistic children "had immediate auditory rote memories as good as or better than those of normal children of similar mental age. However, the recall capacity of the control group improved significantly more when syntactical and meaningfully-related material was presented, than did that of the autistic children. On the other hand, the autistic children showed stronger recency effects than the other groups." Hermelin and O'Connor maintain that autistic children hold information in a relatively 'raw' or unprocessed form due to a central deficiency in the processing of information. They note the tendency of the autistic child to impose simple, repetitive patterns on random as well as on structured input; the autistic child differs from the normal child in lacking the capacity for feature extraction of ordered or structured input. Note however that this applies only to verbal information; autistic children may be extraordinarily skillful in extracting visual–spatial information (see below regarding left and right hemisphere function).

The limitation of central multi-dimensional associational processes in autism was elegantly demonstrated by Churchill (1978) in a study of language in autistic children using a simplified 9-word language (consisting of 3 nouns (block, ring, stick); 3 adjectives (red, yellow, blue) and 3 verbs (give, tap, slide)). Children were first conditioned to utilize each word appropriately in response to stimuli, then higher-order language functions involving combinations of elements were explored. Although the children were worked with for months, when they reached an impasse, "it is usually insurmountable by any degree of extra effort and inventiveness that we have been able to muster." In one illustrative child, the failure was as if he "could master one dimension of the task if all other dimensions were held constant, but if two dimensions of the task were varied simultaneously he was lost." Clearly the child's associative capacity for more than one language element at a time was severely limited and was not enhanced by practice. Another child mastered the 9-word language without difficulty but when Churchill attempted to move from echolalic speech and rote performance to a more functional language, he encountered difficulties similar to those seen in the first child, albeit at a higher level of complexity. Churchill describes the language challenge failed by the second child as a double-classification system: "Once a set is established for talking about what he is doing *or* what I am doing *or* what he has *or* what I have, Jonathan is well able to give correct answers endlessly, even when dozens of different objects or positions are introduced — so long as those objects or positions stay within the *same response set*. But, to talk interchangeably about what he is doing *and* what I am doing *and* what he has *and* what I have leaves him demonstrably incompetent. . . It is as if only two of the four cells exist for Jonathan, while the other two are irretrievable." Churchill's analysis is that "when. . . multiple stimuli come to have syntactical relationships to each other. . . even the highest-functioning autistic child demonstrates incompetence. . . To use discriminative stimuli in two different dimensions or sets simultaneously appears to immediately exceed the linguistic competence of such children. We have seen no evidence that the underlying rules of grammar. . . can be taught. And the autistic child, however good his speech, seems locked into a concrete world in which only one dimension can be responded to at a time." These elegant observations can be interpreted in terms of a limited capacity for higher-order association. Churchill illustrates the double classification task attempted with Jonathan as a four-cell grid; Jonathan's performance utilized only two cells (though it could be any two cells). It was the higher dimensional associative capacity that was limited.

Thus we see a convergence in the description of the deficit in adult amnesia, in anmestic (hippocampectomized) animals, *and in autism*. In all three, the deficit is not so much in memory storage per se as in the kind of information stored, and in the ability to organize, flexibly reorder, and widely associate items of information with other items. A theory of a central associative processing mechanism — allowing for free, wide, flexible, and complex association of information — can account for these observations. Further, the conjunction of the three situations provides strong presumption that the associative processing mechanism resides in the hippocampus.

In autism, further questions are raised, such as whether the stable knowledge (semantic) system is impoverished by deficits from early life in the associational processing system. If so, and it seems inevitable that it would be so, then the semantic deficits in autism would be explained, and this difference from adult amnesia would be resolved.

Unilateral medial temporal lobe lesions in early life: memory after temporal lobectomy for epilepsy

The important subject of unilateral lesions has been extensively studied as a part of the increasing use of temporal lobectomy to treat epilepsy arising, generally, from unilateral mesial temporal sclerosis. Most studies describe young adults, but seizure onset is commonly in childhood and surgery is being performed on progressively younger children, so that the consequences of such surgery for memory are pertinent in a discussion of childhood memory. Lewis, Thompson, Santos et al. (1996) reported results of 23 adolescents age 17 years or less (mean 14.5 years), who had undergone temporal lobectomy with at least one year follow-up. Wechsler memory Scale scores (both semantic and figural) showed no change from pre- to post-operative testing, suggesting that the removed tissue was already dysfunctional. There were no significant differences between pre-operative and post-operative short- or long-term semantic or long-term figural memory as a function of side of operation. However, short-term figural memory was poorer in patients who had right temporal lobectomies both pre- and post-operatively than those with left lobectomies.

Such studies after temporal lobectomy have become increasingly informative (Morris, Abrahams, Baddeley and Polkey, 1995). Helmstaedter, Grunwald, Lehnertz et al. (1997) studied verbal declarative memory pre- and post-operatively after selective hippocampectomy, temporal cortical lesionectomy, or anterior two-third en bloc temporal lobe resection. Their results suggested that verbal declarative memory relies on a synergistic interaction of at least two functionally distinct brain systems: material-specific data acquisition is mediated by neocortical temporal structures, whereas long-term consolidation/retrieval is particularly mediated by temporomesial (hippocampal) structures (the latter not material-specific).

Brockway, Follmer, Preuss et al. (1998) pointed out the severe impairment of complex language function in patients with temporal lobe epilepsy. In a series of patients having medial temporal lobe disorders and subsequent medial temporal lobectomies, the authors sought to mimic the language demands of ordinary everyday situations, by assessing a broad range of pragmatic language-based memory functions. Presurgical testing scores revealed that these patients had significant deficits of both short- and long-term memory. Patients performed worse than normals on recall tasks that involved connected discourse (gist, detail, and the generation of inferences); simple lexical recall tasks; paired associates (picture–picture) recall; face recall; and digit span. The ability to remember and generate connected discourse correlated inversely with the extent of hippocampal damage. During the two-year period after surgery, complex language memory tasks performance improved significantly.

Temporal lobe epilepsy patients (pre-surgery) matched objects as well as normals, but showed significant deficits on object naming recognition tasks. The overwhelming differences between temporal lobe patients and normals, however, were seen in the processing and subsequent reconstruction of connected discourse. Temporal lobe epilepsy patients were largely incapacitated for (1) recalling the gist of a paragraph; (2) generation of causal, deductive, entailment, predictive and/or affective inferences; or (3) recalling pertinent details from the paragraph. In all these respects, temporal lobe patients' performance was remarkably poorer than that of controls, for both left and right temporal cases. This emphasis on the effects of medial temporal lobe damage on language memory is a welcome opening, which promises to yield greater insight into the intimate role of memory in language.

Relation to split-brain data: memory after callosotomy

Particularly interesting is the question of memory differences between the left and right hemispheres. Recent functional magnetic resonance imaging (fMRI) has demonstrated that encoding of words produced left greater than right medial temporal lobe activation; encoding of nameable objects produced equal bilateral medial temporal lobe activation; and encoding of unfamiliar faces or nonsense objects right greater than left medial temporal lobe activation. In each case, however, bilateral activation was seen (Kelley, Miezin, McDermott et al., 1998; Martin, Wiggs and Weisberg, 1997).

The example of post-callosotomy adult patients may have some relevance for memory in autism. In split-brain (post-callosotomy) adult patients, one can study isolated hemisphere memory by feeding information selectively only to one hemisphere (for example via the opposite visual field). Metcalfe, Funnell and Gazzaniga (1995) investigated the specialized character of memory in each cerebral hemisphere after callosotomy (including sectioning the hippocampal commissure) by lateralized stimulus presentation. They concluded that there is a right hemisphere superiority for rote memorization and that the right hemisphere is better able to reject distractors, both verbal and non-verbal, that are similar to the originally presented materials. (Autistic children have been found to resist distractors better than control children in a visual search task [Plaisted et al., 1998].) The left hemisphere interprets and integrates incoming information with existing schemata, making it available to semantic processing but losing some precision in retrieval.

Further, split-brain experience suggests that interhippocampal connections are necessary for optimal semantic learning, especially for language material. Studies of hippocampal patients indicate that the encoding of a whole word resulting from the consolidation of verbal elements does not require right hippocampal structures. However, the integrity of both hippocampal structures is required for normal encoding of associations between words (Jha, Kroll, Baynes and Gazzaniga, 1997). "Words must be available to recombine freely into sentences to provide the generative power of language. . . The encoding of word pairs appears to require the integrity of both hippocampal structures. This was evidenced by the poor performance of both groups of unilateral hippocampal patients on the task. Like the hippocampal patients, callosotomy patients are characterized as having encoding deficits during this task; that is, both are impaired during the initial learning of the word pairs." Likewise, "the integrity of both hippocampal structures is required for normal encoding of pictorial elements; most likely a complete or optimal memory trace is one that combines information from both hemispheres during the binding of pictorial elements into a complete 'gestalt'. . . The performance of callosotomy patients on these. . . tasks was remarkably similar to that of patients with damage to their right hippocampal system. These experiments thus suggest that callosotomy impairs the types of encoding that require callosal integration from the left and right hippocampal structures. . . Callosotomy patients performed not significantly different from hippocampal patients" (Jha et al., 1997).

Lateralized brain function in autism: left and right hemisphere memory

It is a striking fact that idiopathic autistic children (that is, autistic children without evidence of brain damage or known cause for their autism; idiopathic autistic children are the typical autistics) often have very poor language and sequential skills (left hemispheral functions) and near normal visual–spatial and simultaneous skills (right hemispheral functions) (Dawson, 1983). Clearly in such cases the right hemisphere has not assumed the functions of the left. Standard imaging methods have not shown a clear interhemispheral difference in autism. However, such a difference, not evident by other imaging techniques, was dramatically demonstrated by Chugani et al. (1997) with PET scans using a serotonin precursor (alpha-^{11}C-methyltryptophan). This study, of seven autistic boys aged 3–7 years, showed very low serotonin synthesis in the left hemisphere (excepting the occipital lobe) in five, and in the right hemisphere in two; increased activity was seen in the contralateral cerebellar dentate nucleus. There were no clinical differences correlating with the reversed asymmetry. Further studies have shown bilaterally low activity in a series of autistic girls (Chugani et al., 1999). While these findings need to be replicated and expanded, a possible link between these PET observations and the functional defects of autism is supported by our finding that fluoxetine (which increases the synaptic availability of serotonin) improves language and sequential function in some children with autism (DeLong et al., 1998). These observations, provocative but fragile, suggest the idea that it is low serotonin synthesis in the left hemisphere that impairs development of language and related functions without triggering their transfer to the right hemisphere.

Very little is known about the effective triggers permitting right hemisphere assumption of language tasks. This question is clearly a crucial one for autism, because all observations — even leaving aside those discussed in the preceding paragraph — indicate poor left hemisphere function with preserved right hemisphere function in autism (Dawson, 1983). Milner (1973) has the best data, indicating that early damage to the left hemisphere primary speech areas causes the transfer of speech development to the right hemisphere (or perhaps more accurately, causes the latent language function of the right hemisphere to become operational); but that lesions outside the specific speech areas have no effect on the lateralization of speech. Autism may not involve the primary speech areas, in general. Many autistic children can articulate and echo quite well (though the learning of this is delayed, and a proportion of children with autism have language disorders that involve phonology and syntax [Rapin and Dunn, 1997]); it is higher language functions that typically fail (Minshew et al., 1997). Thus we might not expect transfer. In any event, language and language-related cognitive processing (predominantly left hemispheral functions) are impaired in autism, and this deficit is not compensated. The right hemisphere appears to be isolated from the left in such autistic children.

Do the callosotomy findings have relevance for the idiopathic autistic child? In autism, memory is veridical, hyperspecific, rote, and resistant to distractors, as described for isolated right hemisphere memory in split-brain patients (Jha et al., 1997). These split-brain findings suggest the existence of similar information processing deficits in children with autism and persons with complete callosotomy (that is, callosotomy involving interhippocampal connections). In addition, the callosotomy patients have many similarities to patients with hippocampal lesions, as noted previously: the split-brain findings suggest interhippocampal integration is required for optimal language function and optimal pictorial integration.

Fluoxetine treatment, in some autistic children, appears to effect definite improvement in language and related functions. Presumably this reflects improved left hemisphere function. In light of Chugani's PET findings, it is an attractive hypothesis that the increased available serotonin improves left hemisphere function. Correspondingly, if the left hemisphere has been nonfunctional and now becomes functional, interhemispheric communication can improve. If the left hemisphere dysfunction involved both neocortical and hippocampal levels, the potential for improved interhemispheric integration of function would include both structures. Were this true, the autistic child's function would change from one of isolated right hemisphere (neocortical and hippocampal) function to one of left and right hemispheral function and interhemispheral integration at neocortical and hippocampal levels, permitting integration and semantic processing of incoming information. This hypothesis is sketched out in some detail because it is suggested by and consistent with the aforementioned split-brain, PET, and fluoxetine data — and most importantly the great mass of neuropsychological data about language and cognitive function in autism. It is disprovable by detailed quantitative testing of learning before and after fluoxetine treatment, in conjunction with appropriate neuroimaging modalities showing serotonin metabolism and neuropsychological function.

Memory in savants: the savant and autistic savant

One cannot discuss memory in childhood without addressing the question of 'savants.' Savant syndrome is a rare syndrome in which persons with developmental disabilities, especially autistic disorders, have islands of ability or brilliance that stand in marked contrast to otherwise very limited intellectual capacity. The syndrome has been well described by Treffert (1988). He defines it as "an exceedingly rare but remarkable condition in which persons with serious mental handicaps, resulting either from developmental disability or from major mental illness, have spectacular areas of mental ability that stand in stark, markedly incongruous contrast to those handicaps." In some individuals the skill may be remarkable simply in contrast to the handicap; in others the ability would be brilliant even if it occurred in normal persons. It may be congenital or acquired by an otherwise normal individual following brain injury or disease. Premature birth is commonly reported. About half of cases are associated with autism, and (as in autism) the savant syndrome occurs in males more frequently than females (by a ratio of 6 : 1, higher than with autism). We found savant abilities in some children with bipolar disorder, whether or not they were autistic, but bipolar disorder is not necessary for development of savant skills (DeLong and Aldershof, 1988).

The special skills shown by savants occur within a narrow and constant range of human functions, which gives the first clue to understanding them. Tredgold (1914) catalogued the categories of skills possessed by savants, which have simply been confirmed in later writings. They consist of mechanical ability; lightning calculation and mathematical ability; exceptional mnemonic skills; artistic talents; calendar calculating; musical skills (usually piano with perfect pitch); map memorizing; visual measurement; and perfect appreciation of past or passing time without knowledge of a clock face. The skills are predominantly right hemispheric in type: visual–spatial, concrete, artistic, musical, non-symbolic, and directly perceived. Regardless of the particular islands of ability, savants all have in common a phenomenal memory, which is highly focused, specific, concrete, and veridical. Investigators note the 'memory without consciousness' which characterizes savants regardless of their particular individual skills — a phenomenon worthy of further study.

O'Connor and Hermelin (1989) raised two basic questions about savants: whether the specific memory of the savant is categorically organized or not, and whether this memory is IQ independent or IQ related. These authors demonstrated that the outstanding memories of savant calculators and musicians are founded on strategies that are rule based, and which draw on knowledge of the structure of the calendar or of music, for example. They also presented evidence that the eliciting of rules and the development of rule-based strategies tended to be specific to the particular areas of ability of these subjects. For example, calendar calculators were quite poor in addition and subtraction of numbers unrelated to the calendar, and musical memory in a savant was found to be confined to compositions based on familiar tonal structure and did not extend to atonal music.

Newer findings on cerebral lateralization and imaging studies that show left hemisphere damage in some savants suggest the most plausible explanation for the savant syndrome to be left hemisphere dysfunction with isolated right hemisphere function. Whether other factors must be invoked is not clear: presumably native talent and hypertrophy of habit memory may play roles. The savant thus very much resembles the picture outlined in this chapter of the autistic child, with isolated right hemisphere function including memory. It is not surprising that half of savants are autistic. The occurrence of savant features in bipolar children, some of whom were autistic and some not, was mentioned previously. (This conjunction of special abilities, bipolar disorder, and autistic features is one factor supporting an etiologic relation between some cases of autism and familial affective disorder [DeLong and Nohria, 1994]. The occurrence of unusual creative talents in bipolar disorder is well-described [Coryell et al., 1989].)

Memory and language

We must never forget that what we know, in this field, is much less than what we don't know. As I ponder this subject, I am drawn back repeatedly to the question of language. What is the relation of language to memory? What is the relation of memory to cognition, and of cognition to language? There are strong indications that language in humans cannot be discussed separately from memory. There has been great interest in comparing the performance of anmestic human individuals to that of hippocampectomized experimental animals, and the comparisons teach us much. However, such studies cannot tell us about language, and therefore ignore a major aspect of human cognition. The proper study is necessarily of humans. Several studies emphasize the importance of dealing with language directly in studying memory, perhaps especially in childhood:

(1) Above, we described cases in which early-life bilateral mesial temporal sclerosis completely arrested cognitive development, precluding language development almost totally (DeLong and Heinz, 1997).
(2) Extensive neuropsychological investigation of patients with unilateral mesial temporal sclerosis coming to temporal lobectomy revealed a severe deficiency of language function, whether the lesion was right- or left-sided (Brockway et al., 1998, see earlier discussion).
(3) Long-term follow-up of a child sustaining bilateral hippocampal-formation damage at age 8 years showed that the skills arrested by his memory disorder were literacy skills, certain basic language functions and vocabulary development. In contrast, mathematical and logical skills continued to develop to adult levels (Broman et al., 1997, see earlier discussion).

The relations between language comprehension and memory have been reconsidered in an important recent study which re-examines the data on patient HM (MacKay et al., 1998). The prevailing view has been that HM suffers from a pure memory deficit but completely spares other cognitive processes including language comprehension. Such a view postulates separate units and processes for language and memory in sequentially ordered processing modules: comprehension, storage, retrieval, and production. MacKay and collaborators demonstrate that HM's language comprehension, as well as his semantic-level language production, are significantly impaired. They argue that this comprehension deficit contradicts the separation of comprehension, storage, and retrieval postulated in stages-of-processing theories. Rather, they state, their data support an argument for a distributed network, that there is no dividing line between language and memory for verbal materials, and that HM's binding deficits are simultaneously responsible for both his language deficits and his memory deficits. The concept of 'binding' is that new experiences are comprehended by binding with old data, to form new memories. Such binding occurs centrally in the hippocampal formation, as discussed earlier. Someone with a binding deficit, or difficulty in forming new connections, will not be able to comprehend novel aspects of language, because forming new connections is integral to comprehending new ideas. Not all language comprehension requires new connection formation; much of everyday language use requires activation only of familiar nodes and connections.

This formulation of hippocampal memory function is very persuasive. (It is, of course, a restatement of the idea of a hippocampal cognitive processor discussed above. Once the developmental dimension is introduced into memory study, we can't think only of memory as such, but must conceptualize *cognitive processing*. Isolated memory research in the developmental context becomes hollow.) This formulation also goes a long way toward explaining the striking language disabilities seen in young children with unilateral (Brockway et al., 1998) — and much more so bilateral (DeLong and Heinz, 1997) — hippocampal formation lesions. I have applied an essentially similar concept to autism (DeLong, 1992), arguing that autism represents the failure of a central cognitive processor which is necessary for flexible multidimensional association of perceptual experience, memory, and motivational states, and thus for the flexible formation and production of new concepts and new language. The binding function of the hippocampus was postulated "to be necessary for normal development in the child of language syntax, semantics, and pragmatics; the capacity for creativity and generativity in language and behavior, and combinatorial possibilities in general; for the integration of motivational states with experience and learning; and for the construction of a complex, useful, and flexible structure of meaning, of which both language and appropriate purposive behavior are examples. These constructs, once secure and practiced, become independent of the hippocampus for use, but the hippocampus is still required to modify or add to them. Thus the adult amnesiac can still perform well in some respects, utilizing his past construction, but he cannot go forward with new conceptual learning." (DeLong, 1992) This formulation appears to parallel that of MacKay and collaborators closely.

Thus it appears that memory and language can no longer be studied in isolation; certainly not in development, and probably not at all. The intimate interconnection of language with memory — and indeed of the broad range of behavior, in its complex variegated creativity, with memory — is a powerful concept to apply to the study of cognitive function.

A glossary of memory terms

Declarative memory Conscious or explicit memory for new events and facts, including Episodic and Semantic Memories (Squire, 1992).

Cognitive memory Approximately equivalent to Declarative memory, including memory for events and facts.

Propositional memory Approximately the same as Declarative and Cognitive memory.

Episodic memory (equals Event memory) Conscious or explicit memory for events; the explicit consciousness of having experienced remembered events. In episodic memory encoding, hippocampal formation activation is sensitive to the overall degree of novelty, whereas prefrontal activation is sensitive to changes in previously formed connections (Dolan RJ, Fletcher PC. Nature: 388; 582–585, 1997).

Semantic memory (equals Fact memory) Conscious or explicit memory for facts; also the sum of factual memory, constituting a structure of meaning, such as language knowledge and one's entire body of conscious knowledge of the world.

Procedural memory Memory, learning, or attainment of skills that are not conscious and may be learned and retained independently of declarative memory.

Retrograde memory Memory for past events; for events that occurred before the onset of amnesia (loss of retrograde memory is retrograde amnesia).

Anterograde memory Memory for new events; for events occurring after the onset of amnesia (loss of anterograde memory is anterograde amnesia).

Working memory A system for temporary storage and manipulation of information in the brain, a function critical for a wide range of cognitive operations; primarily localized in the prefrontal lobes.

Digit span A type of immediate memory; the number of digits that can be remembered after one hearing. The length of time that memory of the digits is retained is sometimes referred to as "immediate memory".

Short-term memory Declarative memory beyond "immediate memory" (see above), which is subject to forgetting over a period usually measured in minutes to hours.

Long-term memory Declarative memory which is retained for long periods, often life-long. Hippocampal formation function is necessary to lay down long-term memories, but the memories are thought to be stored in neocortex and can be recalled even if the hippocampus is subsequently destroyed.

References

Baddeley A: Working memory. Science 255: 556–9, 1992.

Bolton PF, Griffiths PD: Association of tuberous sclerosis of temporal lobes with autism and atypical autism. Lancet 349: 392–395, 1997.

Boucher J, Warrington EK: Memory deficits in early infantile autism: some similarities to the amnesic syndrome. British Journal of Psychiatry: 67; 73–87, 1976.

Brockway JP, Follmer RL, Preuss LA, Prioleau CE, Burrows GS, Solsrud KA, Cooke CN, Greenhoot JH, Howard J: Memory, simple and complex language, and the temporal lobe. Brain and Language: 61; 1–29, 1998.

Broman M, Rose AL, Hotson G, McCarthy M, Case C: Severe anterograde amnesia with onset in childhood as a result of anoxic encephalopathy. Brain: 120; 417–433, 1997.

Bunsey M, Eichenbaum H: Conservation of hippocampal memory function in rats and humans. Nature: 379; 255–257, 1996.

Chugani HT, Da Silva E, Chugani DC: Infantile spasms: III: prognostic implications of bitemporal hypometabolism in positron emission tomography. Annals of Neurology: 39; 643–649, 1996.

Chugani DC, Musik O, Rothermel R et al: Altered serotonin synthesis in the dentatothalamocortical pathway in autistic boys. Annals of Neurology: 42; 666–669, 1997.

Chugani DC, Muzik O, Behen M, Rothermel R, Janisse JJ, Lee J, Chugani HT: Developmental changes in brain serotonin synthesis capacity in autistic and nonautistic children. Annals of Neurology: 45; 287–295, 1999.

Churchill DW: Language: the problem beyond conditioning. In Rutter M, Schopler E (Eds), Autism. New York: Plenum Press, pp. 73–84, 1978.

Corkin S: Lasting consequences of bilateral medial temporal lobectomy: Clinical course and experimental findings in H.M. Seminars in Neurology: 4; 249–259, 1984.

Coryell W, Endicott J, Keller M, Andreasen N, Grove W, Hirschfeld RM, Scheftner W: Bipolar affective disorder and high achievement: a familial association. American Journal of Psychiatry: 146; 983–988, 1989.

Dawson G: Lateralized brain dysfunction in autism: evidence from the Halstead–Reitan Neuropsychological Battery. Journal of Autism and Developmental Disorders: 13; 269–286, 1983.

DeLong GR: Autism, amnesia, hippocampus, and learning. Neuroscience and Biobehavioral Reviews: 16; 63–70, 1992.

DeLong GR: Autism: New data suggest a new hypothesis. Neurology: 52; 911–916, 1999.

DeLong GR, Aldershof AL: An Association of Special Abilities with Juvenile Manic-Depressive Illness. In Obler LK, Fein D (Eds), The Exceptional Brain. New York: Guilford Press, pp. 387–395, 1988.

DeLong GR, Bean SC, Brown FR: Acquired reversible autistic syndrome in acute encephalopathic illness in children. Archives of Neurology: 38; 191–194, 1981.

DeLong GR, Heinz ER: The syndrome of early-life bilateral hippocampal sclerosis. Annals of Neurology: 42; 11–17, 1997.

DeLong GR, Nohria C: Psychiatric family history and neurological disease in autistic spectrum disorders. Developmental Medicine and Child Neurology: 36; 441–448, 1994.

DeLong GR, Teague LA, Kamran MM: Effect of fluoxetine treatment in young children with idiopathic autism. Developmental Medicine and Child Neurology: 40; 551–562, 1998.

Ehlers S, Nyden A, Gillberg C, Sandbeerg AD, Dahkgren SO, Hjelmquist E, Oden A: Asperger syndrome, autism and attention disorders: a comparative study of the cognitive profiles of 120 children. Journal of Child Psychology and Psychiatry: 38; 207–217, 1997.

Eichenbaum H: How does the brain organize memories? Science: 277; 330–332, 1997.

Fitzgerald JM: A developmental account of early childhood amnesia. Journal of Genetic Psychology: 152; 159–171, 1991.

Gabrieli JDE, Brewer JB, Desmond JE, Glover GH: Separate neural bases of two fundamental memory processes in the human medial temporal lobe. Science: 276; 264–266, 1997.

Geschwind N: Disorders of higher cortical function in children. Clinical Proceedings of the Children's Hospital National Medical Center: 28; 261–272, 1972.

Gilmore RO: Toward a neuropsychology of visual development. In Segalowitz SJ, Rapin I (Eds), Child Neuropsychology, Handbook of Neuropsychology, 2nd Edition, vol. 8, part II. Amsterdam: Elsevier, pp. 417–437, 2003.

Gloor P: The Temporal Lobe and Limbic System. New York: Oxford University Press, 1997.

Grahame-Smith DG: Serotonin in affective disorders. International Clinical Psychopharmacology: 6 Suppl. 4; 5–13, 1992.

Goldman-Rakic PS: Cellular and circuit basis of working memory in prefrontal cortex of nonhuman primates. Progress in Brain Research: 85; 325–336, 1990.

Hampson HE, Simeral JD, Deadwyler SA: Distribution of spatial and nonspatial information in dorsal hippocampus. Nature: 402; 610–614, 1999.

Helmstaedter C, Grunwald T, Lehnertz K, Gleissner U, Elger CE: Differential involvement of left temporolateral and temporomesial structures in verbal declarative learning and memory — evidence from temporal lobe epilepsy. Brain and Cognition: 35; 110–131, 1997.

Hermelin B, O'Connor N: Psychological Experiments with Autistic Children. Oxford: Pergamon Press, pp. 1–142, 1970.

Jha AP, Kroll NEA, Baynes K, Gazzaniga MS: Memory encoding following complete callosotomy. Journal of Cognitive Neuroscience: 9; 143–159, 1997.

Kelley WM, Miezin FM, McDermott KB, Buckner RL, Raichle ME, Cohen NJ, Ollinger JM, Akbudak E, Conturo TE, Snyder AZ, Petersen SE: Hemispheric specialization in human dorsal frontal cortex and medial temporal lobe for verbal and nonverbal memory encoding. Neuron: 20; 927–936, 1998.

Kitchener EG, Hodges JR, McCarthy R: Acquisition of postmorbid vocabulary and semantic facts in the absence of episodic memory. Brain: 121; 1313–1327, 1998.

Lee NS, Radtke RA, Gray L, Burger PC, Montine TJ, DeLong GR, Lewis DV, Oakes WJ, Friedman AH, Hoffman JM: Neuronal migration disorders: Positron emission tomography correlations. Annals of Neurology: 35; 290–297, 1994.

Lewis DV, Thompson RJ Jr, Santos CC, Oakes WJ, Radtke RA, Friedman AH, Lee NS, Swartzwelder H: Outcome of temporal lobectomy in adolescents. Epilepsy: 9; 198–205, 1996.

McDonald RJ, White NM: A triple dissociation of memory systems: hippocampus, amygdala, and dorsal striatum. Behavioral Neuroscience: 107; 3–22, 1993.

MacKay DG, Stewart R, Burke DM: H.M. Revisited: relations between language comprehension, memory, and the hippocampal system. Journal of Cognitive Neuroscience: 10; 377–394, 1998.

Maguire EA, Vargha-Khadem F, Mishkin M: The effects of bilateral hippocampal damage on fMRI regional activations and interactions during memory retrieval. Brain: 124; 1156–1170, 2001.

Malkova L, Mishkin M, Suomi SJ, Bachevalier J: Socioemotional behavior in adult rhesus monkeys after early versus late lesions of the medial temporal lobe. Annals of the New York Academy of Science: 807; 538–540, 1997.

Martin A, Wiggs CL, Weisberg JW: Modulation of human medial temporal lobe activity by form, meaning, and experience. Hippocampus: 7; 587–593, 1997.

Metcalfe JA, Funnell M, Gazzaniga M: Right hemisphere memory superiority: Studies of a split-brain patient. Journal of Gerontology B. Psychological Science and Social Science: 6; 157–164, 1995.

Milner B: Hemispheric specialization: scope and limits. In Schmidt FO, Worden FG (Eds), The Neurosciences: Third Study Program. Cambridge, MA: MIT Press, pp. 75–89, 1973.

Minshew NJ, Goldstein G, Siegel DJ: Neuropsychologic functioning in autism: profile of a complex information processing disorder. Journal of the International Neuropsychological Society: 3; 303–316, 1997.

Mishkin M, Vargha-Khadem F, Gadian DG: Amnesia and the organization of the hippocampal system. Hippocampus: 8; 212–216, 1998.

Morris RG, Abrahams S, Baddeley A, Polkey CE: Doors and People: visual and verbal memory after unilateral temporal lobectomy. Neuropsychology: 9; 464–469, 1995.

O'Connor N, Hermelin B: The memory structure of idiot-savant mnemonists. British Journal of Psychology: 80; 97, 1989.

Ostergaard AL: Episodic, semantic and procedural memory in a case of amnesia at an early age. Neuropsychologia: 25; 341–357, 1987.

Ostergaard A, Squire LR: Childhood amnesia and distinctions between forms of memory: a comment on Wood, Brown, and Felton. Brain and Cognition: 14; 127–133, 1990.

Penfield W, Jasper H: Epilepsy and the Functional Anatomy of the Human Brain. Boston: Little Brown and Co., 1954.

Plaisted K, O'Riordan M, Baron-Cohen S: Enhanced visual search for a conjunctive target in autism: a research note. Journal of Child Psychology and Psychiatry and Allied Disciplines: 39; 777–783, 1998.

Rapin I: Autism. New England Journal of Medicine: 337; 97–104, 1997.

Rapin I, Dunn M: Language disorders in children with autism. Seminars in Pediatric Neurology: 4; 46–92, 1997.

Rolls ET: A theory of hippocampal function in memory. Hippocampus: 6; 601–620, 1996.

Saunders RC, Kolachana BS, Bachevalier J, Weinberger DR: Neonatal lesions of the medial temporal lobe disrupt prefrontal cortical regulation of striatal dopamine. Nature: 393; 169–171, 1998.

Schacter DL: Multiple forms of memory in humans and animals. In Weinberger NM, McGaugh JL, Lynch G (Eds), Memory Systems of the Brain. New York: Guilford Press, pp 351–379, 1985.

Scoville WB, Milner B: Loss of recent memory after bilateral hippocampal lesions. Journal of Neurology, Neurosurgery and Psychiatry: 20; 11–21, 1957.

Squire LR: Memory and the hippocampus: a synthesis from findings with rats, monkeys, and humans. Psychological Reviews: 99; 195–231, 1992.

Squire LR, Zola-Morgan S, Chen KS: Human amnesia and animal models of amnesia: performance of amnesic patients on tests designed for the monkey. Behavioral Neuroscience: 102; 210–221, 1988.

Tesche CD, Karhu J: Interactive processing of sensory input and motor output in the human hippocampus. Journal of Cognitive Neuroscience: 11; 424–436, 1999.

Tredgold AF: Mental Deficiency. New York: William Wood, 1914.

Treffert DA: The idiot savant: a review of the syndrome. American Journal of Psychiatry: 145; 563–572, 1988.

Tulving E, Hayman CA, Macdonald CA: Long-lasting perceptual priming and semantic learning in amnesia: a case experiment. Journal of Experimental Psychology: Learning, Memory and Cognition: 17; 595–617, 1991.

Vargha-Khadem F, Gadian DG, Watkins KD, Connelly A, Van Paesschen W, Mishkin M: Differential effects of early hippocampal pathology on episodic and semantic memory. Science: 277; 376–380, 1997.

Vargha-Khadem F, Isaacs E, Mishkin M: Agnosia, alexia and a remarkable form of amnesia in an adolescent boy. Brain: 117; 683–714, 1994.

Wood FB, Brown IS, Felton RH: Long-term follow-up of a childhood amnesic syndrome. Brain and Cognition: 10; 76–86, 1989.

Young BJ, Otto T, Fox GD, Eichenbaum H: Memory representation within the parahippocampal region. Journal of Neuroscience: 17; 5183–5195, 1997.

Handbook of Neuropsychology, 2nd Edition, Vol. 8, Part II
S.J. Segalowitz and I. Rapin (Eds)

CHAPTER 28

Neuropsychology of attention disorders

Rosemary Tannock [*]

Brain and Behavior Research Program, The Hospital for Sick Children, University of Toronto, 555 University Avenue, Toronto, ON M5G 1X8, Canada

Introduction

The term 'attention' is part of our everyday vocabulary, but its precise definition remains elusive. In part, this is because the term is used to refer to a diverse set of overt behavioral and covert cognitive phenomena that are not readily mapped on to one another. Attention is not a unitary process, but refers to a complex array of cognitive-behavioral processes involved in the reduction and selection of information and in behavioral response control. The development of these processes continues over the course of infancy, childhood, and adolescence, and is associated with marked individual differences.

This chapter is concerned with *disorders* of attention. Difficulties with attention are common during the preschool and school age years. More marked disturbances are evident in a range of childhood conditions, including prematurity, hydrocephalus, epilepsy, phenylketonuria, congenital hyper/hypothyroidism, traumatic brain injury, and various developmental learning disorders (e.g., developmental dyslexia, dyscalculia). In the extreme these disturbances of attention are impairing to the affected individual and disruptive to those around them, at which point they are conceptualized as symptoms of a mental health disorder. Symptoms of inattention are associated with many psychiatric disorders of childhood, including generalized anxiety disorders, Tourette syndrome, and childhood-onset schizophrenia, but they form one defining dimension of attention-deficit/hyperactivity disorder. This chapter focuses on the neuropsychology of attention disorders as manifest in attention-deficit/hyperactivity disorder (ADHD), but also addresses the continuity/discontinuity between the disturbance of attention in ADHD versus that associated with other neurodevelopmental disorders and mental health disorders.

The chapter first provides a brief overview of the conceptualization and measurement of attention, followed by a review of the clinical features of ADHD, current theoretical accounts, and a synopsis of recent advances in the neurobiology and genetic etiology of ADHD (for more extensive reviews of these issues, see Barkley, 1997a,b; Levy and Hay, 2001; Schachar and Tannock, 2002; Solanto, Arnsten and Castellanos, 2001; Tannock, 1998). Next, a critical review of recent neuropsychological studies of ADHD (i.e., since those reviewed in the 1st edition of the *Handbook of Neuropsychology*, 1992) is presented, which indicates the limitations of current interpretations in accounting for the most salient clinical feature (temporal and contextual variability in symptom expression) and the most robust cognitive feature (response variability) of ADHD. The chapter concludes with a discussion of future directions for understanding attentional disorders in neurodeveopmental disorders such as ADHD.

* Corresponding author. Tel.: +1-416-813-7048; Fax: +1-416-813-6565; E-mail: tannock@sickkids.ca

Conceptualization and measurement of attention

Behavioral versus cognitive conceptualization

Attention encompasses both behavioral and cognitive concepts, which has given rise to confusion in developmental psychopathology, primarily because there is little evidence of any direct relationship between the two concepts. As a behavioral descriptor, attention is typically defined in terms of overt action, such as on-task behavior. On-task behavior emphasizes visual fixation to task-relevant stimuli, such as a designated spatial location (e.g., worksheet, text book, blackboard), person (e.g., parent, teacher, speaker), or event (trajectory of ball, onset of stimulus). Conversely, inattentive behavior is defined as off-task behavior and emphasizes the frequency with which the child looks away from the task-relevant stimuli during a specific activity (e.g., assigned work, a conversation or lesson, baseball game, videogame, or computerized cognitive task).

Attention also denotes a complex set of cognitive processes that operate through a series of neural networks to provide self-regulation of sensory input, motor output, and emotion in the service of internal goals (Posner and Rothbart, 1998). In cognitive neuroscience, three major conceptualizations of attention are discernible: selective attention, executive attention, and sustained attention (Parasuraman, 1998). Selective attention refers to the ability to attend to relevant stimuli and ignore irrelevant stimuli, with greatest emphasis given to documenting visual–spatial attention (i.e., control of attention over space). Executive attention refers to control over cognitive processes in general, rather than biasing visual–spatial processing toward the selection of certain stimuli. Many names have been given to this type of attention, including 'central executive' (Baddeley, 1996), 'executive attention' (Posner and Dehaene, 1994), 'supervisory attention' (Shallice and Burgess, 1991), and 'effortful control' (Ruff and Rothbart, 1996). The third conceptualization is that of sustained attention, which refers to control of attention (in the sense of 'energy' or 'cognitive resources') over time (Parasuraman, 1998). Sustained attention is viewed as a continuous process during which resources are depleted by having to maintain focused attention over time.

Numerous models of attention exist, which vary in the relative emphasis given to the three major conceptualizations and in their interpretation. A comprehensive review of each is beyond the scope of this chapter; readers are referred to existing texts and reviews for detailed expositions (e.g., Cohen, 1993; Heilman, Watson, Valenstein et al., 1988; Mesulam, 2000; Mirsky, Anthony, Duncan et al., 1991; Mirsky and Duncan, 2001; Posner and Raichle, 1994). However, a common set of cognitive/behavioral and neural principles may be discerned amongst the various models, which are summarized in Table 1 (for detailed explanation see Cohen, 1993). This review will examine to what extent any one or more of these component processes of attention are impaired in ADHD. However, since all three types of attention are mediated by widespread neuronal networks (e.g., Posner and Raichle, 1994) that are vulnerable to various kinds of damage and dysfunction, any attentional impairments documented in ADHD are likely to be evident also (albeit to various degrees) in other neurodevelopmental disorders (e.g., childhood-onset schizophrenia, autism, language disorders, reading disorder, etc.).

Measurement of attention

Attentive (or conversely, inattentive) behavior can be assessed directly or indirectly. Direct assessment uses systematic observation of the child during various activities (structured, unstructured) and settings (e.g., home, school, clinic). Observation schedules are either event-related (e.g., number of times the child looks away from task during the activity) or epoch-related (e.g., percentage of 15-second observation intervals in which child looked away from task materials for at least 2 seconds). Indirect assessment involves the use of interviews and standardized rating scales with parents and teachers (or others familiar with the child) to rate the frequency of occurrence of these behaviors (e.g., never/rarely; sometimes; often; very often) over a specified time period (e.g., past 6 months, past week). Rating scales commonly used to assess the behavioral construct of attention (as well as other externalizing and internalizing behavioral symptoms), include the *Behavior Assessment System for Children* (Kamphaus and Frick, 1996); *Conners' Rating Scales* (Conners,

TABLE 1

Cognitive/behavioral and neural principles of attention

	Cognitive/behavioral principles		Neural principles
1.	Information reduction	1.	Subserved by non-localized networks
2.	Information selection (prioritization)	2.	Neural substrate reflects functional organization of the brain
3.	Provides interface between sensory/perceptual input and higher-order cognition and behavioral action	3.	Two broad cortical divisions support sensory selection (posterior brain systems) and motor functions (anterior systems)
4.	Provides for the interaction of incoming information with existing memory traces	4.	Hierarchical organization of neural systems (cortical–subcortical) enables attentional control
5.	Spatial distribution permits selection of information from spatial locations	5.	Requires interaction of neural systems with high versus low neural plasticity
6.	Temporal distribution permits selection of information over time, which is variable	6.	Basic behavioral processes (habituation, sensitization, classical conditioning) underlie the attentional response
7.	Temporal character of attention is determined by anticipation, preparation and response delay	7.	Interaction of inhibitory and excitatory processes provide control of attention.
8.	Motivationally determined	8.	Attention is modulated neurochemically (e.g., by neurotransmitters, neuropeptides, CNS drugs)
9.	Capacity/resource limitations	9.	Attention is modulated by neural processing speed
10.	Divided and focused attention	10.	Support by neural cells with specific attentional functions
11.	Automatic versus controlled operations		
12.	Attention is related to conscious awareness		
13.	A by-product of multiple interactive processes		
14.	Attentional processes are dynamic and adaptive		

Adapted from Cohen RA: The Neuropsychology of Attention. New York: Plenum Press, Ch. 22, pp. 459–479, 1993.

1997); *Child Behavior Checklist* and *Teacher's Report Form* (Achenbach, 1991a,b); and *Child Attention Problems* (Barkley, 1988). (For detailed descriptions of these and other rating scales, see resources such as, American Psychiatric Association, 2000, Barkley, 1990.)

Cognitive constructs of attention are inferred from specific psychometric, neuropsychological, or experimental measures. The measures are assumed to have both neurological validity (i.e., reflect the state of the central nervous system) and psychological validity (i.e., reflect meaningfully some aspect of functioning in everyday life). Examples of measures used in a psychometric approach, include the WISC-3 Freedom From Distractibility Index, Coding or Symbol Search, and Digit Span subtests, to index attentional performance, processing speed, and attention span, respectively. The neuropsychological approach may use a fixed battery of tests (e.g., *NEPSY; Cambridge Automated Neuropsychological Test Assessment Battery*) or a range of tests selected to index one or more components of attention. The most commonly used measures for children include standardized continuous performance tests, letter cancellation tasks, Go–NoGo tasks, Stroop Color–Word Test, Trail-making Test, Wisconsin Card Sorting task, Tower of Hanoi or Tower of London, and various response generation tasks, such as controlled word-list-generation tests. These tasks are multifactorial and measure a variety of cognitive processes, which cannot be separated. The experimental approach uses methods derived from information processing theory that involve experimental manipulation of stimulus characteristics, response demands, and reinforcement. By contrast to neuropsychological methods, which only yield measures of accuracy, these experimental methods include measures of response latency and variability, as well as accuracy and permit some distinctions between the various component processes. Measures used in studies of attention in ADHD include novel versions of continuous performance tests (e.g., Halperin, Wolf, Greenblatt et al., 1991), the stop-signal task (e.g., Oosterlaan and Sergeant, 1998; Schachar, Mota, Logan et al., 2000), visual–spatial orienting tasks (e.g. Swanson, Posner, Potkin et al., 1991; Wood, Maruff, Levy et al., 1999), flanker tasks (e.g., Brodeur and Pond, 2001) and anti-saccade tasks (e.g., Castellanos, Marvasti, Ducharme et al., 2000; Munoz, Hampton, Moore et al., 1999).

One potential problem in clinical practice is that the observable inattentive behavior is assumed to reflect problems in the underlying cognitive processes involved in attention. Yet behavioral and cognitive (i.e., overt and covert) manifestations of attention are separable, as illustrated by the fact that the child who is looking out of the classroom window, may still be listening to the teacher or working on the problem presented on the board. Conversely, the child who is looking directly at the teacher may not be attending to or processing any of the teacher's instructions. Moreover, rating scales do not include operational criteria for individual symptoms. The informant is left to decide what observable behavior constitutes the various phenomena such as 'inability to concentrate' and the extent to which it is present (e.g., 'not at all', 'just a little', 'quite a lot'). Even subtle changes in response categories may have a dramatic effect on scores from behavioral rating scales (Woodward, Thomas, Boyle et al., 1989).

By contrast, psychometric and neuropsychological tests purport to measure specific components of attention (e.g., response inhibition, vigilance). However, they typically measure a complex web of distinct processes, as illustrated by the findings from a recent event-related fMRI study that revealed activation of distinct neural circuits during different stages of the Wisconsin Card Sorting Task (Monchi, Petrides, Petre et al., 2001). Table 2 attempts to map various psychometric, neuropsychological, and experimental measures of attention onto the postulated factors and component processes of attention. Many of these tests were developed to assess neuropsychological functioning in adults with various brain lesions, consequently their neurological and psychological validity, and their psychometric properties for pediatric populations are questionable.

Clinical profile of attention-deficit/hyperactivity disorder

Attention-deficit/hyperactivity disorder (ADHD) is a chronic disorder characterized by developmentally inappropriate, persistent, pervasive and impairing levels of inattention, impulsiveness and hyperactivity (American Psychiatric Association, 1994; World Health Organization, 1993). Conservative prevalence estimates suggest that ADHD occurs in 3–6% of all school age children from diverse cultures and geographical regions, with an over-representation in boys (e.g., Anderson, Williams, McGee and Silva, 1987; Baumgartel, Wolraich and Dietrich, 1995; Bird, Canino, Rubio-Stipec et al., 1988; Leung, Luk, Ho et al., 1996; Szatmari, Offord and Boyle, 1989; Wang, Chong, Chou et al., 1993). More permissive criteria yield estimates of up to 17% (Barbaresi, Katusic, Colligan et al., 2002). Moreover, a recent epidemiological study of the prevalence of inattentive behavior in British children, suggests that 1.3% of 7-year-old boys exhibit marked problems of inattention, 2% exhibit problems of overactivity, and 1.7% exhibit a combination of inattention and overactivity (Warner-Rogers, Taylor, Taylor et al., 2000).

The cardinal features of ADHD are extreme inattention and/or excessive motor activity and impulsiveness. These children often have difficulty attending to instructions in academic and social situations; they are easily distracted by other things going on within and outside of the classroom (e.g., rustle of papers, sound of footsteps in hallway, objects in field of view), may look away or 'drift off' when spoken to, require frequent repetition of instructions, and fail to understand the subtle nuances of conversation or the language of instruction in class. Their schoolwork is characterized by low productivity (e.g., a few statements in point form rather than the required one-page logical and coherent argument; four arithmetic problems completed rather than the required set of ten), careless errors and lack of required detail (e.g., papers are handed in without a name or date, with words left out or misspelled). Poor organization is a hallmark of ADHD across the life-span. Evidence includes papers stuffed into a knapsack or desk, rather than filed in a binder; books, papers, lunch wrappings and magazines intermixed and left in a heap on the floor; work presented haphazardly on a crumpled worksheet, with visible erasing and numerous crossings-out. Children with ADHD may 'jump the gun' by starting a designated activity before the instructions are completed, or are the last to start because they cannot find or have not gathered together the necessary materials, or do not know where to start. Yet, they may be the first to claim

TABLE 2

Neuropsychological taxonomy of attention and assessment measures

Attentional factors	Components	Cognitive measures
1. Selective attention		
	Filtering	Negative priming;
	Selection	Stroop interference test; Eriksen's flanker task
	Focusing	
	Automatic shifting	Spatial cuing paradigm
2. Executive attention (response control)		
	Inhibition	Go–NoGo; Stop-Signal task; CPT-Inhibition
	Active shifting	Wisconsin card sorting task; Trail-making test
	Planning	Tower of London/Hanoi
3. Sustained attention (attentional resources)		
Energetic factors	Arousal	
	Motivation	
	Effort	
Structural factors	Memory capacity	Digit span forwards; Corsi-Blocks
	Processing speed	WISC-3 coding and symbol search;
	Temporal dynamics	Variability of response times
	Spatial constraints	Visual patterns test; Static matrices;
Temporal factors	Vigilance	Continuous performance test; Cancellation test

they have finished the work, albeit unchecked, inaccurate and incomplete, because they have forgotten some of the instructions or omitted some necessary steps. On the one hand, children with ADHD tend to shout out replies too loudly and out of turn, interrupt, and appear to need the instant attention of others. However, when called upon to respond, these same children often struggle to retrieve and organize their thoughts, so that their responses tend to be dysfluent, brief, incoherent, and replete with non-specific terms (e.g., 'the thing'). Many appear to be in constant motion; shifting position in their seats, fiddling with any object at hand (pencils, paper clips, tableware, loose threads in sleeve cuffs, elastic in socks, fluff on the carpet); standing up or even leaving their chairs, racing through rooms and hallways.

One most striking clinical characteristic (described by parents and teachers alike as well as being observable in the home, classroom and clinic) is the marked variability and inconsistency in behavioral symptoms and task performance. Symptoms and performance fluctuate moment-to-moment and appear to vary as a function of the cognitive complexity and demand of the specific task or context. Thus, parents and teachers often describe these children as being both too loud and too quiet, too fast and too slow, too distractible yet unable to shift their attention when needed. Rapid, flexible adaptation to changing demands of academic and social situations is rarely observed. Ironically, the critical thresholds for determining symptom presence and severity have been criticized because they are expressed by imprecise terms, such as *often*, *frequently*, or *pretty much*, *most of the time*, without further specification. Yet, these terms capture precisely the essence of ADHD: temporal and contextual variability in symptom expression and behavioral performance.

ADHD is neither transient nor benign. The behavioral symptoms are evident in early childhood and persist across the lifespan, although there are age- and gender-related changes in their manifestation (e.g., Barkley, Fischer, Edelbrock et al., 1990; Biederman, Faraone, Milberger et al., 1996a; Biederman, Mick and Faraone, 2000; Caspi, Moffitt, Newman et al., 1996; Klein and Mannuzza, 1991; Weiss and Hechtman, 1993). ADHD is associated with significant impairments in family and peer relationships, an increased risk for academic underachievement and school failure, accidental injuries and serious driving accidents, underachievement in employment, social isolation, and additional psychopathology (e.g., Barkley, Murphy and Kwasnik,

1996; Biederman, Faraone, Milberger et al., 1996b; Nada-Raja, Langley, McGee et al., 1997; Weiss and Hechtman, 1993; Woodward, Fergusson and Horwood, 2000).

Diagnostic criteria

ADHD is characterized by three core clusters of behavioral symptoms; poor sustained attention, impulsiveness, and hyperactivity (American Psychiatric Association, 1980, 1987; World Health Organization, 1993). However, over the past two decades there have been changes in both the conceptualization and nomenclature of this disorder (for an historical review, see Sandberg and Barton, 1996; Schachar, 1986). The most recent editions of the *Diagnostic and Statistical Manual of the American Psychiatric Association* (DSM-IV; American Psychiatric Association, 1994) and the *International Classification of Diseases* (ICD-10; World Health Organization, 1993) reflect an effort to bring the definitions closer together. These two classification systems have adopted almost identical criteria for the identification of inattentive, hyperactive, and impulsive symptoms. However, as explained below significant differences remain between the North American and European approaches in their diagnostic algorithms (number of criteria in each symptoms cluster required for a diagnosis), the role of inattention, the definition of pervasiveness across situations, and the handling of concurrent disorders (comorbidity).

Notably, the DSM-IV differentiates *two* symptom clusters: an inattention cluster comprising nine symptoms of inattention; and a hyperactive/impulsive cluster comprising three impulsive and six hyperactive symptoms. The diagnostic criteria require that at least six symptoms in either the inattention or the hyperactivity/impulsivity clusters (or both) have persisted for at least 6 months and that some impairment from the symptoms is present in two or more settings (e.g., home, school). Three behavioral subtypes are distinguished (Predominantly Inattentive, Predominantly Hyperactive-Impulsive, Combined Type), which are thought to be distinct in terms of their etiology, clinical course, correlates, response to treatment, and outcome (Lahey, Applegate, McBurnett et al., 1994). By contrast, the ICD-10 differentiates *three* symptom clusters (i.e., inattention, impulsivity, hyperactivity), and the criteria for a diagnosis of Hyperkinetic Disorder (HD) are more demanding than are the DSM-IV criteria for ADHD. For example, not only must the criteria be met for all three symptom clusters, but also *all* of the necessary criteria must be present both at home and at school (or other situations). As a result, the ICD-10 does not recognize either the DSM-IV predominantly inattentive or predominantly hyperactive/impulsive subtypes.

Clinicians and researchers alike face several major challenges to establishing the diagnosis of ADHD/HD One challenge is that neither the DSM-IV nor the ICD-10 diagnostic algorithms provide operational definitions of the specific symptoms of inattention and hyperactivity/impulsivity, so that one problem behavior (e.g., frequently leaves seat) may be used to code several symptoms (e.g., frequently leaves seat; on the go; easily distracted by external stimuli; difficulty sustaining attention). Moreover, although the symptoms of ADHD are not all equal in their ability to predict the diagnosis (e.g., Lahey et al., 1994; Mota and Schachar, 2000; Power, Costigan, Leff et al., 2001), DSM-IV and ICD-10 treat every item equally in making diagnostic decisions. Another challenge is that neither of the diagnostic algorithms provides guidelines for combining information from multiple informants, which is problematic because agreement between parents and teachers is poor with virtually no agreement for individual ADHD subtypes (Mitsis, McKay, Schulz et al., 2000; Offord, Boyle, Racine et al., 1996). Moreover, parent ratings are likely to be more biased than teacher rating (Simonoff, Pickles, Hervas et al., 1998). For example, parent-reports of ADHD symptoms in school have been found to be more highly correlated with their own reports of their child's behavior at home than with teacher reports of their child's behavior in school (Mitsis et al., 2000). These findings highlight the importance of using multiple informants for diagnosis of this clinical entity and suggest that data from studies in which diagnosis of ADHD and its subtypes are based on a single informant (e.g., parent) may be of questionable validity.

Currently, the DSM-IV Combined subtype is considered to be prototypic of the classic ADHD profile, the closest approximation to the ICD-10 category of HD, and the focus of dysinhibitory theories of

ADHD (Barkley, 1997a; Quay, 1997). The risk factor is presumed to reside in the hyperactivity/impulsivity component of ADHD/HD (Barkley, 1997a; Taylor, 1998). By contrast, there is growing recognition on both sides of the Atlantic that the *inattention* symptom cluster is the greatest risk factor for neuropsychological dysfunction and academic impairments (Carlson and Maan, 2000; Chhabildas, Pennington and Willcutt, 2001; Marzocchi, Lucangeli, De Meo et al., 2002; Todd, Sitdhiraksa, Reich et al., 2002; Warner-Rogers et al., 2000). Notably, inattention symptoms are also accorded greater weight in the criteria for HD (at least six of nine symptoms in two or more settings), relative to those for hyperactivity (three of 6 symptom) and impulsivity (one of three symptoms), and relative to the DSM-IV criteria for ADHD.

Heterogeneity and comorbidity

Both the DSM-IV and ICD-10 recognize the marked heterogeneity in ADHD, but one of the most salient difference between these two diagnostic systems is the approach to diagnosis when more than one disorder coexists with ADHD/HD — a phenomenon known as 'comorbidity.' Numerous other psychiatric disorders and neurodevelopmental disorders co-exist with ADHD (and presumably HD). The DSM-IV recognizes all diagnoses that are present (except for schizophrenia and pervasive developmental disorder), whereas the ICD-10, in general, discourages multiple diagnoses. For example, the ICD-10 does not recommend the HD diagnosis in the presence of co-existing internalizing disorders, such as anxiety or mood disorders. The notable exception is the recognition by ICD-10 of comorbid HD and Conduct Disorder, which is labelled 'hyperkinetic conduct disorder.'

Estimates of comorbidity depend on the criteria used to define hyperactivity, the criteria used to define the other disorders, and the sample under study (e.g., clinical versus epidemiological). Comorbidity is the rule rather than the exception in ADHD, as was demonstrated in the Multi-Modal Treatment Study, in which only one-third of the 576 children were deemed to have 'pure' ADHD (Jensen, Hinshaw, Kraemer et al., 2001). Moreover, about 50% of individuals with ADHD meet criteria for at least two comorbid conditions (Szatmari et al., 1989). Oppositional defiant disorder is observed in 35–50% of cases, conduct disorder in 25%, depressive disorder in 15%, and anxiety disorders in 25–30% (Biederman, Newcorn and Sprich, 1991; Jensen, Martin and Cantwell, 1997). Learning disorders occur in 15–40% of children, and appear to be more closely associated with inattentive symptoms rather than with hyperactive/impulsive symptoms (Warner-Rogers et al., 2000; Willcutt, Pennington and DeFries, 2000). Receptive and expressive language impairments are observed in as many as 60% of cases, particularly if the definitions is broadened to include pragmatic disorders (i.e., impairments in the functional use of language) (reviewed by Baker and Cantwell, 1992; Tannock and Schachar, 1996). However, despite the marked overlap in the types of attentional symptoms observed in both schizophrenia and ADHD, the pattern of overlap between these disorders is unclear. For example, retrospective studies indicate that adults with schizophrenia often report a childhood history of many ADHD features, particularly symptoms of inattention (Elman, Sigler, Kroneberg et al., 1998; Gomez, Janowsky and Zetin, 1981), and that those with both current and childhood diagnosis of ADHD exhibited a more insidious course of schizophrenia, a less robust response to neuroleptics, and a poorer outcome, compared to adults with schizophrenia only (Elman et al., 1998). Also, an increased rate of ADHD features have been documented in the offspring of mothers with schizophrenia (Rieder and Nichols, 1979). By contrast, prospective studies have not found that ADHD per se increases the risk for developing schizophrenia (e.g., Biederman et al., 1996b; Rasmussen and Gillberg, 2000). However, continuity between severe behavioral symptoms of inattention in childhood and the negative symptoms or disorganized symptoms of schizophrenia in adulthood is a possibility that has yet to be explored.

Various subtyping approaches have been proposed, in addition to the DSM-IV phenomenological subtypes, in an attempt to identify more genetically homogeneous subtypes of ADHD than afforded by the current DSM-IV or ICD-10 classifications systems. These include the presence or absence of comorbid conditions, persistence of ADHD in young adulthood, familial ADHD, and subtypes derived from latent-class analysis (e.g., Faraone, Biederman and Friedman, 2000; Neuman, Todd, Heath et al., 1999; Todd, Rasmussen, Neuman et al., 2001; Todd et al., 2002). The high rates of comorbidity associated with ADHD (and in HD, although not recognized formally) poses major conceptual and methodological obstacles to attempts to delineate the neuropsychology of ADHD by starting from groups of affected individuals. Many studies have failed to measure or control for comorbidity, so that differences observed between ADHD and comparison groups could be attributable to the co-existing disorder rather than ADHD per se. This chapter considers possible moderating variables, such as comorbidity, age and gender, on the neuropsychological profile of ADHD. However, it is important to recognize that studies are likely to be sampling from overlapping but not identical populations of individuals with ADHD/HD, because the investigators have used different diagnostic criteria (DSM-IV versus ICD-10), obtained the diagnostic information from different informants, and used different approaches to aggregating information from multiple informants.

Etiology and pathophysiology of ADHD

The etiology and pathophysiology of ADHD remain unknown, but converging evidence implicates genetic factors, as well as various structural, functional, and neurochemical brain abnormalities (e.g., see reviews by Castellanos, 1997; Faraone and Doyle, 2000; Filipek, 1999; Levy and Hay, 2001; Swanson, Castellanos, Murias et al., 1998; Swanson, Posner, Cantwell et al., 1998; Swanson, Sergeant, Taylor et al., 1998; Tannock, 1998; Thapar, Holmes, Holmes et al., 1999). In brief, a range of family, adoption and twin studies have provided compelling evidence that genetic factors contribute a substantial portion of the phenotypic variance in the expression of ADHD, with most heritability estimates exceeding 0.70 (for reviews see Faraone and Doyle, 2000; Levy and Hay, 2001, Tannock, 1998). Moreover, preliminary evidence from twin studies suggests that inattentiveness and hyperactivity/impulsivity are genetically separable traits (Levy, McStephen and Hay, 2001; Neuman et al., 1999), which raises the possibility that these two dimensions of ADHD may be associated with different patterns of brain abnormalities (structural, functional, neurochemical) and neuropsychological impairments.

Molecular genetic studies of ADHD, which aim to identify allelic variations of specific genes that are functionally associated with the disorder, have focused on testing candidate genes linked to dopaminergic pathways because animals models, theoretical considerations, and the effectiveness of stimulant treatment, all implicate dopaminergic dysfunction in the pathophysiology of this disorder. On the one hand, studies based on this loosely formulated dopamine hypothesis (e.g., Castellanos, 1997; Levy, 1991) have been remarkably productive. For example, allelic variation in the dopamine transporter gene (*DAT1*) and the dopamine receptor D_4, have been replicated in several independent samples and laboratories (Cook, Stein, Krasowski et al., 1995; Faraone, 2002; Faraone, Doyle, Mick et al., 2001; Madras, Miller and Fischman, 2002; Swanson, Flodman, Kennedy et al., 2000). On the other hand, the effect sizes associated with these candidate alleles are modest, suggesting that the risk of manifesting ADHD appears to be increased by about 20% to 40% for individuals carrying the putative susceptibility genes (Faraone, 2002). Also implicated in ADHD are catechol-*O*-methyl-transferase (COMT), which is an enzyme that metabolizes released dopamine (particularly in prefrontal cortex where dopamine reuptake proteins are sparse) and SNAP-25, which is a synaptic protein involved in the controlled release of neurotransmitters (e.g., Barr, Feng, Wigg et al., 2000; Eisenberg, Mei-Tal, Steinberg et al., 1999; Mill, Curran, Kent et al., 2002). However, findings are inconsistent and each of these candidate gene polymorphisms are widely distributed in the population and many are also associated with other psychiatric disorders (e.g., schizophrenia), suggesting they are not specific to ADHD. Moreover, the first genome-wide scan for loci involved in ADHD failed to confirm many of these candidate genes but identifed genetic linkage on Chromosome 16p13 in a region implicated in autism (Fisher, Francks, McCracken et al, 2002; Smalley, Kustanovich, Minassian et al, 2002), suggesting that additional strategies and methods will be required to identify susceptibility and protective genes of complex behavioral traits such as ADHD, schizophrenia and autism.

Neuroimaging studies provide converging evidence of dysfunction and dysregulation of cerebellar–striatal–prefrontal circuits that are rich in dopaminergic innervation (e.g., Castellanos, 2001). For example, quantitative studies of total brain volume and regional brain volumes using magnetic resonance imaging (MRI) have consistently reported smaller volumes or (areas) of the right prefrontal brain regions, striatum (caudate nucleus, globus pallidus), cerebellar hemispheres, and even more robustly diminished volumes in the posterior–inferior cerebellar vermis (lobules VIII–X) (for reviews, see Castellanos, 2001; Filipek, 1999; Giedd, Blumenthal, Molloy et al., 2001; Tannock, 1998). Notably, the posterior–inferior vermis is the only region in the cerebellum that receives dense dopaminergic innervation (Melchitzky and Lewis, 2000). Moreover, human functional brain imaging studies have documented the sensitivity of the cerebellum, and particularly the vermis, to the effects of psychostimulants (Anderson, Polcari, Lowen et al., 2002; Ernst, Zametkin, Matochik et al., 1997; Schweitzer, Lee, Ely et al., 1998; Volkow, Wang, Fowler et al., 1997). Functional imaging studies using functional magnetic resonance imaging (fMRI), positron emission tomography (PET), also point to functional differences in prefrontal cortex and striatum, although findings have not been consistent (e.g., both under- and over-activation of these brain regions in ADHD relative to controls; Rubia, Overmeyer, Taylor et al., 1999; Vaidya, Austin, Kirkorian et al., 1998). Electrophysiological studies also agree that ADHD involves hypofunction of the catecholaminergic circuits, particularly those projecting to the prefrontal cortex. Cortical slowing and problems in central arousal patterns and underreactivity to stimulation has also been reported in recent electrophysiological studies using quantitative electroencephalography (QEEG) or event-related potentials (ERP) (Klorman, 1991; Lazzaro, Gordon, Li et al., 1999; Monastra, Lubar, Linden, 2000; Monastra, Lubar, Linden et al., 1999). Moreover, several studies using single photon emitted computed tomography (SPECT) techniques with small samples (approximately 10 adults with ADHD) have reported increased density of the dopamine transporter in the striatum, even in those who had not received any stimulant treatment (Dougherty, Bonab, Spencer et al., 1999; Krause, Dresel, Krause et al., 2000), although this was not replicated in another more recent study (Van Dyck, Quinlan, Cretella et al., 2002) and may differ across gender (Mozley, Gur, Mozley et al., 2001).

There is emerging consensus that cortico-striatal-thalamo-cortical circuits are involved in the selection, initiation and execution of complex cognitive and motor responses, and that cerebellar circuits participate in on-line guidance of these functions (e.g., Graybiel, 1998; Jueptner and Weiller, 1998). Thus, it is reasonable to speculate that a variety of genetic polymorphisms lead to brain abnormalities in the cerebello-striatal-prefrontal circuitry, which in turn may underlie the neuropsychological deficits in attention and executive function associated with ADHD. It is further speculated that the cerebellar vermis exerts important regulatory influences on the prefrontal–striatal circuitry via the ventral tegmental area and locus ceruleus (Castellanos and Tannock, 2002). However, most of these brain-imaging studies to date have involved small and heterogenous groups of individuals with ADHD and have been descriptive with the primary goal of detecting differences between the ADHD group and a control group. Theoretically motivated studies involving larger and more homogeneous groups of individuals with ADHD who have not been treated with psychopharmacological agents are needed.

Neuropsychological models of ADHD

The imperative to delineate the genetic and environmental risk factors for ADHD is motivating the search for quantifiable intermediate constructs, termed *endophenotypes* (Almasy and Blangero, 2001). Endophenotypes are heritable quantitative traits that index an individual's liability to develop or manifest a given disease (e.g., serum cholesterol level predicts the risk of cardiovascular disease). As such, they are presumed to be more directly related to etiological factors than to dichotomous diagnostic categories, such as ADHD (Almasy and Blangero, 2001; Morton and Frith, 1995). Accordingly, the past decade has witnessed a shift from a reliance of purely clinical and descriptive approaches to the development of theoretical accounts of ADHD and potential cognitive endophenotypes. One type of account emphasizes executive attention, particularly inhibitory control of behavioral responses (Barkley, 1997a; Nigg, 2001; Quay, 1988, 1997), whereas another incorporates selective, sustained and executive attention (Swanson et al., 1998b). A third type of account focuses on control over allocation of resources over time (energetic factors) (Sergeant, 2000; Todd and Botteron, 2001), whereas yet another account de-emphasizes attention per se and instead highlights motivational factors such as delay aversion or altered reward mechanisms (Sonuga-Barke, 1994, 2002). These various theoretical models of ADHD are summarized below.

Executive attention models of ADHD

Several influential accounts highlight the putative role of inhibitory dysfunction in ADHD (Barkley, 1997a, 2001; Nigg, 2001; Quay, 1988, 1997). Quay's (1988) account is based upon the formulations of Gray (1982) regarding the functioning of two conceptually distinct brain systems: the behavioral inhibition and behavioral activation systems. Problem behavior associated with ADHD is presumed to arise from an underactive inhibition system, whereas Conduct Disorder is associated with an underactive behavioral inhibition system in combination with an overactive activation system (Quay, 1997). Barkley (1997a, 2001) proposes that behavioral inhibition is the *primary* deficit (and a potential endophenotype) for ADHD, which in turn gives rise to secondary impairments in four other executive neuropsychological abilities that are dependent upon behavioral inhibition for their effective execution (Barkley, 1997a,b, 2001). The four executive functions are (i) nonverbal working memory; (ii) verbal working memory; (iii) self-regulation of affect–motivation–arousal; and (iv) reconstitution (Barkley, 2001). This model is not assumed to apply to the subtype of ADHD characterized exclusively by inattention — currently classified as the predominantly inattentive type in the DSM-IV (American Psychiatric Association, 1994). For example, Barkley (1997a) proposes that the type of inattention manifested by the inattentive subtype (typically characterized as daydreaming, spacey, easily confused, in a fog, staring) most likely reflect deficits in speed of information processing and in focused or selective attention. Accordingly, it is presumed to be qualitatively different from the type of inattention manifested by the combined type of ADHD, which is presumed to reflect problems in sustained attention (persistence) and distractibility.

Behavioral inhibition is a multidimensional construct. Barkley (1997a) proposes three interrelated but somewhat distinct processes, which are (1) the ability to inhibit a 'prepotent' response (i.e., a response associated with positive or negative reinforcement) to a stimulus or event so as to create a delay in responding; (2) the ability stop an ongoing response that is rendered inappropriate or inaccurate by sudden or unexpected changes in task demands (i.e., a sensitivity to error); and (3) interference control, which is conceptualized as the sustained protection of a response from disruption by competing events and responses (interference control or resistance to distraction) (Barkley, 1997b). Individuals with ADHD are assumed to show a deficiency in all three of these interrelated aspects of inhibition. An alternate conceptualization of inhibition (Nigg, 2001) distinguishes between *executive processes of inhibition* (deliberate suppression of thought or action to achieve an internally represented goal), *motivational processes of inhibition* (cessation of response or behavior driven largely by anxiety, fear, or uncertainty), and *automatic processes* (suppression of response that proceeds without effort or controlled processing). Nigg (2001) proposes that ADHD is due to such deficits in *executive* processes of inhibition.

Attentional network model of ADHD

Another neuropsychological account (Swanson et al., 1991), which relates ADHD to disorders of attentional systems, is based upon a current theory of attention that proposes distinct neural networks for three component cognitive processes of attention: alerting, orienting, and executive control (Posner, 1978; Posner and Petersen, 1990; Posner and Raichle, 1994). Posner and colleagues have proposed that *alerting*, which refers to the suppression of background neural noise by inhibiting ongoing or irrelevant activity to establish *sustained attention* and be ready to act, is supported primarily by the right dorsolateral prefrontal cortex. By contrast, *orienting,* which is supported primarily by posterior parietal lobes, consists of mobilizing specific neural resources to prepare to establish *selective inhibition*

TABLE 3

Alignment of symptom clusters, attention systems, and neural networks (Swanson et al., 1998b) [a]

Symptom clusters	Attention systems	Neural networks
Inattention-alerting Difficulty sustaining attention Fails to finish Avoids sustained effort	Alerting (sustained attention)	Right frontal
Inattention-orienting Easily distracted Does not seem to listen Fails to give close attention	Orienting (selective attention)	Posterior parietal
Hyperactive/impulsive Blurts out answers Interrupts or intrudes Can't wait turn	Executive control (executive attention)	Anterior cingulate

[a] Modified from Swanson et al., 1998b, Table 20.2.

(e.g., by covert disengagement, shifting, and engaging attention in response to internal or external cues signalling the type of processing required). Whereas, *executive control,* supported by an anterior cingulate network, establishes *divided attention* (by resolving conflict among multiple mental processes and responses). One novel and potentially useful approach in this theoretical formulation is the attempt to link specific clusters of symptoms of ADHD rather than the disorder itself (i.e., the categorical diagnostic entity) with the cognitive processes and neural networks (see Table 3). Clearly, these are testable predictions. Moreover, this approach gives rise to the possibility that individuals with ADHD may exhibit deficits in one, two or all three of the component processes, which would accommodate the marked heterogeneity in the manifestation of ADHD as well as the inconsistencies in findings across studies of specific cognitive deficits associated with the categorical diagnosis of ADHD.

Energetic models of ADHD

The cognitive-energetic model of information processing proposed by Sergeant and colleagues (Sergeant, 2000; Sergeant, Oosterlaan and Van der Meere, 1999; Sergeant and Van der Meere, 1990a) questions that the fundamental problem in ADHD concerns the ability to inhibit responses or involves impairments in attention per se. Rather, as summarized below, it proposes that primary problems in other moderating systems, such as activation or effort, give rise to or contribute to downstream problems in inhibitory control that are observed in ADHD (Sergeant, 2000). This model, which is derived from theories proposed by Pribram and McGuiness (1975), Sanders (1983) and Tucker and Williamson (1984), proposes that the overall efficiency of information processing is determined by both *structural processes* (operations that mediate between stimulus and response, such as stimulus encoding, memory search) and *energetic mechanisms* (effort, arousal, activation) factors, as well as a higher-order management or evaluation mechanism that resembles the more recent construct of executive function. *Arousal* is defined as phasic responding that alerts sensory activity and is time-locked to stimulus processing. Arousal is generally believed to be a right-lateralized process linked with noradrenergic neural networks that respond to stimulus input and enhance the signal-to-noise ration for novelty detection. *Activation* is a left-lateralized process that entails activation of dopaminergic networks. It implicates tonic changes in physiological activity associated with basal ganglia and corpus striatum and is concerned with control of motor readiness (i.e., motor preparation for response output). *Effort* is conceptualized as the required energy to meet the demands of a task and it is influenced by motivational factors such as knowledge of results, pay-off, self-regulation versus external regulation (Pribram and McGuiness, 1975; Sanders, 1983). It is thought to involve a hippocampal system that regulates the balance between arousal and activation. Moreover, different neurotransmitters are associated with the arousal and activation systems: Noradrenaline and serotonin are the primary neurotransmitters in the arousal system, whereas dopamine and acetylcholine are involved in the activation system (Tucker and Williamson, 1984). In experimental studies, arousal, activation, and effort are often indexed by psychophysiological measures, such as increased heart rate, heart-rate deceleration prior to an anticipated go-stimulus, and reduction of heart rate variability, respectively. According to this cognitive-energetic model, the observed problems in inhibition and in motor-response processes in ADHD that manifest typically as slow-inaccurate responding, reflect an underlying dysfunction in energetic (state) mechanisms, particularly in the effort or activation components (e.g., Sergeant, 2000; Van der Meere, 1996). Thus, in terms of the cognitive-energetic model, disinhibition observed in ADHD results from inadequate *activation* of the inhibitory mechanism — it is viewed as a secondary or 'downstream' problem rather than a primary deficit.

By contrast to the preceding energetic model, a recent biologically-based energetic deficiency model of ADHD relates inattention and impulsivity to hypoactivity of catecholamine projection pathways to prefrontal cortical areas, which results in decreased availability of neuronal energy (Todd and Botteron, 2001). Currently, it is believed that the regulation of neuronal activity-dependent energy metabolism is largely controlled by cortical astrocytes (Magistretti and Pellerin, 1999). Cortical astrocytes (positioned between capillaries and cortical neurons) have active transport mechanisms for neurotransmitters, such as glutamate, dopamine, and noradrenaline, which suggests an important role in the termination of neurotransmitter activity via uptake of neurotransmitters released within the synapse. Also, astrocytes take up and convert glucose from blood capillaries to either lactate for immediate use by neurons or to glycogen for long-term storage, and have receptors for a variety of neurotransmitters (including catecholamines), which play active roles in adjusting the availability of energy to neurons via the regulation of glycogenolysis and glycogen synthesis in the astrocytes (Magistretti and Pellerin, 1999). The hypothesis that a disruption of astrocyte-mediated neuronal energy transfer results in decreased and disorganized neuronal function in prefrontal cortical areas is compatible with current genetic findings and evidence of structural and functional brain changes in ADHD, but has yet to be tested.

Motivational accounts

The 'delay aversion model' challenges the preceding interpretations of poor behavioral inhibition as an underlying *cognitive deficit* (e.g., Sonuga-Barke, 1994, 2002). According to this model, it is not the case that children with ADHD are deficient in some psychological (e.g., inhibitory) process. Rather, the model proposes that ADHD is a functional expression of an aversion to time delays (waiting) that is manifested as a desire to escape or avoid delay and reflects *deviance in terms of motivational attitude.* The central construct is a specific aversion to delaying or suppressing responses over time. This aversion is often (but not invariantly) manifest by the choice of smaller immediate rewards rather than larger rewards given later. In contexts that do not permit such choice or in which no choice exists, aversion to delay may also be manifest by attending to non-temporal stimuli within the environment, so that aversion to delay is independent of a preference for immediate reward (Sonuga-Barke, Houlberg and Hall, 1994; Sonuga-Barke, Williams, Hall et al., 1996). In contrast to the neuropsychological models, the delay-aversion formulation is based on analysis of the situational contexts in which children's ADHD symptoms are manifest. In other words, the symptom domains of inattention and impulsivity/hyperactivity can both be conceived as situation-specific attempts to reduce the subjective perception or experience of the delay (Sonuga-Barke, Taylor and Heppenstall, 1992a). In some situations children with ADHD can wait for rewards, even when this requires inhibition, whereas in other situations that do not require inhibition, they will not wait for rewards (Sonuga-Barke et al., 1994, 1996).

A related model is that of *temporal discounting and altered reward mechanisms*, which refers to the extent to which an individual reduces the values of consequences as a function of aversion is thought to be an acquired characteristic (behavioral manifestation) arising from deficits in a biologically-based alteration in reward mechanisms that have been studied extensively in model systems (Schultz, 2001). According to this model, the key behavioral features of ADHD result from dysfunctioning of one of the main branches of the dopamine system (meso-limbo-cortical branch), which alters reinforcement mechanisms and a *shortened delay-of-reinforcement gradient* (Sagvolden, Aase, Zeiner et al., 1998). The latter phenomenon is manifest by a faster decline in the effectiveness of reinforcement as a function of increasing delay between the behavior and reward (Johansen, Aase, Meyer et al., 2002; Sagvolden et al., 1998). The meso-limbo-cortical branch originates in the ventral tegmental area and projects to the prefrontal cortex, nucleus accumbens, and olfactory tubercle. A preference for small immediate rewards over larger delayed rewards has been associated with lesions in the core of the nucleus accumbens (Cardinal, Pennicott, Sugathapala et al., 2001). Intriguingly, fMRI studies suggest that reward anticipation and outcomes may differentially recruit distinct regions that lie along the trajectory of ascending dopamine projections (Knutson, Adams, Fong et al., 2001a; Knutson, Fong, Adams et al., 2001b). For example, both the nucleus accumbens and cerebellar vermis are selectively activated in healthy adults while they were *anticipating* a reward, whereas reward outcomes activated foci in the ventromedial frontal cortex (Knutson et al., 2001a,b). Anatomical studies have not yet been able to measure the volume of the nucleus accumbens in ADHD, but the most prominent decreases in volume are in the posterior–inferior lobules of the cerebellar vermis (Berquin, Giedd, Jacobsen et al., 1998; Castellanos, Giedd, Berquin et al., 2001; Mostofsky, Reiss, Lockhart et al., 1998). Both phasic and tonic dopamine activities are thought to play major roles in reinforcement and extinction processes (Schultz, 1998), For example, reinforcement is associated with dopamine release in the nucleus accumbens, particularly when reinforcement is unpredictable, associated with higher values, or occurs earlier than predicted (Schultz, 1998). Thus, if tonic dopamine levels are reduced in limbic brain regions in ADHD as suggested (e.g., Grace, 2000; Max, Fox, Lancaster et al., 2002), then an increased release of dopamine during phasic activation would be required in order to affect a sufficient number of dopamine-receptor associated ion channels for reinforcement to take place.

Integrative accounts

Each of the preceding theoretical approaches has clearly advanced understanding of ADHD by stimulating research in areas not previously considered. However, each implies that ADHD is a single entity with a single-cause, and the concern is whether disinhibition in ADHD is primary and gives rise to other regulatory problems such as arousal, (Barkley, 1997a), sensitivity to reward (Sonuga-Barke, 1994), or whether it is a secondary feature arising from decreased energetic mechanisms (Sergeant, 2000). One unintended consequence of these single-cause approaches is that the diagnostic category of ADHD has been reified "as an ontological and psychological reality, rather than just a useful clinical construct" (Sonuga-Barke, 2002, p. 29). However, the marked heterogeneity in the clinical expression of ADHD makes it unlikely that ADHD is a unitary construct or that any single unified account will be possible. Thus, the recent presentations of integrative accounts that emphasize the multifactorial etiology and multidimensional nature of ADHD (Castellanos and Tannock, 2002; Pochon, Levy, Fossati et al., 2002; Sonuga-Barke, 2002) are timely and amenable to integrative collaborative approaches that aim to uncover the causes of various components of the clinical construct currently termed 'ADHD.'

One example is the recent *dual-pathway* model (Sonuga-Barke, 2002) that proposes two distinct subtypes of ADHD, which are distinguished at the level of symptoms, cognitive and motivational profiles, genetic and non-genetic origins. One subtype is thought to be characterized by dysregulation of thought and action, resulting from poor inhibitory control associated with the meso-*cortical* branch of the dopamine system projecting to the prefrontal cortex; the other subtype is characterized by an altered delay of reward gradient linked with the meso-*limbic* branch of the dopamine system associated with reward circuits in the nucleus accumbens (Sonuga-Barke, 2002). This dual-pathway model is compatible with a recent neuroscience formulation that postulates that although motivational and cognitive processes are mediated by different neural networks, a specific neural system should exist to link these two essential processes, to reach maximal efficiency (Pochon et al., 2002). Preliminary support for this model is provided by the findings from a small-scale study using fMRI to study brain activation patterns in normal adults performing a working memory task with varying cognitive load that was associated with different levels of monetary reward. The results suggested a balance between activation in cortical cognitive areas and deactivation in the limbic system during ongoing cognitive processing, with the latter representing emotional gating function necessary to maximize the level of cognitive performance (Pochon et al., 2002). This model suggests that dysfunction in any one or more of the component pathways (cognitive, motivational, bridging) would likely result in inefficient cognitive processing and/or emotional dysregulation – which are characteristic of ADHD.

A second example of an integrative account, which is also rooted in the neurosciences, is the recent proposition by Castellanos and Tannock (2002) that multiple etiological factors (e.g., genetic variations, environmental factors as well as gene–gene and gene–environment interactions) are the initial causes of the multiple conditions or dimensions that manifest symptomatically as ADHD. By contrast to many of the preceding accounts, this reconceptualization of ADHD as an interrelated set of clinical conditions with multiple etiologies is rooted in a developmental causal model (Morton and Frith, 1995) in which an endophenotype underlying one or more of the behavioral characteristics of ADHD may arise from several possible causative brain abnormalities resulting from various etiological factors, such as genetic polymorphisms, environmental factors, and gene–environment interactions. Three endophenotypes, in addition to response inhibition, are proposed: a specific abnormality in reward-related circuitry that leads to shortened delay gradients, deficits in temporal processing that result in high intrasubject intertrial variability, and deficits in working memory that lead to impaired visual–spatial attention and distractibility (Castellanos and Tannock, 2002). For example, Fig. 1 presents a schematic causal model of working memory impairments as a candidate endophenotype of the deficits in executive attention and selective attention that are manifested by observable behavioral symptoms of impulsivity and distractibility in ADHD. This figure also illustrates how working memory deficits (perhaps arising from different brain abnormalities and/or different etiological factors) may be an endophenotype of the phonemic awareness deficits associated with the observed decoding difficulties in dyslexia. Thus, this developmental causal model approach demonstrates how neural factors and endophenotypes are likely to cut across neurodevelopmental disorders and provides one explanation for the high rates of comorbidity in ADHD.

Impairments in attention in ADHD: empirical support

A vast number of neuropsychological studies of ADHD might all be relevant to a broad consideration of attentional disorders in ADHD. Here, only studies pertaining to the three main conceptualizations of attention (selective, executive, sustained) and altered reward mechanisms are reviewed for the purpose of evaluating the extant empirical support for each of the theoretical models of ADHD described previously. Existing reviews (e.g., Barkley, 1997b; Nigg, 2001; Oosterlaan, Logan and Sergeant, 1998; Pennington and Ozonoff, 1996; Sergeant, Geurts and Oosterlaan, 2002) are recommended for more detailed and itemized discussion of the studies.

Selective attention

Results of selective attention studies in ADHD have been mixed, in part because of the diversity of methods used to assess the construct. Subtle deficits in selective visual attention (particularly in the right hemisphere) in ADHD are suggested by the burgeoning literature on covert orienting of attention that have used spatial cueing paradigms to investigate covert shifts in allocation of visual attention across space in the absence of saccadic eye movements (Castellanos et al., 2000; McDonald, Bennett, Chambers et al., 1999; Mostofsky, Lasker, Cutting et al., 2001; Nigg, Swanson and Hinshaw, 1997; Novak, Solanto and Abkoff, 1995; Pearson, Yaffee, Love-

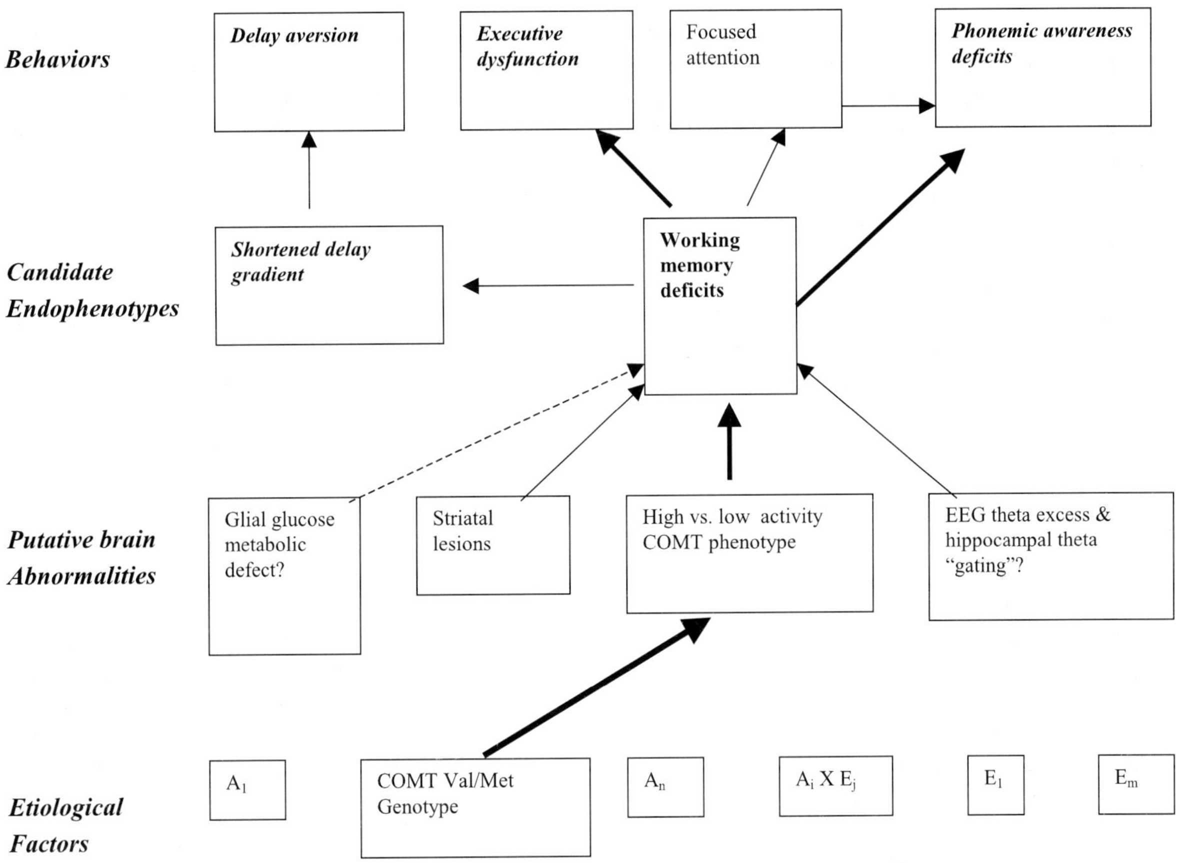

Fig. 1. Schematic causal developmental model (adapted from Castellanos and Tannock, 2002) for working memory as a candidate endophenotype, with impairments in selective attention, executive attention, phonemic awareness and/or delay aversion and as the primary behavioral manifestations, and a functional polymorphism in the catechol-*O*-methyltransferase gene (which results in a four-fold difference in dopamine catabolic efficiency and predicts working memory performance and cerebral activation patterns), as one possible causative factor. Arrows with heavy lines indicate substantial empirical support for that link; standard lines indicate preliminary support for the link; dotted lines indicate potential but unsubstantiated links. $A_{1\text{-}n}$ = additive genetic factors; COMT = catechol-*O*-methyl transferase; $E_{i\text{-}m}$ = environmental factors; $A_i \times E_j$ = gene-environment interaction.

land et al., 1995; Swanson et al., 1991; Tannock, Schachar and Logan, 1995). Evidence of orienting deficits using these paradigms is consistent with the evidence of orienting deficits during performance on the stop-signal and CPT paradigms that are purported measures of response inhibition and sustained attention, respectively (Brandeis, Van Leeuwen, Rubia et al., 1998; Van Leeuwen, Steinhausen, Overtoom et al., 1998). The finding of similar impairments in biological parents is of particular interest, suggesting the influence of genetic factors (Nigg et al., 1997). However, inconsistencies of findings across studies and across child and parent samples do not allow firm conclusions.

Executive attention: inhibition deficits

A wide variety of theoretically distinct tasks have been used to measure different aspects of inhibitory control in ADHD (Kramer, Humphrey, Larish et al., 1994; Nigg, 2001). However, many of these tasks measure multiple related processes, but are not equivalent in terms of their ability to separate inhibition from the other processes.

Inhibition of prepotent responses

Support for deficits in this aspect of inhibition in ADHD comes from experimental studies using the basic (non-motivational) go/no–go task and inhibition versions of continuous performance tasks. These tasks establish a dominant response set by making most trials go-trials that require a response, which must be inhibited on the relatively rare no-go trials. Extensive neuroimaging data support the notion that different brain regions mediate performance on the no-go trials and go-trials, with most studies indicating preferential activation of the prefrontal cortex on the no-go trials (Casey, Trainor, Orendi et al., 1997; Vaidya et al., 1998; Yong, Robaey, Karayanidis et al., 2000). Most studies report an excess of no-go errors (commission errors) in the ADHD samples compared to normal control groups, which is interpreted as evidence of deficits in the ability to inhibit prepotent responses (e.g., see reviews by Pennington and Ozonoff, 1996; Sergeant et al., 2002). Moreover, no-go errors observed in a non-clinical sample of preschoolers were related to teacher ratings of ADHD symptoms, even after controlling for concurrent symptoms of conduct disorder (Berlin and Bohlin, 2002). By contrast, the correlation between response inhibition and conduct problems was not significant when partialling out the effects of ADHD symptoms, suggesting specificity of this inhibition deficit to ADHD (Berlin and Bohlin, 2002). However, since this method cannot functionally isolate inhibition, the failure to inhibit a response on a no-go trial could be due to strong prepotent go-processes, not disinhibition (Schachar, Tannock and Logan, 1993).

Inhibition of ongoing response

One approach used widely throughout North America and Europe is the stop signal paradigm that is based on a well-established theory of response inhibition and purports to measure the ability to stop a planned or ongoing thought and action (Logan, 1994). The stop-signal task requires subjects to respond as quickly and accurately as possible to a primary task (typically a visual choice reaction time task), but to withhold their response to that primary task when presented with an infrequent and unpredictable stop signal (usually a tone). The intervals between the onset of the primary-task stimulus and the stop signal are varied to allow an estimation of the latency of the inhibitory process (known as stop-signal reaction time; SSRT). Data from studies using mathematical modeling, psychophysiological measures (e.g., event-related potentials, lateralized readiness potential), and neuroimaging methods (fMRI) are consistent with the claim that this method separates response output and inhibitory processes (Logan and Cowan, 1984; Rubia et al., 1999a; Van Boxtel, Van der Molen, Jennings et al., 2001).

Virtually all of the 27 stop-signal studies (i.e., with the exception of Kuntsi, Oosterlaan and Stevenson, 2001; Scheres, Oosterlaan and Sergeant, 2001) published to date have reported longer SSRTs in ADHD, indicating a markedly slower inhibitory process compared to controls (Bedard, Ickowicz, Logan et al., 2002; Chhabildas et al., 2001; Epstein, Johnson, Varia et al., 2001; Konrad, Gauggel, Manz et al., 2000b; Manassis, Tannock and Barbosa, 2001; Murphy, 2002; Nigg, Butler, Huang-Pollock et al., 2002; Overtoom, Kenemans, Verbaten et al., 2002; Rubia, Oosterlaan, Sergeant et al., 1998; Rucklidge and Tannock, 2002; Solanto, Abikoff, Sonuga-Barke et al., 2001; also see studies reviewed by Nigg, 2001; Oosterlaan et al., 1998; and Sergeant et al., 2002). Findings of impaired stop-signal inhibition remain robust across various versions of the task using different stimuli, across international laboratories that involve clinical and non-clinical samples of ADHD defined by DSM-III, DSM-III-R, and DSM-IV, across males and females, and across children, adolescents and adults. Most of these studies report an average effect size of about 0.6 (effect size correlation; Cohen, 1988) for the difference in speed of the inhibitory process between ADHD and normal comparison groups (for meta-analyses, see Oosterlaan et al., 1998; Sergeant et al., 2002). Moreover, the preliminary evidence that those children with ADHD who are slow to inhibit are more likely to have first-degree relatives with ADHD, suggests that impaired stop-signal inhibition may provide a potentially useful endophenotype (Crosbie and Schachar, 2001). However, several issues challenge the interpretation that this type of inhibition is a primary deficit in ADHD. First, in addition to the slow inhibitory process, most studies also document slow and highly variable response times to the go-task, with the effect size for the latter being comparable in magnitude to that for the inhibition deficits. For example, two recent studies found that the variability of the go-task response was the strongest predictor of ADHD (Kuntsi et al., 2001; Scheres et al., 2001). These findings not only suggest that it is not an overly strong prepotent go-process that accounts for inhibitory dysfunction (because of this were the case, the go-task response would be fast) but also implicate additional impairments in ADHD. Second, deficits in stop-signal inhibition have been observed in a variety of other disorders, including high functioning autism (Ozonoff and Strayer, 1997), dyslexia (Purvis and Tannock, 2000; Sloot, Licht, Horsley et al., 2000), Tourette syndrome (Johannes, Wieringa, Mantey et al., 2001), traumatic brain injury (Konrad et al., 2000b) and epilepsy (Chevalier, Metz-Lutz and Segalowitz, 2000). Third, typically the inclusion of motivational factors (reinforcements) have been found to eliminate inhibitory control problems in ADHD (Konrad et al., 2000a; Oosterlaan et al., 1998; Slusarek, Velling, Bunk et al., 2001). Notably, a recent study of this type of inhibition during videogame play documented impairments in working memory and other executive functions, but no deficits in inhibition of an ongoing and prepotent response (Lawrence, Houghton, Tannock et al., 2002). By contrast to use of external reinforcement in studies of stop-signal inhibition, videogames are not only intrinsically motivating, but also they developmentally appropriate and are part of children's everyday world.

Interference control

Several reviews have concluded that children with ADHD show greater Stroop interference than comparison groups, which has been interpreted as further support for inhibitory models of ADHD (e.g., Barkley, 1997b; Pennington and Ozonoff, 1996; Sergeant et al., 2002). However, upon closer inspection of this literature, the findings of interference control problems are equivocal. For example, many of the studies that reported Stroop deficits in ADHD reported impairments in the color-word condition, but did not control for the observed impairments in basic naming speed (as measured by the color condition) or reading ability (reflected by performance on the word condition). Studies that have controlled for speed of word reading and color naming have generally failed to find deficits in interference control (e.g., Houghton, Douglas, West et al., 1999; Lawrence et al., 2002; Rucklidge and Tannock, 2002; Willcutt, Pennington, Boada et al., 2001). Moreover, recent evidence that patients with frontal lobe damage exhibit color naming problems on the Stroop, but not greater interference effects (Stuss, Floden, Alexander et al., 2001), suggests either that interference control is not associated with frontal lobe dysfunction or that the Stroop measure of interference control is not sensitive to frontal lobe dysfunction. Recent attempts to explain the Stroop effect suggest that inhibitory control involves memory retrieval processes (Tipper, 2001), and neural activation (MacLeod and MacDonald, 2000).

Inhibition of saccadic eye-movements

Recently, the control of saccadic eye-movements (inhibition of reflexive eye movements and generation of voluntary eye movements) has been investigated as a potential diagnostic marker for various disorders that have been linked with the frontal cortex and basal ganglia, including ADHD (Everling and Fischer, 1998; Munoz et al., 1999; Ross, Hommer, Breiger et al., 1994; Rothlind, Posner and Schaughency, 1991). The limited data available from studies that used different versions of the anti-saccade task, suggest that children with ADHD have more difficulty in accurately controlling visual fixation and in suppressing unwanted saccades compared to controls (Munoz et al., 1999; Ross et al., 1994; Ross, Harris, Olincy et al., 2000; Rothlind et al., 1991). However, numerous clinical populations exhibit difficulties inhibiting reflexive saccades, including schizophrenia, Alzheimer's disease, amyotrophic lateral sclerosis, Huntington's, dyslexia, but not affective disorders, although poor performance may be due to deficits in different underlying subprocesses (Tannock et al., 1995). Furthermore, findings from one study that incorporated ERP measures with the stop signal paradigm, suggested that slow inhibitory processes associated with ADHD could be determined by impairments in the initial orienting of attention, rather than reflecting poor response inhibition per se (Brandeis et al., 1998).

Working memory

Impairments in working memory are predicted by current ADHD theory (e.g., Barkley, 1997a; Levy and Farrow, 2001), but two recent reviews conclude that working memory is not impaired in ADHD (Pennington and Ozonoff, 1996; Welsh, 2002). However, most of the studies included in those reviews focused primarily on auditory–verbal working memory and neither the reviews not the studies therein considered the need to control for comorbid learning disorders, which are themselves associated with working memory impairments. This literature now includes more studies on visual–spatial working memory, which provide stronger evidence for impairments in this aspect of working memory, even after controlling for comorbid learning disorders (e.g., Barnett, Maruff, Vance et al., 2001; Brito, Pereira and Santos-Morales, 1999; Karatekin and Asarnow, 1998a; Kempton, Vance, Maruff et al., 1999; Mariani and Barkley, 1997; Nigg et al., 2002; Williams, Stott, Goodyer et al., 2000). However, preliminary evidence suggests that visual spatial working memory impairments may not be characteristic of ADHD in general, but rather are associated with a more refined behavioral phenotype defined by the presence of pervasive and clinically-severe symptoms of inattention (Martinussen, Bedard, Ickowicz et al., 2002).

Sustained attention (vigilance)

Sustained attention has been measured with a variety of continuous performance tests (CPT) methods that yield measures of response times as well as 'hits' and 'false alarms' (Corkum and Siegel, 1993; Losier, McGrath and Klein, 1996; Sergeant and Van der Meere, 1990a; Van der Meere, 1996). In general, ADHD is associated with inefficient performance (slow, inaccurate) and vigilance decrements (faster than normal decline in performance) that occur with increased demand for effortful processing (Sergeant and Van der Meere, 1990b; Van der Meere, 1996). These impairments in sustained attention are evident across the life span (preschool through adulthood) regardless of comorbidity, but findings are influenced strongly by temporal parameters (interstimulus interval, trial length etc.), stimulus modality, memory load, and context (presence/absence of experimenter, rewards) (Chee, Logan, Schachar et al., 1989; Corkum and Siegel, 1993; Halperin et al., 1991; Losier et al., 1996; Sergeant and Van der Meere, 1990b; Van der Meere, 1996). However, performance impairments on vigilance tasks are exhibited by a wide range of clinical populations, which once again challenges the notion of specificity for ADHD per se (Corkum and Siegel, 1993; Purcell, Maruff, Hyrios et al., 1998). Moreover, according to a recent investigation, performance impairments on an inhibition version of the CPT were associated with RD (reading disability) and not with ADHD (McGee et al., 2000). Furthermore, findings from a recent study that incorporated measures of event-related brain potentials (ERPs) of the electroencephalogram to reveal neurophysiological correlates of poor performance, suggested that the poor performance of children with ADHD (i.e., detection of fewer signals, more false alarms) may be attributable to impairments in preparatory processing of the stimuli (i.e., in orienting to the stimuli), rather than to impairments in later stages of executive-level processing of the stimuli (Van Leeuwen et al., 1998).

Aversion to delay and altered reward mechanisms

Most studies on aversion to delay in ADHD/HD have focused on the willingness to wait for delayed rewards and events. The general finding is that children with ADHD/HD are more likely than controls to choose a small, immediate rewards (e.g., 1 point after 3 s) rather than a larger delayed reward (e.g., 2 points after 30 s) (see review by Sonuga-Barke, 2002). Findings have been replicated in independent laboratories and hold for ADHD and HD (e.g., Kuntsi et al., 2001; Solanto et al., 2001a; Sonuga-Barke et al., 1992a; Sonuga-Barke, Taylor, Sembi et al., 1992b). Aversion to delay is related to longer serial response times (Sonuga-Barke and Taylor, 1992), shorter latency to response on the Matching Familiar Figures Test (Sonuga-Barke et al., 1994), shorter self-selected stimulus exposure times and worse memory recognition (Sonuga-Barke et al., 1992a). Moreover, greater locomotor activity in children with ADHD than in controls was observed only when delays became unavoidable, suggesting that high levels of motor activity and fidgetiness might represent compensatory behavior (Antrop, Roeyers, Van Oost et al., 2000). A recent comparison of aversion to delay and stop-signal inhibition in a large sample of children with ADHD-Combined Type found evidence for both delay aversion and inhibitory deficits, but that children's performance on the key measures from these two tasks was not correlated. This provides preliminary evidence for the independence of the two constructs and suggests that multiple pathways lead to the behavioral symptoms of ADHD/HD.

The pattern of findings suggests that overall delay (as reflected in session length), rather than reward parameters per se (magnitude, rate, pre-reward delay), is the key motivating factor that produced impulsive responding. Such findings are consistent with prior research, which found no robust evidence that children with ADHD/HD differed from normal comparison children in valuation or sensitivity to magnitude of reinforcement (e.g., Douglas and Parry, 1994; Solanto, 1990). However, findings from a more recent study using a variation of a delay-avoidance paradigm indicated that hyperactive children exhibited a systematic tendency to respond before the response window was presented, but had no difficulty inhibiting responses when required. This pattern of findings was interpreted as indicative of impairments in time perception, such as interval discrimination and estimation (Sonuga-Barke, Saxton and Hall, 1998). Notably, deficits in interval discrimination and estimation have been reported in ADHD (Barkley, Koplowitz, Anderson et al., 1997; Smith, Taylor, Warner-Rogers et al., 2002; Toplak, Rucklidge, Hetherington et al., 2002). The continuity of this response style (or potential time perception problem) into adulthood, or its variation with gender or comorbidity is unknown.

Robust but unexplained impairments in processing information

Notwithstanding the growing evidence of a variety of neuropsychological dysfunctions in ADHD, the most striking feature is the *manner* or *process of performance*, rather than the final summed scores of speed and/or accuracy, which invariably indicate poorer performance compared to an age-matched normal comparison group.

One robust but unexpected observation is the marked difficulty with tasks that involve speeded color naming, such as the Stroop Color–Word test (Golden, 1978) and the Rapid Automatized Naming Test (RAN; Denckla and Rudel, 1976). Naming speed has been assumed to be a specific correlate of dyslexia (e.g., Denckla and Cutting, 1999; Denckla and Rudel, 1976; Wolf, 1991, Wolf, O'Rourke, Gidney et al., 2002), not of ADHD (Felton, Wood, Brown et al., 1987; Wood and Felton, 1994). However, recent evidence of slow color naming in ADHD on the Stroop and RAN (Carte, Nigg and Hinshaw, 1996; Houghton et al., 1999; Rucklidge and Tannock, 2002; Semrud-Clikeman, Guy, Griffin et al., 2000; Tannock, Martinussen and Frijters, 2000; Van der Stelt, Van der Molen, Boudewijn Gunning et al., 2001; Willcutt et al., 2001) challenges this tenet. However, the most striking aspect of rapid naming performance in ADHD is not simply the slow naming speed overall, but rather the *process* of naming (particularly colors and objects). The performance of children and adolescents with ADHD is characterized by marked dysfluency (false starts, hesitations, self-corrections) and overt manifestation of behavioral symptoms of ADHD (e.g., fidgeting and squirming in seat, standing up out of seat) during these very brief laboratory-based tasks, each of which can each be completed in less than one minute. Notably, recent evidence that even patients with discrete frontal lobe lesions exhibit color naming impairments but not greater Stroop interference effects (Stuss et al., 2001) challenges a long-standing psychological belief that frontal lobe dysfunction is associated with problems in the ability to inhibit competing stimuli (distractors).

A second robust but unexplained finding is that of excessive trial-by-trial variability (i.e., intra-individual variability), which is found ubiquitously across a variety of speeded reaction time tasks that purport to measure various aspects of attention (e.g., stop-signal task, continuous performance tasks, spatial cueing task, saccade tasks, delay aversion task, time perception task), and across laboratories, and cultures (e.g., Borger and Van der Meere, 2000; Casey et al., 1997; Kuntsi et al., 2001; Kuntsi and Stevenson, 2001; Mostofsky et al., 2001; Munoz et al., 1999; Ross et al., 1994; Rubia, Taylor, Taylor et al., 1999; Scheres et al., 2001; Sonuga-Barke et al., 1998; Swanson et al., 1991; Teicher, Ito, Glod et al., 1996; Zahn, Kruesi and Rapoport, 1991). Response variability appears to reflect a high frequency of responses with very short latency (anticipatory responses) as well as a high frequency of very slow responses (Bedard et al., 2002; Leth-Steensen, Elbaz and Douglas, 2000; Sonuga-Barke et al., 1998; Wada, Yamashita, Matsuishi et al., 2000).

Current models of attention or of ADHD do not account adequately for these robust phenomena. For example, several explanations of response variability are limited to the psychological level, such as 'lapses of attention' (Douglas, 1999); faulty sustained attention (Robertson, Manly, Andrade et al., 1997); transient disruption of a goal directed action system (West and Alain, 2000). Others appeal to energetic models of attention, such as problems in a behavioral 'tonic readiness to respond' (Sanders, 1998); or a non-optimal activation state (Van der Meere, 1996). Similarly, the sole explanations to date of color naming problems are psychological ones that posits underlying deficits in 'effortful, semantic processing' (Tannock et al., 2000) or poor sustained attention (Semrud-Clikeman, Steingard, Filipek et al., 2000). The latter explanation is highly unsatisfactory, given the brief duration of these naming tasks (less than one minute) compared to methods used to evaluate sustained attention and executive attention (typically about 15 minutes or longer).

One problem is that current approaches to measurement and statistical analysis emphasize inter-individual variability and global measures of performance summed across time (e.g., mean response time, total errors) and have ignored trial-by-trial or intra-individual variability, which reflect problems in the moment-by-moment processing of information and decision making during task performance that are the hallmark of ADHD as manifest in both laboratory and real-life contexts. In part, these limitations in measurement, as well as the current conceptualization of the diagnostic category of ADHD reflect the predominant thinking in cognitive and clinical psychology during the past few decades. For example, 'filter' theories of attention were predominant during the 1960s and 1970s, when the inattention symptoms of ADHD/HD gained prominence over the previously emphasized motoric symptoms. Alternate approaches based on new trends in neuroscience, which are described briefly in the final section, might better account for these unexplained phenomena and advance our understanding of disorders of attention in various neurodevelopmental disorders, such as ADHD.

Effects of comorbidity

The high rates of comorbidity between ADHD and other psychiatric and neurodevelopmental disorders raise several important issues for understanding the neuropsychology of ADHD. For example are ADHD, Oppositional Defiant Disorder (ODD), and Conduct Disorder (CD) distinct psychiatric conditions or are they different aspects of the same general phenomenon? Does the presence of comorbid CD or Reading Disorders (RD) alter the neuropsychological profile of individuals with ADHD? Are the observed neuropsychological impairments in ADHD attributable to the comorbid disorder rather than to ADHD per se? Does the comorbid configuration (e.g., ADHD plus RD) represent a heretofore unclassified disorder with an etiology, course, and treatment response that is distinct from those of the component disorders (ADHD, RD)? This section provides a brief overview of the significance of comorbidity of ADHD with RD, CD, and Anxiety Disorders (ANX) in terms of the neuropsychological profile of ADHD. Detailed discussions of comorbidity in ADHD are provided by Brown (2000), Jensen et al. (1997), and Pliszka, Carlson and Swanson (1999).

Comorbid reading disorders

Most studies indicate that comorbidity with reading disorders (RD) *adds to* rather than alters the neuropsychological profile associated with ADHD. For example, children with ADHD+RD are typically found to exhibit the deficits associated with ADHD (i.e., deficits in sustained attention, response inhibition and other executive functions) *and* those associated with RD (i.e., in phonological processing, naming speed, verbal memory deficits), suggesting that ADHD+RD is a hybrid condition (Douglas and Benezra, 1990; Felton and Wood, 1989; Korkman and Pesonen, 1994; Narhi and Ahonen, 1995; Nigg, Hinshaw, Carte et al., 1998; Tannock et al., 2000). By contrast, a few studies indicate that the comorbid group exhibits the cognitive deficits of RD but not of ADHD (e.g., exhibit an impairment in phonological processing but not in executive functions), suggesting that RD leads to secondary symptoms but not the full syndrome of ADHD (i.e., a phenocopy)

(Pennington, Groisser and Welsh, 1993). Alternatively, others have found that the comorbid condition exhibit a different pattern or more marked impairments than either of the single disorders, suggesting that it may reflect a pathophysiologically distinct subtype (Narhi and Ahonen, 1995; Purvis and Tannock, 2000; Seidman, Biederman, Monuteaux et al., 2001; Willcutt et al., 2001). In weighing the evidence, the most parsimonious interpretation is that the neuropsychological impairments discussed in the previous section are associated with ADHD, particularly with the Inattention symptom cluster, and are not an artifact of comorbidity with RD.

Comorbid anxiety disorders

The impact of comorbid anxiety (ANX) on the cognitive profile of ADHD has been subjected to far less scrutiny (for a review, see Tannock, 2000). In general, the findings suggest that children with ADHD+ANX are more impaired on some measures of executive function (e.g., the serial addition task, Trailmaking Test-B, complex display of memory scanning task), but less impaired on others (e.g., continuous performance test) compared to the nonanxious ADHD children (Tannock, 2000). Notably, the tasks on which the ADHD+ANX children are found to be more impaired are cognitively complex and place high demands on short-term or working memory. By contrast, tasks on which children with ADHD+ANX do not show impairments are generally those that require speeded responses or response inhibition, but do not require any appreciable retention of information. Thus, these few studies yield a remarkably consistent pattern of findings and suggest that one effect of comorbid anxiety is to increase (but does not account for) the association between ADHD and problems with working memory and effortful processing. It is unclear whether comorbid anxiety serves to enhance performance on speeded performance in general, to counteract the inhibitory control deficits associated with ADHD or to produce both effects (Barkley, 1997b). Nor is it known whether the impact on cognitive function is attributable primarily to a specific cluster or type of anxiety symptoms (i.e., generalized versus specific anxiety) or to heightened levels of anxiety in general.

Comorbid conduct disorder

According to most population-based studies, the greatest neuropsychological deficits, as well as the poorest long-term outcome, are associated with the comorbid condition of ADHD with Conduct Disorder (ADHD+CD) (Moffitt, 1990; Moffitt and Henry, 1988; Moffitt and Silva, 1988). Given the high rates of comorbidity between ADHD and comorbid CD or Oppositional Defiant Disorder (ODD), particularly in clinical samples and the fact that few clinical studies have controlled for these comorbidities, it is particularly important to determine whether the neuropsychological impairments ascribed to ADHD are in fact confined to the comorbid condition of ADHD+CD or are a feature of ODD/CD rather than ADHD (Biederman et al., 1991; Moffitt, 1990; Nigg et al., 1998). The findings are mixed and the inconsistent findings are likely attributable in part to the small samples as well as to differences in diagnosis and the particular measures used. Briefly, children with ADHD+CD have been found to perform like those with ADHD alone, or like those with CD, to differ from either ADHD or CD, or to exhibit the deficits of both single disorders (Clark, Prior and Kinsella, 2000; Nigg et al., 1998; Schachar and Tannock, 1995; Seidman, Biederman, Faraone et al., 1997; Seidman et al., 2001). Most of the findings indicate that the neuropsychological profile of ADHD+CD more closely resembles that of ADHD than of CD, indicating that the impairments are a correlate of ADHD rather than CD.

Specificity of neuropsychological impairments in ADHD

The preceding review has highlighted a variety of neuropsychological impairments in individuals with ADHD, including deficits in selective, executive, and sustained attention. One critical question is whether any of these impairments is specific to ADHD or to the symptom clusters of inattention and hyperactivity/impulsivity. By contrast to the extensive neuropsychological research involving ADHD and normal comparison groups, studies that provide direct comparisons between ADHD and other psychiatric or neurodevelopmental disorders are comparatively few. Moreover, surprisingly few studies have compared attention in ADHD and schizophrenia, even though both are conceptualized as disorders of attention.

One recent and comprehensive review concluded that deficits in executive function are correlates of ADHD and autism but not of conduct disorder or Tourette's syndrome (Pennington and Ozonoff, 1996). Moreover, both the profile and severity of deficits were found to differ across ADHD and autism. Specifically, impairments in motor response inhibition appeared to be more strongly associated with ADHD than autism, whereas impairments in working memory appeared to be associated with autism rather than ADHD (Pennington and Ozonoff, 1996). That presumptive dissociation has yet to be confirmed empirically. Also, since most of the studies reviewed restricted the comparisons to ADHD versus normal controls, they cannot address the issue of specificity of deficits to ADHD.

Impairments in executive function (including motor inhibition, planning, set-shifting, verbal fluency, and working memory) are evident in other clinical populations, including schizophrenia, obsessive–compulsive disorder, cerebellar cognitive affective syndrome (Barr, 2001; Erlenmeyer-Kimling, Rock, Roberts et al., 2000; Matier-Sharma, Perachio and Newcorn, 1995; Purcell et al., 1998; Schmahmann and Sherman, 1998). However, these studies did not include a sample of individuals with ADHD. Evidence of specificity requires *direct* comparisons between ADHD and at least one other clinical group (ideally controlling for comorbidity) tested under the same conditions and with the same measures. For example, one study using this design found that both schizophrenic and ADHD children exhibited deficits in verbal and spatial working memory (Karatekin and Asarnow, 1998b). By contrast, mild impairments in executive function have been found in boys with childhood ADHD but not in boys of multigenerational alcoholics — a population thought to be at high risk for executive function deficits (Wiers, Gunning and Sergeant, 1998).

Although tests of sustained attention (e.g., CPT, Letter Cancellation Task) distinguish between groups of children with ADHD and normal children, they also distinguish between normal children and groups with other disorders, such as learning disabilities, hydrocephalus, schizophrenia, prematurity, as well as those with prenatal exposure to cocaine, alcohol, or marijuana (e.g., Bandstra, Morrow, Anthony et al., 2001; Brewer, Fletcher, Hiscock et al., 2001; Richardson, Ryan, Willford et al., 2002). Prenatal exposure to such substances is not uncommon in children with ADHD, but these factors are rarely considered when interpreting performance impairments in ADHD samples.

Future directions: a neuroscience perspective

Previous research in ADHD, which has been primarily descriptive and based on dichotomous diagnostic categories, has provided insights into the nature of attention disorders in ADHD. Moreover, it has provided the basis for new integrative and multidisciplinary approaches that incorporate developmental and neuroscience perspectives. An emphasis on delineating endophenotypes that predict disturbances in specific aspects of attention and that are anchored in neuroscience is one promising approach. For example, potentially useful phenotypes include deficits in working memory, specific abnormalities in reward-related circuitry, and deficits in temporal processing (Castellanos and Tannock, 2002). Moreover, given the growing evidence that the behavioral dimensions of inattention and hyperactivity–impulsivity diverge with respect to clinical course (Biederman et al., 2000), associated impairments (Chhabildas et al., 2001; Lahey, Pelham, Stein et al., 1998; Warner-Rogers et al., 2000), and heritability (Levy, McStephen and Hay, 2001; Willcutt et al., 2001), future studies should examine whether individual differences in symptom expression *within* a dimension (i.e., inattention, hyperactivity/impulsivity) are associated with distinct patterns of cognitive impairments.

A second direction necessitates a shift in models of brain function from one that emphasizes neurons as the critical element to a conceptualization that emphasizes the role of oscillatory processes in sensory and cognitive functions. The emergence of oscillatory brain theory, which investigates the brain's natural frequencies, is leading to new understanding of the mechanisms by which the immense number of neurons in the human brain interact to produce the higher cognitive functions (e.g., Basar, 1998; Basar and Bullock, 1992; Freeman, 1998). Oscillatory responses (i.e., changes of ongoing EEG activity related temporally to a defined event, such as a sensory stimulus) have been observed in both cortical and subcortical structures of the brain. The synchronous occurrence of such responses in multiple brain areas suggests the existence of distributed oscillatory systems and parallel processing in the brain, which would facilitate the transfer of information in the brain. Accordingly, any momentary disruptions of oscillatory responses in one or more of these brain structures or networks, would have a transient but deleterious effect on higher cognitive functions, including attention, working memory, and motivation. For example, recent evidence indicates that multisecond oscillations observed in single-unit recordings from basal ganglia output neurons are exquisitely sensitive to dopaminergic tone (Ruskin, Bergstrom, Kaneoke et al., 1999; Ruskin, Bergstrom, Shenker et al., 2001). Thus, alterations in tonic (or phasic) levels of dopamine would influence the oscillatory patterns in the basal ganglia and the synchronization with other oscillatory networks. For example recent evidence suggests that dopamine agonists promote synchronization between multisecond oscillations in basal ganglia and the newly-found multisecond oscillations in theta rhythm strength in forebrain EEG, particularly from the hippocampus (Allers, Ruskin, Bergstrom et al., 2002; Bergstrom, Ruskin, Tierney et al., 2001; Ruskin et al., 2001). These findings are particularly relevant for ADHD, given the evidence of abnormalities in theta rhythm in ADHD (e.g., Clarke, Barry, McCarthy et al., 2001; Lazzaro et al., 1999; Monastra et al., 1999). Notably, stimulants in the therapeutic dose range have prominent effects on multisecond oscillations (frequency < 0.1 Hz) in basal ganglia single-unit recordings (Ruskin, Bergstrom, Tierney et al., 2001). Thus, oscillatory brain theory might accommodate both the hyperdopaminergic and hypodopaminergic models of ADHD, and better account for the intra-individual variability in task performance and drug response than current brain models.

Acknowledgements

Preparation of this chapter was supported in part by a Scientist Award and operating grant (# MT13366) from the Canadian Institutes of Health Research.

References

Achenbach TM: Manual for the Child Behavior Checklist/4–18 and 1991 Profile. Burlington, VT: University of Vermont, 1991a.

Achenbach TM: Manual for the Teacher's Report Form and 1991 Profile. Burlington, VT: University of Vermont, 1991b.

Allers KA, Ruskin DN, Bergstrom DA et al.: Multisecond periodicities in basal ganglia firing rates correlate with theta bursts in transcortical and hippocampal EEG. Journal of Neurophysiology: 87; 1118–22, 2002.

Almasy L, Blangero J: Endophenotypes as quantitative risk factors for psychiatric disease: rationale and study design. American Journal of Medical Genetics: 105; 42–44, 2001.

American Psychiatric Association: Diagnostic and Statistical Manual of Mental Disorders, 3rd edition. Washington, DC: Author, 1980.

American Psychiatric Association: Diagnostic and Statistical Manual of Mental Disorders, 3rd edition, revised. Washington, DC: Author, 1987.

American Psychiatric Association: Diagnostic and Statistical Manual of Mental Disorders, 4th edition. Washington, DC: Author, 1994.

American Psychiatric Association: Task Force for the Handbook of Psychiatric Measures: Handbook of Psychiatric Measures. Washington DC: Author, 2000.

Anderson CM, Polcari AM, Lowen SB et al.: Effects of methylphenidate on functional magnetic resonance relaxometry of the cerebellar vermis in children with ADHD. American Journal of Psychiatry: in press, 2002.

Anderson JC, Williams S, McGee R, Silva PA: DSM-III-R disorders in preadolescent children: prevalence in a large sample from the general population. Archives of General Psychiatry: 44; 69–76, 1987.

Antrop I, Roeyers H, Van Oost P et al.: Stimulation seeking and hyperactivity in children with ADHD. Journal of Child Psychology and Psychiatry: 41; 225–231, 2000.

Baddeley A: Exploring the central executive. Quarterly Journal of Experimental Psychology: 49A; 5–28, 1996.

Baker L, Cantwell DP: Attention deficit disorder and speech/language disorders. Comprehensive Mental Health Care: 2; 3–16, 1992.

Bandstra ES, Morrow CE, Anthony JC et al.: Longitudinal investigation of task persistence and sustained attention in children with prenatal cocaine exposure. Neurotoxicology and Teratology: 23; 545–559, 2001.

Barbaresi WJ, Katusic SK, Colligan IC et al.: How common is attention-deficit/hyperactivity disorder? Incidence in a population-based birth cohort in Rochester, Minn. Archives of Pediatric and Adolescent Medicine: 156; 217–224, 2002.

Barkley RA: Attention. In Tramontana M, Hooper S (Eds), Assessment in Child Neuropsychology: Critical Issues in Neuropsychology. New York: Plenum, pp. 145–176, 1988.

Barkley RA: Attention Deficit Hyperactivity Disorder: A Handbook for Diagnosis and Treatment. New York: Guilford, Ch. 9, pp. 278–326, 1990.

Barkley RA: Behavioral inhibition, sustained attention, and executive functions: constructing a unifying theory of ADHD. Psychological Bulletin: 121; 65–94, 1997a.

Barkley RA: ADHD and the Nature of Self-control. New York: Guilford Press, 1997b.

Barkley RA: The executive functions and self-regulation: an evolutionary neuropsychological perspective. Neuropsychology Review: 11; 1–29, 2001.

Barkley RA, Edwards G, Laneri M et al.: Executive functioning, temporal discounting, and sense of time in adolescents with attention deficit hyperactivity disorder (ADHD) and oppositional defiant disorder (ODD). Journal of Abnormal Child Psychology: 29; 541–556, 2001.

Barkley RA, Fischer M, Edelbrock CS et al.: The adolescent outcome of hyperactive children diagnosed by research criteria: I. An 8-year prospective follow-up study. Journal of the American Academy of Child and Adolescent Psychiatry: 29; 546–557, 1990.

Barkley RA, Koplowitz S, Anderson T et al.: Sense of time in children with ADHD: Effects of duration, distraction, and stimulant medication. Journal of International Neuropsychological Society: 3; 359–369, 1997.

Barkley RA, Murphy KR, Kwasnik D: Motor vehicle driving competencies and risks in teens and young adults with attention deficit hyperactivity disorder. Pediatrics: 98; 1089–1095, 1996.

Barnett R, Maruff P, Vance A et al.: Abnormal executive function in attention deficit hyperactivity disorder: the effect of stimulant medication and age on spatial working memory. Psychological Medicine: 31; 1107–1115, 2001.

Barr CL, Feng Y, Wigg K et al.: Identification of DNA variants in the SNAP-25 gene and linkage study of these polymorphisms and attention-deficit hyperactivity disorder. Molecular Psychiatry: 5; 405–409, 2000.

Barr WB: Schizophrenia and attention deficit disorder. Two complex disorders of attention. Annals of the New York Academy of Science: 931; 239–50, 2001.

Basar E: Brain functions and oscillations. II. Integrative Brain Function, Neurophysiology and Cognitive Processes. New York: Springer, 1998.

Basar E, Bullock TH (Eds): Induced Rhythms in the Brain. Boston, MA: Birkhauser, 1992.

Baumgartel A, Wolraich ML, Dietrich M: Comparison of diagnostic criteria for attention deficit disorders in a German elementary school sample. Journal of the American Academy of Child and Adolescent Psychiatry: 34; 629–638, 1995.

Bedard A-C, Ickowicz A, Logan GD et al.: Selective Inhibition in Children with Attention-Deficit/Hyperactivity Disorder Off and On Stimulant Medication. Manuscript under review, 2002.

Bergstrom DA, Ruskin DN, Tierney PL et al.: Multisecond periodicities in neuronal activity reveal effects of dopamine on functional connectivity between globus pallidus and hippocampus and motor cortex. Society for Neuroscience Abstracts: 27; 177, 2001.

Berlin L, Bohlin G: Response inhibition, hyperactivity, and conduct problems among preschool children. Journal of Clinical Child Psychology: 31; 242–251, 2002.

Berquin PC, Giedd JN, Jacobsen LK et al.: The cerebellum in attention-deficit/hyperactivity disorder: a morphometric study. Neurology: 50; 1087–1093, 1998.

Biederman J, Faraone S, Milberger S et al.: Predictors of persistence and remission of ADHD into adolescence: results from a four-year prospective follow-up study. Journal of the American Academy of Child and Adolescent Psychiatry: 35; 343–351, 1996a.

Biederman J, Faraone S, Milberger S et al.: A prospective 4-year follow-up study of attention-deficit hyperactivity and related disorders. Archives of General Psychiatry: 53; 437–446, 1996b.

Biederman J, Mick E, Faraone SV: Age-dependent decline of symptoms of attention deficit hyperactivity disorder: impact of remission definition and symptom type. American Journal of Psychiatry: 157; 816–8, 2000.

Biederman J, Newcorn J, Sprich S: Comorbidity of attention deficit hyperactivity disorder with conduct, depressive, anxiety and other disorders. American Journal of Psychiatry: 148; 564–577, 1991.

Bird HR, Canino G, Rubio-Stipec M et al.: Estimates of prevalence of childhood maladjustment in a community survey in Puerto Rico. Archives of General Psychiatry: 45; 1120–1126, 1988.

Borger N, Van der Meere J: Visual behaviour of ADHD children during an attention test: an almost forgotten variable. Attention-Deficit Hyperactivity Disorder. Journal of Child Psychology and Psychiatry: 41; 525–32, 2000.

Brandeis D, Van Leeuwen TH, Rubia K et al.: Neuroelectric mapping reveals precursor of stop failures in children with attention deficits. Behaviour Brain Research: 94; 111–25, 1998.

Brito GN, Pereira CC, Santos-Morales TR: Behavioral and neuropsychological correlates of hyperactivity and inattention in Brazilian school children. Developmental Medicine and Child Neurology: 41; 732–739, 1999.

Brewer VR, Fletcher JM, Hiscock M et al.: Attention processes in children with shunted hydrocephalus versus attention deficit-hyperactivity disorder. Neuropsychology: 15; 185–198, 2001.

Brodeur DA, Pond M: The development of selective attention in children with attention deficit hyperactivity disorder. Journal of Abnormal Child Psychology: 29; 229–39, 2001.

Brown TE (Ed): Attention-Deficit Disorders and Comorbidities in Children, Adolescents, and Adults. Washington, DC: American Psychiatric Press, 2000.

Cardinal RN, Pennicott DR, Sugathapala CL et al.: Impulsive choice induced in rats by lesions of the nucleus accumbens core. Science: 292; 2499–2501, 2001.

Carlson CL, Mann M: Attention-deficit/hyperactivity disorder, predominantly inattentive subtype. Child and Adolescent Psychiatric Clinics of North America: 9; 499–510, 2000.

Carte ET, Nigg JT, Hinshaw SP: Neuropsychological functioning, motor speed, and language processing in boys with and without ADHD. Journal of Abnormal Child Psychology: 24; 481–498, 1996.

Casey BJ, Trainor RJ, Orendi JL et al.: A developmental functional MRI study of prefrontal activation during performance of a go–no-go task. Journal of Cognitive Neuroscience: 9; 835–847, 1997.

Caspi A, Moffitt TE, Newman DL et al.: Behavioral observations at age 3 years predict adult psychiatric disorders: Longitudinal evidence from a birth cohort. Archives of General Psychiatry: 53; 1033–1039, 1996.

Castellanos FX: Toward a pathophysiology of attention-deficit/hyperactivity disorder. Clinics in Pediatrics (Philadelphia): 36; 381–393, 1997.

Castellanos FX: Neuroimaging studies of ADHD. In Solanto MV, Arnsten AFT, Castellanos FX (Eds), Stimulant Drugs and ADHD: Basic and Clinical Neuroscience. New York: Oxford University Press, pp. 243–258, 2001.

Castellanos FX, Giedd JN, Berquin PC et al.: Quantitative brain magnetic resonance imaging in girls with attention-deficit/hyperactivity disorder. Archives of General Psychiatry: 58; 289–295, 2001.

Castellanos FX, Marvasti FF, Ducharme JL et al.: Executive function occulomotor tasks in girls with ADHD. Journal of the American Academy of Child and Adolescent Psychiatry: 39; 644–650, 2000.

Castellanos FX, Tannock R: Neuroscience of attention-deficit/hyperactivity disorder: the search for endophenotypes. Nature Reviews/Neuroscience: 3; 1–12, 2002.

Chee P, Logan G, Schachar R et al.: Effects of event rate and display time on sustained attention in hyperactive, normal and control children. Journal of Abnormal Child Psychology: 17; 371–391, 1989.

Chevalier H, Metz-Lutz MN, Segalowitz SJ: Impulsivity and control of inhibition in Benign Focal Childhood Epilepsy (BFCE). Brain and Cognition: 43; 86–90, 2000.

Chhabildas N, Pennington BF, Willcutt EG: A comparison of the neuropsychological profiles of the DSM-IV subtypes of ADHD. Journal of Abnormal Child Psychology: 29; 529–540, 2001.

Clark C, Prior M, Kinsella GJ: Do executive function deficits differentiate between adolescents with ADHD and oppositional defiant/conduct disorder? A neuropsychological study using the Six Elements Test and Hayling Sentence Completion Test. Journal of Abnormal Child Psychology: 28; 403–414, 2000.

Clarke AR, Barry RJ, McCarthy R et al.: Electroencephalogram differences in two subtypes of attention-deficit/hyperactivity disorder. Psychophysiology: 38; 212–221, 2001.

Cohen J: Statistical power analysis for the behavioral sciences (2nd ed.). Hillsdale, NJ: Lawrence Erlbaum, 1988.

Cohen RA: The Neuropsychology of Attention. New York: Plenum Press, 1993.

Conners CK: Conners' Rating Scales — Revised: Technical Manual. New York: Multi-Health Systems, 1997.

Cook EH Jr, Stein MA, Krasowski MD et al.: Association of attention deficit disorder and the dopamine transporter gene. American Journal of Human Genetics: 56; 993–998, 1995.

Corkum PV, Siegel LS: Is the continuous performance task a valuable research tool for use with children with attention-deficit-hyperactivity disorder? Journal of the American Academy of Child and Adolescent Psychiatry: 34; 1217–1239, 1993.

Crosbie J, Schachar R: Deficient inhibition as a marker for familial ADHD. American Journal of Psychiatry: 158; 1884–90, 2001.

Denckla MB, Cutting LE: History and significance of rapid automatized naming. Annals of Dyslexia: 49; 29–42, 1999.

Denckla M, Rudel RG: Rapid automatized naming (RAN): Dyslexia differentiated from other learning disabilities. Neuropsychologia: 14; 471–479, 1976

Dougherty DD, Bonab AA, Spencer TJ et al.: Dopamine transporter density is elevated in patients with attention deficit hyperactivity disorder. Lancet: 354(9196); 2132–2133, 1999.

Douglas VI; Cognitive control processes in ADHD. In Quay HC, Hogan AE (Eds), Handbook of Disruptive Behavior Disorders. New York: Kluwer/Plenum, pp. 105–138, 1999.

Douglas VI, Benezra E: Supraspan verbal memory in attention deficit disorder with hyperactivity, normal and reading disabled boys. Journal of Abnormal Child Psychology: 18; 617–638, 1990.

Douglas VI, Parry PA: Effects of reward and nonreward on frustration and attention in attention deficit disorder. Journal of Abnormal Child Psychology: 22; 281–301, 1994.

Eisenberg J, Mei-Tal G, Steinberg A et al.: Haplotype relative risk study of catechol-*O*-methyltransferase (COMT) and attention deficit hyperactivity disorder (ADHD): association of the high-enzyme activity Val allele with ADHD impulsive–hyperactive phenotype. American Journal of Medical Genetics: 88; 497–502, 1999.

Elman I, Sigler M, Kronenberg J et al.: Characteristics of patients with schizophrenia successive to childhood attention deficit hyperactivity disorder (ADHD). Israel Journal of Psychiatry and Related Sciences: 35; 280–286, 1998.

Epstein JN, Johnson DE, Varia IM et al.: Neuropsychological assessment of response inhibition in adults with ADHD. Journal of Clinical Experimental Neuropsychology: 23; 362–71, 2001.

Erlenmeyer-Kimling L, Rock D, Roberts SA, Janal M, Kestenbaum C, Cornblatt B, Adamo UH, Gottesman II: Attention, memory, and motor skills as childhood predictors of schizophrenia-related psychoses: the New York High-Risk Project. American Journal of Psychiatry: 157; 1416–1422, 2000.

Ernst M, Zametkin AJ, Matochik JA et al.: Intravenous dextroamphetamine and brain glucose metabolism. Neuropsychopharmacology: 17; 391–401, 1997.

Everling S, Fischer B: The antisaccade: a review of basic research and clinical studies. Neuropsychologia: 36; 885–899, 1998.

Faraone SV: Report from the third international meeting of the Attention-Deficit Hyperactivity Disorder Molecular Genetics Network. American Journal of Medical Genetics: 114; 272–276, 2002.

Faraone SV, Biederman J, Friedman D: Validity of DSM-IV subtypes of attention-deficit/hyperactivity disorder: a family perspective. Journal of the American Academy of Child and Adolescent Psychiatry: 39; 300–307, 2000.

Faraone SV, Doyle AE: Genetic influences on attention deficit hyperactivity disorder. Current Psychiatry Reports: 2; 143–146, 2000.

Faraone SV, Doyle AE, Mick E et al.: Meta-analysis of the association between the 7-repeat allele of the dopamine D4 receptor gene and attention deficit hyperactivity disorder. American Journal of Psychiatry: 158; 1052–1057, 2001.

Felton RH, Wood FB: Cognitive deficits in reading disability and attention deficit disorder. Journal of Learning Disabilities: 22; 3–13, 1989.

Felton RH, Wood FB, Brown IS et al.: Separate verbal memory and naming deficits in attention deficit disorder and reading disability. Brain and Language: 31; 171–184, 1987.

Filipek PA: Neuroimaging in the developmental disorders: the state of the science. Journal of Child Psychology and Psychiatry: 40; 113–128, 1999.

Fisher SE, Francks C, McCracken JT et al.: A genomewide scan for loci involved in attention-deficit/hyperactivity disorder. American Journal of Human Genetics: 70; 1183–1196, 2002.

Freeman WJ: Foreward. In Basar E, Brain Function and Oscillations, Vol. I and II. New York: Springer, 1998.

Giedd JN, Blumenthal J, Molloy E et al.: Brain imaging of attention deficit/hyperactivity disorder. Annals of the New York Academy of Sciences: 931; 33–49, 2001.

Golden CJ: Stroop color and word test: A manual for clinical and experimental use. Chicago: Stoelting, 1978,

Gomez RL, Janowsky D, Zetin M: Adult psychiatric diagnosis and symptoms compatible with hyperactive child syndrome: a retrospective study. Journalof Clinical Psychiatry: 42; 389–394, 1981.

Grace AA: Gating of information flow within the limbic system and the pathophysiology of schizophrenia. Brain Research. Brain Research Reviews: 31; 330–41, 2000.

Gray JA: The Neuropsychology of Anxiety: An Enquiry into the Functions of the Septo-hippocampal System. New York: Oxford University Press, 1982.

Graybiel AM: The Basal Ganglia and Chunking of Action Repertoires. Neurobiology of Learning and Memory: 70; 119–136, 1998.

Halperin JM, Wolf LE, Greenblatt ER et al.: Subtype analysis of commission errors on the continuous performance test in children. Developmental Neuropsychology: 7; 207–217, 1991.

Heilman KM, Watson RT, Valenstein E et al.: Attention: behavior and neural mechanisms. Attention: 11; 461–481, 1988.

Houghton S, Douglas G, West J et al.: Differential patterns of executive function in children with attention-deficit hyperactivity disorder according to gender and subtype. Journal of Child Neurology: 14; 801–5, 1999.

Jensen PS, Hinshaw SP, Kraemer HC et al.: ADHD comorbidity findings from the MTA study: comparing comorbid subgroups. Journal of the American Academy of Child and Adolescent Psychiatry: 40; 147–58, 2001.

Jensen PS, Martin BA, Cantwell DP: Comorbidity in ADHD: Implications for research, practice, and DSM-IV. Journal of the American Academy of Child and Adolescent Psychiatry: 36; 1065–1079, 1997.

Johannes S, Wieringa BM, Mantey M et al.: Altered inhibition of motor responses in Tourette syndrome and Obsessive-Compulsive Disorder. Acta Neurologica Scandinavica: 104; 36–43, 2001.

Johansen EB, Aase H, Meyer A et al.: Attention deficit/hyperactivity disorder behavior explained by dysfunctional reinforcement and extinction processes. Behavioural Brain Research: 130; 37–45, 2002.

Jueptner M, Weiller C: A review of differences between basal ganglia and cerebellar control of movements as revealed by functional imaging studies. Brain: 121; 1437–1449, 1998.

Kamphaus RW, Frick PJ: Clinical Assessment of Child and Adolescent Personality and Behavior. Needham Heights, MA: Allyn and Bacon, 1996.

Karatekin C, Asarnow RF: Working memory in childhood-onset schizophrenia and attention-deficit/hyperactivity disorder. Psychiatry Research: 80; 165–76, 1998a.

Karatekin C, Asarnow RF: Components of visual search in childhood-onset schizophrenia and attention-deficit/hyperactivity disorder. Journal of Abnormal Child Psychology: 26; 367–380, 1998b.

Karatekin C, Asarnow RF: Exploratory eye movements to pictures in childhood-onset schizophrenia and attention-deficit/hyperactivity disorder (ADHD). Journal of Abnormal Child Psychology: 27; 35–49, 1999.

Kempton S, Vance A, Maruff P et al.: Executive function and attention deficit hyperactivity disorder: stimulant medication and better executive function performance in children. Psychological Medicine: 29; 527–38, 1999.

Klein RG, Mannuzza S: Long-term outcome of hyperactive children: A review. Journal of the American Academy of Child and Adolescent Psychiatry: 30; 383–387, 1991.

Klorman R: Cognitive event-related potentials in attention deficit disorder. Journal of Learning Disabilities: 24; 130–140, 1991.

Konrad K, Gauggel S, Manz A et al.: Lack of inhibition: a motivational deficit in children with attention deficit/hyperactivity disorder and children with traumatic brain injury. Neuropsychological Development Cognition Sect C Child Neuropsychology: 6; 286–96, 2000a.

Konrad K, Gauggel S, Manz A et al.: Inhibitory control in children with traumatic brain injury (TBI) and children with attention deficit/hyperactivity disorder (ADHD). Brain Injury: 14; 859–75, 2000b.

Korkman M, Pesonen AE: A comparison of neuropsychological test profiles of children with attention deficit-hyperactivity disorder and/or learning disabilities. Journal of Learning Disabilities: 27; 383–392, 1994.

Knutson B, Adams CM, Fong GW et al.: Anticipation of increasing monetary reward selectively recruits nucleus accumbens. Journal of Neuroscience: 21; RC159, 2001a.

Knutson B, Fong GW, Adams CM et al.: Dissociation of reward anticipation and outcome with event-related fMRI. Neuroreport: 12; 3683–73687, 2001b.

Kramer AF, Humphrey DG, Larish JF et al.: Aging and inhibition: beyond a unitary view of inhibitory processing in attention. Psychological Aging: 9; 491–512, 1994.

Krause KH, Dresel SH, Krause J et al.: Increased striatal dopamine transporter in adult patients with attention deficit hyperactivity disorder: effects of methylphenidate as measured by single photon emission computed tomography. Neuroscience Letters: 285; 107–110, 2000.

Kuntsi J, Oosterlaan J, Stevenson J: Psychological mechanisms in hyperactivity: I. Response inhibition deficit, working memory impairment, delay aversion, or something else? Journal of Child Psychology and Psychiatry: 42; 199–210, 2001.

Kuntsi J, Stevenson J: Psychological mechanisms in hyperactivity: II. The role of genetic factors. Journal of Child Psychology and Psychiatry: 42; 211–219, 2001.

Lahey BB, Applegate B, McBurnett K et al.: DSM-IV field trials for attention deficit/hyperactivity disorder in children and adolescents. American Journal of Psychiatry: 151; 1673–1685, 1994.

Lahey B, Pelham WE, Stein MA et al.: Validity of DSM-IV attention-deficit/hyperactivity disorder for younger children. Journal of the American Academy of Child and Adolescent Psychiatry: 37; 695–702, 1998.

Lawrence V, Houghton S, Tannock R et al.: ADHD outside the laboratory: Boys' executive function performance on tasks in videogame play and on a visit to the zoo. Journal of Abnormal Child Psychology: in press, 2002.

Lazzaro I, Gordon E, Li W et al.: Simultaneous EEG and EDA measures in adolescent attention deficit hyperactivity disorder. International Journal of Psychophysiology: 34; 123–134, 1999.

Leth-Steensen C, Elbaz ZK, Douglas VI: Mean response times, variability, and skew in the responding of ADHD children: a response time distributional approach. Acta Psychologica (Amsterdam): 104; 167–90, 2000.

Leung PW, Luk SL, Ho TP et al.: The diagnosis and prevalence of hyperactivity in Chinese schoolboys. British Journal of Psychiatry: 168; 486–496, 1996.

Levy F: The dopamine theory of attention deficit hyperactivity disorder (ADHD). Australian and New Zealand Journal of Psychiatry: 25; 277–283, 1991.

Levy F, Farrow M: Working memory in ADHD: prefrontal/parietal connections. Current Drug Targets: 2; 347–352, 2001.

Levy F, Hay D (Eds): Attention, Genes, and ADHD. Philadelphia, PA: Taylor and Francis, 2001.

Levy F, Hay DA, Wood C et al.: Attention-deficit hyperactivity disorder: A category or a continuum? Genetic analysis of a large-scale twin study. Journal of the American Academy of Child and Adolescent Psychiatry: 36; 737–744, 1997.

Levy F, McStephen M, Hay DA: The diagnostic genetics of ADHD symptoms and subtypes. I: Levy F, Hay D (Eds), Attention, Genes, and ADHD. Philadelphia, PA: Taylor and Francis, pp. 35–57, 2001.

Logan GD: On the ability to inhibit thought and action: A users' guide to the stop-signal paradigm. In Carr DD, Carr TH (Eds), Inhibitory Processes in Attention, Memory, and Language. San Diego, USA: Academic Press, pp. 189–239, 1994.

Logan GD, Cowan WB: On the ability to inhibit thought and action: A theory of act and control. Psychological Review: 91; 295–327, 1984.

Losier BJ, McGrath PJ, Klein RM: Error patterns on the Continuous Performance Test in non-medicated and medicated samples of children with and without ADHD: A meta-analytic review. Journal of Child Psychology and Psychiatry: 37; 971–987, 1996.

MacLeod CM, MacDonald PA: Interdimensional interference in the Stroop effect: uncovering the cognitive and neural anatomy of attention. Trends in Cognitive Science: 4; 383–391, 2000.

Madras BK, Miller GM, Fischman AJ: The dopamine transporter: relevance to attention deficit hyperactivity disorder (ADHD). Behavioural Brain Research: 130; 57–63, 2002.

Magistretti PJ, Pellerin L: Astrocytes Couple Synaptic Activity to Glucose Utilization in the Brain. News Physiological Science: 14; 177–182, 1999.

Manassis K, Tannock R, Barbosa J: Dichotic listening and response inhibition in children with comorbid anxiety disorders and ADHD. Journal of the American Academy of Child and Adolescent Psychiatry: 39; 1152–1159, 2001.

Mariani MA, Barkley RA: Neuropsychological and academic functioning in preschool boys with Attention Deficit Hyperactivity Disorder. Developmental Neuropsychology: 13; 111–129, 1997.

Martinussen R, Bedard A-C, Ickowicz A et al.: Characterization of a theoretically-derived inattentive phenotype of attention-deficit hyperactivity disorder. Manuscript under review, 2002.

Marzocchi GM, Lucangeli D, De Meo T et al.: The disturbing effect of irrelevant information on arithmetic problem solving in inattentive children. Developmental Neuropsychology: 21; 73–92, 2002.

Matier-Sharma K, Perachio N, Newcorn J: Differential diagnosis of ADHD. Child Neuropsychiatry: 1; 118–127, 1995.

Max JE, Fox PT, Lancaster JL et al.: Putamen lesions and the development of attention-deficit/hyperactivity symptomatology. Journal of the American Academy of Child and Adolescent Psychiatry: 41, 563–71, 2002.

McDonald S, Bennett K, Chambers H et al.: Covert orienting and focusing of attention in children with attention deficit hyperactivity disorder. Neuropsychologia: 37; 345–356, 1999.

McGee RA, Clark SE, Symons DK: Does the Conners' Continuous Performance Test aid in ADHD diagnosis? Journal of Abnormal Child Psychology: 28; 415–24, 2000.

Melchitzky DS, Lewis DA: Tyrosine hydroxylase- and dopamine transporter-immunoreactive axons in the primate cerebellum. Evidence for a lobular- and laminar-specific dopamine innervation. Neuropsychopharmacology: 22; 466–472, 2000.

Mesulam MM: Principles of Behavioral and Cognitive Neurology. New York: Oxford University Press, 2000.

Mill J, Curran S, Kent L et al.: Association study of a SNAP-25 microsatellite and attention deficit hyperactivity disorder. American Journal of Medical Genetics: 114; 269–71, 2002.

Mirsky AF, Anthony BJ, Duncan CC et al.: Analysis of the elements of attention: a neuropsychological approach. Neuropsychology Review: 2; 109–45, 1991.

Mirsky AF, Duncan CC: A nosology of disorders of attention. Annals of the New York Academy of Sciences: 931; 17–32, 2001.

Mitsis EM, McKay KE, Schulz KP et al.: Parent-teacher concordance for DSM-IV attention-deficit/hyperactivity disorder in a clinic-referred sample. Journal of the American Academy of Child and Adolescent Psychiatry: 39; 308–313, 2000.

Moffitt TE: Juvenile delinquency and attention-deficit disorder: Developmental trajectories from age 3 to 15. Child Development: 61; 893–910, 1990.

Moffitt TE, Henry B: Neuropsychological assessment of executive functions in self-reported delinquents. Development and Psychopathology: 1; 105–118, 1988.

Moffitt TE, Silva P: Self-reported delinquency, neuropsychological deficit, and history of attention deficit disorder. Journal of Abnormal Child Psychology: 16; 553–569, 1988.

Monastra VJ, Lubar JF, Linden M et al.: Assessing attention deficit hyperactivity disorder via quantitative electroencephalography: an initial validation study. Neuropsychology: 13; 424–433, 1999.

Monastra VJ, Lubar JF, Linden M: The development of a QEEG scanning process for ADHD: reliability and validity studies. Neuropsychology: 15; 136–144, 2000.

Monchi O, Petrides M, Petre V et al.: Wisconsin card sorting revisited: Distinct neural circuits participating in different stages of the task identified by event-related functional magnetic resonance imaging. Journal of Neurocience: 21; 7733–7741, 2001.

Morton J, Frith U: Causal modeling A structural approach to developmental psychopathology. In Cicchetti D, Cohen DJ (Eds), Developmental Psychopathology. New York: John Wiley, pp. 357–390, 1995.

Mostofsky SH, Lasker AG, Cutting LE et al.: Oculomotor abnormalities in attention deficit hyperactivity disorder: a preliminary study. Neurology: 57; 423–30, 2001.

Mostofsky SH, Reiss AL, Lockhart P et al.: Evaluation of cerebellar size in attention-deficit hyperactivity disorder. Journal of Child Neurology: 13; 434–439, 1998.

Mota VL, Schachar RJ: Reformulating attention-deficit/hyperactivity disorder according to signal detection theory. Journal of the American Academy of Child and Adolescent Psychiatry: 39; 1144–1151, 2000.

Mozley LH, Gur RC, Mozley PD et al.: Striatal dopamine transporters and cognitive functioning in healthy men and women. American Journal of Psychiatry: 158; 1492–1499, 2001.

Munoz DP, Hampton KA, Moore KD et al.: Control of purposive saccadic eye movements and visual fixation in children with attention-deficit/hyperactivity disorder. In Becker W, Deubel H, Mergner T (Eds), Current Occulomotor Research: Psychological and Physiological Aspects. New York: Plenum, pp. 415–424, 1999.

Murphy P: Inhibitory control in adults with attention-deficit/hyperactivity disorder. Journal of Attention Disorders: 6; 1–4, 2002.

Nada-Raja S, Langley JD, McGee R et al, 1997.: Inattentive and hyperactive behaviors and driving offences in adolescence. Journal of the American Academy of Child and Adolescent Psychiatry: 36; 515–522, 1997.

Narhi V, Ahonen T: Reading disability with and without attention deficit hyperactivity disorder: Do attentional problems make a difference? Developmental Neuropsychology: 11; 337–350, 1995.

Neuman RJ, Todd RD, Heath AC et al.: Evaluation of ADHD typology in three contrasting samples: A latent class approach. Journal of the American Academy of Child and Adolescent Psychiatry: 38; 25–33, 1999.

Nigg JT: Is ADHD a disinhibitory disorder? Psychological Bulletin: 127; 571–598, 2001.

Nigg JT, Butler KM, Huang-Pollock CL et al.: Inhibitory processes in adults with persistent childhood onset ADHD. Journal of Consulting and Clinical Psychology: 70; 153–157, 2002.

Nigg JT, Hinshaw SP, Carte ET et al.: Neuropsychological correlates of childhood attention deficit hyperactivity disorder: Explainable by comorbid disruptive behavior or reading problems? Journal of Abnormal Psychology: 107; 468–480, 1998.

Nigg JT, Swanson J, Hinshaw SP: Covert visual attention in boys with attention deficit hyperactivity disorder: Lateral effects, methylphenidate response, and results for parents. Neuropsychologia: 35; 165–176, 1997.

Novak G, Solanto M, Abkoff A: Spatial orienting and focused attention in attention deficit hyperactivity disorder. Psychophysiology: 32; 546–559, 1995.

Offord DR, Boyle MH, Racine Y et al.: Integrating assessment data from multiple informants. Journal of the American Academy of Child and Adolescent Psychiatry: 35; 1078–1085, 1996.

Oosterlaan J, Logan GD, Sergeant JA: Response inhibition in AD/HD, CD, comorbid AD/HD+CD, anxious and control children: a meta-analysis of studies with the stop task. Journal of Child Psychology and Psychiatry: 39; 411–426, 1998.

Oosterlaan J, Sergeant JA: Effects of reward and response cost on response inhibition in AD/HD, disruptive, anxious, and normal children. Journal of Abnormal Child Psychology: 26; 161–74, 1998.

Overtoom CC, Kenemans JL, Verbaten MN et al.: Inhibition in children with attention-deficit/hyperactivity disorder: a psychophysiological study of the stop task. Biological Psychiatry: 51; 668–676, 2002.

Ozonoff S, Strayer DL: Inhibitory function in nonretarded children with autism. Journal of Autism and Developmental Disorders: 27; 59–77, 1997.

Parasuraman R: The attentive brain: Issues and prospects. In Parasuraman R (Ed), The Attentive Brain. Cambridge, MA: MIT Press, pp. 3–15, 1998.

Pearson DA, Yaffee LS, Loveland KA et al.: Covert visual attention in children with attention deficit hyperactivity disorder: Evidence for developmental immaturity? Development and Psychopathology: 7; 351–167, 1995.

Pennington BF, Groisser D, Welsh MC: Contrasting cognitive deficits in attention deficit hyperactivity disorder versus reading disability. Developmental Psychology: 29; 511–523, 1993.

Pennington BF, Ozonoff S: Executive functions and developmental psychopathology. Journal of Child Psychology and Psychiatry: 37; 51–87, 1996.

Pliszka SR, Carlson CL, Swanson JM: ADHD with Comorbid Disorders: Clinical Assessment and Management. New York: Guilford Press, 1999.

Pochon JB, Levy R, Fossati P et al.: the neural system that bridges reward and cognition in humans: an fMRI study.

Proceedings of the National Academy of Sciences: 99; 5669–5674, 2002.

Posner MI: Chronometric Explorations of Mind. Hillsdale, NJ: Lawrence Erlbaum, 1978.

Posner MI, Dehaene S: Attentional networks. Trends in Neuroscience: 17; 75–79, 1994.

Posner MI, Petersen SE: The attention system of the human brain. Annual Review of Neuroscience: 13; 25–42, 1990.

Posner MI, Raichle ME: Images of Mind. New York: Scientific American Library, 1994.

Posner MI, Rothbart MK: Attention, self-regulation and consciousness. Philosophical Transactions of the Royal Society of London [B]: 353; 1915–1927, 1998.

Power TJ, Costigan TE, Leff SS et al.: Assessing ADHD across settings: contributions of behavioral assessment to categorical decision making. Journal of Clinical Child Psychology: 30; 399–412, 2001.

Pribram KH, McGuiness D: Arousal, activation and effort in the control of attention. Psychological Review: 82; 116–149, 1975.

Purcell R, Maruff P, Hyrios M et al.: Neuropsychological deficits in obsessive-compulsive disorder: A comparison with unipolar depression, panic disorder, and normal controls. Archives of General Psychiatry: 55; 415–423, 1998.

Purvis KL, Tannock R: Phonological processing, not inhibitory control, differentiates ADHD and reading disability. Journal of the American Academy of Child and Adolescent Psychiatry: 39; 485–94, 2000.

Quay HC: Attention-deficit disorder and the behavioral inhibition system: The relevance of the neuropsychological theory of Jeffrey A Gray. In Bloomingdale LM, Sergeant J (Eds), Attention-deficit Disorder: Criteria, Cognition, Intervention. New York: Pergamon Press, pp. 117–126, 1988.

Quay HC: Inhibition and attention deficit hyperactivity disorder. Journal of Abnormal Child Psychology: 25; 7–13, 1997.

Rasmussen P, Gillberg C: Natural outcome of ADHD with developmental coordination disorder at age 22 years: A controlled longitudinal, community-based study. Journal of the American Academy of Child and Adolescent Psychiatry: 39; 1424–1431, 2000.

Richardson GA, Ryan C, Willford J et al.: Prenatal alcohol and marijuana exposure. Effects on neuropsychological outcomes at 10 years. Neurotoxicology and Teratology: 24; 309–320, 2002.

Rieder RO, Nichols PL: Offspring of schizophrenics. III. Hyperactivity and neurological soft signs. Archives of General Psychiatry: 36; 665–674, 1979.

Robertson IH, Manly T, Andrade J et al.: 'Oops!': performance correlates of everyday attentional failures in traumatic brain injured and normal subjects. Neuropsychologia: 35; 747–758, 1997.

Ross RG, Harris JG, Olincy A et al.: Eye movement task measures inhibition and spatial working memory in adults with schizophrenia, ADHD, and a normal comparison group. Psychiatry Research: 95; 35–42, 2000.

Ross RG, Hommer D, Breiger D et al.: Eye movement task related to frontal lobe functioning in children with attention deficit disorder. Journal of the American Academy of Child and Adolescent Psychiatry: 33; 869–874, 1994.

Rothlind JC, Posner MI, Schaughency EA: Lateralized control of eye movements in attention deficit hyperactivity disorder. Journal of Cognitive Neuroscience: 3; 374–393, 1991.

Rubia K, Oosterlaan J, Sergeant JA et al.: Inhibitory dysfunction in hyperactive boys. Behavioural Brain Research: 94; 25–32, 1998.

Rubia K, Overmeyer S, Taylor E et al.: Hypofrontality in attention deficit hyperactivity disorder during higher-order motor control: a study with functional MRI. American Journal of Psychiatry: 156; 891–896, 1999a.

Rubia K, Taylor A, Taylor E et al.: Synchronization, anticipation, and consistency in motor timing of children with dimensionally defined attention deficit hyperactivity behaviour. Perceptual and Motor Skills: 89; 1237–1258, 1999b.

Rucklidge J, Tannock R: Neuropsychological Profiles of Adolescents with ADHD: Effects of Reading Disabilities and Gender. Journal of Child Psychology and Psychiatry: in press, 2002.

Ruff HA, Rothbart MK: Attention in Early Development. New York: Oxford University Press, 1996.

Ruskin DN, Bergstrom DA, Kaneoke Y et al.: Multisecond oscillations in firing rate in the basal ganglia; Robust modulation by dopamine receptor activation and anesthesia. Journal of Neurophysiology: 81; 2046–2055, 1999.

Ruskin DN, Bergstrom DA, Shenker A et al.: Drugs used in the treatment of attention deficit/hyperactivity disorder affect postsynaptic firing rate and oscillation without preferential autoreceptor action. Biological Psychiatry: 49; 340–350, 2001.

Ruskin DN, Bergstrom DA, Tierney P et al.: Dopamine agonists organize phase relationships of multisecond oscillations in basal ganglia and hippocampal activity. Society for Neuroscience Abstracts: 27; 177, 2001.

Sagvolden T, Aase H, Zeiner P et al.: Altered reinforcement mechanisms in attention-deficit/hyperactivity disorder. Behavioural Brain Research: 94; 61–71, 1998.

Sandberg S, Barton J: Historical development. In Sandberg S (Ed), Hyperactivity Disorders of Childhood. Cambridge: Cambridge University Press, pp. 1–25. 1996.

Sanders AF: Towards a model of stress and performance. Acta Psychologica: 53; 61–97, 1983.

Sanders AF: Elements of human performance: reaction processes and attention in human skill. Mahwah, NJ: Lawrence Erlbaum, 1998.

Schachar RJ: The History of Hyperkinetic Syndrome. In Taylor E (Ed), The Hyperkinetic Child. London: Spastics International Publications, Heinman, pp. 19–40, 1986.

Schachar R, Mota VL, Logan GD et al.: Confirmation of an inhibitory control deficit in attention-deficit/hyperactivity disorder. Journal of Abnormal Child Psychology: 28; 227–235, 2000.

Schachar R, Tannock R: A test of four hypotheses for the comorbidity of attention deficit hyperactivity disorder and conduct disorder. Journal of the American Academy of Child and Adolescent Psychiatry: 34; 639–648, 1995.

Schachar R, Tannock R: Syndromes of hyperactivity and attention deficit. In Rutter M, Taylor E (Eds), Childhood and

Adolescent Psychiatry 4th edition. Oxford, UK: Blackwell, pp. 399–418, 2002.

Schachar R, Tannock R, Logan G: Inhibitory control, impulsiveness and Attention Deficit Hyperactivity Disorder. Clinical Psychology Review: 13; 721–739, 1993.

Scheres A, Oosterlaan J, Sergeant JA: Response execution and inhibition in children with AD/HD and other disruptive disorders: the role of behavioural activation. Journal of Child Psychology and Psychiatry: 42; 347–357, 2001.

Schmahmann JD, Sherman JC: The cerebellar cognitive affective syndrome. Brain: 121; 561–579, 1998.

Schultz W: Predictive reward signal of dopamine neurons. Journal of Neurophysiology: 80; 1–27, 1998.

Schultz W: Reward signaling by dopamine neurons. Neuroscientist: 7; 293–302, 2001.

Schweitzer JB, Lee DO, Ely TD et al.: The effects of methylphenidate on the functional neuroanatomy of working memory in ADHD. Society for Neuroscience Abstracts: 24; 958 (abstract), 1998.

Seidman LJ, Biederman J, Faraone SV et al.: Toward defining a neuropsychology of attention deficit-hyperactivity disorder: Performance of children and adolescents from a large clinically referred sample. Journal of Consulting and Clinical Psychology: 65; 150–160, 1997.

Seidman LJ, Biederman J, Monuteaux MC et al.: Learning disabilities and executive dysfunction in boys with attention-deficit/hyperactivity disorder. Neuropsychology: 15; 544–556, 2001.

Semrud-Clikeman M, Guy K, Griffin JD et al.: Rapid naming deficits in children and adolescents with reading disabilities and attention deficit hyperactivity disorder. Brain and Language: 74; 70–83, 2000.

Semrud-Clikeman M, Steingard RJ, Filipek P et al.: Using MRI to examine brain–behavior relationships in males with attention deficit disorder with hyperactivity. Journal of the American Academy of Child and Adolescent Psychiatry: 39; 477–84, 2000.

Sergeant J: The cognitive-energetic model: an empirical approach to attention-deficit/hyperactivity disorder. Neuroscience and Biobehavioral Reviews: 24; 7–12, 2000.

Sergeant JA, Geurts H, Oosterlaan J: How specific is a deficit of executive functioning for attention-deficit/hyperactivity disorder? Behavioural Brain Research: 130; 3–28, 2002.

Sergeant JA, Oosterlaan J, Van der Meere J: Information processing and energetic factors in attention deficit/hyperactivity disorder. In Quay HC, Hogan AE (Eds), Handbook of Disruptive Behavior Disorders. New York: Plenum, pp. 75–104, 1999.

Sergeant J, Van der Meere J: Additive factor method applied to psychopathology with special reference to childhood hyperactivity. Acta Psychologica (Amsterdam): 74; 277–295, 1990a.

Sergeant JA, Van der Meere JJ: Convergence of approaches in localizing the hyperactivity deficit. In Lahey BB, Kazdin AE (Eds), Advances in Clinical Psychology. New York: Plenum Press, pp. 207–246, 1990b.

Shallice T, Burgess P: Higher-order cognitive impairments and frontal lobe lesions in man. In Levin HS, Eisenberg HM, Benton AL (Eds), Frontal Lobe Function and Dysfunction. New York: Oxford University Press, pp. 125–138, 1991.

Simonoff E, Pickles A, Hervas A et al.: Genetic influences on childhood hyperactivity: contrast effects imply parental rating bias, not sibling interaction. Psychological Medicine: 28; 825–371, 1998.

Sloot Van der M, Licht R, Horsley TM et al.: Inhibitory Deficits in Reading Disability Depend on Subtype: Guessers but not Spellers. Neuropsychology, development, and cognition. Section C, Child neuropsychology: a Journal on Normal and Abnormal Development in Childhood and Adolescence: 6; 297–312, 2000.

Slusarek M, Velling S, Bunk D et al.: Motivational effects on inhibitory control in children with ADHD. Journal of the American Academy of Child and Adolescsent Psychiatry: 40; 355–63, 2001.

Smalley SL, Kustanovich V, Minassian SL et al: Genetic linkage of attention-deficit/hyperactivity disorder on chromosome 16p13, in a region implicated in autism. American Journal of Human Genetics: 71, 959–963, 2002.

Smith A, Taylor E, Warner-Rogers J et al.: Evidence for a pure time perception deficit in children with ADHD. Journal of Child Psychology and Psychiatry: 43; 529–542, 2002.

Solanto MV: The effects of reinforcement and response cost a delayed response task in children with attention deficit hyperactivity disorder: a research note. Journal of Child Psychology and Psychiatry: 31; 803–808, 1990

Solanto MV, Abikoff H, Sonuga-Barke E et al.: The ecological validity of delay aversion and response inhibition as measures of impulsivity in AD/HD: a supplement to the NIMH multimodal treatment study of AD/HD. Journal of Abnormal Child Psychology: 29; 215–28, 2001a.

Solanto MV, Arnsten AFT, Castellanos FX (Eds): Stimulant Drugs and ADHD: Basic and Clinical Neuroscience. New York: Oxford University Press, 2001b.

Sonuga-Barke EJS: On dysfunction and function in psychological theories of childhood disorder. Journal of Child Psychology and Psychiatry: 35; 801–815, 1994.

Sonuga-Barke EJS: Psychological heterogeneity in AD/HD — a dual pathway model of behaviour and cognition. Behavioural Brain Research: 130; 29–36, 2002.

Sonuga-Barke EJS, Houlberg K, Hall M: When is 'impulsiveness' not impulsive? The case of hyperactive children's cognitive style. Journal of Child Psychology and Psychiatry: 35; 1247–1253, 1994.

Sonuga-Barke EJS, Saxton T, Hall M: The role of interval underestimation in hyperactive children's failure to suppress responses over time. Behavioural Brain Research: 94; 45–50, 1998.

Sonuga-Barke EJS, Taylor E: The effect of delay on hyperactive and non-hyperactive children's response times. Journal of Child Psychology and Psychiatry: 33; 1091–1096, 1992.

Sonuga-Barke EJS, Taylor E, Hepenstall E: Hyperactivity and delay aversion-II: the effects of self versus externally imposed stimulus presentation periods on memory. Journal of Child Psychology and Psychiatry: 33; 399–409, 1992a.

Sonuga-Barke EJS, Taylor E, Sembi S et al.: Hyperactivity and delay aversion I: the effect of delay on choice. Journal of Child Psychology and Psychiatry: 33; 387–398, 1992b.

Sonuga-Barke EJS, Williams E, Hall M et al.: Hyperactivity and delay aversion III: the effects on cognitive style of imposing delay after errors. Journal of Child Psychology and Psychiatry: 37; 189–194, 1996.

Stuss DT, Floden D, Alexander MP et al.: Stroop performance in focal lesion patients: dissociation of processes and frontal lobe lesion location. Neuropsychologia: 39; 771–86, 2001.

Swanson J, Castellanos FX, Murias M et al.: Cognitive neuroscience of attention deficit hyperactivity disorder and hyperkinetic disorder. Current Opinion in Neurobiology: 8; 263–271, 1998a.

Swanson JM, Flodman P, Kennedy J et al.: Dopamine genes and ADHD. Neuroscience Biobehavioral Review: 24; 21–25, 2000.

Swanson J, Posner MI, Cantwell D et al.: Attention-deficit/hyperactivity disorder: symptom domains, cognitive processes, and neural networks. In Parasuraman R (Ed), The Attentive Brain. Cambridge, MA: MIT Press, pp. 445–460, 1998b.

Swanson JM, Posner MI, Potkin S et al.: Activating tasks for the study of visual–spatial attention in ADHD children; a cognitive anatomic approach. Journal of Child Neurology: 3; S119–S127, 1991.

Swanson J, Sergeant J, Taylor E et al.: Attention deficit hyperactivity disorder and hyperkinetic disorder. The Lancet: 351; 429–433, 1998c.

Szatmari P, Offord DR, Boyle MH: Ontario Child Health Study: Prevalence of attention deficit disorder with hyperactivity. Journal of Child Psychology and Psychiatry: 30; 219–230, 1989.

Tannock R: Attention deficit hyperactivity disorder: advances in cognitive, neurobiological, and genetic research. Journal of Child Psychology and Psychiatry: 39; 65–99, 1998.

Tannock R: Attention deficit disorders with anxiety disorders. In Brown TE (Ed), Attention Deficit Disorders and Comorbidities in Children, Adolescents and Adults. Washington, DC: American Psychiatric Press, pp. 125–170, 2000.

Tannock R, Martinussen R, Frijters I: Naming speed performance and stimulant effects Indicate controlled processing deficits in Attention-Deficit Hyperactivity Disorder. Journal of Abnormal Child Psychology: 28; 237–252, 2000.

Tannock R, Schachar R: Executive dysfunction as an underlying mechanism of behavior and language problems in attention deficit hyperactivity disorder. In Beitchman JH, Cohen N, Konstantareas MM, Tannock R (Eds), Language, Learning and Behaviour Disorders: Developmental, Biological, and Clinical Perspectives. Cambridge, UK: Cambridge University Press, pp. 128–155, 1996.

Tannock R, Schachar R, Logan G: Methylphenidate and cognitive flexibility: dissociated dose effects in hyperactive children. Journal of Abnormal Child Psychology: 23; 235–266, 1995.

Teicher MH, Ito Y, Glod CA et al.: Objective measurement of hyperactivity and attentional problems in ADHD. Journal of the American Academy of Child and Adolescent Psychiatry: 35; 334–42, 1996.

Thapar A, Holmes J, Poulton K et al.: Genetic basis of attention deficit and hyperactivity. British Journal of Psychiatry: 174; 105–111, 1999.

Tipper SP: Does negative priming reflect inhibitory mechanisms? A review and integration of conflicting views. Quarterly Journal of Experimental Psychology A: 54; 321–43, 2001.

Todd RD, Botteron KN: Is attention-deficit/hyperactivity disorder an energy deficiency syndrome? Biological Psychiatry: 50; 151–158, 2001.

Todd RD, Rasmussen EK, Neuman RJ et al.: Familiality and heritability of ADHD subtypes in a population of female twins. American Journal of Psychiatry: 158; 1891–189, 2001.

Todd RD, Sitdhiraksa N, Reich W et al.: Discrimination of DSM-IV and latent class attention-deficit/hyperactivity disorder subtypes by educational and cognitive performance in a population-based sample of child and adolescent twins. Journal of the American Academy of Child and Adolescent Psychiatry: 41; 820–828, 2002.

Toplak ME, Rucklidge JJ, Hetherington R et al.: Time perception deficits in attention-deficit/hyperactivity disorder and comorbid reading difficulties in child and adolescent samples. Manuscript under review, 2002.

Tucker DM, Williamson PA: Asymmetrical neural control systems in human self-regulation. Psychological Review: 91; 185–215, 1984.

Van Leeuwen TH, Steinhausen HC, Overtoom CC et al.: The continuous performance test revisited with neuroelectric mapping: impaired orienting in children with attention deficits. Behavioural Brain Research: 94; 97–110, 1998.

Van der Meere JJ: The role of attention. In Sandberg ST (Ed), Monographs in Child and Adolescent Psychiatry. Hyperactivity Disorders of Childhood. Cambridge: Cambridge University Press, pp. 109–146, 1996.

Van der Stelt O, Van der Molen M, Boudewijn Gunning W et al.: Neuroelectrical signs of selective attention to color in boys with attention-deficit hyperactivity disorder. Brain Research. Cognitive Brain Research: 12; 245–264, 2001.

Vaidya CJ, Austin G, Kirkorian G et al.: Selective effects of methylphenidate in attention deficit hyperactivity disorder: a functional magnetic resonance study. Proceeding of the National Academy of Sciences: 95; 14494–14499, 1998.

Van Boxtel GJM, Van der Molen MW, Jennings JR et al.: A psychophysiological analysis of inhibitory motor control in the stop-signal paradigm. Biological Psychology: 58; 229–262, 2001.

Van Dyck CH, Quinlan DM, Cretella LM et al.: Unaltered dopamine transporter availability in adult attention deficit hyperactivity disorder. American Journal of Psychiatry: 159; 309–312, 2002.

Volkow ND, Wang GJ, Fowler JS et al.: Effects of methylphenidate on regional brain glucose metabolism in humans: relationship to dopamine D2 receptors. American Journal of Psychiatry: 154; 50–55, 1997.

Wada N, Yamashita Y, Matsuishi T et al.: The test of variables of attention (TOVA) is useful in the diagnosis of Japanese male children with attention deficit hyperactivity disorder. Brain Development: 22; 378–382, 2000.

Wang YC, Chong MY, Chou WJ et al.: Prevalence of attention deficit hyperactivity disorder in primary school children in Taiwan. Journal of the Formosan Medical Association: 9; 133–138, 1993.

Warner-Rogers J, Taylor A, Taylor E et al.: Inattentive behavior in childhood: Epidemiology and implications for development. Journal of Learning Disabilities: 33; 520–536, 2000.

Weiss G, Hechtman LT: Hyperactive Children Grown Up: ADHD in Children, Adolescents, and Adults. New York: The Guilford Press, 1993.

Welsh MC: In Molfese DL, Molfese VJ (Eds), Developmental Variations in Learning: Applications to Social, Executive Function, Language, and Reading Skills. Mahwah, NJ: Lawrence Erlbaum, pp. 139–185, 2002.

West R, Alain C: Evidence for the transient nature of a neural system supporting goal-directed action. Cerebral Cortex: 10; 748–52, 2000.

Wiers RW, Gunning B, Sergeant JA: Is a mild deficit in executive functions in boys related to childhood ADHD or to parental multigenerational alcoholism? Journal of Abnormal Child Psychology: 26; 415–430, 1998.

Willcutt EG, Pennington BF, Boada R et al.: A comparison of the cognitive deficits in reading disability and attention-deficit/hyperactivity disorder. Journal of Abnormal Psychology: 110; 157–172, 2001.

Willcutt EG, Pennington BF, DeFries JC: Twin study of the etiology of comorbidity between reading disability and attention-deficit/hyperactivity disorder. American Journal of Medical Genetics (Neuropsychiatric Genetics): 96; 293–30, 2000.

Williams D, Stott CM, Goodyer IM et al.: Specific language impairment with or without hyperactivity: neuropsychological evidence for frontostriatal dysfunction. Developmental Medicine and Child Neurology: 42; 368–375, 2000.

Wolf M, Bowers P, Biddle K: Naming-speed processes, timing, and reading: A conceptual review. Journal of Learning Disabilities: 33; 387–407, 2000.

Wolf M, O'Rourke AG, Gidney C et al.: The second deficit: An investigation of the independence of phonological and naming-speed deficits in developmental dyslexia. Reading and Writing: 15; 43–72, 2002.

Wood C, Maruff P, Levy F et al.: Covert orienting of visual spatial attnetion in attention deficit hyperactivity disorder: Does comorbidity make a difference? Archives of Clinical Neuropsychology: 14; 179–189, 1999.

Wood FB, Felton RH: Separate linguistic and attentional factors in the development of reading. Topics in Language Disorders. Special Issue: ADD and its Relationship to Spoken and Written Language: 14; 42–57, 1994.

Woodward CA, Thomas HB, Boyle MH et al.: Methodologic note for child epidemiological surveys: the effects of instructions on estimates of behavior prevalence. Journal of Child Psychology and Psychiatry and Allied Disciplines: 30; 919–924, 1989.

Woodward LJ, Fergusson DM, Horwood LJ: Driving outcomes of young people with attentional difficulties in adolescence. Journal of the American Academy of Child and Adolescent Psychiatry: 39; 627–34, 2000.

World Health Organization: The ICD-10 Classification of Mental and Behavioral Disorders: Diagnostic Criteria for Research. Geneva, Switzerland: Author, 1993.

Yong LG, Robaey P, Karayanidis F et al.: ERPs and behavioral inhibition in a go/no-go task in children with attention-deficit hyperactivity disorder. Brain and Cognition: 43; 215–220, 2000.

Zahn TP, Kruesi MJ, Rapoport JL: Reaction time indices of attention deficits in boys with disruptive behavior disorders. Journal of Abnormal Child Psychology: 19; 233–252, 1991.

Handbook of Neuropsychology, 2nd Edition, Vol. 8, Part II
S.J. Segalowitz and I. Rapin (Eds)

CHAPTER 29

Executive functioning in normal and abnormal development

Loisa Bennetto [a,*] and Bruce F. Pennington [b]

[a] *Clinical and Social Sciences in Psychology, Meliora Hall, University of Rochester, Rochester, NY 14627, USA*
[b] *Department of Psychology, Frontier Hall, University of Denver, Denver, CO 80208, USA*

Introduction

Executive function (EF) is a term used by neuropsychologists to refer to a wide range of skills that are goal directed and future oriented. These skills include organization, planning, working memory, inhibiting inappropriate responses, and switching flexibly from one task or strategy to another. A common feature of EFs is that they allow an individual to disengage from the current situation or context, and use a mental representation to guide future responding. These abilities are clearly important for many complex human behaviors, and particularly for those that require an individual to process constantly changing input and environmental contingencies.

The construct of EF has provided a promising model for understanding many aspects of both normal and abnormal development. On the one hand, developmental research has identified EF as a key component underlying a variety of changes in cognitive development in both childhood and aging. On the other hand, deficient EF has been cited as a primary impairment in several developmental disorders, including attention-deficit/hyperactivity disorder (ADHD), autism, and Tourette syndrome. EF deficits have also been found in several psychiatric disorders, including conduct disorder and schizophrenia, as well as neurological disorders with known genetic etiologies, such as fragile X syndrome and early-treated phenylketonuria. Not only do patients with these various disorders typically perform poorly on traditional EF tests, but a number of theoretical models have linked EF and the development, or at least presence of some of the social and behavioral symptoms that characterize these disorders.

The fact that EF deficits have been found in so many disorders is also the root of the problem in using EF as a model for various forms of psychopathology. Because globally conceived EF deficits appear to be present across a wide range of complex behavioral disorders, they consequently hold very little explanatory power for any one of them. In other words, how can disorders with clearly different behavioral characteristics share the same neuropsychological underpinnings? In this chapter, we will explore several solutions to this problem of discriminant validity. In our discussion, we will address conceptual issues related to EF, as well as empirical issues related to its measurement. Next, we will explore the role of EF in several neurodevelopmental disorders. We will focus our discussion on autism, as a paradigm of our model for understanding executive dysfunction in psychopathology. We will also discuss how this model applies to both ADHD and fragile X syndrome. Finally, we will conclude by examining what this developmental psychopathology approach can tell us about the construct of EF for both normal and abnormal development.

* Corresponding author. E-mail: bennetto@psych.rochester.edu

Conceptual and empirical issues

EFs are often described as a unitary construct. This perspective is due, in part, to their association with the frontal lobes. Since at least the time of Harlow's (1868) report of Phineas Gage, the frontal lobes have been associated with planning and other aspects of higher order cognition. Much of the early work that followed suggested that this region of the brain was broadly responsible for 'supervisory' aspects of behavior (e.g., Brickner, 1934; Goldstein, 1941), but played little role in the specifics of general intellectual functioning (Hebb, 1945). Although more recent research demonstrates the nonequipotentiality of the frontal cortices (discussed below), the tendency persists to lump together the functions of the frontal lobes.

Components of EF

The unitary nature of EF has also been sustained by the use of traditional, broadly defined neuropsychological tests that tap a range of executive abilities (Pennington, Bennetto, McAleer and Roberts, 1996). Recent studies that employ more precise tasks suggest that EF may instead be composed of a set of unique and dissociable components, including cognitive flexibility, planning, working memory, and inhibition (e.g., Baddeley, 1986; Burgess, 1997; Duncan, Burgess and Emslie, 1995; Pennington, 1997; Robbins, 1998).

Cognitive flexibility refers to the ability to shift one's thoughts or behavior to adapt to the changing demands of a situation (Lezak, 1995). To solve a novel problem, one often needs to shift from an ineffective strategy to a new one. In a social situation, one may need to change conversation topics if one's partner seems disinterested. Cognitive flexibility is also evident in a concrete or literal interpretation of language. To understand idioms and sarcasm, one must shift from the literal meaning of the word to its intended meaning. Individuals who have problems with flexibility may engage in perseverative responding, or the continued use of a previously correct behavior even though that behavior is no longer appropriate. Similarly, they may appear to utilize concrete or rigid approaches to problem solving because they are unable to generate novel strategies that take into account feedback about performance or new aspects of a situation.

Working memory is a construct that was first proposed by Baddeley and Hitch (1974) to refer to the simultaneous processing and storage of information during complex cognitive tasks. Individuals with limited working memory have difficulty holding ideas or choices in their minds as they evaluate and select the most appropriate course of action. Similarly, poor working memory can impair one's ability to remember and complete several steps of a task in the correct order. More recently, working memory has been described as critical for integrating short-lived, context-specific information from diverse sources (Pennington, 1994), and thus provides a theoretical tie between EF and social interactions. Effective social interaction depends on the integration of multiple, constantly changing cues that are often much more subtle and complex than the types of cues used in neuropsychological studies.

Another component of EF is the ability to inhibit thoughts and actions. Inhibition may involve stopping oneself from processing irrelevant details in one's environment, or from executing a well-practiced, habitual response in a situation where that response is not appropriate or adaptive. Poor inhibition may also lead to repetitive behaviors or patterns of responding (Turner, 1997a).

Several models have been proposed to explain these apparent components within the EF domain (see Roberts, Robbins and Weiskrantz, 1998 for a comprehensive review of EF models). For example, Baddeley (1986; Baddeley and Hitch, 1974) proposed a complex system composed of a central executive and two specialized subsidiary systems, the phonological loop and the visuospatial scratchpad. According to this model, the central executive is responsible for the attentional control of working memory and for allocating cognitive resources. More recent work in this area has identified subcomponent processes within the central executive, such as the ability to selectively attend to stimuli versus switch attention flexibly from one stimulus to another (Baddeley, 1996). Shallice (1988) proposed a similar model, in which a Supervisory Attentional System (SAS) exerts higher level control over more automatic, modular processing systems. Again, more recent accounts of this theory have begun to fractionate the SAS into subcomponents, such as working memory, strategy generation, and monitoring (Shallice and Burgess, 1998). Roberts and Pennington (1996) conceptualize EF processing as a dynamic interaction between working memory resources, the working memory demands of a task, and the strength of competing response alternatives. In this model, inhibition is intrinsic to the working memory demands of a task; increases in working memory resources inhibit the activation of prepotent but incorrect response choices. In general, these models support dissociations within the EF domain, and may help explain performance differences across age or between disorders.

Several empirical approaches have also been used to identify components or dimensions of EF. First, factor analytic approaches suggest that batteries of EF tests do not have a unitary factor structure (Levin, Eisenberg and Benton, 1991; Pennington, 1997; Welsh, Pennington and Groisser, 1991). For example, Pennington (1997) conducted factor analyses on the performance of a large sample of twins, including both children with and without reading disabilities, on a range of EF tasks. Their analyses identified at least three distinguishable factors. A version of the Continuous Performance Task (AX) and the Stopping Task (Logan, Cowan and Davis, 1984) loaded onto the first factor, Inhibition. The second factor, Set-shifting, included the Wisconsin Card Sorting Test (Heaton, Chelune, Talley et al., 1993), the Contingency Naming Test (Taylor, 1988), the Stroop Test, and two measures of intelligence. A third Working Memory factor also emerged; tasks that loaded onto this factor were two verbal working memory span tasks and a digit span task.

A second approach to identifying components of EF is to compare performance differences across developmental disorders with globally defined EF deficits (e.g., Ozonoff, 1997; Ozonoff and Jensen, 1999; Pennington, 1997). This line of research has provided further confirmation that individual tasks are measuring distinct abilities within the broader domain of executive functioning. For example, Ozonoff and Jensen (1999) found that children with autism performed significantly worse on tests of flexibility and planning than age-matched children with Tourette syndrome, ADHD, and normal controls, after covarying group differences in Full Scale IQ. In contrast, children with ADHD performed poorly on a test of inhibition, but not on tests of flexibility or planning. Pennington (1997) compared individuals with autism, fragile X syndrome, and ADHD, and found a similar differentiation of abilities across specific EF tasks.

Neurobiological evidence for EF components

This componential approach to EF has been largely supported by neurobiological research. As mentioned above, early theories assumed equipotentiality of the frontal cortex. But recent research suggests that different areas of the prefrontal cortex are required for distinct functions. For example, fMRI studies with both adults (Braver, Cohen, Nystrom et al., 1997; Cohen, Forman, Braver et al., 1994) and children (Casey, Cohen, Jezzaard et al., 1995) have demonstrated reliable activity in the dorsolateral prefrontal cortex during a working memory task. In contrast, an fMRI study of inhibition in both adults and children demonstrated increased activation in the anterior cingulate, inferior and middle frontal gyri, and orbitofrontal gyri (Casey, Trainor, Orendi et al., 1997).

Other studies have begun to differentiate these subcomponent processes even further. For example, several behavioral studies have demonstrated a dissociation between working memory involving phonological versus visuospatial information (e.g., Cornoldi, Vecchia and Tressoldi, 1995; Shah and Miyake, 1996). Neurobiological studies also support distinctions within EF components. Goldman-Rakic and her colleagues have examined the working memory domain in primate models. They demonstrated dissociations between spatial versus featural aspects of the to-be-remembered stimulus, which mapped onto the dorsolateral and inferior regions of the prefrontal cortex, respectively (Wilson, Scalaidhe and Goldman-Rakic, 1993). Dias, Robbins and Roberts (1996) similarly distinguish two types of set shifting: attentional (shifting from one perceptual dimension of a stimulus to another) versus affective (shifting between stimulus-reward associations). In a lesion study of marmoset monkeys, they demonstrated that attentional shifts were controlled by the lateral prefrontal cortex, whereas affective shifts were controlled by the orbitofrontal region.

Thus, there is increasing evidence that distinct regions within the prefrontal cortex serve different components of EF. This provides a possible solution to the discriminant validity problem, in that different disorders may have developmental lesions that affect very specific areas within the prefrontal cortex. It may also be the case that disorders differ in their connectivity between the prefrontal cortex and other cortical or subcortical regions.

Age-related variations in frontal lobe development may also influence different patterns of EF deficits across disorders. The maturation of the human prefrontal cortex is quite protracted, and thus critical changes in its functional development continue to occur through adolescence (see Casey, Giedd and Thomas, 2000 for a review). Synaptic density in the prefrontal cortex shows relatively large increases through age 2 (e.g., Huttenlocher, 1990), which is considerably later than when peak density is reached in posterior regions. Similarly, the pruning phase is prolonged in prefrontal compared to posterior (e.g., visual) cortex (Huttenlocher, 1990, 1997). Metabolic activity in the prefrontal cortex is consistent with this time course of synaptogenesis and pruning, and does not reach adult levels until late adolescence (Chiron, Raynaud, Maziere et al., 1992; Chugani, Phelps and Mazziotta, 1987). Maturation of neurotransmitter systems, and particularly serotonin synthesis may also play a role in developmental changes in prefrontal function. In typically developing children, serotonin synthesis capacity in the brain increases between ages 2 and 5 to nearly twice that of normal adult levels, then declines to adult levels before puberty (Chugani, Muzik, Behen et al., 1999). Since serotonin levels have been shown to modulate neuronal differentiation and synaptic connectivity in animal models, this developmental increase is likely to play an important role in postnatal brain development. In summary, given the extended maturation of the prefrontal regions, this area of the brain may be more sensitive to individual differences and/or susceptible to developmental insults.

A related issue is that different neurocognitive tasks may rely on different regions of the brain depending on the age of the individual. For example, Casey, Trainor, Orendi et al. (1997) examined the neural bases of inhibition in both children (7–12 years old) and young adults using fMRI. Their results showed that children and adults activated similar regions of the brain for Go–No Go tasks, but that adults showed less activation overall (perhaps following the decrease in synapses discussed above, or as a function of increased inhibition). Their findings also suggest that children may be less selective in which prefrontal regions they use for various tasks, or that children rely on different strategies than adults to perform the same tasks. Primate studies have demonstrated that performance on a standard delayed-response task relies on the dorsolateral prefrontal cortex in adult animals, but appears to depend on different regions during infancy, with increasing involvement of the dorsolateral regions over time (e.g., Alexander and Goldman, 1978). Thus, changes in performance may depend not only on maturation of specific brain regions, but also on increased integration of neural circuitry.

These observations may help to explain EF performance differences within, as well as across disorders. As we will discuss below, one challenge to an EF model of autism is that not all studies of young children have found autism-specific impairments on EF tasks. If different brain regions serve these functions at young ages, it is possible that what appear to be 'frontal' impairments may not be evident until children are older.

Measurement issues

It is also important to discuss the measurement problems inherent in some existing EF tests. To the extent that traditional EF tests tend to be complex tasks that assess multiple interacting processes, performance on them can be disrupted in many different ways. Tests like the Wisconsin Card Sorting Test (WCST) may tap multiple aspects of executive functioning, as well as nonexecutive components that are unlikely to be related to the functioning of the prefrontal cortex. In the WCST, four 'key' cards are placed in front of the subject. The cards have patterns on them that vary in terms of color (e.g., red, green), form (e.g., circle, triangle), and number (e.g., 1 shape, 2 shapes). The subject is given a stack of cards and asked to match them to one of the four key cards. The subject is not told how to match the cards (i.e., according to shape, color, or number), but is told after each match whether it was 'right' or 'wrong.' After 10 correct trials, the experimenter changes the sorting rule without telling the subject. Since the old rule no longer works, the subject must shift his or her strategy to discover the new one. Thus, performance on the WCST requires active strategy formation, maintenance in working memory of the current category and most recently reinforced response, and inhibition of the previously reinforced, but incorrect category. In addition, knowledge and salience of the individual categories themselves can affect performance. A child who has not yet attained the category of number could sort only to color and form, and would thus be more likely to perseverate to these categories. The WCST may also involve aspects of social processing, as the experimenter identifies whether each sort was right or wrong, and deceives the subject by changing the sorting rule without warning. Ozonoff (1995) compared performance on experimenter- versus computer-administered versions of the WCST, and found that children with autism were significantly better on the computer-administered version than the standard version of this task.

Newer instruments for measuring EF may help to address this issue. For example, the Cambridge Neuropsychological Test Automated Battery (CANTAB; Robbins et al., 1994, 1998) is becoming an increasingly popular method for assessing EF in neurological and psychiatric populations. The battery contains tests measuring a range of EF components (i.e., set shifting, working memory, planning), as well as visual memory and learning tasks. All tests are nonverbal and administered with a computerized touch screen, so they are ideal for testing both children and individuals with developmental disorders. In addition to batteries that tap multiple aspects of EF, there is a clear need for tasks that employ within-subjects controls for nonessential processes (e.g., number concept, memory, language, motor skills).

Finally, complex EF tasks may have problems with specificity and sensitivity. For example, the WCST has failed to discriminate patients with focal frontal damage from patients with diffuse damage or with focal nonfrontal damage (Anderson, Damasio, Jones and Tranel, 1991; Axelrod, Goldman, Heaton et al., 1996; see Heaton et al., 1993, for a review). On the other hand, some patients with documented frontal lesions and dramatic organizational problems in everyday life perform within normal limits on the WCST (Damasio, Tranel and Damasio, 1991).

In the sections below, we will outline what has been learned in studies examining EF in autism, ADHD, and fragile X syndrome. In this review, we will include empirical studies that utilized appropriately matched comparison groups (i.e., matched on both age and IQ, unless otherwise noted). Because the componential approach outlined above has been helpful in understanding EFs across disorders, we will organize the review when possible by performance on key components of EF including cognitive flexibility, working memory, and inhibition.

Executive functions in autism

Autism is a neurodevelopmental disorder that involves impairments in social relatedness and communication, as well as restricted or repetitive patterns of behavior. In recent years, considerable attention has focused on the possible role of executive dysfunction in both the cognitive and the behavioral profiles of this disorder. Many individuals with autism have difficulty with change, tend to focus on specific topics or interests, and may adhere strictly to routines. This tendency to persist with a particular response or behavior, even despite feedback that the response is incorrect, is a central feature of executive dysfunction.

Many early descriptive papers on autism documented evidence consistent with EF impairment, including difficulties with abstract thinking (Scheerer, Rothman and Goldstein, 1945), tendencies toward perseverative response patterns (e.g., Hermelin and O'Conner, 1970), and stimulus overselectivity (Lovaas and Schreibman, 1971). It was not until the mid-1980's, however, that empirical work directly addressing this issue was conducted (Rumsey, 1985; Steel, Gorman and Flexman, 1984). Since then, many research centers have examined EF in children, adolescents, and adults with autism (see Pennington and Ozonoff, 1996 for a review). The majority of these tasks have found EF deficits compared to appropriately matched control groups, which has led researchers to propose that the symptoms of autism are due to a core deficit in EF (Ozonoff, Pennington and Rogers, 1991; see Russell, 1997 for a review).

Cognitive and behavioral flexibility in autism

Impaired flexibility in both thoughts and behavior is a common feature of autism, and research in this area has consistently documented difficulties. One of the most frequently used tasks of EF, the WCST, is typically considered a measure of cognitive flexibility (Lezak, 1995). Individuals with autism often have great difficulty shifting to a new sorting strategy on this test. Instead, they often make 'perseverative responses' by continuing to sort cards according to the old strategy, despite the fact that they are repeatedly told their responses are incorrect. In our experience, it is not uncommon for individuals with autism to make over 50 consecutive perseverative responses, even though they are clearly trying to, and may eventually find the new rule.

The WCST was first employed in a research study by Rumsey (1985), who found that high-functioning adults with autism made significantly more perseverative responses than a control sample matched on age and Performance IQ. Since that time, the WCST has been used in many studies of autism, including studies of both adults (e.g., Ciesielski and Harris, 1997; Rumsey and Hamburger, 1990) and children (e.g., Ozonoff et al., 1991; Prior and Hoffman, 1990). Of the studies reported thus far, only three have failed to find impaired WCST performance in autism (Minshew, Goldstein, Muenz and Payton, 1992; Minshew, Goldstein and Siegel, 1997; Schneider and Asarnow, 1987). In addition, Liss, Fein, Allen et al. (2001) found that children with high-functioning autism were impaired on the WCST relative to controls with developmental language disorder matched on Full Scale IQ, Nonverbal IQ, and age. However, this group difference was no longer significant after accounting for the effects of Verbal IQ. Finally, a three-year longitudinal study of adolescents with high-functioning autism found that impaired flexibility on the WCST appears to be stable over time (Ozonoff and McEvoy, 1994). In general, research on the WCST suggests it is a sensitive indicator of perseverative behavior in autism, but also points to some degree of variability within the EF domain.

Although the WCST clearly tests flexibility, poor performance may be influenced by a number of other variables, including concept formation, understanding of the category of number, and encoding social feedback. To address this lack of specificity, Hughes, Russell and Robbins (1994) examined the performance of subjects with autism on the intra-dimensional/extra-dimensional (ID/ED) set-shifting task from the CANTAB. This is a simplified version of the set-shifting component of the WCST and allows for more valid assessment of a greater range of ability levels. Their results suggested that subjects with autism were differentially impaired in attentional set shifting relative to control subjects.

Working memory in autism

Working memory refers to the online processing and storage of information during complex tasks. This type of active maintenance and control of memory appears to be distinct from rote, factual memory and recognition memory (e.g., Shimamura, Janowsky and Squire, 1991). Since the latter are often a strength for individuals with autism (e.g., Bennetto, Pennington and Rogers, 1996), the concept of working memory may help explain why individuals with autism can demonstrate such marked discrepancies between memory for specific, rote information and memory for multi-step, verbal directions. Similarly, impairments in working memory may account for the difficulties that individuals with autism have in processing social information.

Several studies have examined working memory skills in children and adolescents with autism. Bennetto et al. (1996) examined verbal working memory in a group of high-functioning adolescents with autism, compared to a control group matched on age and Verbal IQ. They utilized two verbal span tasks designed to measure concurrent storage and processing of information, as well as a comprehensive battery of traditional memory tasks. The subjects with autism demonstrated a pattern of strengths and weaknesses consistent with impairment in working memory, but not rote memory. In particular, they demonstrated intact rote memory, short- and long-term recognition, and cued recall, but significant impairments on verbal working memory, temporal order memory, and source memory. Russell, Jarrold and Henry (1996) also examined working memory in children with autism. Using Baddeley and Hitch's (1974) model of working memory, they designed tasks to measure both the articulatory loop (i.e., the system that updates information through articulatory rehearsal) and the central executive (i.e., the limited-capacity processing space, which utilizes information held in the articulatory loop). They compared lower functioning children with autism to control groups of children with moderate learning disabilities matched on verbal mental age (MA) and normally developing children matched on verbal MA. Their results suggested that at least verbal children with autism have an intact articulatory loop, which is consistent with typically reported good performance on rote memory tasks. However, compared to the subjects with moderate learning disabilities, the subjects with autism did not demonstrate impairments on tasks designed to measure central executive functioning. In fact, both children with autism and children with moderate learning disability were impaired relative to the normally developing children in this domain. This raises the question of whether general or diffuse neurological dysfunction is more likely to disrupt the pathways required for working memory tasks, and thus whether working memory can be a core impairment in autism or any neurological disorder.

A related question is whether individuals with autism are impaired on nonverbal working memory tasks. Neither working memory task in the Bennetto et al. (1996) study, and only one of the tasks in the Russell et al. (1996) study was nonverbal, and one could argue that verbal working memory is more difficult for individuals with autism simply because of the verbal demands. Turner (1997b) addressed this question by administering two spatial working memory tasks to individuals with autism and matched clinical control subjects. On both tasks, she found that subjects with autism were significantly worse than control subjects when they were required to devise, or even simply implement strategies to enhance their performance. This difficulty appeared to hold for both high-functioning and low-functioning subjects with autism, when compared to appropriate controls. In contrast, Ozonoff and Strayer (2001) administered three nonverbal working memory tasks to children with high-functioning autism, children with Tourette syndrome, and typically developing children, matched on age and IQ. They found no group differences on any of the tasks.

In summary, the results on working memory in autism are inconclusive. Although working memory deficits appear to be present in some individuals with autism, it may be the case that impaired working memory is a manifestation of any type of neurological involvement. Thus, while attention to poor working memory may be useful in devising treatment programs, it may not provide answers to the etiology of autistic symptoms.

Inhibition in autism

Inhibition has been measured in subjects with autism utilizing a variety of neuropsychological and cognitive paradigms. The Stroop Color–Word Test (Stroop, 1935) is a traditional neuropsychological task that is often used to measure inhibition (Lezak, 1995). Subjects are first asked to read a list of printed words (e.g., 'red,' 'blue'). Next, they are asked to name the ink color of a series of colored non-word stimuli. In the final condition, subjects are asked to name the ink color of a series of color words that are printed in incongruent colors (e.g., 'red' printed in blue ink). This latter condition requires subjects to inhibit the automatic response of reading printed words. Two studies have examined the performance of high-functioning individuals with autism using variations on the Stroop paradigm (Bryson, 1983; Eskes, Bryson and McCormick, 1990). The results of the two studies were similar: subjects with autism demonstrated a normal 'Stroop interference effect,' which suggested that they were able to represent the semantic context of the words in the task. They did not, however, show a differentially greater interference effect than controls, which suggests that their inhibition was no better or worse than expected.

Ozonoff, Strayer, McMahon and Filloux (1994) compared the inhibitory skills of a group of high-functioning children with autism and matched comparison groups of children with Tourette syndrome and normally developing children. They utilized the Go–No Go task, which was designed to test increasingly complex types of inhibition (i.e., inhibition of a neutral response, inhibition of a habitual response, and cognitive flexibility between different response patterns). The authors found that subjects with autism were unimpaired on neutral inhibition, but made significantly more errors on the habitual responding and flexibility conditions. These results suggest that impaired cognitive set shifting, rather than simple motor inhibition, may underlie EF deficits in autism.

Ozonoff and Strayer (1997) further examined inhibitory processes in high-functioning children with autism on tasks measuring motor and cognitive inhibition. On the first task, subjects were tested on their ability to inhibit a motor response to neutral and prepotent stimuli, which placed relatively little demand on cognitive set shifting. On a second task, the authors measured negative priming, which was thought to involve a more central cognitive inhibitory process. The authors found that, compared to matched controls, subjects with autism were unimpaired on both measures of inhibition.

Finally, Hughes (1996) examined the performance of children with autism, children with learning difficulties, and normal controls on a task designed to assess inhibitory control of hand gestures, a task which had previously been shown to be difficult for patients with frontal lesions. A second task measured the ability to delay gratification by inhibiting a smaller short-term reward in favor of a larger delayed reward. On both tasks, children with autism were less able to inhibit prepotent responses than control subjects, which may be the result of poor inhibitory control, impaired flexibility, or difficulty using language to mediate self-control strategies.

In summary, individuals with autism appear to have intact inhibition on relatively simple cognitive and motor tasks. However, they may have more difficulty when required not only to inhibit, but also to shift their attention or cognitive set to a new stimulus.

EF deficits in young children with autism

While the above studies have documented varying degrees of impairment on EF tasks in older children, adolescents, and adults with autism, EF deficits in preschoolers have not been as consistently documented. McEvoy, Rogers and Pennington (1993) examined EF in a group of young children with autism (mean age of 64 months), compared to both matched clinical and typical comparison groups. They found significantly worse performance in the autism group on a Spatial Reversal task, which involves both shifting set and inhibiting a previously reinforced response. However, a near-replication of this study in a younger group of children (mean age 51 months) did not find autism-specific deficits on Spatial Reversal or any of a number of other EF tasks (Griffith, Pennington, Wehner and Rogers, 1999). Lack of group differences in preschoolers with autism on EF tasks was also reported by Barth, Fein and Waterhouse (1995). However, Dawson, Meltzoff, Osterling and Rinaldi (1998) reported that compared to both matched clinical and typical controls, preschoolers with autism performed worse on a delayed response task, thought to tap dorsolateral prefrontal functioning, but also performed worse a delayed nonmatching-to-sample task thought to measure medial temporal lobe functioning. In general, these studies raise questions about whether executive deficits are present early in the development of children with autism, and whether EF is therefore a reasonable candidate for a primary deficit.

Neurological evidence of EF impairment in autism

EF impairment is typically associated with patients who have prefrontal lobe lesions. Such patients often have difficulties with organization and planning, exhibit repetitive behaviors and speech, display a lack of insight and poor understanding of social rules, and often, but not always perform poorly on traditional tests of EF (Stuss and Benson, 1986). Thus, patients with frontal lobe damage share many similarities to individuals with autism. However, diffuse brain damage (e.g., Heaton et al., 1993), injury to subcortical structures connected to the frontal lobes (e.g., Cummings, 1993), and damage to attention systems such as the cerebellum (e.g., Courchesne, Townsend, Akshoomoff et al., 1994) can also produce EF impairment. Thus, while patients with prefrontal lobe lesions may provide a good analogy for understanding some of the characteristics of autism, poor performance on EF tasks does not mean that individuals with autism have frontal lobe dysfunction. In recent years, there has been considerable progress in understanding the neuropathology of autism (for reviews see Bailey, Phillips and Rutter, 1996; Robbins, 1997). There are several studies that bear specifically on EF deficits, which we will discuss briefly below.

Zilbovicius, Garreau, Tzourio et al. (1992) measured regional cerebral blood flow in a group of 5 to 11 year old children with autism. They found no evidence of localized cortical dysfunction or delayed maturation compared to age-matched controls with language delays. Zilbovicius, Garreau, Samson et al. (1995) later conducted a longitudinal study of metabolic maturation of the frontal cortex in a group of children with autism and age-matched controls. They measured single photon emission computed tomography (SPECT) between the ages of 3 and 4, and again between ages 6 and 7. The authors found that at 3–4 years, children with autism showed a pattern of normal posterior and global cortical values, but significantly lower blood flow in frontal cortex. This frontal hypoperfusion is similar to the pattern reported in much younger normal children. By the age of 6–7, however, the frontal cerebral blood flow of children with autism had increased to normal levels, which was consistent with their earlier findings. These two studies suggest a delayed postnatal maturation of frontal cortex in autism, and have significant implications for the EF theory of autism. Metabolically active frontal lobes are obviously important for cognitive development, and delays in maturation may help to explain the findings discussed above. A further implication is that normal metabolic activity during critical periods is thought to be important in postnatal synaptogenesis and neuronal pruning. Thus it is possible that abnormal frontal input during early years may have altered the connectivity of neural structures in autism. This idea is consistent with findings of decreased metabolic connectivity between frontal and parietal cortex (Horwitz, Rumsey, Grady and Rapoport, 1988) and abnormal phospholipid metabolism in dorsolateral prefrontal cortex (Minshew, Goldstein, Dombrowski et al., 1993). These findings also underscore the fact that EF tasks do not share a one-to-one correspondence with frontal functioning. Because the frontal lobes share extensive reciprocal connections with other brain regions, damage to other areas or in the pattern of connectivity between areas may also produce EF-type deficits (e.g., Ciesielski, Harris, Hart and Pabst, 1997).

A related area of research in autism involves differences in expected developmental changes of neurotransmitter levels. Chugani et al. (1999) have recently documented that the normal period of high serotonin synthesis in the brain (typically through age 5) continues even longer in autism, through age 15. In addition, they have observed focal abnormalities in serotonin synthesis in the frontal cortex, thalamus, and cerebellum (Chugani, Muzik, Rothermel et al., 1997). This protracted period of increased brain serotonin levels may lead to disruptions in synaptogenesis.

Limitations of the EF model of autism

For a neuropsychological deficit to be a primary cause of a disorder, it should be present in all individuals with the disorder, and be specific to that disorder and not others. Although the majority of studies have found EF deficits in autism, not all studies have confirmed this finding (e.g., Minshew et al., 1997; Schneider and Asarnow, 1987). In addition, much of the neuropsychological research in autism has been conducted with high-functioning subjects, and may not be generalizable to individuals with autism who also have mental retardation. For example, as discussed above, research on components of EF has demonstrated working memory impairments in subjects with high-functioning autism relative to IQ-matched controls (e.g., Bennetto et al., 1996; Turner, 1997b), but not in low-functioning subjects relative to matched controls with mental retardation (e.g., Griffith et al., 1999; Russell et al., 1996; Turner, 1997b). These findings could indicate that EF impairment is not present in all individuals with autism and therefore cannot be a primary cause of the disorder. Conversely, the EF tasks used in these studies may not be sensitive enough to detect impairment in individuals across the lifespan or the full range of IQs.

Executive functions in attention-deficit/hyperactivity disorder

ADHD is one of the most common, chronic disorders of childhood. It is diagnosed by the presence of one or both of two distinct, yet correlated behavioral dimensions: inattention and hyperactivity-impulsivity. These symptoms have an early onset, are inconsistent with a child's developmental level, and are present across multiple situations. Deficits in EF have long been thought to be integral to ADHD, in part because of their apparent value in explaining the behavioral symptoms of the disorder. A recent review of EF in ADHD reported that 15 of 18 published studies found significantly worse performance in subjects with ADHD compared to controls on one or more EF measures (Pennington and Ozonoff, 1996). A total of 60 EF tasks were used across all studies reviewed; subjects with ADHD showed relative deficits on 40 of these. In contrast, none of the tasks was a significant strength in the ADHD group.

Like children with autism, those with ADHD tend to perform poorly on molar tests of EF. For example, the majority of studies employing the Tower of Hanoi in ADHD have found them to be impaired relative to controls (Aman, Roberts and Pennington, 1998; Pennington, Groisser and Welsh, 1993; Weyandt and Willis, 1994), though some studies have not found significant group differences (Ozonoff and Jensen, 1999). The Tower of Hanoi and its variants are disk-transfer problems that broadly assess planning, but also require abstract thinking, goal maintenance, working memory, and inhibition. Although individuals with autism and ADHD often perform poorly on the Tower of Hanoi, a componential analysis of their EF deficits begins to reveal distinct patterns of intact and impaired abilities. While individuals with autism showed the clearest evidence for deficits in set shifting, individuals with ADHD demonstrate consistent impairments on tasks involving inhibition or delay of behavioral responses.

A core deficit in inhibition has been supported by a number of researchers in this area (e.g., Barkley, 1997; Conners and Wells, 1986; Douglas, 1983; Schachar, Tannock and Logan, 1993; see Tannock, 2003, this volume, for a comprehensive review). Individuals with ADHD have demonstrated clear impairments on tests of relatively pure motor inhibition in the majority of studies reported in the literature. One commonly used task, the Stop Signal Task (Logan et al., 1984) measures voluntary motor inhibition by teaching a subject a particular response, then later requiring them to inhibit that same response on trials on which they hear a tone or beep. A recent meta-analysis of the Stop Signal task (Oosterlaan and Sergeant, 1998) reported consistent deficits in ADHD groups on this type of motor inhibition. Studies employing other motor inhibition tasks, such as the Go–No Go and Anti-Saccade tasks, have also reported ADHD-specific deficits relative to controls (e.g., Aman et al., 1998). Similarly, the majority of studies using inhibition measures with a cognitive component, such as the Stroop Color–Word and Matching Familiar Figures tests, have found performance to be worse in subjects with ADHD (e.g., Grodzinsky and Diamond, 1992; Ozonoff and Jensen, 1999; see Pennington and Ozonoff, 1996 for a review).

There is increasing evidence that motor inhibition may be related to the underlying biology of ADHD. For example, Aman et al. (1998) demonstrated that ADHD-specific deficits on the Stop Signal task were normalized when children were given methylphenidate. Casey and colleagues (Casey, Castellanos, Giedd et al., 1997) tested children with ADHD and age-matched controls on three inhibition tasks. Subjects with ADHD performed significantly worse on all three tasks. Furthermore, performance on these tasks was correlated with MRI-based volumetric measurements of right frontostriatal circuitry that has previously been shown to be abnormal in ADHD, including the prefrontal cortex, caudate nucleus, and globus pallidus (e.g., Castellanos, Giedd, Eckburg et al., 1994; Castellanos, Giedd, Marsh et al., 1996; Zametkin, Nordahl, Gross et al., 1990).

In contrast to tests of inhibition, subjects with ADHD are less consistently impaired on tests involving cognitive flexibility or set shifting. In the Pennington and Ozonoff (1996) review, only 4 out of 10 studies reported deficient performance in children with ADHD on the WCST. In fact, two studies that specifically compared tests of inhibition and set shifting in children with ADHD found clear differences on tests of inhibition, but intact performance on tests involving set shifting (Grodzinsky and Diamond, 1992; Ozonoff and Jensen, 1999).

Less attention has been paid to working memory deficits in ADHD, but preliminary studies suggest that this is not an area of impairment. Siegel and Ryan (1989) compared children with ADHD and typical controls on two verbal working memory span tasks. They found that the 9–10 year old ADHD group performed similarly to matched controls on both tasks; 7–8 year old children showed intact performance on one of the two tasks, but lower scores on the other. Recently, we compared working memory and inhibition skills across three samples: children with ADHD ($n = 15$), children with autism ($n = 19$), and women with fragile X syndrome ($n = 20$) (Bennetto and Pennington, 1999). Each group was matched to its own control group on age and IQ. On two verbal working memory span tasks (similar to those used in Siegel and Ryan, 1989), subjects with autism and fragile X syndrome were significantly impaired relative to their controls, while subjects with ADHD demonstrated intact performance. In contrast, subjects with ADHD were impaired on measures of inhibition (Stroop Color–Word task), while the other groups were not.

Comorbidity and subtypes of ADHD

Over half of children who meet diagnostic criteria for ADHD qualify for a comorbid diagnosis (Biederman, Faraone, Keenan et al., 1992), which can include conduct disorder, Tourette syndrome, oppositional defiant disorder, and reading disorder. EF deficits have previously been documented in the first two of these comorbid conditions, which may impact the strength of EF findings in heterogeneous ADHD samples. Thus, studies that control for or examine the effects of comorbid conditions will be most helpful in specifying the nature of EF deficits in ADHD (e.g., Klorman, Hazel-Fernandez, Shaywitz et al., 1999; Moffitt and Henry, 1989).

A related issue involves heterogeneity within the ADHD diagnosis. Several studies have found different patterns of EF functioning when comparing children with the predominantly inattentive, predominantly hyperactive–impulsive, or combined subtype of ADHD (e.g., Barkley, 1998; Houghton, Douglas, West et al., 1999; Klorman et al., 1999), with children diagnosed with the combined subtype typically showing the strongest EF deficits.

Executive functions in fragile X syndrome

Fragile X syndrome (FXS) is the leading inherited cause of mental retardation in males (see Hagerman and Cronister, 1996, for a review). It is associated with an abnormal gene at the Xq27.3 location, characterized by an unstable CGG trinucleotide repeat sequence. In the normal population, the Fragile X Mental Retardation (*FMR1*) gene contains between 6 and 50 CGG repeats. In individuals with a FXS premutation, the size of the amplification can range from 50 to 200 repeats. Individuals with this premutation typically do not exhibit the cognitive characteristics of the FXS phenotype. A full mutation contains over 200 trinucleotide repeats, and is usually associated with hypermethylation of the *FMR1* gene and the adjacent CpG island, which prevents transcription of the *FMR1* gene. Reduced or absent amounts of the RNA binding protein (FMRP) coded for by this gene have general effects on gene transcription, which lead to the phenotypic effects of FXS, including mental retardation in most males.

Studies of females with a FXS full mutation have identified a wider spectrum of involvement, with an average IQ roughly one standard deviation below population norms, as well as neuropsychological deficits in several areas (see Bennetto and Pennington, 1996 for a review). The greater variation in the phenotypic expression in females is due, in part, to the normal process of X inactivation. Females have two X chromosomes, one of which is randomly inactivated to prevent over-production of proteins coded by X chromosome genes. Since a full mutation female only has the FXS mutation on one of her X chromosomes, the other X chromosome has a normal *FMR1* gene that can produce FMRP. Measuring the proportion of normal X chromosomes that are active thus provides a link between the underlying biology and neurocognitive characteristics of this disorder. In addition, because roughly two-thirds of females with a full mutation have cognitive skills in the normal to borderline range of intelligence, they provide a unique opportunity to study a titrated form of this mental retardation syndrome. By examining these milder forms of FXS, we can use a greater range of tests to identify specific effects of the *FMR1* mutation on brain functions, apart from the nonspecific effects on overall developmental level.

Neuropsychological research on FXS has focused primarily on determining whether EF impairment is a core part of the phenotype, and is only beginning to shift toward looking at components within the EF domain. A deficit in EF is consistent with some of the behavioral problems often observed in males with FXS. These problems include poor attentional control, impulsivity, and difficulty with transitions or shifting from one activity to another. A deficit in EF would also help to explain some of the deviant performance in language and memory. For example, perseverative thinking, difficulty with topic maintenance, and tangential conversational style are all common manifestations of an EF deficit.

EF in males with fragile X syndrome

Preliminary neurocognitive evidence for a deficit in EF came from the pattern of impairments that males with FXS show on the K-ABC, in which their performance on the Sequential Processing score is typically worse than performance on the Simultaneous Processing score. Tasks of sequential processing, such as imitating sequential hand movements, often rely on an individual's ability to hold a sequence of actions on line in working memory and formulate a motor plan to execute a response. Other tasks of motor sequencing have been shown to be sensitive to frontal lobe deficits (Kolb and Whishaw, 1996).

Cornish, Munir and Cross (2001) examined EF in a group of 15 adult males with FXS, compared to age- and verbal MA-matched males with Down syndrome, and normally-developing control subjects matched on verbal MA. On a shortened version of the WCST, which measures cognitive set shifting and concept formation, the subjects with FXS made significantly more perseverative errors than both the Down syndrome and normal control groups.

Munir, Cornish and Wilding (2000) examined inhibition in a group of 25 boys with FXS compared to age and verbal MA-matched boys with Down syndrome. The subjects with FXS had significantly more difficulty inhibiting a simple, practiced motor response, but were relatively better than subjects with Down syndrome on an inhibition task that required shifting from one response strategy to another. The authors also administered several measures of attention. On a task of selective attention, in which subjects had to search for specific targets in a field of distractors, the boys with FXS found fewer correct targets than subjects with Down syndrome. They also made more false alarms, which suggests difficulty in inhibition. On a task of divided attention, both groups found a similar number of targets. Further analysis, however, revealed that the FXS group employed less efficient search strategies. Finally, on a task of sustained attention, subjects with FXS again found as many correct targets as subjects with Down syndrome, but made significantly more false alarms. These results suggest that males with FXS have impairments in neuropsychological measures of set shifting and inhibition relative to control subjects with developmental delays. In addition, they suggest a specific profile of attentional abilities within the FXS sample, which appears to be characterized by difficulties with inhibition across a range of tasks.

Recent studies of males with a FXS premutation have begun to examine specificity within their neurocognitive profile. A study by Hills, Wilson, Sobesky et al. (2002) suggests that these deficits in EF may be present in a more titrated form in males with a premutation. The authors compared three groups of premutation males: 6 boys, 15 adults, and 5 elderly men. The first two groups were matched on age and Verbal IQ with groups of control subjects. The authors found that, overall, the males with FXS made more perseverative errors than controls on the WCST. Moreover, there appeared to be a developmental trend in their EF skills. The younger group demonstrated only borderline weaker performance than their controls, but by adulthood, the males with FXS showed significant impairments. The authors compared the performance of the elderly group to published norms for subjects of their age, and found they were significantly lower than one would predict based on their age and IQ.

EF in females with Fragile X syndrome

One of the most consistent neuropsychological findings in studies of females with a FXS full mutation is a specific deficit in EF (e.g., Bennetto, Pennington, Porter et al., 2001; Mazzocco, Hagerman, Cronister-Silverman and Pennington, 1992; Mazzocco, Hagerman and Pennington, 1992; Mazzocco, Pennington and Hagerman, 1993; Sobesky, Taylor, Pennington et al., 1996; Thompson, Gulley, Rogeness et al., 1994). Unlike most studies of males with FXS, studies of high-functioning females (IQ > 70) are able to utilize standard clinical tasks that are sensitive to frontal lobe functioning.

In their study of neuropsychological performance of women with FXS, Mazzocco et al. (1993) reported their most consistent and strongest group differences on tasks of EF. Compared to both carrier women and controls, and after covarying IQ, women with FXS were significantly impaired on relevant variables from the WCST, the Contingency Naming Test (which measures set shifting and inhibition), and the Visual–Verbal Test (which measures concept formation and flexible thinking).

Hinton, Halperin, Dobkin et al. (1995) also examined EF skills in their neuropsychological study of non-retarded women with a FXS full mutation, a premutation, and non-FXS controls. They used a version of the Continuous Performance Test, which taps both attention and inhibition. A series of 4-digit numbers appears briefly on a computer screen, and subjects are instructed to press a key whenever a number is repeated immediately after its presentation. After covarying age and IQ, the full mutation women were significantly more likely to miss the targets, which is thought to reflect poor attentional skills. However, they did not make more false alarms (a measure of inhibition), which differs from the pattern reported in males with FXS, who appear to have more trouble with inhibition than attention (Munir et al., 2000).

Sobesky et al. (1996) examined EF in a sample of 29 women with a full mutation, compared to women with a premutation, and non-FXS controls. They found that the full mutation women showed significant deficits in EF, as measured by the WCST and the Contingency Naming Test, even after covarying age and IQ. Analysis of molecular data found a significant relationship between X activation ratio and EF.

Finally, Bennetto et al. (2001) found significant EF deficits (as measured by the WCST and Contingency Naming Test) in a sample of full mutation women, even after covarying age and IQ. The authors also provide the clearest evidence of the specificity of EF deficits in women with FXS, by replicating their initial findings in a second study in which women with FXS were compared to age and IQ-matched controls with mild learning disabilities. Finally, EF skills were significantly related to the underlying biology of the disorder, as measured by the X activation ratio.

There is converging evidence that many women with the full mutation have deficits in EF, and that this area of functioning may be particularly sensitive to the effects of the *FMR1* mutation. Preliminary research on component processes further suggests that individuals with FXS have difficulties with cognitive flexibility, and at least males with this disorder show impairments in some aspects of inhibition. Further research linking neurocognitive functioning to molecular variables will help to better define variations in the phenotype of FXS as well as the role of biological variables in the normal development of EF. Deficits in EF may also help to explain some of the other areas of weakness observed in individuals with FXS. For example, pragmatics, organizational aspects of memory, and behavioral problems such as hyperactivity or impulsivity may be manifestations of a more general deficit in EF.

Concluding remarks

In this chapter, we have examined several dimensions of EF as a way of understanding both similarities and differences across neurodevelopmental disorders. Although the three disorders discussed above all typically present with general EF deficits, a componential analysis reveals some specificity within their unique EF profiles. Individuals with autism show the clearest evidence for deficits in cognitive flexibility, but appear to have less difficulty on tasks of simple response inhibition. In contrast, individuals with ADHD demonstrate an opposite pattern of impaired inhibition but relatively spared set shifting. Although the research on EF in FXS is still in a preliminary phase, individuals with this disorder appear to have some difficulties with both flexibility and inhibition. In the case of all three disorders, further research that specifies individual components of EF as well as diagnostic classifications will likely clarify what, if any, components of EF are primary to the phenotypes of each disorder.

A componential approach to EF deficits in psychopathology also shows promise for revealing phenotypic differences within diagnostic groups. For example, research on ADHD suggests that individuals diagnosed with different subtypes of this disorder demonstrate different patterns of impairment across EF tasks. In research on autism, EF deficits appear more consistent in high-functioning, older individuals compared to younger children with both autism and mental retardation.

Although many of the tasks presented above appear to draw strongly on one or another of the EF components, one could argue that many of them still require both multiple executive and nonexecutive skills. A better test for specificity within the EF domain is provided by research designs that employ within-task manipulations of executive skills. For example, Aman et al. (1998) examined motor inhibition by contrasting performance on an Anti-Saccade task with a Pro-Saccade task; the latter task retained all the elements of the executive task without the demand for inhibition. Children with ADHD were differentially worse than controls in the Anti-Saccade compared to Pro-Saccade condition, which provides a convincing argument for the validity of an inhibition deficit in this population.

Finally, one of the goals of studying neurocognitive deficits in developmental psychopathology is to provide clues to the developmental processes that ultimately lead to the symptoms of a particular disorder. In the case of EF, there is often an assumption that deficits on EF tasks are manifestations of underlying pathology in prefrontal circuitry. As we discussed above, this assumption may be flawed, particularly in the case of developmental disorders. A related goal of neurocognitive research is to understand something about the direction of effects in the pathogenesis of a disorder. In the case of syndromes with clear genetic etiologies, such as FXS or phenylketonuria, identifying an underlying neurocognitive deficit may provide a fairly direct link between the genotype and behavioral phenotype of the disorder. The relationship between EF and X activation ratio in FXS provides some support for this hypothesis (Bennetto et al., 2001; Sobesky et al., 1996). In contrast to this direct effect model, EF deficits could be a secondary effect of an altered developmental trajectory caused by a primary deficit in another neuropsychological domain. For example, a basic deficit in imitation skills in autism (e.g., Meltzoff and Gopnik, 1993; Rogers and Pennington, 1991) could disconnect a child from the early infant-caregiver interactions that enculturate us as social beings and shape our attention and executive processes (Donald, 1995, 2001). According to this model, EF deficits in autism would be due to environmental deprivation, rather than a direct effect of a genetic etiology on neural development, as may be the case in FXS. So, across these two syndromes, a similar pattern of EF deficits (even at the component level) may be reached through two distinct developmental pathways. A neuropsychological approach can thus allow for a broader examination of causal pathways in developmental psychopathology.

References

Alexander GF, Goldman PS: Functional development of the dorsolateral prefrontal cortex: an analysis utilizing reversible cryogenic depression. Brain Research: 143; 233–249, 1978.

Aman CJ, Roberts RJ, Pennington BF: A neuropsychological examination of the underlying deficit in ADHD: The frontal lobe vs. right parietal lobe theories. Developmental Psychology: 34; 956–969, 1998.

Anderson SW, Damasio H, Jones RD, Tranel D: Wisconsin card sorting test performance as a measure of frontal lobe damage. Journal of Clinical and Experimental Neuropsychology: 13; 909–992, 1991.

Axelrod BN, Goldman RS, Heaton RK, Curtiss G, Thompson LL, Chelune GJ, Kay GG: Discriminability of the Wisconsin card sorting test using the standardization sample. Journal of Clinical and Experimental Neuropsychology: 18; 338–442, 1996.

Baddeley A: Working Memory. Oxford: Clarendon Press, 1986.

Baddeley AD: Exploring the central executive. Quarterly Journal of Experimental Psychology: 49A; 5–28, 1996.

Baddeley AD, Hitch GJ: Working memory. In Bower GH (Ed), The Psychology of Learning and Motivation. New York: Academic Press, Vol. 8, pp. 47–89, 1974.

Bailey A, Phillips W, Rutter M: Autism: Towards an integration of clinical, genetic, neuropsychological, and neurobiological perspectives. Journal of Child Psychology and Psychiatry: 37; 89–126, 1996.

Barkley RA: Behavioral inhibition, sustained attention, and executive functions: Constructing a unifying theory of ADHD. Psychological Bulletin: 121; 65–94, 1997.

Barkley RA: Attention-Deficit Hyperactivity Disorder (2nd ed.). New York: Guilford, 1998.

Barth C, Fein D, Waterhouse L: Delayed match-to-sample performance in autistic children. Developmental Neuropsychology: 11; 53–69, 1995.

Bennetto L, Pennington BF: The neuropsychology of fragile X syndrome. In Hagerman RJ, Cronister AC (Eds), Fragile X Syndrome: Diagnosis, Treatment, and Research (2nd ed.). Baltimore, MD: Johns Hopkins University Press, pp. 210–248, 1996.

Bennetto L, Pennington BF: Dissociating components of executive functioning across developmental disorders. Presented at the Biennial Meeting of the Society for Research in Child Development, Albuquerque, NM, April, 1999.

Bennetto L, Pennington BF, Porter D, Taylor AK, Hagerman RJ: Profile of cognitive functioning in women with the fragile X mutation. Neuropsychology: 15; 290–299, 2001.

Bennetto L, Pennington BF, Rogers SJ: Intact and impaired memory functions in autism. Child Development: 67; 1816–1835, 1996.

Biederman J, Faraone SV, Keenan K, Benjamin J, Krifcher B, Moore C, Sprich-Buckminster S, Ugalglia K, Jelinek MS, Steingard R, Spencer T, Norman D, Kolodny R, Draus I, Perrin J, Keller MB, Tsuang MT: Further evidence for family-genetic risk factors in attention deficit hyperactivity disorder: Patterns of comorbidity in probands and relatives in psychiatrically and pediatrically referred samples. Archives of General Psychiatry: 49; 728–738, 1992.

Braver TS, Cohen JD, Nystrom LE, Jonides J, Smith EE, Noll DC: A parametric study of prefrontal cortex involvement in human working memory. Neuroimage: 5; 49–62, 1997.

Brickner RM: An interpretation of frontal lobe function based upon the study of a case of partial bilateral frontal lobectomy. In Orton ST, Fulton JF, Davis TK (Eds), Localization of Function in the Cerebral Cortex. Baltimore: Williams and Wilkins, pp. 259–351, 1934.

Bryson SE: Interference effects in autistic children: Evidence for the comprehension of single stimuli. Journal of Abnormal Psychology: 92; 250–254, 1983.

Burgess PW: Theory and methodology in executive function research. In Rabbitt P (Ed), Methodology of Frontal and Executive Functions. Hove: Psychology Press, 1997.

Casey BJ, Castellanos FX, Giedd JN, Marsh WL, Hamburger SD, Schubert AB, Vauss YC, Vaituzis AC, Dickstein DP, Sarfatti SE, Rapoport JL: Implication of right frontal striatal circuitry in response inhibition and attention-deficit/hyperactivity disorder. Journal of the American Academy of Child and Adolescent Psychiatry: 36; 374–383, 1997.

Casey BJ, Cohen JD, Jezzaard P, Turner R, Noll DC, Trainor RJ, Giedd J, Kaysen D, Hertz-Pannier L, Rapoport JL: Activation of prefrontal cortex in children during a nonspatial working memory task with functional MRI. Neuroimage: 2; 221–229, 1995.

Casey BJ, Giedd JN, Thomas KM: Structural and functional brain development and its relation to cognitive development. Biological Psychology: 54; 241–257, 2000.

Casey BJ, Trainor RJ, Orendi JL, Schubert AB, Nystrom LE, Giedd JN, Castellanos FX, Haxby JV, Noll DC, Cohen JD, Forman SD, Dahl RE, Rapoport JL: A developmental functional MRI study of prefrontal activation during performance of a go–no-go task. Journal of Cognitive Neuroscience: 9; 835–847, 1997.

Castellanos FX, Giedd JN, Eckburg P, Marsh WL, Vaituzis AC, Kaysen D, Hamburger SD, Rapoport JL: Quantitative morphology of the caudate nucleus in attention deficit hyperactivity disorder. American Journal of Psychiatry: 151; 1791–1796, 1994.

Castellanos FX, Giedd JN, Marsh WL, Hamburger SD, Vaituzis AC, Dickstein DP, Sarfatti SE, Vauss YC, Snell JW, Lange N, Kaysen D, Krain AL, Ritchie GF, Rajapakse JC, Rapoport JL: Quantitative brain magnetic resonance imaging in attention-deficit hyperactivity disorder. Archives of General Psychiatry: 53; 607–616, 1996.

Chiron C, Raynaud C, Maziere B, Zilbovicius M, Laflamme I, Masure M-C, Dulac O, Bourguignon M, Syrota A: Changes in regional cerebral blood flow during brain maturation in children and adolescents. Journal of Nuclear Medicine: 33; 696–703, 1992.

Chugani DC, Muzik O, Behen M, Rothermel R, Janisse JJ, Lee J, Chugani HT: Developmental changes in brain serotonin synthesis capacity in autistic and nonautistic children. Annals of Neurology: 45; 287–295, 1999.

Chugani DC, Muzik O, Rothermel R, Behen M, Chakraborty P, Mangner T, da Silva EA, Chugani HT: Altered serotonin synthesis in the dentatothalamocortical pathway in autistic boys. Annals of Neurology: 14; 666–669, 1997.

Chugani HT, Phelps MF, Mazziotta JC: Positron emission tomography study of human brain functional development. Annals of Neurology: 22; 487–497, 1987.

Ciesielski KT, Harris RJ: Factors related to performance failure on executive tasks in autism. Child Neuropsychology: 3; 1–12, 1997.

Ciesielski KT, Harris RJ, Hart BL, Pabst HF: Cerebellar hypoplasia and frontal lobe cognitive deficits in disorders of early childhood. Neuropsychologia: 35; 643–655, 1997.

Cohen JD, Forman SD, Braver TS, Casey BJ, Servan-Schreiber D, Noll DC: Activation of prefrontal cortex in nonspatial working memory task with functional MRI. Human Brain Mapping: 1; 293–304, 1994.

Conners CK, Wells KC: Hyperkinetic Children: A Neuropsychological Approach. Beverly Hills: Sage, 1986.

Cornish KM, Munir F, Cross G: Differential impact of the FMR-1 full mutation on memory and attention functioning: A neuropsychological perspective. Journal of Cognitive Neuroscience: 13; 144–150, 2001.

Cornoldi C, Vecchia RD, Tressoldi PE: Visuo-spatial working memory limitation in low visuo-spatial high verbal intelligence children. Journal of Child Psychology and Psychiatry: 36; 1053–1064, 1995.

Courchesne E, Townsend J, Akshoomoff NA, Saitoh O, Yeung-Courchesne R, Lincoln AJ, James HE, Haas RH, Schreibman L, Lau L: Impairment in shifting attention in autistic and cerebellar patients. Behavioral Neuroscience: 108; 848–865, 1994.

Cummings JL: Frontal-subcortical circuits and human behavior. Archives of Neurology: 50; 873–880, 1993.

Damasio AR, Tranel D, Damasio HC: Somatic markers and the guidance of behavior: theory and preliminary testing. In Levin HS, Eisenberg HM, Benton AL (Eds), Frontal Lobe Function and Dysfunction. New York: Oxford University Press, pp. 217–220, 1991.

Dawson G, Meltzoff AN, Osterling J, Rinaldi J: Neuropsychological correlates of early symptoms of autism. Child Development: 69; 1276–1285, 1998.

Dias R, Robbins TW, Roberts AC: Dissociation in prefrontal cortex of affective and attentional shifts. Nature: 380; 69–72, 1996.

Donald M: The neurobiology of human consciousness: An evolutionary approach. Neuropsychologia: 33; 1087–1102, 1995.

Donald M: Mind so Rare: The Evolution of Human Consciousness. New York: WW Norton, 2001.

Douglas VI: Attention and cognitive problems. In Rutter M

(Ed), Developmental Neuropsychiatry. New York: Guilford, pp. 280–329, 1983.

Duncan J, Burgess PW, Emslie J: Fluid intelligence after frontal lobe lesions. Neuropsychologia: 33; 261–268, 1995.

Eskes GA, Bryson SE, McCormick TA: Comprehension of concrete and abstract words in autistic children. Journal of Autism and Developmental Disorders: 20; 61–73, 1990.

Goldstein K: The mental changes due to frontal lobe damage. Journal of Psychology: 17; 187–208, 1941.

Grodzinsky GM, Diamond R: Frontal lobe functioning in boys with attention-deficit hyperactivity disorder. Developmental Neuropsychology: 8; 427–445, 1992.

Griffith EM, Pennington BF, Wehner EA, Rogers SJ: Executive function in young children with autism. Child Development: 70; 817–832, 1999.

Hagerman RJ, Cronister AC (Eds): Fragile X syndrome: Diagnosis, Treatment, and Research (2nd ed.). Baltimore, MD: Johns Hopkins University Press, 1996.

Harlow JM: Recovery from the passage of an iron bar through the head. Publication of the Massachusetts Medical Society: 2; 337–346, 1868.

Heaton RK, Chelune GJ, Talley JL, Kay GG, Curtiss G: Wisconsin Card Sorting Test manual: Revised and expanded. Odessa, FL: Psychological Assessment Resources, 1993.

Hebb DO: Man's frontal lobes: a critical review. Archives of Neurology and Psychology: 54; 10–24, 1945.

Hermelin B, O'Conner N: Psychological Experiments with Autistic Children. New York: Pergamon, 1970.

Hills JL, Wilson R, Sobesky W, Harris SW, Grigsby J, Butler E, Loesch D, Huggins R, Hagerman RJ: Executive functioning deficits in males with the fragile X premutation: an emerging phenotype. Manuscript in review, 2002.

Hinton VJ, Halperin JM, Dobkin CS, Ding XH, Brown WT, Miezejeski CM: Cognitive and molecular aspects of fragile X. Journal of Clinical and Experimental Neuropsychology: 17; 518–528, 1995.

Horwitz B, Rumsey J, Grady C, Rapoport S: The cerebral metabolic landscape in autism: Intercorrelations of regional glucose utilization. Archives of Neurology: 45; 749–755, 1988.

Houghton S, Douglas G, West J, Whiting K, Wall M, Langsford S, Powell L, Carroll A: Differential patterns of executive function in children with attention-deficit hyperactivity disorder according to gender and subtype. Journal of Child Neurology: 14; 801–805, 1999.

Hughes C: Control of action and thought: Normal development and dysfunction in autism: A research note. Journal of Child Psychology and Psychiatry: 37; 229–236, 1996.

Hughes C, Russell J, Robbins TW: Evidence for a central executive dysfunction in autism. Neuropsychologia: 32; 477–492, 1994.

Huttenlocher PR: Morphometric study of human cerebral cortex development. Neuropsychologia: 28; 517–527, 1990.

Huttenlocher PR: Regional difference in synaptogenesis in human cerebral cortex. Journal of Comparative Neurology: 387; 167–168, 1997.

Klorman R, Hazel-Fernandez LA, Shaywitz SE, Fletcher JM, Marchione KE, Holahan JM, Stuebing KK, Shaywitz BA: Executive functioning deficits in attention-deficit/hyperactivity disorder are independent of oppositional defiant disorder or reading disorder. Journal of the American Academy of Child and Adolescent Psychiatry: 38; 1148–1155, 1999.

Kolb B, Whishaw IQ: Fundamentals of Human Neuropsychology (4th ed). New York: WH Freeman, 1996.

Levin HS, Eisenberg HM, Benton AL: Frontal Lobe Function and Dysfunction. New York: Oxford University Press, 1991.

Lezak J: Neuropsychological Assessment (3rd ed). New York: Oxford University Press, 1995.

Liss M, Fein D, Allen D, Dunn M, Feinstein C, Morris R, Waterhouse L, Rapin I: Executive functioning in high-functioning children with autism. Journal of Child Psychology and Psychiatry: 42; 261–270, 2001.

Logan GD, Cowan WB, Davis KA: On the ability to inhibit simple and choice reaction time responses: a model and a method. Journal of Experimental Psychology, 10; 276–291, 1984.

Lovaas OI, Schreibman L: Stimulus over-selectivity of autistic children in a two stimulus situation. Behavior Research and Therapy: 9; 305–310, 1971.

Mazzocco MMM, Hagerman RJ, Cronister-Silverman A, Pennington BF: Specific frontal lobe deficits among women with the Fragile X gene. Journal of the American Academy of Child and Adolescent Psychiatry: 31; 1141–1148, 1992.

Mazzocco MMM, Hagerman RJ, Pennington BF: Problem solving limitations among cytogenetically expressing Fragile X women. American Journal of Medical Genetics: 43; 78–86, 1992.

Mazzocco MMM, Pennington BF, Hagerman RJ: The neurocognitive phenotype of female carriers of Fragile X: Additional evidence for specificity. Developmental and Behavioral Pediatrics: 14; 328–334, 1993.

McEvoy RE, Rogers S, Pennington BF: Executive function and social communication deficits in young autistic children. Journal of Child Psychology and Psychiatry: 34; 563–578, 1993.

Meltzoff A, Gopnik A: The role of imitation in understanding persons and developing a theory of mind. In Baron-Cohen S, Tager-Flusberg H, Cohen DJ (Eds), Understanding Other Minds. Oxford: Oxford University Press, pp. 335–366, 1993.

Minshew NJ, Goldstein G, Dombrowski SM, Panchalingam K, Pettegrew JM: A preliminary 31P-MRS study of autism: Evidence for undersynthesis and increased degradation of brain membranes. Biological Psychiatry: 33; 762–773, 1993.

Minshew NJ, Goldstein G, Muenz LR, Payton JB: Neuropsychological functioning in nonmentally retarded autistic individuals. Journal of Clinical and Experimental Neuropsychology: 14; 749–761, 1992.

Minshew NJ, Goldstein G, Siegel DJ: Neuropsychologic functioning in autism: Profile of a complex information processing disorder. Journal of the International Neuropsychological Society: 3; 303–316, 1997.

Moffitt TE, Henry B: Neuropsychological assessment of executive functions in self-reported delinquents. Development and Psychopathology: 1; 105–118, 1989.

Munir G, Cornish KM, Wilding J: A neuropsychological profile of attention deficits in young males with fragile X syndrome. Neuropsychologia: 38; 1261–1270, 2000.

Oosterlaan J, Sergeant JA: Response inhibition in ADHD, CD, comorbid ADHD+CD, anxious and normal children: A meta-analysis of studies with the stop task. Journal of Child Psychology and Psychiatry: 39; 411–426, 1998.

Ozonoff S: Reliability and validity of the Wisconsin Card Sorting Test in studies of autism. Neuropsychology: 9; 491–500, 1995.

Ozonoff S: Components of executive function in autism and other disorders. In Russell J (Ed), Autism as an Executive Disorder. New York: Oxford University Press, pp. 179–211, 1997.

Ozonoff S, Jensen J: Brief report: Specific executive function profiles in three neurodevelopmental disorders. Journal of Autism and Developmental Disorders: 29; 171–177, 1999.

Ozonoff S, McEvoy RE: A longitudinal study of executive function and theory of mind development in autism. Development and Psychopathology: 6; 415–431, 1994.

Ozonoff S, Pennington BF, Rogers SJ: Executive function deficits in high-functioning autistic individuals: Relationship to theory of mind. Journal of Child Psychology and Psychiatry: 32; 1081–1105, 1991.

Ozonoff S, Strayer DL: Inhibitory function in nonretarded children with autism. Journal of Autism and Developmental Disorders: 27; 59–77, 1997.

Ozonoff S, Strayer DL: Further evidence of intact working memory in autism. Journal of Autism and Developmental Disabilities: 31; 257–263, 2001.

Ozonoff S, Strayer DL, McMahon WM, Filloux F: Executive function abilities in autism and Tourette syndrome: An information processing approach. Journal of Child Psychology and Psychiatry: 35; 1015–1032, 1994.

Pennington BF: The working memory function of the prefrontal cortices: Implications for developmental and individuals differences in cognitive. In Haith MM, Benson J, Roberts R, Pennington BF (Eds), The Development of Future Oriented Processes. Chicago: University of Chicago Press, pp. 243–289, 1994.

Pennington B: Dimensions of executive functions in normal and abnormal development. In Krasnegor NA, Lyon GR, Goldman-Rakic PS (Eds), Development of the Prefrontal Cortex: Evolution, Neurobiology, and Behavior. Baltimore, MD: Paul H. Brooks Publishing Co., Inc., pp. 265–281, 1997.

Pennington BF, Bennetto L, McAleer O, Roberts RJ: Executive functions and working memory: Theoretical and measurement issues. In Lyon GR, Krasnegor NA (Eds), Attention, Memory and Executive Function. Baltimore, MD: Paul H. Brookes, pp. 327–348, 1996.

Pennington BF, Groisser D, Welsh MC: Contrasting cognitive deficits in attention deficit hyperactivity disorder versus reading disability. Developmental Psychology: 29; 511–523, 1993.

Pennington BF, Ozonoff S: Executive functions and developmental psychopathology. Journal of Child Psychology and Psychiatry: 37; 51–87, 1996.

Prior M, Hoffman W: Brief Report: Neuropsychological testing of autistic children through an exploration with frontal lobe tests. Journal of Autism and Developmental Disabilities: 20; 581–590, 1990.

Robbins TW: Integrating the neurobiological and neuropsychological dimensions of autism. In Russell J (Ed), Autism as an Executive Disorder. New York: Oxford University Press, pp. 21–53, 1997.

Robbins TW: Dissociating executive functions of the prefrontal cortex. In Roberts AC, Robbins TW, Weiskrantz L (Eds), The Prefrontal Cortex: Executive and Cognitive Functions. Oxford: Oxford University Press, pp. 117–130, 1998.

Robbins TW, James M, Owen AM, Sahakian BJ, Lawrence AD, McInnes L, Rabbitt PMA: A study of performance on test from the CANTAB battery sensitive to frontal lobe dysfunction in a large sample of normal volunteers: Implications for the theories of executive functioning and cognitive aging. Journal of the International Neuropsychological Society: 4; 474–490, 1998.

Robbins TW, James M, Owen AM, Sahakian BJ, McInnes L, Rabbit P: Cambridge Neuropsychology Test Automated Battery (CANTAB): A factor analytic study of a large sample of normal elderly volunteers. Dementia: 5; 266–281, 1994.

Roberts AC, Robbins TW, Weiskrantz L (Eds): The Prefrontal Cortex: Executive and Cognitive Functions. Oxford: Oxford University Press, 1998.

Roberts RJ, Pennington BF: An interactive framework for examining prefrontal cognitive processes. Developmental Neuropsychology: 12; 105–126, 1996.

Rogers SJ, Pennington BF: A theoretical approach to the deficits in infantile autism. Development and Psychopathology: 3; 137–162, 1991.

Rumsey JM: Conceptual problem-solving in highly verbal, nonretarded autistic men. Journal of Autism and Developmental Disorders: 15; 23–36, 1985.

Rumsey JM, Hamburger SD: Neuropsychological divergence of high-level autism and severe dyslexia. Journal of Autism and Developmental Disorders: 20; 155–168, 1990.

Russell J: How executive disorders can bring about inadequate 'theory of mind.' In Russell J (Ed), Autism as an Executive Disorder. New York: Oxford University Press, pp. 256–304, 1997.

Russell J, Jarrold C, Henry L: Working memory in children with autism and with moderate learning disabilities. Journal of Child Psychology and Psychiatry: 37; 673–686, 1996.

Schachar RJ, Tannock R, Logan G: Inhibitory control, impulsiveness, and attention deficit hyperactivity disorder. Clinical Psychology Review: 13; 721–739, 1993.

Scheerer M, Rothman E, Goldstein K: A case of 'idiot savant': An experimental study of personality organization. Psychological Monographs: 58; 1–63, 1945.

Schneider SG, Asarnow RF: A comparison of cognitive/neuropsychological impairments of nonretarded autistic and schizophrenic children. Journal of Abnormal Child Psychology: 15; 29–45, 1987.

Shah P, Miyake A: The separability of working memory resources for spatial thinking and language processing: an individual differences approach. Journal of Experimental Psychology: General: 125; 4–27, 1996.

Shallice T: From Neuropsychology to Mental Structure. Cambridge: Cambridge University Press, 1988.

Shallice T, Burgess P: The domain of supervisory processes and the temporal organization of behaviour. In Roberts AC, Robbins TW, Weiskrantz L (Eds), The Prefrontal Cortex: Executive and Cognitive Functions. Oxford: Oxford University Press, 1998.

Shimamura AP, Janowsky JS, Squire LR: What is the role of frontal damage in memory disorders? In Levin HS, Eisenberg HM, Benton AL (Eds), Frontal Lobe Function and Dysfunction. New York: Oxford University Press, pp. 173–195, 1991.

Siegel LS, Ryan EB: The development of working memory in normally achieving and subtypes of learning disabled children. Child Development: 60; 973–980, 1989.

Sobesky WE, Taylor AK, Pennington BF, Riddle J, Hagerman RJ: Molecular/clinical correlations in females with fragile X. American Journal of Medical Genetics: 64; 340–345, 1996.

Steel JG, Gorman R, Flexman JE: Neuropsychiatric testing in an autistic mathematical idiot savant: evidence for nonverbal abstract capacity. Journal of the American Academy of Child Psychiatry: 23; 704–707, 1984.

Stroop JR: Studies of interference in serial verbal reactions. Journal of Experimental Psychology: 18; 643–662, 1935.

Stuss DT, Benson DF: The Frontal Lobes. New York: Raven Press, 1986.

Tannock R: Neuropsychology of attention disorders. In Segalowitz SJ, Rapin I (Eds), Child Neuropsychology, Handbook of Neuropsychology, 2nd Edition, vol. 8, part II. Amsterdam: Elsevier, pp. 753–784, 2003.

Taylor G: Leaning disabilities. In Mash EJ, Terdal LG (Eds), Behavioral Assessment of Childhood Disorders. 2nd ed. New York: Guilford Press, pp. 402–450, 1988.

Thompson NM, Gulley ML, Rogeness GA, Clayton RJ, Johnson C, Hazelton B, Cho CG, Zellmer VT: Neurobehavioral characteristics of CGG amplification status in fragile X females. American Journal of Medical Genetics: 54; 378–383, 1994.

Turner M: Toward an executive dysfunction account of repetitive behavior in autism. In Russell J (Ed), Autism as an Executive Disorder. New York: Oxford University Press, pp. 57–100, 1997a.

Turner M: Working memory and strategy use in high-functioning and learning disabled individuals with autism. Paper presented at the Biennial Meeting of the Society for Research in Child Development. Washington, DC, April, 1997b.

Welsh MC, Pennington BF, Groisser DB: A normative-developmental study of executive function: a window on prefrontal function in children? Developmental Neuropsychology: 7; 131–149, 1991.

Weyandt LL, Willis WG: Executive functions in school-aged children: Potential efficacy of tasks in discriminating clinical groups. Developmental Neuropsychology: 10; 27–38, 1994.

Wilson FAW, Scalaidhe SP, Goldman-Rakic PS: Dissociation of object and spatial processing domains in primate prefrontal neurons. Science: 260; 1955–1958, 1993.

Zametkin AJ, Nordahl TE, Gross M, King AC, Semple WE, Rumsey J, Hamburger S, Cohen RM: Cerebral glucose metabolism in adults with hyperactivity of childhood onset. New England Journal of Medicine: 323; 1361–1366, 1990.

Zilbovicius M, Garreau B, Samson Y, Remy P, Barthelemy C, Syrota A, Lelord G: Delayed maturation of the frontal cortex in childhood autism. American Journal of Psychiatry: 152; 248–252, 1995.

Zilbovicius M, Garreau B, Tzourio N, Mazoyer B, Bruck B, Martinot J-L, Raynaud C, Samson Y, Syrota A, Lelord G: Regional cerebral blood flow in childhood autism: A SPECT study. American Journal of Psychiatry: 49; 924–930, 1992.

Handbook of Neuropsychology, 2nd Edition, Vol. 8, Part II
S.J. Segalowitz and I. Rapin (Eds)

CHAPTER 30

A frontal activation model of emotion regulation: developmental implications

Louis A. Schmidt [a,*], Shari R. Waldstein [b] and Diane L. Santesso [a]

[a] *Department of Psychology, McMaster University, Hamilton, ON L8S 4K1, Canada*
[b] *Department of Psychology, University of Maryland, Baltimore County, and Division of Gerontology, Department of Medicine, University of Maryland School of Medicine and Geriatrics Research Education and Clinical Center, Baltimore Veterans Affairs Medical Center, Baltimore, MD, USA*

Introduction

Emotions are ubiquitous phenomena that play an important role in the motivational, communicative, and adaptive aspects of human social behavior. Moreover, the root of many forms of psychopathology can be traced in some way to the dysregulation of emotion. Since the last publication of this Handbook more than a decade ago, significant progress has been made in the study of the neuropsychology of emotion. While emotions have traditionally been viewed rather disparagingly in the scientific community, there has been a renewed interest in the study of emotion. This progress is due largely to recent theoretical and methodological advances in the field of neuroscience. These inroads — mainly credited to the nonhuman work of LeDoux and Panksepp (see LeDoux, 1996 and Panksepp, 1998 for reviews) and the human work of Damasio and Davidson (see Damasio, 1999 and Davidson, 2000 for reviews) — have provided some of the most reliable evidence to date concerning the neural circuitry of emotion. Moreover, if the current extant literature is one measure by which to index revival, then the last decade is to emotion research what the 1960's–80's were to cognitive psychology, with major publications in the field including two editions of the *Handbook of Emotion*, Oxford University Press' *Series in Affective Science*, and the launching of American Psychological Association's new journal, *Emotion*.

Although there has been a burgeoning amount of interest and research attention directed towards the study of emotion in the last decade, much of this research has been done with nonhuman animals and adult humans. There has been comparatively little work directed towards the study of emotion in children in general, and even less examining the neuropsychology of emotional development in particular. In this chapter, we discuss a model that involves the active participation or inhibition of both the left and right frontal lobes in the regulation of emotion, and how this model can account for individual differences in normal affective style, on the one hand, and developmental psychopathology, on the other.

A frontal activation model of emotion regulation and dysregulation

Development of a model

Evidence from a variety of sources has shown that the frontal cortex plays an active role in several key aspects of emotional experience, including the mo-

* Corresponding author. Fax: +1-905-529-6225;
E-mail: schmidtl@mcmaster.ca

tor expression of emotion, the cognitive appraisal of emotion, and the regulation of emotion (see Fox, 1991, 1994 for reviews). Data from studies of individuals who suffered unilateral cerebral injury or who have undergone sodium amobarbital (Wada) testing (where one hemisphere is temporarily anesthetized by a barbiturate) for identification of an epileptic focus suggest that the left anterior region in adults is associated with the expression and experience of positive emotion, while the right anterior region is associated with the expression and experience of negative emotion (see Davidson, 1993, 2000; Fox, 1991, 1994 for reviews). Although alternative interpretations of these data have been offered (Borod, 1993), the findings indicate that the frontal region is involved in the experience and expression of emotion, whereas the posterior region is involved in emotion perception (see, e.g., Heller, 1993).

The expression and regulation of emotion involves multiple complex behaviors including cognitive, motor, and autonomic responses. No single region of the cortex or sub-cortical area is responsible for the integration of these various components of emotion. However, the frontal region is indeed unique in its integrative function, as it has inputs from all regions of the cortex as well as from those sub-cortical areas thought to be directly involved in the expression of emotion (see LeDoux, 1996).

A number of studies utilizing regional EEG measures to index frontal activation have corroborated the importance of the frontal lobe in emotion. These studies have used changes in EEG alpha power as their index of activation and examined the relative difference between activation in the two frontal lobes as a measure of asymmetry. Schmidt and Trainor (2001), for example, found that in adults the presentation of pleasant music was associated with greater relative left frontal EEG activation, while the presentation of unpleasant music was related to greater relative right frontal EEG activation. Davidson and his colleagues (Davidson, Ekman, Saron et al., 1990) reported differences in frontal EEG activation in adults that were a function of the type of emotion expressed on the face. Negative affect facial expressions were associated with greater relative right frontal EEG activity, while positive affect facial expressions were associated with greater relative left frontal activity. Importantly, these two studies noted a similar pattern of frontal EEG asymmetry for emotional valence regardless of the stimulus sensory modality differences.

Fox and Davidson (1988) found similar relations between frontal EEG patterns and facial expression of positive and negative emotion in normal infants. Negative facial affective expressions were related to greater relative right frontal EEG activation, while positive facial expressions were associated with greater relative left frontal EEG activation. As well, Fox and Davidson (1987) also noted changes in the pattern of frontal EEG during stress. Infants exhibited greater relative right frontal EEG activation in response to the approach of a stranger and maternal separation than during neutral conditions.

Further evidence to support the notion that the frontal lobe plays an important role in emotion comes from work that measures individual differences in frontal activation using continuous EEG, and then relating these patterns of resting frontal EEG activity to affective style. There are individuals whose modal response to mild stress or novelty is one of positive emotion while other individuals display negative emotions. There are also differences within these groups of individuals in the intensity of expression of emotion and in the ability of the individual to modulate that expression. These differences are mediated by different brain systems, with a tendency to express negative emotions associated with right frontal activation, and the tendency to express positive emotions with left frontal activation. The patterns of frontal EEG activity may be a marker reflecting the tendency to express positive or negative emotions in response to novelty or mild stress (Davidson, 1993, 2000). For example, individuals exhibiting greater right frontal EEG activation are known to be more likely to express negative affect in response to novel or mildly stressful events, while individuals exhibiting greater left frontal EEG activation are more likely to express positive affect. Davidson and his colleagues noted that adults who displayed stable right frontal EEG activation were more likely to rate video-tapes that varied in emotional content in a negative manner than adults who exhibited stable left frontal activation (Tomarken, Davidson and Henriques, 1990, and replicated by Jones and Fox, 1992). In addition, Davidson and Fox (1989) noted a similar relation between the pattern of frontal EEG asymmetry and affective expression in infants. Infants exhibiting greater relative right frontal EEG activation during baseline conditions were more likely to cry to maternal separation than infants displaying greater relative left activation at baseline. It seems plausible then to speculate that resting asymmetry in favor of the right reflects a negative bias in response to stress. This bias may, over time, reinforce negative perceptions about the self, ultimately affecting adaptive behavior.

The pattern of EEG activity measured from the frontal region may also be viewed as reflecting a dynamic process of affect regulation (e.g., Fox, 1991, 1994). Individuals will use multiple strategies, including the expression of different discrete emotions, use of verbal strategies and manipulation of attention in order to modulate their positive or negative affective states. The frontal lobes are intimately involved in the expression of these different emotion regulatory strategies. As such, during periods of affective challenge, the pattern of frontal activity may reflect the individual's attempt to regulate emotional arousal.

A model

The model considered here revolves around the active participation or inhibition by either the left or right sides of the prefrontal cortex and relates this dynamic balance to emotion regulation (see, Fox, 1994). Schematically, it can be represented by a 2×2 matrix in which each of the four quadrants in Fig. 1 is defined by the active participation or inhibition of activity of either the left or right frontal region, with the consequent emotion regulatory behaviors and personality styles within each cell (see Fig. 1). Thus, for example, the active participation of the left frontal region would affect the expression of positive affect, those responses involved in approach, and would characterize individuals who are sociable and outgoing. Active participation of the right frontal region would affect the expression of negative affect, those responses involved in withdrawal, and would characterize individuals who are shy. Lack of active participation of the left frontal region would produce an absence of approach or positive affect and would characterize individuals who are depressed and withdrawn. Lack of active participation of the right frontal region might produce an absence of withdrawal and an inability to experience the consequences of negative affect, those responses seen in impulsive and aggressive individuals. Thus, by considering the dynamic balance of activity in the two frontal hemispheres, we might be able to account for a number of individual differences in affective styles. We have represented in Fig. 1 four different affective styles of a number of possible consequences of left and right resting frontal activation.

To date, the model has been tested primarily with young adults using continuous EEG as an index of frontal activation. It is important to point out that, traditionally, frontal EEG asymmetry scores have been computed by subtracting right frontal EEG power *minus* left frontal EEG power, with negative scores reflecting greater relative right activation. Using this metric, there are at least two ways one can display asymmetry producing greater right frontal activation, and at least two ways one can exhibit asymmetry producing greater left frontal activation. *Relative right frontal EEG activation* could result from (1) a reduction in EEG power in the right electrode site, with EEG power in the left site remaining constant (an example of right EEG hyperactivation) or (2) EEG power in the right site could remain constant, with an increase in EEG power in the left site (an example of left EEG hypoactivation). *Relative left frontal EEG activation* could result from (1) a reduction in EEG power in the left site, with EEG power in the right remaining constant (an example of left EEG hyperactivation) or (2) EEG power in the left remaining constant, with an increase in EEG power in the right site (an example of right EEG hypoactivation). The manner by which one displays these varying patterns of frontal EEG asymmetry is not trivial, as they appear to have different psychological meanings.

The evidence

There have been at least two empirical studies to date testing the model. For example, Henriques and Davidson (1991) found a pattern of greater relative right frontal EEG activation in depressed adults; the asymmetry was a function of left-hypoactivation. Henriques and Davidson (1991) speculated that left frontal EEG hypoactivation in depression may reflect lack of approach and an absence of positive affect rather than the presence of heightened negative af-

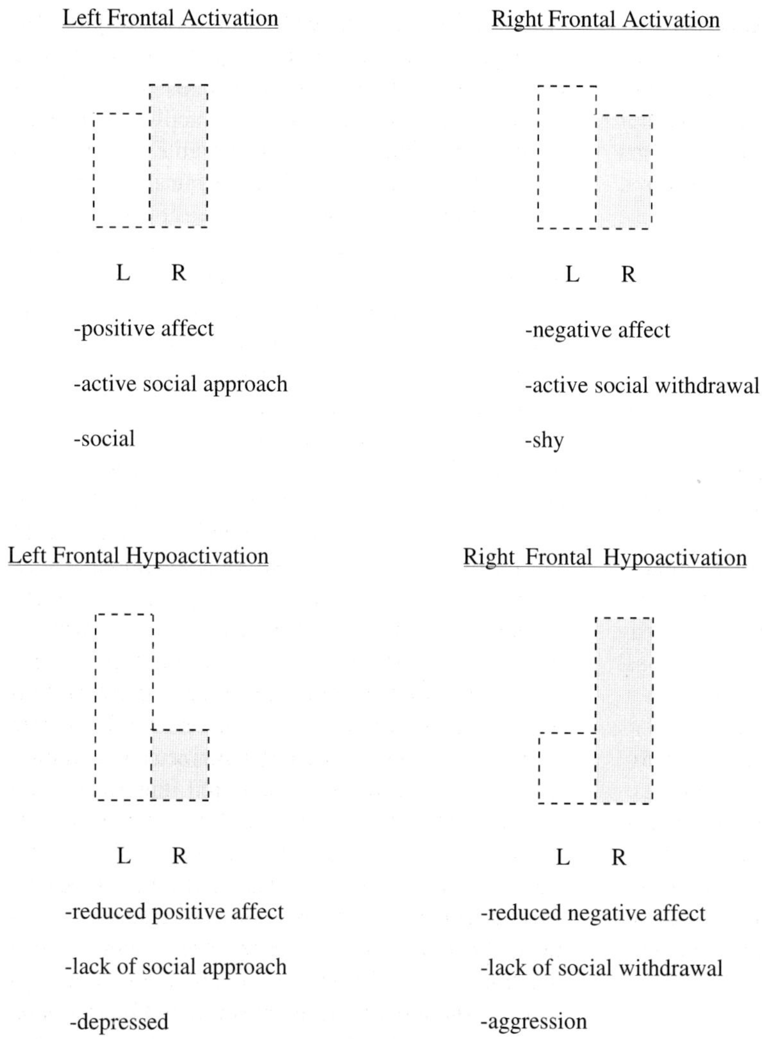

Fig. 1. At least four possible consequences of dynamic balances of left (L) and right (R) frontal EEG power (adapted from Fox, 1994). Note that EEG power is thought to be inversely related to activation, with lower power reflecting greater cortical activation (Davidson and Tomarken, 1989).

fect. Schmidt (1999), more recently, has used this model in order to understand individual differences in social behavior in adults. He examined the pattern of resting frontal EEG activation in a group of undergraduates, some of whom self-reported high and low shyness *and* sociability. He found that, although high shy/high social and high shy/low social subjects both exhibited a pattern of greater relative right frontal EEG activation, the two subtypes were distinguishable based upon the pattern of activity only in the left frontal site. High shy/high social subjects exhibited significantly more activation on the left site compared with high shy/low social subjects. He speculated that the pattern of frontal EEG activation in both hemispheres in the high shy/high social subjects may reflect an approach-avoidance conflict manifested by an inability to regulate the experience of intense positive and negative emotions. Together, these data provide empirical support for the theoretical model and suggest that not only the pattern of resting frontal activity, but the balance in frontal activity in both hemispheres as well may distinguish individual differences in personality. There have been relatively few studies that have used the frontal activation model to understand individual differences in affective style in normal development. We now turn to review some of the developmental studies of individual differences in affective style in normal and atypical development in which we describe how the model might help to understand some of these differences.

Frontal activation model in understanding developmental psychopathology

In this section, we focus our discussion on how this model can be applied to understand the origins and maintenance of two broad band categories of childhood behavioral disorders: internalizing- and externalizing-related problems. Current thinking suggests that the origins and maintenance of internalizing and externalizing problems are linked in some way to an inability to regulate emotion (see Davidson, 2000; Davidson, Putman and Larson, 2000). For many internalizing problems, it appears that the roots of these behaviors are linked to an inability to regulate the emotion of fear and anxiety; for other externalizing problems, it appears that these behaviors are linked to an inability to regulate anger. Although there have been relatively few studies examining the psychophysiological correlates of childhood psychological and behavioral problems, there is converging evidence to suggest that the frontal lobes play an important role in the maintenance of these childhood problems.

Internalizing-related problems

Behavioral inhibition

Prior to the last two decades, the study of childhood temperament in North America waxed and waned during the preceding 50 years or so. Allport (1937) defined temperament as the characteristic phenomena of an individual's emotional nature, comprising susceptibility to emotional stimulation, strength and speed of response, the quality of his prevailing mood, and fluctuation and intensity in mood. However, it was not until the 1960's that the New York Longitudinal Study conducted by Thomas and Chess (Thomas and Chess, 1981; Thomas, Chess and Birch, 1968) revived scientific interest in this issue. This now classic study examined temperamental differences in newborn infants and provided descriptions of their behavior patterns along nine dimensions of temperament: activity level, rhythmicity, approach/withdrawal, adaptability, intensity, sensory threshold, mood, distractibility, attention span/persistence. The authors suggested that these temperamental differences remained relatively stable throughout development while at the same time interacted with environmental influences to shape later personality. Furthermore, these temperamental and environmental interactions placed individuals at differential risk for developing subsequent behavioral problems and affective disorders.

During the last two decades, there has been a renewed interest in the issue of temperamental contributions to social behavior and developmental psychopathology and systematic investigation of the issues described by Thomas and Chess (1981). This work has stemmed primarily from the work of Jerome Kagan and his colleagues at Harvard. At birth, infants exhibit individual differences in temperament: they vary in approach or withdrawal tendencies, inhibition to the unfamiliar, and the degree to which they are aroused by environmental stimuli. The cohort of infants and children that Kagan and the Harvard group have been following longitudinally are all healthy, normally developing, primarily Caucasian and of middle-class backgrounds. Kagan and his colleagues (Kagan, 1997; Kagan and Snidman, 1991a,b) have suggested that infants' early reactions to novelty may be predictive of developmental outcome and later personality. For example, some infants exhibit a high degree of motor activity and distress in response to the presentation of novel auditory and visual stimuli; others exhibit a high degree of motor activity and positive affect in response to these stimuli; and still other infants exhibit relatively low levels of motor activity and affect in response to these stimuli. The interesting point here is that these three temperamental groups of infants are distinguishable on physiological indices and social behavior during the first four years of life, as we will see below. Kagan (1994, 1999) speculated that individual differences in infant reactivity to novelty may be linked to sensitivity in forebrain circuits involved in the processing and regulation of emotion. He has argued that children who become easily distressed during the presentation of novel stimuli may have a lower threshold for arousal in forebrain areas, particularly the central nucleus of the amygdala. This hypothesis is based largely on findings from studies of animals in which the amygdala plays an important role in the regulation and maintenance of conditioned fear. We have used measures of frontal EEG activity and the startle eyeblink response to test Kagan's speculation (see Schmidt and Fox, 1999, for a review). These two measures are thought to index forebrain limbic and frontal cortical areas involved in the regulation of emotion.

Using a design identical to that reported by Kagan and Snidman (1991b), Fox and his colleagues (Calkins, Fox and Marshall, 1996) examined the behavioral and psychophysiological antecedents of shyness in a group of infants selected at age 4 months for temperamental constellations thought to predict behavioral inhibition and shyness in early childhood. Eighty-one healthy infants were selected at age 4 months from a larger sample of 207 infants. The infants were observed in their homes at age 4 months and videotaped as they responded to novel auditory and visual stimuli. The 81 infants were selected based upon their frequency of motor activity and degree of positive and negative affect displayed in response to these novel stimuli, and three reactivity groups were formed: *negative reactive* ($n = 31$) comprised infants who displayed both high amounts of motor activity and negative affect and low amounts of positive affect; *positive reactive* ($n = 19$) comprised infants who displayed both high amounts of motor activity and positive affect and low amounts of negative affect; and *low reactive* ($n = 31$) comprised infants who displayed low amounts of motor activity and low amounts of both positive and negative affect. The infants were then seen in the laboratory at 9, 14, and 24 months, at which time regional brain electrical activity (EEG) was recorded using a lycra stretch cap while the infant was seated, alert, and attentive. EEG was recorded from the left and right anterior and posterior brain regions. The startle eyeblink response was recorded during a stranger approach situation at 9-months of age. Startle eyeblink responses were measured from two miniature electrodes placed around the infant's right eye. Infants were presented with a 95 dB burst of white noise for 50 ms during a baseline condition and an approaching stranger. In addition, behavioral responses to the presentation of unfamiliar social and nonsocial stimuli were recorded at 14 and 24 months. We found that infants classified as *negative reactive* at 4 months exhibited a significantly greater startle amplitude to an approaching stranger at 9 months compared with infants in the other two 4-month reactivity groups (Schmidt and Fox, 1998). The negative reactive infants were also more likely to exhibit greater relative right frontal EEG activity at 9 months (Calkins et al., 1996) and 24 months (Fox, Calkins and Bell, 1994), and more inhibition to novel stimuli at age 14 and 24 months (Calkins et al., 1996; Fox et al., 1994) than the other two 4-month reactivity groups. These findings were consistent with Kagan's predictions. It is seems plausible, then, to suggest that the frontal EEG and startle measures are indexing individual differences in forebrain sensitivity given the dense connections between the frontal cortex and forebrain limbic areas. These findings were also consistent with the frontal activation model: behavioral inhibition is conceptually linked to active withdrawal and right frontal hyperactivation at 9 and 24 months (see Fig. 1).

It is important to point out that behaviorally inhibited children may also be more likely to develop anxiety-related disorders later in life as a result of hypersensitivity to environmental cues. For example, a subset of children classified as behaviorally inhibited at 21 months and who remained inhibited at 4, 4.5, and 7.5 years had higher rates of anxiety disorders than children who were not consistently inhibited (Hirshfeld, Rosenbaum, Biederman et al., 1992). Parents of these children also had higher rates of multiple childhood anxiety disorders and a continuing history of anxiety disorder (Beiderman, Rosenbaum, Bolduc-Murphy et al., 1990). These studies suggest that in normally developing children temperamental variation may be due to how the child regulates emotion and is predictive of social behavior and developmental psychopathology during the early school age years. The frontal activation model predicts that behaviorally inhibited children at risk for anxiety would exhibit active withdrawal and extreme right frontal hyperactivation and low amounts of left frontal involvement.

Environmental effects on the development of behavioral inhibition and frontal EEG activity. Lack of parental care and attachment security is also associated with the development of internalizing disorders. Researchers seem to agree that separation distress may be one of the earliest forms of anxiety experienced by an infant, and variations in maternal care and infant attachment can have deleterious effects on infant development (see Sroufe, 1996 for a review). Secure attachments are often a result of effective responding and sensitivity of the caregiver to the infant's needs. By receiving this care, the infant develops a sense of trust that their signals of distress will be answered, and they will be protected from harm. If, however, the caregiver fails to respond effectively or consistently, infants may lower their threshold for distress and intensify their distress signals in an attempt to gain the caregiver's attention (Warren, Huston, Egeland and Sroufe, 1997). By doing so, infants become frequently anxious and behaviorally inhibited even in mildly stressful situations.

While there have been relatively fewer studies examining the psychophysiology of behavioral inhibition in children that resulted from poor attachment, there have been studies that have examined the psychophysiological correlates in non-normative mother–child relationships. In a series of studies, Tiffany Field and her colleagues have noted that depressed mothers and their infants exhibit atypical behavioral and frontal EEG patterns. Depressed mothers are known to display less positive affect and reduced levels of stimulation when interacting with their infants (Cohn, Matias, Tronick et al., 1986; Cohn and Tronick, 1989; Field, 1986; Field, Healy, Goldstein et al., 1988) and these behavioral symptoms are apparently transmitted to the infant. For example, infants of depressed mothers are known to display less positive affect and increased irritability (Cohn et al., 1986; Cohn and Tronick, 1989; Field, 1986; Field, Sandberg, Garcia et al., 1985), and greater relative right frontal EEG activity (a marker of stress) (Dawson, Grofer Klinger, Panagiotides et al., 1992; Field, Fox, Pickens and Nawrocki, 1995) compared with infants of non-depressed mothers. This frontal EEG asymmetry can develop as early as one month of age (Jones, Field, Fox et al., 1997).

The influence of temperament-attachment interaction on the development of behavioral inhibition and its physiology. Kagan and Snidman (1991a) suggest that temperament directly influences attachment based on the evidence that highly reactive (or 'difficult') infants may be less likely to have secure attachments by virtue of their irritability and inability to be soothed. In line with this view, Van den Boom (1989, 1994) reported that highly reactive and irritable infants were less sociable with their mother and were anxiously attached one year later whereas low reactive infants were more sociable and tended to be securely attached. Calkins and Fox (1992) later reported that infants who displayed a high degree of irritability and negative affect during early infancy were likely to display insecure attachments with their caregiver and inhibited social behavior later in life. However, a difficult temperament is not the only factor affecting later social adjustment.

Another possibility is that temperament modifies maternal responsiveness to the infant and, in turn, affects attachment. For example, researchers report that infant levels of irritability and their mothers' level of attentiveness are related (Van den Boom, 1989, 1994). Mothers interact less with their highly reactive infants during their first year than low reactive infants (Belsky and Vondra, 1989). Similarly, insecurely attached infants of depressed mothers develop interpersonal difficulties with family and peers. By age 5, these children exhibit high amounts of withdrawal and passivity when observed interacting with peers in a free play session (Rubin, Booth, Zahn-Waxler et al., 1991). In each case, these authors argue that insecurely attached infants fail to develop social competence and a sense of efficacy and therefore tend to avoid potentially rewarding social encounters contributing to social inhibition later in life (Calkins and Fox, 1992). For example, Warren and colleagues demonstrated that insecure attachment in infants was associated with anxiety disorders 16 years later (Warren, Huston, Egeland and Sroufe, 1997). Despite the apparent interplay between constitutionally-based factors and the environment, few studies have examined more direct physiological correlates of behavioral inhibition produced by this combination. One study by Gunnar and her colleagues noted that the interaction of temperamental inhibition and insecure attachment was a more robust predictor of salivary cortisol levels (a marker of stress) than the main effect of either component (Nachmias, Gunnar, Mangelsdorf et al., 1996).

Clearly, future research needs to consider the interaction of both temperament and environmental factors on the developing brain and emotional development.

Shyness

A number of researchers have suggested that early behavioral inhibition may predispose individuals to develop shyness and social anxiety by increasing sensitivity specifically to social evaluation and social novelty (Kagan, 1994, 1999; Kagan, Reznick, Snidman et al., 1987, 1988; Kerr, Lambert, Stattin and Klackenberg-Larson, 1994; Stemberger, Turner, Beidel and Calhoun, 1995). Caspi and Silva (1995) found that children inhibited at age 3 lacked effective social skills, were submissive, and not fond of leadership roles at age 18. In another study, these authors found that 34% of the children originally classified as behaviorally inhibited developed social anxiety disorder compared to 9% of those who were uninhibited (Caspi, Henry, McGee et al., 1995). Temperamentally shy children appear less socially competent (Fox, Rubin, Calkins et al., 1995), show social skills deficits, long speech latencies, poor voice tone, poor facial gaze, and fail to maintain meaningful social discourse (see Beidel and Turner, 1998 for a review). Again, a long history of social inhibition/avoidance will likely prevent that individual from encountering opportunities for learning adequate social skills (Antony, 1997) thus exacerbating social inhibition. There are, in addition, a number of distinct patterns of psychophysiological responses evidenced in temperamentally shy children that are linked to frontal lobe processes.

We have found that the pattern of physiological and behavioral responses seen in temperamentally reactive infants appears to be preserved into the preschool and early school age years and is predictive of shyness. In a series of studies of preschoolers and early school age children, Fox and Schmidt and their colleagues have noted that preschoolers who displayed a high proportion of shy behavior during peer play groups at age four exhibited significantly greater resting right frontal activation (Fox, Henderson, Rubin et al., 2001; Fox, Schmidt, Calkins et al., 1996; Fox et al., 1995) and higher morning basal salivary cortisol levels (Schmidt, Fox, Rubin et al., 1997) compared with children displaying relatively less shy behavior at age four. As well, children displaying a high degree of observed shy behavior during peer play were rated as shy at age four by their mothers and a significant proportion of them were likely to have been in the *negative reactive* temperamental group at age four months (Schmidt et al., 1997). Kagan and his colleagues (Kagan et al., 1987, 1988; Snidman and Kagan, 1994) had also noted earlier that temperamentally shy children were characterized by elevated morning basal cortisol levels, a high and stable heart rate, and exaggerated startle responses compared with their nonshy counterparts. More recently, Schmidt, Fox, Schulkin and Gold (1999a) found that temperamentally shy children exhibited a distinct pattern of physiological responses across different physiological measures in response to stress. They noted that, compared with their nonshy counterparts, temperamentally shy seven year-olds exhibited a significantly greater increase in right, but not left, frontal EEG activation and a significantly greater increase in heart rate during a self-presentation task as the task became more demanding. These physiological responses were paralleled by an increase in overt signs of behavioral anxiety. We also noted that children who were classified as low in social competence (a feature of shyness) exhibited a significantly greater change in salivary cortisol reactivity in response to the self-presentation task compared with socially competent children (Schmidt, Fox, Sternberg et al., 1999b). These data suggest that children who are classified as temperamentally shy during the preschool and early school age years exhibit a distinct pattern of frontal brain activity, heart rate, and salivary cortisol levels during baseline conditions and in response to stress, and are likely to have been highly reactive infants. These shy children are also at risk for social withdrawal and problems with anxiety and depression (see Rubin, Stewart and Coplan, 1995).

Social phobia

Social inhibition may be a predispositional factor for social phobia, a more extreme form of social anxiety. For example, Stemberger et al. (1995) noted that approximately 72% of socially phobic individuals report a childhood history of shyness compared with 52% of normal controls. The cognitive, physiological, and behavioral processes exhibited by socially phobic individuals are quite similar to those seen in shyness. For example, social phobics have negative thoughts (self-statements) during social encounters; negatively evaluate their social performance; engage in excessive self-monitoring; and are preoccupied with peer evaluation (Purdon, Antony, Monteiro and Swinson, 2001; Turner, Beidel and Townsley, 1990). These individuals also appear to have poor social skills, long speech latencies, increased gaze aversion, and nonassertiveness (see Beidel and Turner, 1998). Similar somatic and physiological symptoms include increased right frontal EEG activation, heart rate, and cortisol levels during baseline conditions and in response to public speaking/self-presentation tasks in children and adults who are shy (Schmidt, 1999; Schmidt and Fox, 1994; Schmidt et al., 1999a,b).

Social phobia may be unique to shyness in several ways. First, social phobia is chronic whereas shyness is transitory. Retrospective adult data indicate that early childhood onset of social phobia predicts nonrecovery in adulthood (Davidson, Hughes, George and Blazer 1993). Second, social phobics are more likely to suffer from traumatic social conditioning. Stemberger et al. (1995) noted that 44% of socially phobic individuals reported a history of traumatic conditioning. Third, studies show that the right dorsal-lateral prefrontal cortex and left parietal cortex are uniquely activated by the experience of anxiety in social phobia. These areas may be related to planning affective responses and to awareness of body position (Bell, Malazia and Nutt, 1999), an important characteristic of social phobia. fMRI data reveal significant bilateral amygdala activation to neutral faces by social phobics compared with control subjects (Birbaumer, Wolfgang, Diedrich et al., 1998). These differences may account, in part, for the unique symptoms of social phobia. Shyness and social phobia often precede depressive disorders. This is due, in part, because of concomitant social withdrawal, negative self-statements, and self-blame.

Depression

A growing literature emphasizes the role of the frontal cortex in depression. As noted earlier, studies have shown greater relative right frontal EEG activation in depression, even when the depression is in remission (Henriques and Davidson, 1990), and the pattern of asymmetry tends to result from a reduction in activity in the left frontal area, i.e. left hypoactivation (Henriques and Davidson, 1991; see Fig. 1). PET studies also show left frontal decreases in cerebral blood flow or metabolism in depressed subjects compared with controls (Little, Ketter, Kimbrell et al., 1996; Rush, Sclesser, Stokely et al., 1982). Together these findings suggest that depressive symptoms may be a consequence of heritable temperamental profiles and distinct neurophysiological symptoms, particularly frontal lobe involvement in some individuals.

Generalized anxiety disorder and panic disorder

Recent studies have revealed that the neurobiological basis for anxiety disorders in adults is similar to those seen in childhood behavioral inhibition and may be equated with the inability to regulate fear (see Schmidt and Schulkin, 1999). There also appear to be significant brain activation correlates associated with anxiety. For example, right frontal hyperactivity during rest has been noted in anxious and depressed patients (e.g., Henriques and Davidson, 1990); as well, anxious adults at rest or during induced states of anxious arousal/panic show greater right than left parietal activation (Bruder, Fong, Tenke et al., 1997; Heller, Nitschke, Etienne and Miller, 1997). EEG studies also show that patients with Panic Disorder (an anxiety disorder) exhibit increased right frontal brain activity when exposed to anxiety-relevant stimuli (Weidemann, Pauli, Dengler et al., 1999). Repeated episodes of childhood physical and sexual abuse, which gradually lowers the threshold for activation, can predispose for the development of panic disorder, and generalized anxiety disorder (Portegijs, Jeuken, Van der Horst et al., 1996; Stein, Walker, Anderson et al., 1996).

Externalizing-related problems

Although childhood externalizing problems are particularly costly to the child, peers, families, and society, there have been relatively few studies examining the development of such problems in children. Moreover, there have been still fewer studies examining the role of emotion and its psychophysiological basis in childhood externalizing problems. Current thinking suggests that the origins of aggressive, impulsive, and violent behavior are due to an inability to regulate negative emotion (particularly anger) (see Davidson et al., 2000), and the frontal lobe once again is the primary locus for the maintenance of these behaviors.

Temperament and arousal perspectives

A small subset of infants (approximately 10%) may inherit an underactive amygdala or a propensity to raise their threshold for activation (Kagan, 1997; Raine, 1993). These individuals, unlike inhibited children, display low levels of fear or fail to respond to the same degree of fear/anxiety as normal individuals and seek out stimulation. These tendencies are manifested in lack of constraint, appropriate control, and aggressive and antisocial acts (Caspi et al., 1995).

Kochanska (1993) notes that temperament, specifically fear and effortful control, contribute to compliance and appropriate behavioral conduct. That is, infants must be able to effectively regulate their emotional responses and frustration in order to internalize societal standards for conduct. Infants who are easily frustrated and fail to modulate their emotions may respond with noncompliance and employ this strategy in subsequent situations of emotional arousal. Stifter, Spinrad and Braungart-Rieker (1999) examined compliance in groups of infants classified by reactivity and emotional regulatory skills. This group found that infants who exhibited high levels of reactivity and low levels of regulation at 5 months displayed more defiance/noncompliance than all other infants. Infants characterized as low reactive/high regulation or low reactive/low regulation were likely to use passive noncompliance (i.e., ignoring requests) while infants who were high reactive/high regulation were the least defiant. Furthermore, these tendencies remained relatively stable over the first two years after birth.

There have been few studies that have examined the psychophysiology of childhood aggression and externalizing problems. Studies indicate that low resting heart rate may be the most robust biological marker of antisocial and aggressive behavior in children and adolescents (Raine, 1996). Recently, Raine, Venables and Mednick (1997) demonstrated a bi-directional effect between the relationship of low heart rate and aggression. In this study, not only did aggressive individuals display low heart rates, but low resting heart rate at age 3 was predictive of aggressive behavior at age 11. This suggests that temperamental predispositions toward aggression occur very early in life and remain relatively stable across development. These findings are in line with Caspi and Silva (1995) who found children characterized by an undercontrolled temperament at age 3 were more likely at age 18 to score high on personality measures of aggression and danger-seeking.

Raine (1996) suggests lack of fear may lead individuals to antisocial and violent behavior because the associated behaviors (e.g., fighting) require a certain degree of fearlessness to perform. Children or adults who contemplate committing violent acts will not experience the usual feeling (shame, guilt, anxiety) that accompanies anticipation of the consequences and provide an effective restraint on their action (Kagan, 1997). The lack of such feelings appear early in childhood and have been consistently observed in children aged 9–12 exhibiting low resting heart rates and increased fighting from 5–12 years old (Kindlon, Tremblay, Mezzacappa et al., 1995).

Childhood aggression and frontal lobe functioning

Our studies of the relation between patterns of activity in the prefrontal region and motor and negative affect are based upon the notion that there are two motivational systems underlying emotional behavior — one being an approach system, and the other reflective of withdrawal. The initial formulation of this model was that behaviors associated with the expression and/or experience of positive affect would be influenced by activation in the left frontal region, while the expression and/or experience of negative affect is related to activation in the right frontal region (see Davidson, 1993, 2000; Fox, 1991, 1994). Recently, we have attempted to expand this model to understand the role of emotion regulation. Our thinking is that motor responses, affect expressions, and cognitive processes all serve to modulate emotional behavior, and that the larger role of the prefrontal cortex in emotion is linked to the regulation of emotions, perhaps as much as to the actual expression of discrete emotions. This has obvious implications for the study of aggressive behaviors.

Although most of the studies on the psychophysiology of childhood antisocial behavior have relied primarily on measures of peripheral nervous system activity (e.g., heart rate and electrodermal responses), one recent study by our lab group has focused on the use of EEG measures to understand childhood aggression. We examined differences in baseline regional EEG (Shahinfar, Schmidt and Fox, 2001), heart rate, and behavior during dyadic play in a group of toddlers, some of whom were selected for high proportions of aggressive behavior. Baseline EEG and heart rate data were collected continuously for 3 min at age 27 months while the toddler attended to a novel visual stimulus. Each toddler was also unobtrusively observed during a dyadic play session while interacting with a peer, and during a task designed to elicit empathy. We view aggressive behaviors, in part, as a manifestation of dysregulated anger responses that may be linked to perceived threat by the individual. There is strong evidence from the developmental literature that certain forms of childhood aggression are a function of perceived threat by the child (see Dodge, 1990). However, it is the inappropriate nature of the response on which we focus. Specifically, we would expect that most individuals would inhibit their aggressive responses, modulating both motor and affective behaviors. Individuals who are aggressive, however, may express their anger with little ability to modulate that response. We found that toddlers classified as aggressive exhibited a higher percentage of aggressive interactions, a lower frequency of social withdrawal, and less overall empathy in response to experimenter simulation of distress than their nonaggressive peers during the dyadic play session. Aggressive toddlers also exhibited greater relative left frontal baseline EEG activity that was a function of less activity in the right frontal site (i.e., right frontal hypoactivation) compared with nonaggressive toddlers consistent with our frontal activation model (see Fig. 1). There were no differences in resting heart rate between the two groups. Thus, right frontal hypoactivation may reflect an inability to regulate negative affect and its consequences in some aggressive children.

Summary

The evidence reviewed above suggests that the origins of two broad-band categories of childhood behavioral and psychological problems are linked to dysregulation of emotion. More specifically, many internalizing-related problems are linked to the dysregulation of fear and anxiety, while many externalizing-related problems are linked to the dysregulation of anger. There are, in addition, significant behavioral and psychophysiological correlates associated with the dysregulation of these affects in these problem behaviors, and we believe that the inability to regulate such emotion is strongly linked to specific patterns of activation in the frontal cortex. Furthermore, the origins of these childhood disorders might be linked to the balance of activity in the two frontal lobes. Early temperamental profiles by themselves, however, may be insufficient to result in psychopathology. Rather, it is a complex interplay between constitution and environmental factors the shape the developing brain, behavior, and outcomes.

Conclusions and future directions

Emotions are the elements of consciousness and the foundation on which the human condition is based. They pervade our daily lives, and our literatures, theologies, music, philosophies and arts. Yet, although they are such ubiquitous phenomena, there has been relatively little scientific study of them, particularly developmentally. It seems plausible that individual differences in emotion regulatory processes may give rise to different personality styles and that these differences can be expressed in the dynamic balance that exists between activation and regulation of the two frontal hemispheres. Future research should consider using the dynamic balance in frontal EEG activation to explain individual variation in affective style in normal and atypical development. Future research should also examine whether the frontal activation model described in this chapter also holds true during conditions of affective challenge and other environmental influences.

Acknowledgements

Preparation of this chapter was supported in part by grants from the Natural Science and Engineering Research Council of Canada (NSERC 203710-99, 203710-00) and the Social Sciences and Humanities

Research Council of Canada (SSHRC 410-99-1206) awarded to LAS and the National Institute of Aging (1R29AG15112) awarded to SRW.

References

Allport G: Personality: A Psychological Interpretation. New York: Holt, 1937.

Antony MM: Assessment and treatment of social phobia. Canadian Journal of Psychiatry: 42; 826–834, 1997.

Beidel DC, Turner SM: Shy Children, Phobic Adults. Washington, DC: American Psychological Association, 1998.

Beiderman J, Rosenbaum JF, Bolduc-Murphy E, Farone S, Chaloff J, Hirshfeld D, Kagan J: Psychiatric correlates of behavioral inhibition in young children of parents with and without psychiatric disorders. Archives of General Psychiatry: 47; 21–26, 1990.

Bell CJ, Malazia A, Nutt D: The neurobiology of social phobia. European Archives of Psychiatry and Clinical Neuroscience: 249(Suppl 1); S11–S18, 1999.

Belsky J, Vondra J: Lessons from child abuse: The determinants of parenting. In Cicchetti D, Carlson V (Eds), Child Maltreatment: Theory and Research on the Causes and Consequences of Child Abuse and Neglect. New York: Cambridge University Press, pp. 153–202, 1989.

Birbaumer N, Wolfgang G, Diedrich O, Klose U, Erb M, Lotze M, Schneider F, Flor H: fMRI reveals amygdala activation to human faces in social phobics. Neuroreport: 9; 1223–1226, 1998.

Borod JC: Cerebral mechanisms underlying facial, prosodic, and lexical emotional expression: A review of neuropsychological studies and methodological issues. Neuropsychology: 7; 445–463, 1993.

Bruder GE, Fong R, Tenke CE, Leite P, Towey JP, Stewart JE, McGarth PJ, Quitkin FM: Regional brain asymmetries in major depression with or without an anxiety disorder: A quantitative electroencephalographic study. Biological Psychiatry: 41; 939–948, 1997.

Calkins SD, Fox NA: The relations among infant temperament, security of attachment, and behavioral inhibition at 24 months. Child Development: 63; 1456–1472, 1992.

Calkins SD, Fox NA, Marshall TR: Behavioral and physiological antecedents of inhibited and uninhibited behavior. Child Development: 67; 523–540, 1996.

Caspi A, Henry B, McGee R, Moffitt T, Silva P: Temperamental origins of child and adolescent behavior problems: From age 3 to age 15. Child Development: 66; 55–68, 1995.

Caspi A, Silva PA: Temperamental qualities at age three predict personality traits in young adulthood: Longitudinal evidence from a birth cohort. Child Development: 66; 486–498, 1995.

Cohn JF, Matias R, Tronick EZ, Connell D, Lyons-Ruth D: Face-to-face interactions of depressed mothers and their infants. In Tronick EZ, Field T (Eds), Maternal Depression and Infant Disturbance. San Francisco, CA: Jossey-Bass, pp. 31–45, 1986.

Cohn JF, Tronick EZ: Specificity of infant's response to mothers' affective behavior. Journal of the American Academy of Child and Adolescent Psychiatry: 28; 242–248, 1989.

Damasio AR: The Feeling of What Happens: Body and Emotion in the Making of Consciousness. New York: Harcourt Brace, 1999.

Davidson RJ: The neuropsychology of emotion and affective style. In Lewis M, Haviland JM (Eds), Handbook of Emotion. New York: Guilford, pp. 143–154, 1993.

Davidson RJ: Affective style, psychopathology, and resilience: Brain mechanisms and plasticity. American Psychologist: 55; 1196–1214, 2000.

Davidson RJ, Ekman P, Saron CD, Senulis JA, Friesen WV: Approach/withdrawal and cerebral asymmetry: Emotional expression and brain physiology I. Journal of Personality and Social Psychology: 58; 330–341, 1990.

Davidson RJ, Fox NA: The relation between tonic EEG asymmetry and ten-month-old emotional response to separation. Journal of Abnormal Psychology: 98; 127–131, 1989.

Davidson JR, Hughes DL, George LK, Blazer DG: The epidemiology of social phobia: findings from the Duke Epidemiological Catchment Area Study. Psychological Medicine: 23(3); 709–718, 1993.

Davidson RJ, Putnam KM, Larson CL: Dysfunction in the neural circuitry of emotion regulation: A possible prelude to violence. Science: 289; 591–594, 2000.

Davidson RJ, Tomarken AJ: Laterality and emotion: An electrophysiological approach. In Boller F, Grafman J (Eds), Handbook of Neuropsychology. Amsterdam: Elsevier Science, pp. 419–441, 1989.

Dawson G, Grofer Klinger L, Panagiotides H, Hill D, Spieker S: Frontal lobe activity and affective behavior in infants of mothers with depressive symptoms. Child Development: 63; 725–737, 1992.

Dodge KA: The structure and function of reactive and proactive aggression. In Pepler D, Rubin KH (Eds), The Development and Treatment of Childhood Aggression. Hillsdale, NJ: Erlbaum, pp. 201–218, 1990.

Field T: Models of reactive and chronic depression in infancy. In Tronick EZ, Field T (Eds), Maternal Depression and Infant Disturbance. San Francisco, CA: Jossey-Bass, pp. 47–60, 1986.

Field T, Fox NA, Pickens J, Nawrocki T: Relative right frontal EEG activation in 3- to 6-month-old infants of depressed mothers. Developmental Psychology: 31; 358–363, 1995.

Field T, Healy B, Goldstein S, Perry S, Bendall D, Schanberg S, Zimmerman E, Kuhn C: Infants of depressed mothers show 'depressed' behavior even with nondepressed adults. Child Development: 59; 1569–1579, 1988.

Field T, Sandberg D, Garcia R, Vega-Lahr N, Goldstein S, Guy L: Prenatal problems, post-partum depression, and early mother–infant interaction. Developmental Psychology: 12; 1152–1156, 1985.

Fox NA: If it's not left, it's right: Electroencephalogram asymmetry and the development of emotion. American Psychologist: 46; 863–872, 1991.

Fox NA: Dynamic cerebral processes underlying emotion regulation. In Fox NA (Ed), The development of emotion regulation:

Behavioral and biological considerations. Monographs of the Society for Research in Child Development, pp. 152–166, 59, (2–3, Serial No. 240), 1994.

Fox NA, Calkins SD, Bell MA: Neural plasticity and development in the first two years of life: Evidence from cognitive and socioemotional domains of research. Development and Psychopathology: 6; 677–696, 1994.

Fox NA, Davidson RJ: Electroencephalogram asymmetry in response to the approach of a stranger and maternal separation in 10-month-old infants. Developmental Psychology: 23; 233–240, 1987.

Fox NA, Davidson RJ: Patterns of brain electrical activity during facial signs of emotion in 10-month-old infants. Developmental Psychology: 24; 230–236, 1988.

Fox NA, Henderson HA, Rubin KH, Calkins SD, Schmidt LA: Continuity and discontinuity of behavioral inhibition and exuberance: Psychophysiological and behavioral influences across the first four years of life. Child Development: 72; 1–21, 2001.

Fox NA, Rubin KH, Calkins SD, Marshall TR, Coplan RJ, Porges SW, Long JM, Stewart S: Frontal activation asymmetry and social competence at four years of age. Child Development: 66; 1770–1784, 1995.

Fox NA, Schmidt LA, Calkins SD, Rubin KH, Coplan RJ: The role of frontal activation in the regulation and dysregulation of social behavior during the preschool years. Development and Psychopathology: 8; 89–102, 1996.

Heller W: Neuropsychological mechanisms of individual differences in emotion, personality, and arousal. Neuropsychology: 7; 476–489, 1993.

Heller W, Nitschke JB, Etienne MA, Miller GA: Patterns of regional brain activity differentiate types of anxiety. Journal of Abnormal Psychology: 106(3); 376–385, 1997.

Heller W, Nitschke JB, Lindsay DL: Neuropsychological correlates of arousal in self-reported emotion. Cognition and Emotion: 11; 383–402, 1997.

Henriques JB, Davidson RJ: Regional brain electrical asymmetries discriminate between previously depressed and healthy controls. Journal of Abnormal Psychology: 99; 22–31, 1990.

Henriques JB, Davidson RJ: Left frontal hypoactivation in depression. Journal of Abnormal Psychology: 100; 535–545, 1991.

Hirshfeld DR, Rosenbaum JF, Biederman J, Bolduc EA, Faraone SV, Snidman N, Reznick JS, Kagan J: Stable behavioral inhibition and its association with anxiety disorder. Journal of the American Academy of Child and Adolescent Psychiatry: 31; 103–111, 1992.

Jones NA, Field T, Fox NA, Lundy B, Davalos M: EEG activation in 1-month-old infants of depressed mothers. Development and Psychopathology: 9; 491–505, 1997.

Jones NA, Fox NA: Electroencephalogram asymmetry during emotionally evocative films and its relation to positive and negative affectivity. Brain and Cognition: 20; 280–299, 1992.

Kagan J: Galen's Prophecy: Temperament in Human Nature. New York: Basic Books, 1994.

Kagan J: Temperament and the reactions to unfamiliarity. Child Development: 68; 139–143, 1997.

Kagan J: The concept of behavioral inhibition. In Schmidt LA, Schulkin J (Eds), Extreme Fear, Shyness, and Social Phobia: Origins, Biological Mechanisms, and Clinical Outcomes. New York: Oxford University Press, pp. 3–13, 1999.

Kagan J, Reznick JS, Snidman N: The physiology and psychology of behavioral inhibition in children. Child Development: 58; 1459–1473, 1987.

Kagan J, Reznick JS, Snidman N: Biological basis of childhood shyness. Science: 240; 167–171, 1988.

Kagan J, Snidman N: Temperamental factors in human development. American Psychologist: 46; 856–862, 1991a.

Kagan J, Snidman N: Infant predictors of inhibited and uninhibited profiles. Psychological Science: 2; 40–44, 1991b.

Kerr M, Lambert W, Stattin H, Klackenberg-Larson I: Stability of inhibition in a Swedish longitudinal sample. Child Development: 65; 138–146, 1994.

Kindlon DJ, Tremblay RE, Mezzacappa E, Earls F, Laurent D, Schaal B: Journal of American Academic Child and Adolescent Psychiatry: 34; 371–377, 1995.

Kochanska G: Toward a synthesis of parental socialization and child temperament in early development of conscience. Child Development: 64; 325–347, 1993.

LeDoux JE: The Emotional Brain. New York: Simon and Schuster, 1996.

Little JT, Ketter TA, Kimbrell TA, Danielson A, Benson B, Willis M, Eng M, Post RM: Venlafaxine or bupropion responders but not nonresponders show baseline prefrontal and paralimbic hypometabolism compared with controls. Psychopharmalogical Bulletin: 32; 629–635, 1996.

Nachmias M, Gunnar M, Mangelsdorf S, Hornik Parritz R, Buss K: Behavioral inhibition and stress reactivity: The moderating role of attachment security. Child Development: 67; 508–522, 1996.

Panksepp J: Affective Neuroscience: The Foundations of Human and Animal Emotions. New York: Oxford University Press, 1998.

Portegijs PJM, Jeuken FMH, Van der Horst FG, Kraan HF, Knottnerus JA: A troubled youth: Relations with somatization, depression, anxiety in adulthood. Family Practice: 13; 1–11, 1996.

Purdon C, Antony MM, Monteiro S, Swinson RP: Social anxiety in college students. Journal of Anxiety Disorders: 15; 203–215, 2001.

Raine A: The Psychopathology of Crime: Criminal Behavior as a Clinical Disorder. San Diego: Academic Press, 1993.

Raine A: Autonomic nervous system factors underlying disinhibited, antisocial, and violent behavior: Biosocial perspectives and treatment implications. Annals of the New York Academy of Sciences: 794; 46–59, 1996.

Raine A, Venables P, Mednick S: Low resting heart rate at age 3 predisposes to aggression at age 11 years: Evidence from the Mauritius Child Health Project. Journal of American Child and Adolescent Psychiatry: 36; 1457–1464, 1997.

Rubin KH, Booth L, Zahn-Waxler C, Cummings EM, Wilkinson M: Dyadic play behaviors of children of well and depressed mothers. Development and Psychopathology: 3; 243–251, 1991.

Rubin KH, Stewart SL, Coplan RJ: Social withdrawal in childhood: Conceptual and empirical perspectives. In Ollendick T, Prinz R (Eds), Advances in Clinical Child Psychology. Vol. 17, New York: Plenum Press, pp. 157–196, 1995.

Rush AJ, Sclesser MA, Stokely EM et al: Cerebral blood flow in depression and mania. Psychopharmacological Bulletin: 18; 6–8, 1982.

Schmidt LA: Frontal brain electrical activity in shyness and sociability. Psychological Science: 10; 316–320, 1999.

Schmidt LA, Fox NA: Patterns of cortical electrophysiology and autonomic activity in adults' shyness and sociability. Biological Psychology: 38; 183–198, 1994.

Schmidt LA, Fox NA: Fear-potentiated startle responses in temperamentally different human infants. Developmental Psychobiology: 32; 113–120, 1998.

Schmidt LA, Fox NA: Conceptual, biological, and behavioral distinctions among different categories of shy children. In Schmidt LA, Schulkin J (Eds), Extreme Fear, Shyness, and Social Phobia: Origins, Biological Mechanisms, and Clinical Outcomes. New York: Oxford University Press, pp. 47–66, 1999.

Schmidt LA, Fox NA, Rubin KH, Sternberg EM, Gold PW, Smith C, Schulkin J: Behavioral and neuroendocrine responses in shy children. Developmental Psychobiology: 30; 127–140, 1997.

Schmidt LA, Fox NA, Schulkin J, Gold PW: Behavioral and psychophysiological correlates of self-presentation in temperamentally shy children. Developmental Psychobiology: 35; 119–135, 1999a.

Schmidt LA, Fox NA, Sternberg EM, Gold PW, Smith C, Schulkin J: Adrenocortical reactivity and social competence in seven year-olds. Personality and Individual Differences: 26; 977–985, 1999b.

Schmidt LA, Schulkin J (Eds): Extreme Fear, Shyness, and Social Phobia: Origins, Biological Mechanisms, and Clinical Outcomes. New York: Oxford University Press, 1999.

Schmidt LA, Trainor LJ: Frontal brain electrical activity (EEG) distinguishes valence and intensity of musical emotions. Cognition and Emotion: 15; 487–500, 2001.

Shahinfar A, Schmidt LA, Fox NA: Behavioral and psychophysiological correlates of aggressive toddlers. Manuscript submitted for publication, 2002.

Snidman N, Kagan J: The contribution of infant temperamental differences to acoustic startle response. [Abstract]. Psychophysiology: 31; S92, 1994.

Sroufe LA: Emotional Development. New York: Cambridge University Press, 1996.

Stein M, Walker JR, Anderson G, Hazen A, Ross C, Eldridge G et al: Childhood physical and sexual abuse in patients with anxiety disorders in a community sample. American Journal of Psychiatry: 153; 275–277, 1996.

Stemberger RM, Turner SM, Beidel DC, Calhoun KC: Social phobia: An analysis of possible developmental factors. Journal of Abnormal Psychology: 104; 526–531, 1995.

Stifter CA, Spinrad TL, Braungart-Rieker JM: Toward a developmental model of child compliance: The role of emotion regulation in infancy. Child Development: 70; 21–32, 1999.

Thomas A, Chess S: The Reality of Difficult Temperament. Merrill-Palmer Quarterly: 28; 1–19, 1981.

Thomas A, Chess S, Birch: Temperament and Behavior: Disorders in Children. New York: New York University Press, 1968.

Tomarken AJ, Davidson RJ, Henriques JB: Resting frontal brain asymmetry predicts affective responses to films. Journal of Personality and Social Psychology: 59; 791–801, 1990.

Turner SM, Beidel DC, Townsley RM: Social phobia: Relationship to shyness. Behaviour Research and Therapy: 28; 497–505, 1990.

Van den Boom D: Neonatal irritability and the development of attachment. In Kohnstamm G, Baltes J, Rothbart M (Eds), Temperament in Childhood. New York: John Wiley and Sons, pp. 299–318, 1989.

Van den Boom D: The influence of temperament and mothering on attachment and exploration: An experimental manipulation of sensitive responsiveness among lower-class mothers with irritable infants. Child Development: 65; 1457–1477, 1994.

Warren S, Huston L, Egeland B, Sroufe LA: Child and adolescent anxiety disorders and early attachment. Journal of American Academy of Child and Adolescent Psychiatry: 36; 637–644, 1997.

Weidemann G, Pauli P, Dengler W, Lutzenberger W, Birbaumer N, Buchkremer G: Frontal brain asymmetry as a biological substrate of emotions in patients with panic disorder. Archives of General Psychiatry: 56; 78–84, 1999.

Handbook of Neuropsychology, 2nd Edition, Vol. 8, Part II
S.J. Segalowitz and I. Rapin (Eds)

CHAPTER 31

Neurobiological and developmental influences on the addiction to psychotropic drugs

Kristine Erickson [a,*], Kamal Habib [b] and Jay Schulkin [c]

[a] *Mood and Anxiety Disorders Program, NIMH, Bethesda, MD 20892, USA*
[b] *Clinical Neuroendrocrinology Branch, NIMH, Bethesda, MD 20892, USA*
[c] *Department of Physiology and Biophysics, Georgetown University, School of Medicine, Washington, DC 20007, USA*

Introduction

Substance abuse disorders in children, adolescents, and adults are associated with a number of biological and behavioral factors. How these various facets of the individual interact to create addiction is under debate. Environment can play a key role in forming addictions, making prediction of pathological development rocky at best. As young children mature, there is no single reason some end up using and becoming addicted to licit and illicit drugs. Perhaps those who continue their involvement for long periods have some innate vulnerability, or perhaps environmental circumstances are present during development, such as excessive physical or psychological abuse throughout their childhood, that contribute to drug use beyond experimentation. However, these hypothetical circumstances do not explain the wide range of individuals who become enmeshed in drug abuse and dependence.

Conversely, simple exposure to addictive psychotropic drugs is not sufficient to create drug dependency. Many people experiment with drug use and never become dependent upon or addicted to any particular drug. Some individuals sample drugs on only a single occasion, do not enjoy the experience, and never use any drug again. Alcohol is an example of a potentially addictive legal substance that a majority of adults use on a regular basis without developing abuse or dependence upon that drug. These realizations transformed theories of drug addiction from the early situational theories, based primarily on peer influence and availability, into the current working theories encompassing hypotheses of individual vulnerability. Some research on contributions to addiction vulnerability, including temperament, genetic factors, and environmental conditions, are outlined in Table 1. We will return to these issues later in the chapter.

The United States National Research Council reported that a quarter of Americans over the age of fifteen have a physiological dependence on at least one addictive substance. Cigarettes, alcohol, or addictive drugs caused a quarter of all deaths in 1995 (McGinnis and Foege, 1999). Twenty-one percent of deaths in Canada in 1992 were the result of tobacco, alcohol, or drug use (Single, Robson, Rehm and Xie, 1999). Substance use is a problem in Mexico (Medina-Mora, Tapia, Rascon et al., 1990), Australia (Hall, Teesson, Lynskey and Degenhardt, 1999), China (Wang, 1999), and throughout Europe (European Monitoring Centre for Drugs and Drug Addiction, 1999). Substance use also accounts for a large amount of economic burden and social costs to families and communities, including crime, birth defects, family violence, and divorce. These issues make the need to understand addiction clear. If we

* Corresponding author. E-mail: ericksok@intra.nimh.nih.gov

TABLE 1

Predictive risk factors in childhood for addiction from recent selected studies

Risk factor	Study	Findings
Behavior, affect, temperament	McMahon, 1994	Conduct disorder, oppositional defiant disorder, and attention-deficit/hyperactivity disorder; difficult temperament, including moodiness, negativity, poor compliance
	Friedman, Kramer, et al., 1996	Violent behavior
	Brook, Whiteman, et al., 1996	Childhood aggression
	Brook et al., 1998	Quality of parent–child attachment
	McBurnett et al., 2000	Childhood aggression
	Masse and Tremblay, 1997	Novelty-seeking behaviors in childhood
Genetics	Kendler et al., 1992	Genetic risk for alcohol abuse
	Pickens et al., 1991	Genetic risk for alcohol abuse
	Merikanjas et al., 1992	Genetic risk for opiate abuse
Sex	Jang, Livesley and Vernon, 1997	Risk more prevalent in men than women
	Van den Bree et al., 1998	Risk more prevalent in men than women
Environment	Wilsnack et al., 1997	Childhood sexual abuse in women
	Fleming et al., 1998	Childhood sexual abuse in women
	Spak, Spak and Allebeck, 1998	Childhood sexual abuse in women
	Epstein et al., 1998	Childhood sexual abuse in women + post-traumatic stress disorder
	Clark, Lesnick and Hegedus, 1997	Childhood sexual abuse in women
		Childhood physical abuse in men
	Hill et al., 1997	Socioeconomic stress

can explain the underlying reasons for the behaviors, perhaps we can discover an effective solution to the problem. Understanding drug use and addiction is important for child neuropsychologists because of (1) the prevalence of substance use in the general population (2) the predisposing genetic factors that manifest behaviorally (3) the predisposing environmental factors in childhood that affect brain development and (4) the critical age of drug initiation occurring in pre-adolescence and adolescence, which makes it likely that child neuropsychologists will see clients with substance use problems.

In this essay we discuss the relationship between stress and substance abuse. The activity of the neuropeptide CRH (corticotropin releasing hormone) and its relationship to dopamine systems in the brain characterize this relationship. We describe central motive states that underlie the need of the individual to regulate an internal sense of well being. This is particularly relevant to children who are at-risk for substance abuse. To provide an understanding of the relevant activity at the cellular level, the essay continues with an outline of the CRH and dopamine systems, the sites of drug action within the brain, mechanisms of reward, and the relationship between stress responses and CRH. We review the animal and human research into stress, motivation, and addiction in terms of genetic and environmental vulnerability and implications for the developing child.

Central motive states

Addiction is a paradigmatic example of central motive states (Koob, 1999), which are states of the brain linked to a desire, that result in appetitive behaviors (the search for the desired object or condition) and consummation of that desire (Lashley, 1938). Motivational states modulate emotional responses and are inherently information-processing (Lang, Bradley and Cuthbert, 1998). Hence, motivational states are cognitive. Central motive states underlie our behavioral responses (Lashley, 1938; Stellar, 1954), and are restrained by neurobiology (Nader, Bechara and Van der Kooy, 1997). Hormones associated with a particular central motive state prepares the individual to perceive relevant environmental stimuli necessary for obtaining the desired outcome (Schulkin, 1999). These may be mediated through approach and avoidance systems, two primary emotional and motivational circuits in the brain (Davidson and Rickman, 1999). Systems in the brain that generate approach and withdrawal behavior events are becoming more clear (Davidson, Ekman, Saron et al., 1990; Schnierla, 1959).

The appetitive activities of central motive states are mediated by the approach systems (Davidson and Rickman, 1999). Approach systems include prefrontal cortex, basal ganglia, amygdala, and hypothalamus. Human imaging and electroencephalographic studies show that appetitive emotions at the cortical level may be lateralized to the left frontal cortex in humans (Davidson, 1998; Harmon-Jones and Allen, 1998). Note that this left-sided lateralization is related to approach, appetitive, or goal-directed emotion, and not necessarily to 'positive' emotion in general (Harmon-Jones and Allen, 1998). The basal ganglia are important for initiating and terminating movement, and for the anticipation of reward (Kelley, 1999). The prefrontal cortex encompasses two separate and important stages of the approach system. The dorsolateral prefrontal cortex may be important for representation of the goal state in working memory, while the medial prefrontal cortex may play a role in retaining the reinforcement contingencies in working memory (Thorpe, Rolls and Maddison, 1983). The medial prefrontal cortex also projects to the nucleus accumbens, which is part of the dopaminergic reward system and will be discussed in more detail below.

The amygdala is linked to both approach (Adolphs, Tranel, Hamann et al., 1999; Davidson, 1998; Stellar and Stellar, 1985) and to withdrawal from objects and withdrawal-related negative affects (LeDoux, Cicchetti, Xagoraris and Romanski, 1990; Smith, DeVito and Astley, 1990). Fear and disgust are emotions associated with withdrawal from objects or situations. Imaging studies show increased activation in the amygdala when individuals are shown fearful facial expressions (withdrawal affect), while happy facial expressions (approach af-

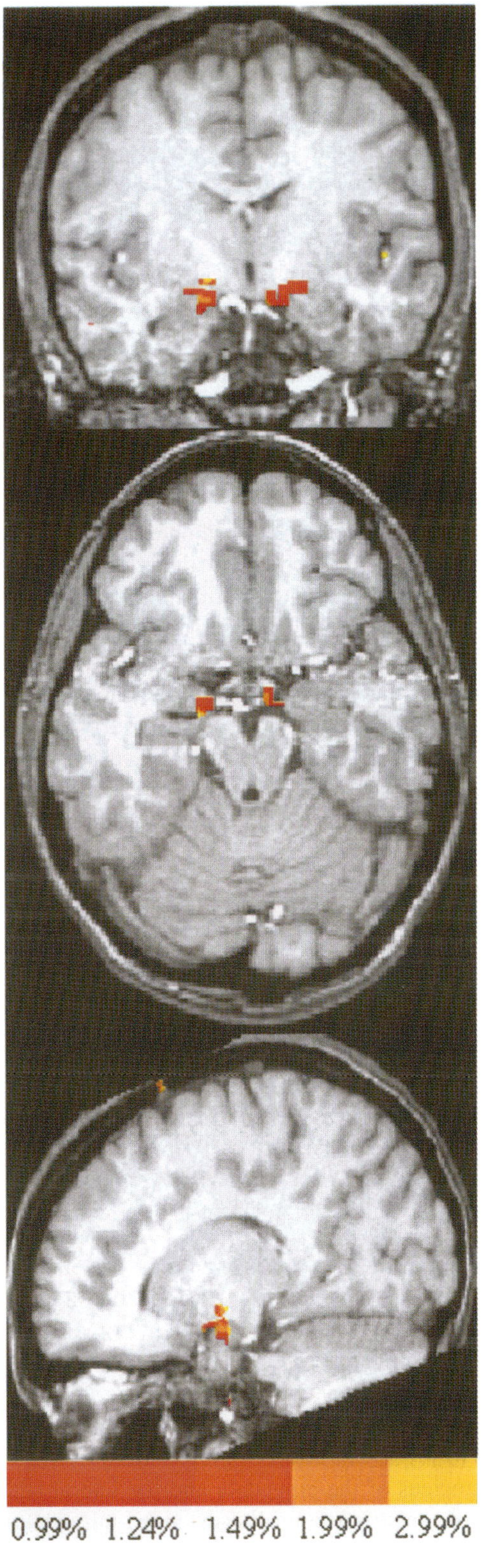

Fig. 1. Group data showing bilateral activation in the amygdala detected with fMRI in response to aversive compared with neutral pictures. From Irwin et al. (1996).

fect) lead to decreased amygdala activation (Morris, Frith, Perrett et al., 1996). Fig. 1 illustrates amygdala activation in response to viewing aversive pictures, when compared to neutral pictures. Cortical structures involved in withdrawal affect are the temporal region (Blair, Morris, Frith et al., 1999; Reiman, Fusselman, Fox and Raichle, 1989) and prefrontal cortex (Davidson, Abercrombie, Nitschke and Putnam, 1999; Heilman, 1997). The cortical activity related to withdrawal affect may be more lateralized to the right frontal cortex (Blair et al., 1999; Davidson et al., 1990). However, the left amygdala appears to show more activation relative to the right amygdala in response to fearful stimuli (Breiter, Etcoff, Whalen et al., 1996; Ketter, Andreason, George et al., 1996; Morris et al., 1996).

Corticotropin releasing hormone (CRH) and dopamine are a neuropeptide and a neurotransmitter, respectively, that are located in the brain areas associated with both approach and withdrawal behaviors. The following sections outline the distribution of CRH and dopamine in the brain. Other neurotransmitters such as serotonin are also mentioned later in the text.

CRH distribution and regulation by cortisol

CRH is widely distributed in the brain (see Fig. 2). CRH neurons are located in the paraventricular nucleus (PVN) of the hypothalamus and in the amygdala. Some CRH neurons are also located in other hypothalamic areas, and in the cingulate cortex and prefrontal cortex. CRH receptor sites are distributed throughout the brain (Schulkin, 1999). Primary sites include the hippocampus, septum, amygdala, neocortex, ventral thalamus, medial hypothalamus, cerebellum, and some in the PVN and pituitary glands.

Two CRH systems are affected by glucocorticoids (see Table 2). One system is the hypothalamic–pituitary–adrenal (HPA) axis, and this system exhibits rapid and specific restraint upon the activity of CRH in order to maintain important homeostatic functions (Sawchenko, 1987). The second system, and the one with which we are most concerned here, is the extrahypothalamic CRH system and its relationship to stress. The effect of glucocorticoids in the central nucleus of the amygdala and the lateral bed nucleus of the stria terminalis (extended amygdala) is an increase in CRH gene expression (Makino, Gold and Schulkin, 1994; Swanson and Simmon, 1989; Watts and Sanchez-Watts, 1995). When CRH is elevated in these areas, there is increased anxiety and cautious avoidance, and CRH facilitates hyperarousal (Kalin, 1985; Koob et al., 1993).

Dopamine in the brain

Dopamine is also widely distributed in the brain. Although dopamine is a major transmitter implicated in the brain's reward system, dopamine is involved with other regulatory and cognitive systems. Three primary clusters of dopaminergic cell bodies are located in the brain: within the arcuate nucleus of the hypothalamus, important for neuroendocrine regulation; within the substantia nigra, important for subcortical movement; and within the ventral tegmental area, important for aspects of reward (Hyman and Nestler, 1993). From these major cell body clusters, dopamine cells project to numerous areas (see Fig. 3). The third cluster (the mesocorticolimbic dopamine system) includes the brain system important for food, drink, drug, social, and other reward (Berridge and Robinson, 1998). Dopamine projections from the ventral tegmental area terminate in various brain areas, including the nucleus accumbens, stria terminalis, amygdala, prefrontal cortex, anterior cingulate, and limbic areas of the striatum (Byne, Kemether, Jones et al., 1999; Hyman and Nestler, 1993).

But naturally, the dopamine reward system does not exist in a vacuum. Neurons in the nucleus accumbens receive input from the hippocampus, brainstem serotonin neurons and glutamate neurons from the cortex and thalamus. Neurons within the nucleus accumbens contain receptors for many other neurotransmitters (Hyman, 1999). Destruction of dopamine pathways in animals leads not only to movement deficits but also to failure to work for a reward (Wise, 1982; Wise, Spindler, deWit and Gerberg, 1978). PET and MRI imaging show changes in the dopamine projection sites of nucleus accumbens, neostriatum, and prefrontal cortex during various reward activities in humans (Fowler, Volkow, Malison and Gatley, 1999; Nestler, 1999).

The realization that the neurotransmitters for movement and motivation are one and the same led

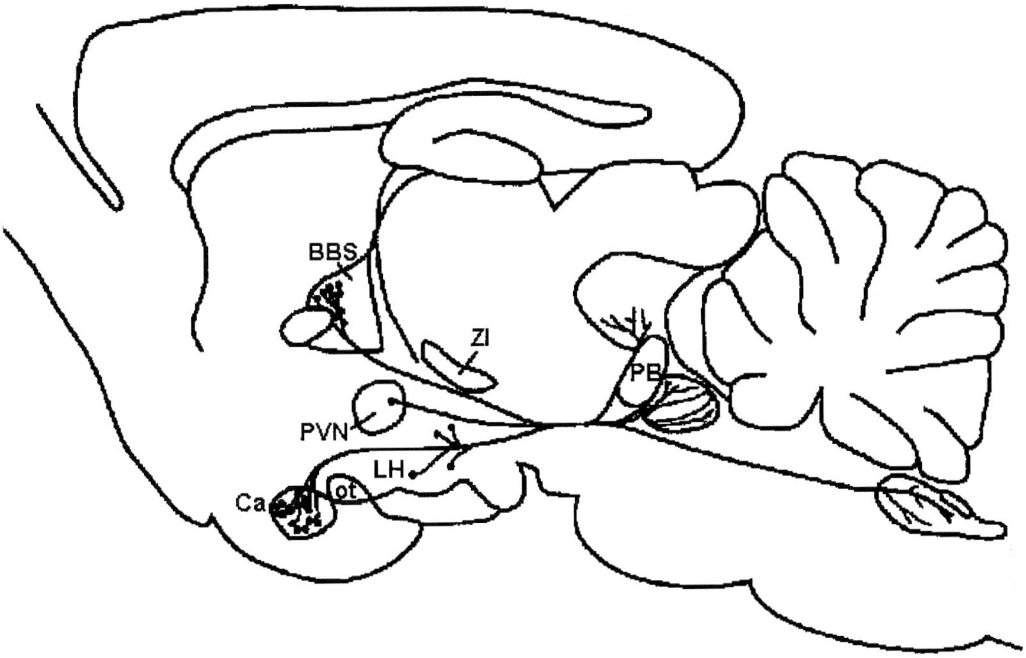

Fig. 2. CRH sites in the brain. Abbreviations: *BBS*, bed nucleus of the stria terminalis; *Ce*, central nucleus of the amygdala; *LH*, lateral hypothalamus; *ot*, optic tract; *PB*, parabrachial nucleus; *PVN*, paraventricular nucleus of the hypothalamus; *ZI*, zona incerta. (From Gray, 1990.)

TABLE 2

Relationships between CRH and glucocorticoids

Term	Alternative term	Definition	Point of origin	Effect
Corticotropin releasing hormone (CRH)	Corticotropin releasing factor (CRF)	Neuropeptide	Hypothalamus (HPA system)	Homeostatic regulation
			Amygdala (extra-hypothalamic system)	Fear and anxiety responses
Adrenocorticotropic hormone (ACTH)		Peripheral hormone	Anterior pituitary	Activates glucocorticoids
Glucocorticoids	Corticosterone (in rats)	Peripheral hormone	Adrenal glands	Restrains CRH expression in hypothalamus
	Cortisol (in primates)			Facilitates CRH expression in amygdala

to theoretical links between motivation and muscle. The nucleus accumbens, within the basal ganglia, may be a primary ganglion for the organization of action within the brain. Some time ago, Nauta (1961) suggested that the nucleus accumbens is an important link between the amygdala (Fig. 4) and the organization of action (Mogenson, 1987). Translation of motivational output from the amygdala to the behavioral outputs of the basal ganglia is via the connectivity to the nucleus accumbens (Kelley, 1999; Mogenson, Jones and Yim, 1980).

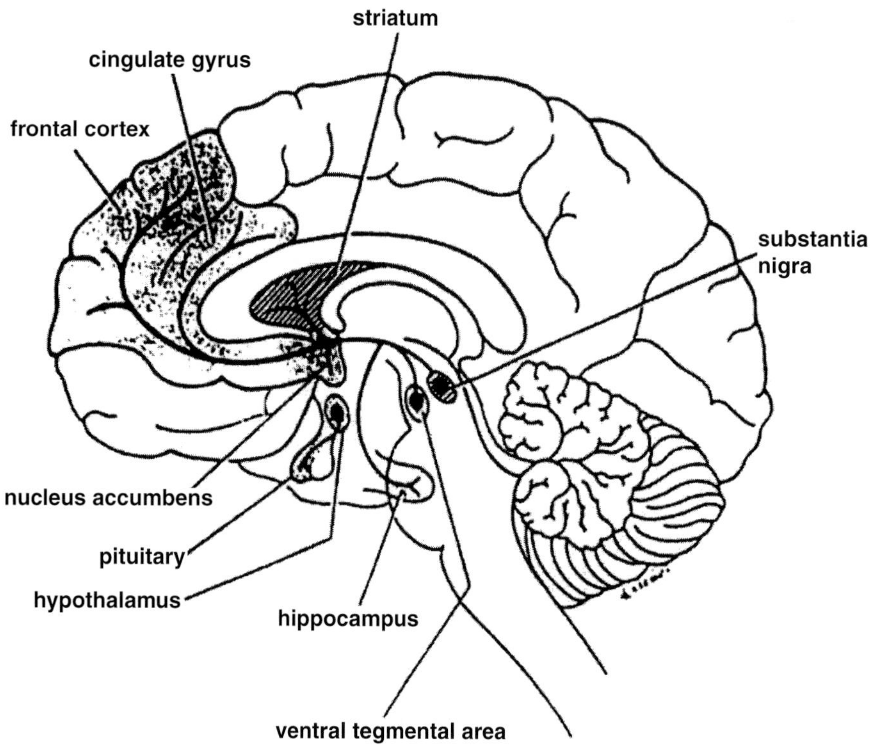

Fig. 3. Dopamine distribution in the human brain. (From Hyman and Nestler, 1993.)

Sites of drug action

One extensively studied drug is cocaine, which has a very fast uptake rate and clearance rate. Cocaine's acute effects are mediated by the dopamine system, and the reinforcement and motivation to search for the drug is dependent upon the activity of the nucleus accumbens (Chang, Sawyer, Lee and Woodward, 1994). Studies with rats show there is anticipatory neuronal activity in the nucleus accumbens just prior to lever presses to receive cocaine. Another group of neurons in the nucleus accumbens responds immediately following cocaine infusion and is presumably the activity of the reinforcing effects of the drug. Injection of a dopamine antagonist directly into the shell of the nucleus accumbens and the central nucleus of the amygdala effectively decreases cocaine self-administration in rats (Caine, Heinrich, Coffin and Koob, 1995). Positron emission tomography imaging studies of cocaine and human brain activation show that the nucleus accumbens is one among many areas of increased activation (Breiter, Gollub, Weisskoff et al., 1997). Many neurotransmitter systems and brain areas are engaged during drug use and abuse. Each drug of abuse involves a different constellation of systems and sites; dopamine is one system involved across the various drug families.

Animal and human research support the involvement of frontal cortex in the rewarding aspects of drug use. For example, rats work for cocaine injections administered directly into the medial prefrontal cortex (Carlezon and Wise, 1996). Cue-induced craving in human crack cocaine addicts are associated with activation of left dorsolateral prefrontal cortex (Maas, Lukas, Kaufman et al., 1998), and orbitofrontal cortex (Grant, London, Newlin et al., 1996); a positive correlation exists between cortical activation and self-reported levels of craving (Maas et al., 1998). Chronic alcoholics who are neurologically normal show metabolic abnormalities in both mediofrontal cortex and left dorsolateral prefrontal cortex (Dao-Castellana, Samson, Legault et al., 1998). From the prefrontal cortex, there are direct dopamine projections to the nucleus accumbens.

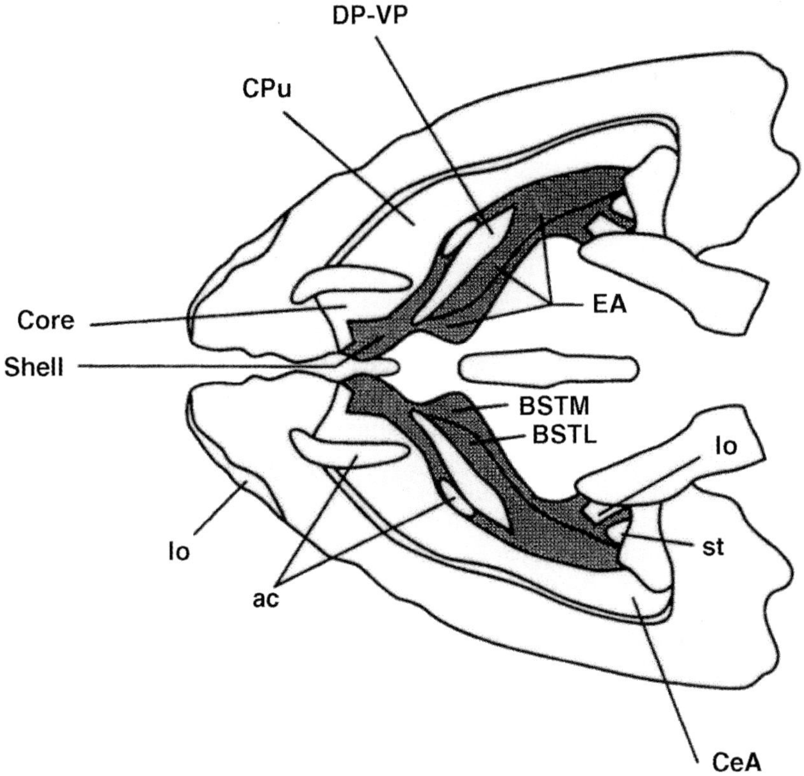

Fig. 4. Nucleus accumbens and amygdala. Horizontal section of a rat brain depicting the principal structures of the bed nucleus of the stria terminalis. These structures include the central nucleus of the amygdala, the shell part of the nucleus accumbens, and the bed nucleus of the stria terminalis. Abbreviations: *Cpu*, Caudate-putamen; *DP-VP*, Dorsal/ventral pallidum; *lo*, Lateral olfactory tract; *ac*, anterior conunissure; *CeA*, central nucleus of the amygdala; *st*, stria terminalis; *ol*, optic tract; *EA*, extended amygdala; *BSTM*, medial bed nucleus of the stria terminalis; *BSTL*, lateral bed nucleus of the stria terminalis. (From Alheid et al., 1996.)

Once rats receive prolonged exposure to an addictive substance, there are changes in the dendrites of prefrontal cortex (Robinson and Kolb, 1997).

Drugs of addiction affect cerebral blood flow and glucose metabolisms, and the distribution of these changes can give insights into the areas associated with addiction. Regional cerebral blood flow and glucose metabolism usually return to normal levels after sustained periods of abstinence. Imaging studies of abstinent opioid addicts show that asymmetrical cerebral blood flow is related to depression and antisocial behavioral traits and not necessarily to the substance abuse history (Gerra, Calbiani, Zaimovic et al., 1998). Human studies indicate that there are changes in the metabolic activity of addicted subjects in orbitofrontal cortex (Volkow, Fowler, Wolf et al., 1991), temporal cortex, cingulate gyrus, and prefrontal cortex (Volkow, Hitzemann, Wang et al., 1992).

A history of chronic stress interacts with the dopaminergic reward system. An increase in dopamine release occurs in the frontal cortex of rats exposed to chronic stress, while rats without a chronic stress history do not show as much frontal cortex dopamine release when put in the same stressful situation (Cuadra, Zurita, Lacerra and Molina, 1999). Chronic stress also leads to a decrease in dopamine in the nucleus accumbens (Gambarana, Ghiglieri, Masi et al., 1999).

Drug use and reward

One of the primary reasons for using drugs of abuse is the pleasurable feeling derived from the drug use.

TABLE 3

Relationship of addiction components and behavioral constructs

Addictive component	Operational construct
Pleasure	Positive reinforcement
Self-medication	Negative reinforcement
Habit	Conditioned positive reinforcement
Habit	Conditioned negative reinforcement

Adapted from Koob (2000).

However, there are many negative consequences to substance use, and research into addiction attempts to delineate the behavioral and physiological correlates of the components of abuse and dependence. Pathways to addiction may vary between individuals. Table 3 describes the behavioral components of addiction (Koob, 1999). The positive reinforcement model of addiction states that drug use is no different from sexual gratification. The drug's effects are desirable and motivation for continued use is dependent only upon those effects. The negative reinforcement model of addiction states that drug use is the result of a need to alleviate negative states. This is a self-medication model, and the compulsive nature of drug addiction results from the need for the drug to feel normal. The self-medication aspect can stem from illness, grief, depression, anxiety, or poverty (Weiss, 1999).

Conditioned positive and negative reinforcement are relevant to both continued drug abuse and to relapse after prolonged abstinence. If substance use was based purely in unconditioned positive and negative reinforcement (and their underlying neural substrates), then relapse after extended abstinence should not be the social problem that it is in our society. One habit-forming aspect of compulsive drug use is the result of the associated euphoria. Examples of conditioned positive reinforcement exist in the animal and human research literature. Animal studies suggest that the amygdala and ventral striatum, including the nucleus accumbens, are important for acquiring the conditioned reinforcing effects of stimuli associated with addiction (Altman, Everitt, Glautier et al., 1996; Robbins, Cador, Taylor and Everitt, 1989; Robbins and Everitt, 1999). Heroine addicts find injections of saline pleasurable because the conditioned positive reinforcement of the injection is associated with heroin injections. The motivation to continue drug use in order to avoid the negative affective and physiological consequences of withdrawal is a negatively reinforcing aspect of dependence (Koob, 1999). Conditioned negative reinforcement is relevant to internal physiological changes in drug set point, on which we will elaborate when we describe allostasis.

Dopamine and reward. Dopamine is important for the wanting of drugs, the salience of associations, and, to some degree, for the liking of drugs (Berridge and Robinson, 1998). Dopamine also plays a role in integrating stress and environmental stimuli with homeostatic mechanisms such as cardiovascular regulation (Van den Buuse, 1997).

The behavioral consequences of introducing dopamine antagonists, which constrain the activity of dopamine in the brain, is a reduction in the self-administration of amphetamine, cocaine, nicotine, and morphine (Phillips, Robbins and Everitt, 1994). But there is also a body of literature that suggests dopamine depletion does not interfere with food consummatory palatability judgements (Berridge and Robinson, 1998). In other words, blocking the activity of the dopamine reward system does not axiomatically result in not liking the food; rather, dopamine antagonists block the wanting of or desire for the food.

Recent animal and human studies assessing the hedonic and incentive characteristics of dopamine within the reward pathways show interesting results that are relevant to addiction. Dopamine antagonists decrease the 'wanting' of a drug. Rats do not self-administer psychoactive drugs when an antagonist is present, but behavioral observation of tongue movements and paw licks show that the rats still 'like' the food or drug (Berridge and Robinson, 1998). In contrast, dopamine agonists cause rats to 'want' the drug, but behavioral observation shows that, although the rats are self-administering the drug, they have an aversive reaction, or 'dislike', for that drug. Dopamine is apparently relevant for craving, but is not relevant for the hedonic value of a drug. A distinction between wanting and liking is evoked; you can want something without liking it, and the mechanisms that underlie these cognitive states appear to be different (Berridge and Robinson, 1998).

Human studies parallel the findings reported in the animal literature. When human subjects make self-reports of 'liking' amphetamine (Brauer and De Wit, 1997) or cocaine (Ohuoha, Maxwell, Thomson et al., 1997), subjective ratings of 'liking' are unaffected. Subjects felt the pleasurable effects of the drugs whether the antagonists were present or absent. Subjective ratings of 'wanting' (or craving) decreased in both studies when dopamine antagonists were present. Apparently, the neural substrates of 'liking' are located elsewhere in the brain. Opiates like morphine can enhance the hedonic liking of food, and the shell of the nucleus accumbens may be an opioid 'liking' site (Pecina and Berridge, 1996). Destruction of opiate receptors within this area results in an aversion to food (Berridge, 1996).

In terms of the extensive energy output in addiction, the dopamine pathways involved in wanting are important for the motivational craving experienced by the individual. Whether the individual received hedonic pleasure from the drug use is no longer important. For most individuals, the hedonic value of the drug is only important during the initial experience of a drug. Once addicted, the appetitive motivational state is only concerned with satisfying the craving induced by the activity of dopamine.

Glucocorticoids and CRH

Both glucocorticoids and central CRH are elevated under a number of conditions. Food consumption is generally a rewarding activity, and measuring CRH levels using microdialysis showed that CRH is elevated during rewarding activities such as food consumption (Merali, McIntosh, Kent et al., 1998). Drug use is also a rewarding experience, and microdialysis studies showed elevated CRH within the central nucleus of the amygdala and the hypothalamus of rats during self-administration of psychotropic drugs. Elevated CRH levels are present in the central nucleus of the amygdala and the bed nucleus of the stria terminalis during nicotine infusion (Matta, Valentine and Sharp, 1997). Corticotropin releasing hormone continues to release during the consummatory phase of cocaine consumption in rats engaged in chronic cocaine administration (Richter, Pich, Koob and Weiss, 1995).

The relationship between glucocorticoids and drug use is more complicated than elevation and release during rewarding experiences. These hormones facilitate cocaine and alcohol administration in rats (Fahlke, Engel, Eriksson et al., 1994; Piazza, Maccari, Deminiere et al., 1991). Corticosterone, under some conditions, may also be intrinsically reinforcing. Rats will self-administer corticosterone, and the dose response curve is similar to that of an addicting drug (Piazza, Deroche, Deminiere et al., 1993). Rats who are high responders to corticosterone also tend to be high responders to novelty and to psychotropic drugs, and this has implications for some children's biological vulnerability to addiction. Children and adults who find increased levels of corticosterone during stressful situations intrinsically rewarding may be more vulnerable to drug addiction.

Corticotropin releasing hormone levels are elevated during both positive and negative experiences (Richter et al., 1995). Expression of corticotropin releasing hormone in the brain increases the salience of environmental stimuli (Rosen and Schulkin, 1998), and has implications for situational learning both in addiction and during a child's development. In addiction, this is relevant in terms of search and acquisition of the desired object. The actions of glucocorticoids might also be adaptable mechanisms for reducing overactivity of physiological stress systems, allowing the animal to cope more effectively with the stressful situation (Piazza and Le Moal, 1996). This is relevant for children as well as animals. In chronic stress situations, hippocampal deterioration takes place (Magarinos, McEwen, Flugge and Fuchs, 1996).

Both glucocorticoids and CRH have psychomotor effects, as does dopamine. Cocaine is considered a psychomotor stimulant. The psychomotor and euphoric effects resulting from cocaine consumption may reflect activation of the neuropeptide CRH and neurotransmitter dopamine and their regulation by glucocorticoids (Koob, 1999; Piazza et al., 1993; Schulkin, Gold and McEwen, 1998). Cocaine activates the pituitary adrenal axis in both rats and nonhuman primates; CRH is activated in both hypothalamic and extrahypothalamic areas during cocaine consumption (Koob, 1999). After three weeks of binge cocaine administration, rats show higher basal corticosterone levels when compared to rats in the no-cocaine placebo group (Sarnyai, Dhabhar, McEwen and Kreek, 1998). Increases in CRH activity during cocaine consumption, along with mesolimbic dopaminergic activity, may increase the salience of cocaine and stimuli associated with cocaine use.

The effects of drug consumption interact with individual stress responses, and may be relevant to both the initiation and maintenance of drug abuse. Individual differences in biological response to stress are measurable in the laboratory. Rats can be categorized as low responders and high responders to stress by measuring corticosterone release and locomotor reactivity in response to stressful situations. Most animals and humans avoid stressful situations because those situations are unpleasant; however, some animals and humans can be described as stress-seeking (Piazza et al., 1993). Animal research shows that these individuals are more likely to self-administer and are more sensitive to the effects of psychostimulants. Young children who show novelty-seeking characteristics may have a similar vulnerability (see human vulnerability section below).

Once within the cycle of addiction, individual biology is not as relevant to the animal's interpretation of the environment. One result of cocaine binge administration in rats is the diminution of individual differences in corticosterone hormone response to stress (Sarnyai et al., 1998). Rats that showed high levels of corticosterone release in response to stress and those that show low levels of release were put in binge cocaine and saline/control conditions. The individual differences were maintained in animals injected with saline over 3- and 6-week periods. However, the differences in response to stress between low-responders and high-responders disappeared in the rats treated with cocaine during the same time periods (Sarnyai et al., 1998).

From the animal literature, we can hypothesize that adolescents who show high corticosterone release in response to stress and who are exposed to chronic stressful situations may initially find some relief during drug use. However, one corollary to this chapter is studying central nervous system levels of CRH and related substances in human beings is quite difficult. When we refer to levels of cortisol and ACTH in humans, we are referring to peripheral levels of these substances as measured in saliva, blood or urine. From the animal literature, researchers can make inferences about the CNS activity of CRH and glucocorticoids.

Vulnerability: animal studies

Genetic vulnerability

An individual's inborn characteristics can have mediating effects upon both response to stress and reactions to drugs. Animals can be selectively bred to have higher basal levels of corticosterone. Similarly, strains of animals that prefer specific drugs, and are more likely to respond to specific drugs, can be bred in laboratories. Behavioral and physiological characteristics of selectively bred animals can give insights into characteristics of human vulnerability.

Many studies demonstrate that rats with higher glucocorticoid levels are more likely to self-administer a number of psychotropic agents (Piazza et al., 1993). In different strains of rats that have different genetically based levels of corticosterone, the corticosterone levels are related to the likelihood of self-administration of psychotropic drugs. Rats with higher levels of corticosterone are more likely to self-administer cocaine, heroin and amphetamines. In other words, the greater the level of corticosterone that circulates within the central nervous system, the greater the probability of rats self-administering these agents (Erb, Shaham and Stewart, 1996; Piazza, Deminiere, Le Moal and Simon, 1989; Piazza et al., 1993).

The vulnerability story is more complex than cortisol, corticosterone, or CRH levels. One line of research also implicates the serotonin neurotransmitter system and its relationship to impulse control. There are serotinergic projections from the brainstem raphe to the nucleus accumbens. Decreased serotonin levels are correlated with impaired impulse control and with increased drug self-administration, and is one of the neurotransmitters implicated in Type II, adolescent-onset, alcoholism, which is characterized by impulsivity and aggressive behavior. Non-human primates with low levels of serotonin are more aggressive than those with normal serotonin levels (Mehlman, Higley, Faucher et al., 1994). Rats who lack the serotonin 5-HT1B receptor have a greater response to the effects of cocaine, and are more motivated to self-administer cocaine (Rocha, Scearce-Levie, Lucas et al., 1998).

Environmental vulnerability

Environment can impact the biology of an individual. Animal research allows the manipulation of key variables and allows extreme control over the animals' environments. As a result, we are learning the environmental conditions that might create vulnerability to self-administration of drugs in animals that are not genetically vulnerable.

CRH and early life stress

Recent research suggests that even prenatal stress can have lifelong effects. When cortisol is elevated in both mother and fetus, CRH levels in the amygdala are significantly higher in the offspring when they become young adults (Cratty, Ward, Johnson et al., 1995). Additionally, CRH injections to the mother during pregnancy increase the fear responses of the offspring when they are provoked as adults. Prenatal stress also impairs future motor development in primates (Schneider, Coe and Lubach, 1992).

Research groups are studying stress and early social development in some detail using nonhuman primates (Habib, Weld, Schulkin et al., 1999; Higley, Linnoila and Suomi, 1994; Higley, Suomi and Linnoila, 1996a,b). Parental deprivation is an important variable for predicting later vulnerability to stress among non-human primates. Plasma cortisol levels quickly increase in rhesus infants when they are separated from their mothers and peers (Higley, Suomi and Linnoila, 1992). Rhesus monkeys maternally deprived during development tend to have higher systemic levels of cortisol than mother-reared monkeys. Rhesus monkey infants subjected to short-term maternal separation and isolation exhibit higher cortisol levels; those rhesus infants reared by surrogate mothers and with limited peer contact do not show as high a cortisol response to isolation (Shannon, Champoux and Suomi, 1998).

Experiences of various stressful events, including prenatal events, elevate glucocorticoid levels in an individual. Links between early life stress and subsequent effects on the mesolimbic dopamine system are emerging in the animal literature. Perinatal stress in the form of birth complications has long-lasting effects on dopamine release in response to stress. Later in life, animals that experienced birth complications show longer-lasting dopamine release in the nucleus accumbens than animals that experienced no birth complications (Brake, Noel, Boksa and Gratton, 1997).

Early life experience with food availability is another stressor with long-lasting consequences. Studies using non-human primates indicate that experience of variable food availability during development results in greater CRH levels in the CSF during adulthood, and greater fear-related behavioral responses (Coplan, Trost, Owens et al., 1998). The changes in the stress system as a result of early trauma stem from lack of predictability and the extreme demands upon the CRH system.

Stress and drug use

Stressful events, which lead to higher glucocorticoid levels, also induce an increased likelihood of self-administration of drugs at higher rates. When rats are exposed to non-contingent shock, they self-administer cocaine at much higher rates than rats who are exposed to contingent shock or no shock (Goeders, 1998). The non-contingent shock rats were more responsive to lower cocaine doses than the rats in the other shock groups, who required two times the dosage amount before engaging in significant amounts of cocaine self-administration. Plasma corticosterone in the non-contingent shock rats was much higher than the levels in the other rats.

Maternally deprived macaques have both higher plasma cortisol concentrations and higher central CRH in the CSF as young mature adults (Habib et al., 1999; Higley et al., 1992, 1996). Behaviorally, peer-reared macaques show higher baseline rates of alcohol consumption compared to mother-reared macaques. However, when subjected to social separation, mother-reared monkeys increase their alcohol consumption during social separation until the consumption is equal to that of peer-reared macaques, as illustrated in Fig. 5 (Higley, Hasert, Suomi and Linnoila, 1991; Kraemer and McKinney, 1985). Mother-reared macaques also have larger increases in ACTH than peer-reared macaques during social separation (Clarke, 1993). Macaques separated from their mothers and raised by peers are more socially inept, more aggressive, engage in more deviant behaviors,

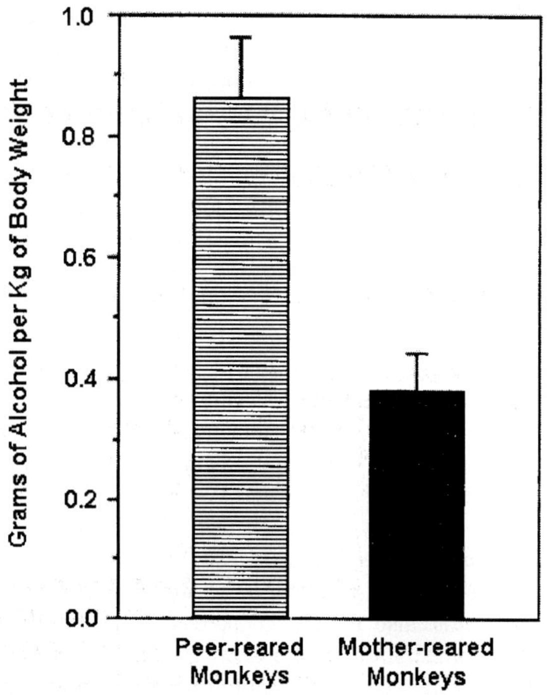

Fig. 5. Effects of early rearing experiences and social separation on alcohol consumption. Bars represent average alcohol consumption per kg of body weight for both rearing groups. Average alcohol consumption over 10 days in home cage. Peer-reared monkeys consume significantly more alcohol than mother-reared monkeys. (From Higley et al., 1991.)

and consume more alcohol than their mother-reared counterparts (Fig. 5; Higley et al., 1996a, b).

Environmental early life stress influences serotonin levels. Low levels of cerebrospinal fluid 5-HIAA, a marker of central nervous system serotonin concentrations, correlate with impaired impulse control. Rhesus monkeys who undergo maternal separations have both of these characteristics (Higley et al., 1996b). Reduced serotonin and impaired impulse control are stable from childhood to adulthood, and these rhesus monkeys consume higher rates of alcohol than other monkeys (Higley et al., 1996a).

Vulnerability: human studies

Genetic vulnerability

A family history of alcoholism is one clear marker of vulnerability to alcohol and drug abuse. Both adoption and twin studies support a genetic risk for alcoholism (Kendler, Heath, Neale et al., 1992; Merikanjas, 1990; Pickens, Svikis, McGue et al., 1991). Survey, adoption and twin studies also report increased risk of substance use in people with a family history of alcoholism. One finding reported by Merikanjas, Rounsaville and Prusoff (1992) stated that 90% of opiate addicts' siblings who experimented with any addictive drug developed a substance abuse problem. This is convincing correlational evidence for an inborn biological vulnerability to drug abuse. The identification of physiological and behavioral markers gleaned from those who are genetically vulnerable to addiction can be useful because animal research indicates that environmental factors may induce similar states in those not genetically vulnerable.

Twin studies investigating the genetic and environmental influences on substance use show that genetic vulnerability is more pronounced in men than in women (Jang, Livesley and Vernon, 1997; Van den Bree, Johnson, Neale and Pickens, 1998). Presence of first- and second-degree alcoholic relatives and multi-generational alcoholism are strongly associated with alcoholism. However, not all children of alcoholics become alcoholics, and not all alcoholics have a family history of alcoholism. For example, one adoption study concluded that the incidence of alcoholism in men with genetic and environmental risk factors of Type 1 adult-onset alcoholism is 11.4%, compared to a general population rate of about 3.0%; the incidence of alcoholism in men with genetic risk factors of Type 2 adolescent-onset alcoholism is 10.7%, compared to a rate of 2.0% in the general population (Sigvardsson, Bohman and Cloninger, 1996).

One correlate of substance abuse is lowered peripheral cortisol levels in individuals with childhood onset of conduct disorders. These children are more aggressive and impulsive than those with adolescent onset conduct disorder, and their lowered cortisol levels correlate with more conduct disorder symptoms (McBurnett, Lahey, Frick et al., 1991; McBurnett, Lahey, Rathouy and Loeber, 2000). When other diagnoses are present in a child, or when conduct disorder symptoms do not include overtly aggressive behaviors, the relationship between lower cortisol levels and conduct disorder diagnosis is weaker

(McBurnett et al., 1991). Children with conduct disorder and co-occurring depression are at risk for substance abuse, though those with depression alone are not at risk (Miller-Johnson, Lochman, Coie et al., 1998). High CNS levels of CRH are associated with increased fear-related behavioral responses and increased drug self-administration in animals. If the lowered cortisol levels of children with conduct disorder is an accurate measure of CNS CRH activity, the low cortisol levels and presence of risk-taking behaviors are a logical association. The biological vulnerability of these children to addiction might be similar to that of rats who are high responders to novelty and who self-administer psychotropic drugs.

Type II alcoholism is associated with impulsivity and low levels of the serotonin neurotransmitter. Studies of sensation-seeking behavior in children prior to the onset of pathological behavior and in adults after onset of pathological behavior show a relationship with impulsivity. The characteristics are derived from the tridimensional theory of personality of Cloninger (1987), which includes a novelty-seeking (impulsivity) dimension. Although research inconsistently supports the correlative and predictive value of the other theory dimensions, the usefulness of the novelty-seeking/impulsivity dimension is upheld consistently (Fergusson and Lynskey, 1996; Howard, Kivlahan and Walker, 1997; Johnson, Waid and Anton, 1997; Sax and Strakowski, 1998). Evidence from animal research indicates that these relationships are probably related to (dys)function of the reward system of the limbic-medial prefrontal cortex, and involve the dopamine circuitry within this system (Piazza et al., 1993).

Novelty-seeking characteristics, like early signs of aggressive behavior in childhood, appear to be predictive, though not necessarily causal, of pathology in late childhood and adolescence (Masse and Tremblay, 1997; Wills, Windle and Cleary, 1998). High rates of impulsivity and novelty-seeking behavior in children as young as six years old are stable across childhood and are predictive of early alcohol, tobacco, and drug use. Kindergartners who are impulsive and who show little anxiety are much more likely to engage in risk-taking behaviors later on than children who do not show these two characteristics (Masse and Tremblay, 1997).

High rates of novelty-seeking behaviors exist in individuals suffering from alcoholism and other substance use disorders. There are characteristic signs of 'frontal dysfunction' on neuropsychological test batteries (Dao-Castellana et al., 1998). One problem with drawing predictive conclusions from this research is that substance use can have a causal effect on novelty-seeking behavior (Sax and Strakowski, 1998). Also, impulse control problems may contribute to the likelihood of engaging in risk-taking behaviors, such as substance use, without being an explicit cause.

Environmental vulnerability: childhood trauma

Animal research shows that maternal separation and other stress-inducing or traumatic events can affect responses to later stressful experiences and responses to addictive substances. More recently, the role of early life stress in humans on subsequent alcohol and drug addiction is the topic of a small body of research. Although the effects are not as strong and clear-cut as those found in the animal research, there is a relationship between childhood trauma and future substance use, and the childhood trauma is linked to certain characteristics of the CRH system. Most research focuses on the experiences of women, but in several studies men are also included in the early life stress samples.

Childhood sexual abuse is a contributor to alcohol abuse and cigarette smoking in women (Anda, Croft, Felitti et al., 1999; Clark, Lesnick and Hegedus, 1997; Epstein, Saunders, Kilpatrick and Resnick, 1998; Flemming, Mullen, Sibthorpe et al., 1998; Miller, Downs, Gondoli and Keil, 1987; Spak, Spak and Allebeck, 1998; Yama, Tovey, Fogas and Teegarden, 1992). An early study reported that a history of childhood sexual abuse predicted a woman's status in the alcoholic group, and lack of abuse history predicted status in the non-alcohol-abusing group (Miller et al., 1987). Routine childhood abuse histories taken in drug treatment centers revealed 42% of teenaged boys and 71–90% of teenaged girls reported a history of child abuse (Rohsenow, Corbett and Devine, 1988). Sixty-five percent of another substance abuse treatment sample reported a history of childhood physical or sexual abuse, and over 25% met posttraumatic stress disorder (PTSD) criteria (Ellason, Ross, Sainton and Mayran, 1996).

Subsequent research investigated mediating factors that influence future substance abuse. Perceptions of family members and beliefs about alcohol have a mediating impact on alcohol use (Flemming et al., 1998). Development of PTSD symptoms following childhood rape also has a mediating effect on future substance abuse, with more PTSD symptoms correlated with more severe substance abuse patterns (Epstein et al., 1998). The trauma does not need to be sexual in nature; victims of physical assault in childhood have more PTSD and substance abuse than those without an assault history (Duncan, Saunders, Kilpatrick et al., 1995).

The presence of PTSD symptoms following childhood trauma has a definite impact on both physiology and behavior in adulthood. Brain imaging shows that brain volume correlated with both age of onset of physical abuse and with the duration of abuse during childhood (DeBellis, Keshavan, Clark et al., 1999). Subsequent symptoms, such as intrusive thoughts, avoidance behavior, hyperarousal, and dissociation are positively correlated with ventricular volume and negatively correlated with corpus callosum size. Corpus callosum size is smaller in all regions except in areas involving motor function (DeBellis et al., 1999). Hippocampal volumes are smaller in adult survivors of childhood abuse and abuse-related PTSD (Bremner, Randall, Vermetten et al., 1997), but see Bonne, Brandes, Gilboa et al. (2001).

Urinary dopamine, norepinephrine and urinary-free cortisol are elevated in children with PTSD (DeBellis, Baum, Birmaher et al., 1999), though studies of adults with PTSD generally report decreased cortisol concentrations (see Yehuda, 2002 for review). Children who are both depressed and abused show increased ACTH secretion compared to non-abused depressed and normal children (Kaufman, Birmaher, Perel et al., 1997). This pattern continues into adulthood, with victims of childhood sexual abuse who also suffer from PTSD showing elevated daily levels of norepinephrine, epinephrine and dopamine. Victims without PTSD symptoms do not show elevated levels of these molecules (Lemieux and Coe, 1995). Basal cortisol responses to stressful or traumatic situations in adulthood are lowered in individuals with a history of childhood trauma (Smith, Davidson, Ritchie et al., 1989; Stein, Yehuda, Koverola and Hanna, 1997; Yehuda, Resnick, Schmeidler et al., 1998). These individuals hypersecrete central CRH on a daily basis; there are increased CRH peptide and neurotransmitter levels on a constant basis.

The timing of the trauma experience is an important factor in subsequent development of substance abuse. Abuse prior to age thirteen is a critical factor (Pedersen and Skrondal, 1996; Spak et al., 1998). Abuse prior to age thirteen, but not a lifetime history of abuse, is related to higher measures of anxiety and alcohol abuse in adulthood (Spak et al., 1998). Alcohol consumption during middle-teen years is found in childhood sex victims, and a significant rise in alcohol-related problems appears by the end of the teen years (Pedersen and Skrondal, 1996). Sexual abuse after the age of thirteen is related to promiscuous behavior, but not necessarily to alcohol abuse (Pedersen and Skrondal, 1996). There may be two separate groups of female alcoholics; one with a family history of alcoholism and one with sexual abuse histories, and these two contributions to alcoholism in women do not interact (Yama et al., 1992).

Parent–child attachment and the stability of that attachment throughout childhood has a mediating effect on the future development of substance use problems (Brook, Cohen and Jaeger, 1998; Brook, Nomura and Cohen, 1989; Brook, Whiteman, Finch and Cohen, 1998). Not all adolescent girls who have a family history of alcoholism and are exposed to high levels of stress are predestined to have substance use problems. The ability to use positive coping strategies is a buffer between stress and substance use in older adolescent girls (Johnson and Pandina, 1993).

The effects of childhood trauma on subsequent substance use may be more obvious in women because of the weaker link between family history and drug use in this population. Sexual abuse in women is associated with increased depression, anxiety, suicide attempts, and PTSD (Gil-Rivas, Fiorentine, Anglin and Taylor, 1997). Trauma in childhood might be related to adolescent and adult drug use in men, but there is little information available in the literature. Childhood sexual abuse is rarer among men (Gil-Rivas, Fiorentine and Anglin, 1996), but physical abuse and other forms of victimization do happen to male children, and may be related to adolescent drug use (Clark et al., 1997). An increased number of substance dependence disorders were associated with childhood trauma experiences in male war veterans (Triffleman, Marmar, Delucchi and Ronfeldt, 1995). Childhood sexual abuse in boys is linked to anxiety in adulthood, while childhood physical abuse is associated with depression, anxiety, suicidal ideation, and PTSD in men (Gil-Rivas et al., 1997).

Loss of a loved one or close friend during childhood is related to future substance use. The nature of the loss and the nature of the relationship may affect the future outcome. A twin study found that loss of a parent through separation, but not through death, is related to future alcohol use (Kendler, Neale, Prescott et al., 1996). Adolescents in substance abuse treatment programs often report death of a close friend in their histories (Clark et al., 1997). Interestingly, geographical relocation during childhood has been associated with substance use. This may be a form of loss: leaving childhood friends and being forced to make new friends, or be friendless, is stressful. Moves prior to age sixteen are related to adolescent use of marijuana, hallucinogens, cocaine, crack, and prescribed drugs (DeWitt, 1998).

Anxiety and substance use

There is some speculation about the role of anxiety disorders in the development of substance use disorders. Adult measures of anxiety and anxiety disorders are related to childhood trauma (Gil-Rivas et al., 1997; Stein et al., 1996). Both male and female patients with anxiety disorders have a higher incidence of physical and sexual abuse in childhood. Sixty percent of women with panic disorder reported a history of childhood sexual abuse (Stein et al., 1996). It is possible that the anxiety associated with these childhood experiences is a risk factor in adult substance use. For example, cigarette smoking in women is strongly associated with adverse childhood experiences, and stress-reduction is one frequently-cited reason teenaged girls give for smoking (Anda et al., 1999; Nichter, Nichter, Vuckovic et al., 1997). As early as the fourth grade, smoking and the intent to smoke is associated with stress (Coogan, Adams, Geller et al., 1998).

A high correlation between certain types of anxiety disorders and substance abuse exists. Panic disorder with or without agoraphobia, social phobia, and specific phobias usually precede substance abuse in patients with co-occurring anxiety disorders and substance use disorders, while generalized anxiety disorder usually emerges following the initiation of substance use (Kushner, Sher and Beitman, 1990).

Children with anxiety disorders can have higher salivary cortisol levels (McBurnett et al., 1991). One mediating factor between childhood stress and later drug dependence is the presence of social phobia (DeWit, MacDonald and Offord, 1999). Social phobia is characteristic of extremely shy children and adults, although social phobia is certainly not limited to shy temperaments. The mediation of childhood stress by social phobia may reflect a temperamental variable that affects substance use.

Mediation by environmental factors

Family history of alcoholism, childhood trauma, and mediating early environmental experiences (unrelated to trauma) interact with one another to strengthen or weaken vulnerability to substance use. Family conflict and dysfunction are forms of environmental stress related to adolescent alcohol and substance abuse (Barnes and Windle, 1987; Clark et al., 1997; McKay, Murphy, Rivinus and Maisto, 1991). Environmental stress is a moderator in people with a family history of alcoholism (Turnbull, 1994), but the presence of paternal alcoholism is a much more predictive variable among this population (Chassin, Rogosch and Barrera, 1991). According to one study, socioeconomic stress and family history of alcoholism have independent effects on future substance use behavior, and both variables impact males and females equally (Hill, Ross, Mudd and Blow, 1997).

Environmental factors can mediate future substance use in cases of early childhood trauma. Growing up in a supportive environment can protect against the effects of trauma and other forms of environmental stress, just as family dysfunction and emotional unavailability can contribute to adolescent substance use. This is shown in cases of parental separation (Kendler et al., 1996) and in cases of child sexual abuse (Flemming et al., 1998). Children with parents who spend more time and communicate more frequently with them have lower onset rates of tobacco and alcohol use. Monitoring by parents, and positive relationships between parents and their children protect against risk factors for tobacco and alcohol use (Cohen, Richardson and LaBree, 1994).

A model of genetic vulnerability to early life stressors proposed by Chrousos (1997) predicts outcomes of prenatal and early life stress (see Fig. 6). On a continuum of genetic resiliency and genetic vulnerability, vulnerable children require very little stress to develop long-lasting externalizing and internalizing disorders. Externalizing disorders include oppositional-defiant disorder, conduct disorder, and substance use disorders, while internalizing disorders include anxiety disorders and mood disorders. Outcomes for children with a genetic vulnerability include anxiety disorders, depression, alcoholism and substance abuse, eating disorders, personality and conduct disorders, and psychosomatic diseases. Chrousos (1997) envisions a continuum of genetic predisposition to stressful events, with the children most vulnerable on one end and those most resilient on the other end of this continuum. Those children on the extreme vulnerability end of the continuum require very little prenatal or early life stress to develop any one of the comorbid states. Other children are much more resilient to prenatal and early life

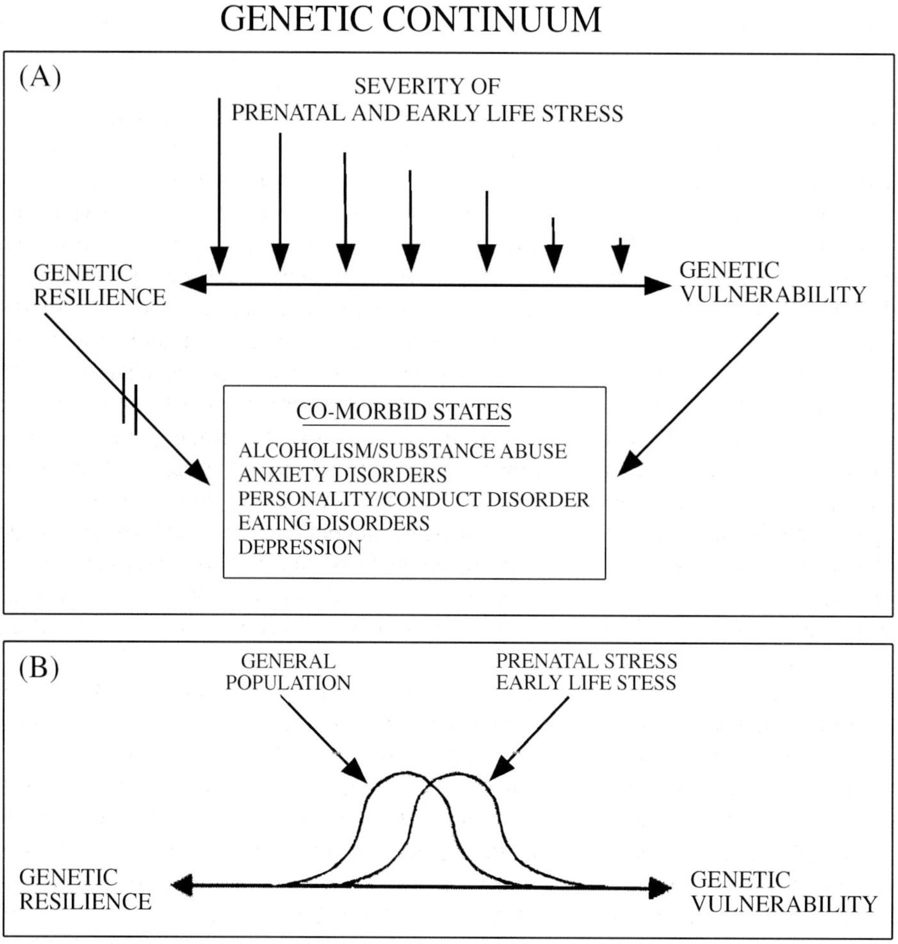

Fig. 6. Genetic continuum that defines resiliency and vulnerability to early life stress. (A) The genetic continuum of genetic resilience and vulnerability to prenatal and early life stress. Those who are genetically more resilient require more severe stress early in life to develop behavioral or psychiatric disorders, while those who are less resilient require less stress to develop the same disorders. (B) The normal population continuum of vulnerability and a superimposed population of those who are affected by prenatal or early life stressors. (Adapted from Chrousos, 1997.)

stress (Chrousos, 1997). Those children far to the resilience end of the continuum require a large amount of stress early in life to develop the associated psychological conditions.

Any combination of factors, including genetic predisposition, early life trauma, stressful childhood environment, and temperament, can play a role in the individual backgrounds of substance users. Regardless of the initial reasons for engaging in substance use, the person becomes caught in the cycle of addiction. Awareness of the initial causes may help in the treatment process, but the addiction itself must be treated as a separate entity.

Neuropsychological performance and substance use

Few predictive neuropsychological markers of future drug use are known. The exceptions are children with disruptive behavior disorders who engage in novelty-seeking behaviors. These children are characterized by low levels of self-regulation (Wills et al., 1998) and some impairment on sustained attention tasks (Kruesi, Schmidt, Donnelly et al., 1989). A second group of at-risk children who have a defined neuropsychological profile are children of alcoholics. There is overlap between these two groups of at-risk children. Children of alcoholics tend to have deficits characterized by impulsivity, aggressiveness, reward-seeking behavior, and, in some cases, conduct disorders (Wiers, Sergeant and Gunning, 1994). Also, adolescent substance abusers with conduct disorder symptoms that occur independently of drug use have a poorer clinical outcome following drug treatment (Brown, Gleghorn, Schuckit et al., 1996).

Substance abuse has direct effects on visuoperceptual, memory and executive function performance (Beatty, Katzung, Moreland and Nixon, 1995; Berry, Van Gorp, Herzberg et al., 1993; Van Gorp, Wilkins, Hinkin et al., 1999). Alcoholics and polysubstance abusers tend to perform more poorly than cocaine abusers in these areas (Selby and Azrin, 1998). Some addicting substances can have long-lasting cognitive and neuropsychological effects. However, the performance deficits manifested in long-term substance abusers under 40 years of age on cognitive measures usually improve with abstinence (Mann, Gunther, Stetter and Ackermann, 1999; Mearns and Lees-Haley, 1993; Rourke and Grant, 1999). The findings may not be relevant to the relatively short-term use found in most adolescents.

Adolescents who use substances like cannabis have difficulties with short term verbal and nonverbal memory (Schwartz, Gruenewald, Klitzner and Fedio, 1989; Williams and Haut, 1995). Some report the deficits caused by cannabis use are short-term, with no lasting effects (Fant, Heishman, Bunker and Pickworth, 1998; Heishman, Huestis, Henningfield and Cone, 1990; Wert and Raulin, 1986), but at least one study reported cognitive deficits in adolescents after six weeks of abstinence (Schwartz et al., 1989). Adolescent alcoholics have lower verbal IQs and academic achievement than nonalcoholic adolescents, but do not show the memory and executive function deficits usually reported in adult alcoholics (Moss, Kirisci, Gordon and Tarter, 1994). Findings of mild cognitive deficits in adolescent substance users may reflect interference with cognitive development instead of the general cognitive decline found in older substance users (Bernal, Ardila and Bateman, 1994). Another possible explanation is that cognitive deficits in adolescence as a result of substance use may be delayed and manifest only after continued persistent use (Scheier and Botvin, 1995). However, one recent report suggests that deficits in attention and executive functioning during adolescence may be predictive of future substance use (Tapert, Baratta, Abrantes and Brown, 2002).

A possible moderator of the relationship between drug or alcohol use and neuropsychological performance is the experience of withdrawal. Experience with drug or alcohol withdrawal may be a predictor of neuropsychological deficits in early-onset substance abuse (Tapert and Brown, 1999). Elevated glucocorticoid and CRH levels characterize withdrawal from drugs of abuse. Drugs that produce a pattern of elevated glucocorticoids and CRH in the paraventricular nucleus of the hypothalamus and the central nucleus of the amygdala during withdrawal conditions include ethanol (Adinoff, Anton, Linnoila et al., 1996; Pich, Lorang, Yeganeth et al., 1995), cocaine (Richter and Weiss, 1999; Sarnyai et al., 1998), morphine (Fig. 7), cannabis (Rodriguez de Fonseca, Carrera, Navarro et al., 1997), and even nicotine (Rasmussen, 1998). Deficits in the areas of visuospatial abilities were associated with a history

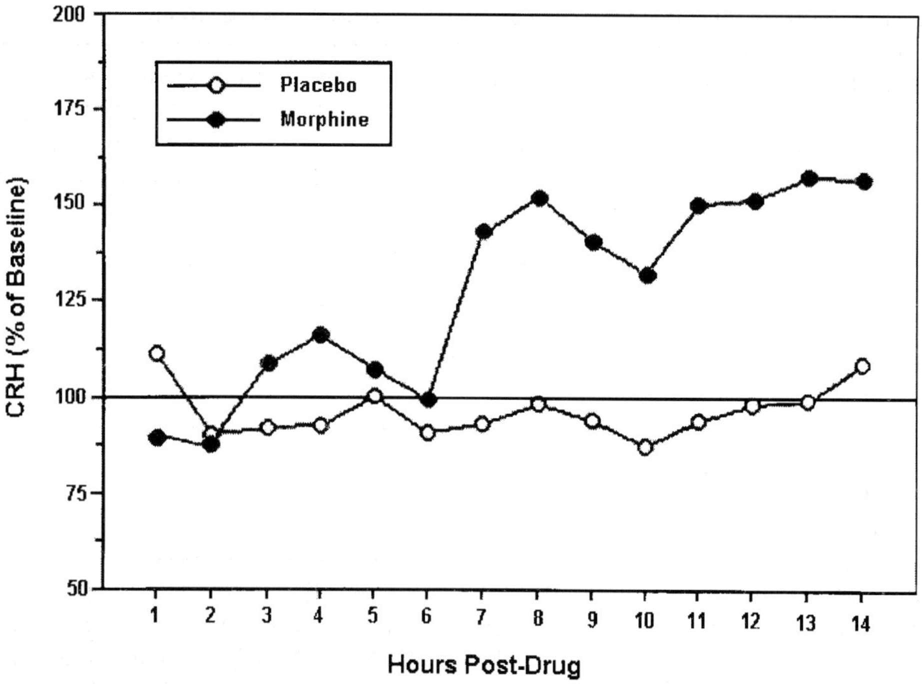

Fig. 7. Morphine withdrawal. Effect of morphine withdrawal on CRH release in the rat amygdala measured through dialysis. CRH concentrations were transformed into percentagof baseline values during pre-withdrawal period. Animals treated with morphine had an extreme rise in CRH values during hour seven post-withdrawal. (Unpublished data, Richter, Weiss, Shulkin et al.)

of withdrawal from drugs or alcohol in adolescents (Brown, Tapert, Granholm and Delis, 2000; Tapert and Brown, 1999). Additionally, a history of alcohol withdrawal in adolescents was associated with deficits in verbal and nonverbal retrieval (Brown et al., 2000). Physiologically, CSF concentrations of CRH are elevated during the first day of abstinence from alcohol, and levels decrease over the next three weeks in humans (Adinoff et al., 1996). These effects may be due to the interaction of glucocorticoids and dopamine during use of or withdrawal from addictive substances.

Allostatic overload

The lifestyle of drug abuse, with its illegal, viral, and other health-related consequences, is a run-down state. Addicts spend most of their time thinking of how to procure the next fix. The actual time of pleasure decreases as the addiction takes hold. It requires more of a drug to produce the desired effect, the effect may not last long, and the dominance of the obsession takes hold of the individual.

Physiological systems can be described as homeostatic or allostatic. Homeostasis refers to stability through holding parameters constant. Negative feedback mechanisms exist throughout the brain and body in which a change in a system's state triggers an automatic response, bringing the system back to a basal level of functioning. Allostasis refers to the principle of 'stability through change'; there is no consistent 'set point' (Sterling and Eyer, 1981). The organism responds to the demands of the external environment by changing its internal 'set points'. This is evident in blood pressure changes during the course of an individual day; blood pressure rises in response to stressful, arousing situations that are psychologically experienced as pain, fear or rage.

When an animal is in a state of relaxation, the body is able to repair damaged tissue and rebuild energy stores. However, when an organism is in a state of psychological arousal, the body begins breaking down metabolic compounds to produce energy. States of arousal are associated with a number of physiological responses including increased blood pressure, increased breakdown of carbohydrate, fat, and protein, and decreased production of immune system cells. There are increased levels of a number of hormones, including cortisol, vasopressin, angiotensin, and endogenous opiates.

An advantage of allostatic mechanisms is an increased efficiency in dealing, physiologically, with changing environmental demands (Schulkin et al., 1998). Moving from a state of complete relaxation to a state of complete alertness is difficult for a homeostatic system because of the great leap in energy demand. When an animal exists in an environment that frequently requires arousal states, allostatic mechanisms allow the body to physiologically change the basal 'set points' of various systems to meet the arousal requirements. This allows the organism to maintain a constant state of alertness. However, there is a price to pay for this allostatic adjustment: increased energy demands upon the body compromise other important functions, such as the immune system.

Allostatic overload is relevant in terms of traumatic childhood experiences. When allostatic load is introduced during childhood, i.e., long-standing socioeconomic stress or traumatic experiences, the way in which physiological systems respond later in life can be affected. Multiple novel stressors, which can manifest through unpredictable environmental situations, is one type of allostatic load. Fig. 8 illustrates some hypothetical examples of normal and abnormal physiological response to stress. In terms of cortisol activity and allostatic overload, the inadequate response to stress is directly applicable. Normal adaptation can result in abnormal responses to traumatic events later in life. For example, women who experience childhood sexual abuse have blunted physiological responses to subsequent rape experiences (Smith et al., 1989; Stein et al., 1997; Yehuda et al., 1998).

Maintaining an addiction is like maintaining glucose levels or calcium levels. There is a homeostatic element involved. The homeostatic nature of addiction is a popular concept (Koob, 1999). The body requires the drug in order to maintain equilibrium and to avoid getting sick. The negatively reinforcing effects of drugs take hold. Central motive states are elicited, and both approach and consummatory behaviors are expressed.

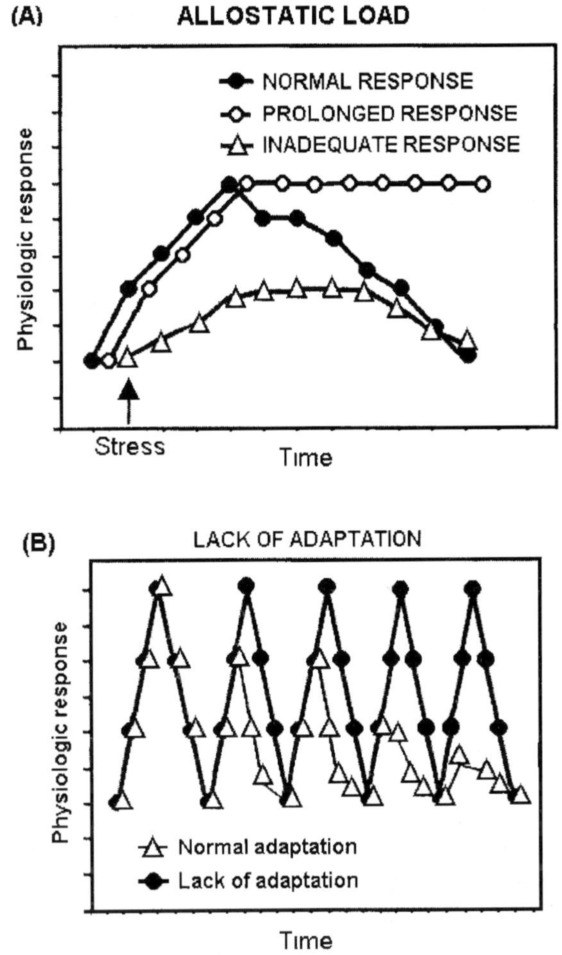

Fig. 8. Allostatic overload. (A) illustrates three possible responses to stress. In the normal response, the body reacts to a stressor and them compensates after a period of time, bringing levels back to baseline. During a prolonged response, the body reacts to the stressor but is unable to bring levels back to baseline. An inadequate response is when the body does not react sufficiently to an environmental stressor. (B) illustrates normal adaptation to a repeated stressor, and lack of adaptation to a repeated stressor. (Adapted from McEwen, 1998.)

One hypothesis is that allostasis is more descriptive of the addicted state (Koob and Le Moal, 2001). As psychological and physical tolerance develops, the consummatory phase is less and less satisfying. When an individual becomes drug-dependent, there are changes in the internal drug set points; there is an allostatic reaction to the constant presence of a drug such as cocaine, heroin, or alcohol. In rats, a limited period of daily access to a drug leads to maintaining the same levels of intake from one session to the next. An increased period of daily access (six hours) leads to increased self-administration of the drug (Ahmed and Koob, 1998). A higher level of intake is required to gain the same hedonic effect of the drug (Koob, 1999).

More of the drug is used more frequently, and physical health deteriorates in the addict because of extended wear and tear upon the physical body. Deterioration of health, associated with drug abuse, is evident even in adolescence and young adulthood (Aarons, Brown, Coe et al., 1999). At one level the event is homeostatic (Cannon, 1929) and the behavior serves the physiology (Richter and Weiss, 1999). At another level, the behavior is allostatic, a term that includes, in part, anticipatory responses and not just reactive responses (see also Sterling and Eyer, 1981).

At least two allostatic responses function within the addicted person. One is the change in drug set point: more drug is required to maintain an internal equilibrium. Animal models reflect this allostatic change in drug hedonic set point (Ahmed and Koob, 1998). The second response is in response to stress: The addict's life, characterized by chronic worry, is replete with anticipatory angst, and both glucocorticoids and central CRH should be elevated (Schulkin et al., 1998).

Allostatic overload is the chronic over-arousal of basic physiological and psychological mechanisms in which there is no clear set point of equilibrium. Allostatic overload refers to the wear and tear on the body in response to constant over-arousal (McEwen, 1998; McEwen and Stellar, 1993; Schulkin, 2003). Chronic allostatic overload exists when both glucocorticoids and central CRH are elevated; the body is unable to reduce the levels. There is a breakdown of normal inhibitory response. Maintaining high levels of glucocorticoids for long periods of time, which is the normal state of the addict, has many consequences. The breakdown of tissue, along with the associated addicted lifestyles, leads to increased risk of many diseases, including HIV and hepatitis. Compromised immune function, bone deterioration, and impaired memory functions (McEwen, 1998) are a few of the results of maintaining high-energy arousal states over a long period. For example, high levels of glucocorticoids facilitate hippocampal deterioration (McEwen and Magarinos, 1997). Increase in depression or anxiety are psychological consequences of maintaining increased glucocorticoids and central CRH. Early-onset adolescent drug use is associated with more severe health problems in girls and boys (Aarons et al., 1999).

Social and psychological responsibility and future research

The neurobiology of learning and memory in addiction, addressed through animal experimentation and neuroimaging research, is giving clues into brain areas associated with the motivational and emotional experiences of drug craving in humans (Everitt, 1999). We are learning more about the neurotransmitters that influence addiction in this age of molecular biology. The molecular substrates underlying craving, reinforcement, and withdrawal are being laid open. However, these discoveries must be couched in terms of the social milieu in which addicts function. Methadone blocks both reward and withdrawal from opiates, but that is only part of the solution. Corticotropin releasing hormone and serotonin are other examples of the ambiguity involved in defining correlations among neurobiological substrates. Low serotonin levels and impulsivity do not cause substance abuse; serotonin agonists will not solve drug abuse problems. Similarly, cortisol levels and stress do not cause substance abuse; CRH blockers also will not solve the substance abuse problems. The human connectedness factor must be addressed (Jaspers, 1913, 1997).

Temperament may play a role in some aspects of vulnerability. Individuals who are impulsive and show the aggressive characteristics of conduct disorder as children are more likely to become addicted in adolescence and adulthood. However, this type of individual engages in an array of risk-taking behaviors, and drug experimentation is only one aspect of the behavior. Do lower serotonin levels mean that these individuals respond differently to drugs? Perhaps, but this group is only a subset of those suffering from drug addiction.

Early life trauma and blunted cortisol response are associated with later substance use. However, these samples are necessarily taken from clinical populations. Patients in treatment for anxiety disorders and substance use disorders might only be a portion of those who suffered early life trauma. Do relatively large proportions of people who suffer early traumas maintain relatively normal lives, socially and biochemically?

Perhaps consistent, positive human touch and contact can mediate the long-term effects of trauma, and perhaps the pathways influenced are directly related to CRH activity (Liu, Diorio, Tannenbaum et al., 1997). Successful drug rehabilitation programs often employ social contact as a vehicle towards mental health (Ouimette, Ahrens, Moos and Finney, 1998). The idea of 'reaching out' to others in order to maintain abstinence is certainly not new. The effectiveness of this approach might be related to the reduced stress levels and, consequently, reduced CRH levels within the recovering individual. Perhaps those who do not relapse into drug use are those who maintain the social contacts, while those who experience relapse are those who refuse social support and are too impulsive to stay on the course of recovery.

References

Aarons GA, Brown SA, Coe MT, Myers MG, Garland AF, Ezzet-Lofstram R, Hazen AL, Hough RL: Adolescent alcohol and drug abuse and health. Journal of Adolescent Health: 24(6); 412–421, 1999.

Adinoff B, Anton R, Linnoila M, Guidotti A, Nemeroff CB, Bissette G: Cerebrospinal fluid concentrations of corticotropin-releasing hormone (CRH) and diazepam-binding inhibitor (DBI) during alcohol withdrawal and abstinence. Neuropsychopharmacology: 15(3); 288–295, 1996.

Adolphs R, Tranel D, Hamann S, Young AW, Calder AJ, Phelps EA, Anderson A, Lee GP, Damasio AR: Recognition of facial emotion in nine individuals with bilateral amygdala damage. Neuropsychologia: 37; 1111–1117, 1999.

Ahmed SH, Koob GF: Transition from moderate to excessive drug intake: change in hedonic set point. Science: 282(5387); 298–300, 1998.

Alheid GG, deOlmos J, Beltramino CA: Amygdala and extended amygdala. In Paxinos G (Ed), The Rat Nervous System, 2nd ed. Academic Press: San Diego, 1996.

Altman J, Everitt BJ, Glautier S, Markou A, Nutt D, Oretti R, Phillips GD, Robbins TW: The biological, social and clinical bases of drug addiction: commentary and debate. Psychopharmacology: 125(4); 285–345, 1996.

Anda RF, Croft JB, Felitti VJ, Nordenberg D, Giles WH, Williamson DF, Grovino GA: Adverse childhood experiences and smoking during adolescence and adulthood. Journal of the American Medical Association: 282(17); 1652–1658, 1999.

Barnes GM, Windle M: Family factors in adolescent alcohol and drug abuse. Pediatrician: 14(1–2); 13–18, 1987.

Beatty WW, Katzung VM, Moreland VJ, Nixon SJ: Neuropsychological performance of recently abstinent alcoholics and cocaine abusers. Drug and Alcohol Dependence: 37(3); 247–253, 1995.

Bernal B, Ardila A, Bateman JR: Cognitive impairments in adolescent drug-abusers. International Journal of Neuroscience: 75(3–4); 203–212, 1994.

Berridge KC: Food reward: brain substrates of wanting and liking. Neuroscience and Biobehavioral Reviews: 20(1); 1–25, 1996.

Berridge KC, Robinson TE: What is the role of dopamine in reward: hedonic impact, reward learning, or incentive salience? Brain Research: Brain Research Reviews: 28(3); 309–369, 1998.

Berry J, Van Gorp WG, Herzberg DS, Hinkin C, Boone K, Steinman L, Wilkins JN: Neuropsychological deficits in abstinent cocaine abusers: preliminary findings after two weeks of abstinence. Drug and Alcohol Dependence: 32(3); 231–237, 1993.

Blair RJ, Morris JS, Frith CD, Perrett DI, Dolan RJ: Dissociable neural responses to facial expressions of sadness and anger. Brain: 122(Pt 5); 883–893, 1999.

Bonne O, Brandes D, Gilboa A, Gomori JM, Shenton ME, Pitman RK, Shalev AY: Longitudinal MRI study of hippocampal volume in trauma survivors with PTSD. American Journal Of Psychiatry: 158(8); 1248–1251, 2001.

Brake WG, Noel MB, Boksa P, Gratton A: Influence of perinatal factors on the nucleus accumbens dopamine response to repeated stress during adulthood: an electrochemical study in the rat. Neuroscience: 77(4); 1067–1076, 1997.

Brauer LH, De Wit H: High dose pimozide does not block amphetamine-induced euphoria in normal volunteers. Pharmacology, Biochemistry, and Behavior: 56(2); 265–72, 1997.

Breiter HC, Etcoff NL, Whalen PJ, Kennedy WA, Rauch SL, Buckner RL, Strauss MM, Hyman SE, Rosen BR: Response and habituation of the human amygdala during visual processing of facial expression. Neuron: 17(5); 875–887, 1996.

Breiter HC, Gollub RL, Weisskoff RM, Kennedy DN, Makris N, Berke JD, Goodman JM, Kantor HL, Gastfriend DR, Riorden JP, Mathew, RT, Rosen BR, Hyman SE: Acute effects of cocaine on human brain activity and emotion. Neuron: 19(3); 591–611, 1997.

Bremner JD, Randall P, Vermetten E, Staib L, Bronen RA, Mazure C, Capelli S, McCarthy G, Innis RB, Charney DS: Magnetic resonance imaging-based measurement of hippocampal volume in posttraumatic stress disorder related to childhood physical and sexual abuse - a preliminary report. Biological Psychiatry: 41(1); 23–32, 1997.

Brook JS, Cohen P, Jaeger L: Developmental variations in factors related to initial and increased levels of drug involvement. Journal of Genetic Psychology: 159(2); 179–194, 1998.

Brook JS, Nomura C, Cohen P: Prenatal, perinatal, and early childhood risk factors and drug involvement in adolescence. Genetic, Social, and General Psychology Monographs: 115(2); 221–241, 1989.

Brook JS, Whiteman M, Finch S, Cohen P: Mutual attachment, personality, and drug use: pathways from childhood to young adulthood. Genetic, Social, and General Psychology Monographs: 124(4); 492–510, 1998.

Brown SA, Gleghorn A, Schuckit MA, Myers MG, Mott MA: Conduct disorder among adolescent alcohol and drug abusers. Journal of Studies on Alcoholism: 57(3); 314–324, 1996.

Brown SA, Tapert SF, Granholm E, Delis DC: Neurocognitive functioning of adolescents: effects of protracted alsohol use. Alcoholism, Clinical and Experimental Research: 24(2); 164–171, 2000.

Byne W, Kemether E, Jones L, Haroutunian V, Davis KL: The neurochemistry of schizophrenia. In Charney DS, Nestler EJ, Bunney BS (Eds), Neurobiology of Mental Illness. New York: Oxford University Press, 1999.

Caine SB, Heinrich SC, Coffin VL, Koob GF: Effects of the dopamine D-1 antagonist SCH 23390 microinjected into the accumbens, amygdala or striatum on cocaine self-administration in the rat. Brain Research: 692(1–2); 47–56, 1995.

Carlezon WA, Wise RA: Rewarding actions of phencyclidine and related drugs in nucleus accumbens shell and frontal cortex. Journal of Neuroscience: 16(9); 3112–3122, 1996.

Chang JY, Sawyer SF, Lee RS, Woodward DJ: Electrophysiological and pharmacological evidence for the role of the nucleus accumbens in cocaine self-administration in freely moving rats. Journal of Neuroscience: 14(3 Pt. 1); 1224–1244, 1994.

Chassin L, Rogosch F, Barrera M: Substance use and symptomatology among adolescent children of alcoholics. Journal of Abnormal Psychology: 100(4); 449–463, 1991.

Chrousos GP: The future of pediatric and adolescent endocrinology. Annals of the New York Academy of Science, June 17: 816; 4–8, 1997.

Clark DB, Lesnick L, Hegedus AM: Traumas and other adverse life events in adolescents with alcohol abuse and dependence. Journal of the American Academy of Child and Adolescent Psychiatry: 36(12); 1744–1751, 1997.

Clarke AS: Social rearing effects on HPA axis activity over early development and in response to stress in rhesus monkeys. Developmental Psychobiology: 26(8); 433–446, 1993.

Cloninger CR: Neurogenetic adaptive mechanisms in alcoholism. Science: 236(4800); 410–416, 1987.

Cohen DA, Richardson J, LaBree L: Parenting behaviors and the onset of smoking and alcohol use: a longitudinal study. Pediatrics: 94(3); 368–375, 1994.

Coogan PF, Adams M, Geller AC, Brooks D, Miller DR, Lao RA, Koh HK: Factors associated with smoking among children and adolescents in Connecticut. American Journal of Preventative Medicine: 15(1); 17–24, 1998.

Coplan JD, Trost RC, Owens MJ, Cooper TB, Gorman JM, Nemeroff CB, Rosenblum LA: Cerebrospinal fluid concentrations of somatostatin and biogenic amines in grown primates reared by mothers exposed to manipulated foraging conditions. Archives of Genral Psychiatry: 55(5); 473–477, 1998.

Cratty MS, Ward HE, Johnson EA, Azzaro AJ, Birkle DL: Prenatal stress increases corticotropin-releasing factor (CRF) content and release in rat amygdala minces. Brain Research: 675(1–2); 297–302, 1995.

Cuadra G, Zurita A, Lacerra C, Molina V: Chronic stress sensitizes frontal cortex dopamine release in response to a subsequent novel stressor: reversal by naloxone. Brain Research Bulletin: 48(3); 303–308, 1999.

Dao-Castellana MH, Samson Y, Legault F, Martinot JL, Aubin HJ, Crouzel C, Feldman L, Barrucand D, Rancurel G, Feline A, Syrota A: Frontal dysfunction in neurologically normal chronic alcoholic subjects: metabolic and neuropsychological findings. Psychological Medicine: 28(5); 1039–1048, 1998.

Davidson RJ: Anterior electrophysiological asymmetries, emotion, and depression: conceptual and methodological conundrums. Psychophysiology: 35(5); 607–14, 1998.

Davidson RJ, Abercrombie H, Nitschke JB, Putnam K: Regional brain function, emotion and disorders of emotion. Current Opinions in Neurobiology: 9(2); 228–234, 1999.

Davidson RJ, Ekman P, Saron CD, Senulis JA, Friesen WV: Approach-withdrawal and cerebral asymmetry: emotional expression and brain physiology. I. Journal of Personality and Social Psychology: 58(2); 330–341, 1990.

Davidson RJ, Rickman M: Behavioral inhibition and the emotional circuitry of the brain: stability and plasticity during the early childhood years. In Schmidt LA, Schulkin J (Eds), Extreme Fear, Shyness, and Social Phobia. New York: Oxford University Press, 1999.

DeBellis MD, Baum AS, Birmaher B, Keshavan MS, Eccard CH, Boring AM, Jenkins FJ, Ryan ND: A.E. Bennett Research Award. Developmental traumatology. Part I: biological stress systems. Biological Psychiatry: 45(10); 1259–1270, 1999.

DeBellis MD, Keshavan MS, Clark DB, Casey BJ, Giedd JN, Boring AM, Frustaci K, Ryan ND: A.E. Bennett Research Award. Developmental traumatology. Part II: brain development. Biological Psychiatry: 45(10); 1271–1284, 1999.

DeWitt DJ: Frequent childhood geographic relocation: its impact on drug use initiation and the development of alcohol and other drug-related problems among adolescents and young adults. Addictive Behavior: 23(5); 623–34, 1998.

DeWit DJ, MacDonald K, Offord DR: Childhood stress and symptoms of drug dependence in adolescence and early adulthood: social phobia as a mediator. American Journal of Orthopsychiatry: 69(1); 61–72, 1999.

Duncan RD, Saunders BE, Kilpatrick DG, Hanson RF, Resnick HS: Childhood physical assault as a risk factor for PTSD, depression, and substance abuse: findings from a national survey. American Journal of Orthopsychiatry: 66(3); 437–448, 1995.

Ellason JW, Ross CA, Sainton K, Mayran LW: Axis I and II comorbidity and childhood trauma history in chemical dependency. Bulletin of the Menninger Clinic: 60(1); 39–51, 1996.

Epstein JN, Saunders BE, Kilpatrick DG, Resnick HS: PTSD as a mediator between childhood rape and alcohol use in adult women. Child Abuse and Neglect: 22(3); 223–234, 1998.

Erb S, Shaham Y, Stewart J: Stress reinstates cocaine-seeking behavior after prolonged extinction and a drug-free period. Psychopharmacology: 128(4); 408–412, 1996.

European Monitoring Centre for Drugs and Drug Addiction:

Implementation, follow-up, and analysis of cohort studies on mortality among drug users in European Union member States. Lisbon: EMCDDA, 1999.

Everitt B: Craving cocaine cues: cognitive neuroscience meets drug addiction research. Cognitive Sciences: 1; 1–2, 1999.

Fahlke C, Engel JA, Eriksson CJP, Hard E, Soderpalm B: Involvement of corticosterone in the modulation of ethanol consumption in the rat. Alcohol: 11(3); 195–202, 1994.

Fant RV, Heishman SJ, Bunker EB, Pickworth WB: Acute and residual effects of marijuana in humans. Pharmacology, Biochemical, and Behavior: 60(4); 777–784, 1998.

Fergusson DM, Lynskey MT: Adolescent resiliency to family adversity. Journal of Child Psychology and Psychiatry: 37(3); 281–292, 1996.

Flemming J, Mullen PE, Sibthorpe B, Attewell R, Bammer G: The relationship between childhood sexual abuse and alcohol abuse in women: a case-control study. Addiction: 93(12); 1787–1798, 1998.

Fowler JS, Volkow ND, Malison R, Gatley SJ: Neuroimaging studies of substance abuse disorders. In Charney DS, Nestler EJ, Bunney BS (Eds), Neurobiology of Mental Illness. New York: Oxford University Press, 1999.

Friedman AS, Kramer S, Kreisher C, Granick S: The relationships of substance abuse to illegal and violent behavior, in a community sample of young adult African American men and women (gender differences). Journal of Substance Abuse: 8(4); 379–402, 1996.

Gambarana C, Ghiglieri O, Masi F, Scheggi S, Tagliamonte A, De Montis MG: The effects of long-term administration of rubidium or lithium on reactivity to stress and on dopamine output in the nucleus accumbens in rats. Brain Research: 826(2); 200–209, 1999.

Gerra G, Calbiani B, Zaimovic A, Sartori R, Ugolotti G, Ippolito L, Delsignore R, Rustichelli P, Fontanesi B: Regional cerebral blood flow and comorbid diagnosis in abstinent opioid addicts. Psychiatry Research: 83(2); 117–126, 1998.

Gil-Rivas V, Fiorentine R, Anglin MD: Sexual abuse, physical abuse, and posttraumatic stress disorder among women participating in outpatient drug abuse treatment. Journal of Psychoactive Drugs: 28(1); 95–102, 1996.

Gil-Rivas V, Fiorentine R, Anglin MD, Taylor E: Sexual and physical abuse: do they compromise drug treatment outcomes? Journal of Substance Abuse Treatment: 14(1); 351–358, 1997.

Goeders NE: Stress, the hypothalamic-pituitary–adrenal axis, and vulnerability to drug abuse. NIDA Research Monograph: 169; 83–104, 1998.

Grant S, London ED, Newlin DB, Villemagne VL, Liu X, Contoreggi C, Phillips RL, Kimes AS, Margolin A: Activation of memory circuits during cue-elicited cocaine craving. Proceedings of the National Academy of Sciences, USA: 93(21); 12040–12045, 1996.

Gray TS: The organization and possible function of amygdaloid corticotropin-releasing factor pathways. In: DeSousa EB, Nemeroff CB (Eds), Corticotropin-releasing Factor: Basic and Clinic Studies of a Neuropeptide. Boca Raton: CRC Press, 1990.

Habib KE, Weld KP, Schulkin J, Pushkas J, Listwak S, Champoux M, Shannon C, Chrousos GP, Suomi S, Gold PW, Higley JD: Cerebrospinal fluid levels of corticotropin-releasing hormone positively correlate with acute and chronic social stress in non-human primates. Presented at Society for Neuroscience Annual Meeting, Miami Beach, Florida, 1999.

Hall W, Teesson M, Lynskey M, Degenhardt L: The 12-month prevalence of substance use disorders in Australian adults: findings from the National Survey of Mental Health and Well-Being. Addiction: 94(10); 1541–1550, 1999.

Harmon-Jones E, Allen JJ: Anger and frontal brain activity: EEG asymmetry consistent with approach motivation despite negative affective valence. Journal of Personality and Social Psychology: 74(5); 1310–1316, 1998.

Heilman KM: The neurobiology of emotional experience. Journal of Neuropsychiatry and Clinical Neuroscience: 9(3); 439–448, 1997.

Heishman SJ, Huestis MA, Henningfield JE, Cone EJ: Acute and residual effects of marijuana: profiles of plasma THC levels, physiological, subjective, and performance measures. Pharmacology, Biochemistry, and Behavior: 37; 561–565, 1990.

Higley JD, Hasert MF, Suomi SJ, Linnoila M: Nonhuman primate model of alcohol abuse: effects of early experience, personality, and stress on alcohol consumption. Proceedings of the National Academy of Sciences: 88(16); 7261–7265, 1991.

Higley JD, Linnoila M, Suomi SJ: Ethological contributions: experiential and genetic contributions to the expression and inhibition of aggression in primates. In: Hersen M, Ammerman RT, Sisson L (Eds), Handbook of Aggressive and Destructive Behavior in Psychiatric Patients. New York: Plenum Press, 1994.

Higley JD, Suomi SJ, Linnoila M: A longitudinal assessment of CSF monoamine metabolite and plasma cortisol concentrations in young rhesus monkeys. Biological Psychiatry: 32(2); 127–145, 1992.

Higley JD, Suomi SJ, Linnoila M: A nonhuman primate model of Type II excessive alcoholism? Part 1. Low cerebrospinal fluid 5-hydroxyindoleacetic acid concentrations and diminished social competence correlate with excessive alcohol consumption. Alcoholism, Clinical and Experimental Research: 20(4); 629–642, 1996a.

Higley JD, Suomi SJ, Linnoila M: A nonhuman primate model of Type II alcoholism? Part 2. Diminished social competence and excessive aggression correlates with low cerebrospinal fluid 5-hydroxyindoleacetic acid concentrations. Alcoholism, Clinical and Experimental Research: 20(4); 643–650, 1996b.

Hill EM, Ross LT, Mudd SA, Blow FC: Adulthood functioning: the joint effects of parental alcoholism, gender and childhood socio-economic stress. Addiction: 92(5); 583–596, 1997.

Howard MO, Kivlahan D, Walker RD: Cloninger's tridimensional theory of personality and psychopathology: applications to substance use disorders. Journal of Studies on Alcoholism: 58(1); 48–66, 1997.

Hyman SE, Nestler E: The Molecular Foundations of Psychiatry. Washington, DC: American Psychiatric Press, 1993.

Hyman SE, Malenka RC: Addiction and the brain: the neurobiology of compulsion and its persistence. Nature Reviews Neuroscience: 2(10); 695–703.

Irwin W, Davidson RJ, Lowe MJ, Mock BJ, Sorenson JA, Turski PA: Human amygdala activation detected with echo-planar functional magnetic resonance imaging. NeuroReport: 7(11); 1765–1769, 1996.

Jang KL, Livesley WJ, Vernon PA: Gender-specific etiological differences in alcohol and drug problems: a behavioral genetic analysis. Addiction: 92(10); 1265–1276, 1997.

Jaspers K: General Psychopathology. Baltimore: Johns Hopkins University Press, 1913.

Jaspers K: General Psychopathology. Baltimore: Johns Hopkins University Press, 1997.

Johnson DE, Waid LR, Anton RF: Childhood hyperactivity, gender, and Cloninger's personality dimensions in alcoholics. Addictive Behavior: 22(5); 649–653, 1997.

Johnson V, Pandina RJ: A longitudinal examination of the relationships among stress, coping strategies, and problems associated with alcohol use. Alcoholism, Clinical and Experimental Research: 17(3); 696–702, 1993.

Kalin NH: Behavioral effects of ovine corticotropin-releasing factor administered to rhesus monkeys. Federal Proceedings: 44(1 Pt. 2); 249–253, 1985.

Kaufman J, Birmaher B, Perel J, Dahl RE, Moreci P, Nelson B, Wells W, Ryan ND: The corticotropin-releasing hormone challenge in depressed abused, depressed nonabused, and normal control children. Biological Psychiatry: 42(8); 679–699, 1997.

Kelley AE: Functional specificity of ventral striatal compartments in appetitive behaviors. Annals of the New York Academy of Sciences, June 29: 877; 71–90, 1999.

Kendler KS, Heath AC, Neale MC, Kessler RC, Eaves LJ: A population-based twin study of alcoholism in women. Journal of the American Medical Association: 268(14); 1877–1882, 1992.

Kendler KS, Neale MC, Prescott CA, Kessler RC, Heath AC, Corey LA, Eaves LJ: Childhood parental loss and alcoholism in women: a causal analysis using a twin-family design. Psychological Medicine: 26(1); 79–95, 1996.

Ketter TA, Andreason PJ, George MS, Lee C, Gill DS, Parekh PI, Willis MW, Herscovitch P, Post RM: Anterior paralimbic mediation of procaine-induced emotional and psychosensory experiences. Archives of General Psychiatry: 53(1); 59–69, 1996.

Koob GF: The role of the striatopallidal and extended amygdala systems in drug addiction. Annals of the New York Academy of Science, Jun 29: 877; 445–460, 1999.

Koob GF: Neurobiology of addiction. Toward the development of new therapies. Annals of the New York Academy of Sciences: 909; 170–185, 2000.

Koob GF, Le Moal M: Drug addiction, dysregulation of reward, and allostasis. Neuropsychopharmacology: 24(2); 97–129, 2001.

Koob GF et al: The role of corticotropin releasing hormone in behavioral responses to stress. In Chadwick K, Marshj J, Ackrill K (Eds), Corticotropin-Releasing Factor. Wiley: New York, 1993.

Kraemer GW, McKinney WT: Social separation increases alcohol consumption in rhesus monkeys. Psychopharmacology (Berl): 86(1–2); 182–189, 1985.

Kruesi MJ, Schmidt ME, Donnelly M, Hibbs ED, Hamburger SD: Urinary free cortisol output and disruptive behavior in children. Journal of the American Academy of Child and Adolescent Psychiatry: 28(3); 441–443, 1989.

Kushner MG, Sher KJ, Beitman BD: The relation between alcohol problems and the anxiety disorders. American Journal of Psychiatry: 147(6); 685–695, 1990.

Lang PJ, Bradley MM, Cuthbert BN: Emotion, motivation, and anxiety: brain mechanisms and psychophysiology. Biological Psychiatry: 44(12); 1248–1263, 1998.

Lashley KS: An experimental analysis of instinctive behavior. Psychological Review: 45; 445–471, 1938.

LeDoux JE, Cicchetti P, Xagoraris A, Romanski LM: The lareral amygdaloid nucleus: sensory interface of the amygdala in fear conditioning. Journal of Neuroscience: 10(4); 1062–1069, 1990.

Lemieux AM, Coe CL: Abuse-related posttraumatic stress disorder: evidence for chronic neuroendocrine activation in women. Psychosomatic Medicine: 57(2); 105–115, 1995.

Liu D, Diorio J, Tannenbaum B, Caldji C, Francis D, Freedman A, Sharma S, Pearson D, Plotsky PM, Meaney MJ: Maternal care, hippocampal glucocorticoid receptors, and hypothalamic–pituitary–adrenal responses to stress. Science: 277(5332); 1659–1662, 1997.

Maas LC, Lukas SE, Kaufman MJ, Weiss RD, Daniels SL, Rogers VW, Kukes TJ, Renshaw PF: Functional magnetic resonance imaging of human brain activation during cue-induced cocaine craving. American Journal of Psychiatry: 155(1); 124–126, 1998.

Magarinos AM, McEwen BS, Flugge G, Fuchs E: Chronic psychosocial stress causes apical dendritic atrophy of hippocampal CA3 pyramidal neurons in subordinate tree shrews. Journal of Neuroscience: 16(10); 3534–3540, 1996.

Makino S, Gold PW, Schulkin J: Corticosterone effects on corticotropin-releasing hormone mRNA in the central nucleus of the amygdala and the parvocellular region of the paraventricular nucleus of the hypothalamus. Brain Research: 640(1–2); 105–112, 1994a.

Makino S, Gold PW, Schulkin J: Effects of corticosterone on CRH mRNA and content in the bed nucleus of the stria terminalis; comparison with the effects in the central nucleus of the amygdala and the paraventricular nucleus of the hypothalamus. Brain Research: 657(1–2); 141–149, 1994b.

Mann K, Gunther A, Stetter F, Ackermann K: Rapid recovery from cognitive deficits in abstinent alcoholics: a controlled test-retest study. Alcohol and Alcoholism: 34(4); 567–574, 1999.

Masse LC, Tremblay RE: Behavior of boys in kindergarten and the onset of substance use during adolescence. Archives of General Psychiatry: 54(1); 62–68, 1997.

Matta SG, Valentine JD, Sharp BM: Nicotinic activation of CRH neurons in extrahypothalamic regions of the rat brain. Endocrine: 7(2); 245–253, 1997.

McBurnett K, Lahey BB, Frick PJ, Risch C, Loeber R, Hart EL, Christ MA, Hanson KS: Anxiety, inhibition, and conduct disorder in children: II. Relation to salivary cortisol. Journal of the American Academy of Child and Adolescent Psychiatry: 30(2); 192–196, 1991.

McBurnett K, Lahey BB, Rathouy PJ, Loeber R: Low salivary cortisol and persistent aggression in boys referred for disruptive behavior. Archives of General Psychiatry: 57(1); 38–43, 2000.

McEwen BS: Protective and damaging effects of stress mediators. New England Journal of Medicine: 338(3); 171–179, 1998.

McEwen BS, Magarinos AM: Stress effects on morphology and function of the hippocampus. Annals of the New York Academy of Science, June 21: 821; 271–284, 1997.

McEwen BS, Stellar E: Stress and the individual: mechanisms leading to disease. Archives of Internal Medicine: 153(18); 2093–3101, 1993.

McGinnis JM, Foege WH: Mortality and morbidity attributable to use of addictive substances in the United States. Proceedings of the Association of American Physicians: 111(2); 109–118, 1999.

McKay JR, Murphy RT, Rivinus TR, Maisto SA: Family dysfunction and alcohol and drug use in adolescent psychiatric inpatients. Journal of the American Academy of Child and Adolescent Psychiatry: 30(6); 967–972, 1991.

McMahon RJ. Diagnosis, assessment, and treatment of externalizing problems in children: the role of longitudinal data. Journal of Consulting and Clinical Psychology: 62(5); 901–917, 1994.

Medina-Mora ME, Tapia CR, Rascon ML, Solache G, Otero BR, Lazcano F, Marino MC: Epidemiologic status of drug abuse in Mexico. Bulletin of the Pan American Health Organization: 24(1); 1–11, 1990.

Mearns J, Lees-Haley PR: Discriminating neuropsychological sequelae of head injury from alcohol-abuse-induced deficits: a review and analysis. Journal of Clinical Psychology: 49(5); 714–720, 1993.

Medina-Mora ME, Tapia CR, Rascon ML, Solache G, Otero BR, Lazcano F, Marino MC: Epidemiologic status of drug abuse in Mexico. Bull Pan Am Health Organ: 24(1); 1–11, 1990.

Mehlman P, Higley JD, Faucher I, Lilly AA, Taub DM, Vickers J, Suomi SF, Linnoila M: Low CSF 5-HIAA concentrations and severe aggression and impaired impulse control in nonhuman primates. American Journal of Psychiatry: 151(10); 1485–1491, 1994.

Merikanjas KR: The genetic epidemiology of alcoholism. Psychological Medicine: 20(1); 11–22, 1990.

Merikanjas KR, Rounsaville BJ, Prusoff BA: Familial factors in vulnerability to substance abuse. In Glantz M, Pickens R (Eds), Vulnerability to Drug Abuse. Washington, DC: American Psychiatric Association Press, 1992.

Miller BA, Downs WR, Gondoli DM, Keil A: The role of childhood sexual abuse in the development of alcoholism in women. Violence and Victims: 2(3); 157–172, 1987.

Miller-Johnson S, Lochman JE, Coie JD, Terry R, Hyman C: Comorbidity of conduct and depressive problems at sixth grade: substance use outcomes across adolescence. Journal of Abnormal Child Psychology: 26(3); 221–232, 1998.

Mogenson GJ: Limbic-motor integration. In Epstein AN, Sprague J (Eds), Progress in Psychobiology and Physiological Psychology. New York: Academic Press, 1987.

Mogenson GJ, Jones DL, Yim CY: From motivation to action: functional interface between the limbic system and the motor system. Progress in Neurobiology: 14(2–3); 69–97, 1980.

Merali Z, McIntosh J, Kent P, Michaud D, Anisman H: Aversive and appetitive events evoke the release of corticotropin-releasing hormone and bombesin-like peptides at the central nucleus of the amygdala. Journal of Neuroscience: 18(12); 4758–4766, 1998.

Morris JS, Frith CD, Perrett DI, Rowland D, Young AW, Calder AJ, Dolan RJ: A differential neural response in the human amygdala to fearful and happy facial expressions. Nature: 383(6603); 812–815, 1996.

Moss HB, Kirisci L, Gordon HW, Tarter RE: A neuropsychologic profile of adolescent alcoholics. Alcoholism, Clinical and Experimental Research: 18(1); 159–163, 1994.

Nader K, Bechara A, Van der Kooy D: Neurobiological constraints on behavioral models of motivation. Annual Review of Psychology: 48; 85–114, 1997.

Nauta JH: Fibre degeneration following lesions of the amygdaloid complex in the monkey. Journal of Anatomy: 95; 516–531, 1961.

Nestler EJ: Cellular and molecular mechanisms of addiction. In Charney DS, Nestler EJ, Bunney BS (Eds), Neurobiology of Mental Illness. New York: Oxford University Press, 1999.

Nichter M, Nichter M, Vuckovic N, Quintero G, Ritenbaugh C: Smoking experimentation and initiation among adolescent girls: qualitative and quantitative findings. Tobbaco Control: 6(4); 285–295, 1997.

Ohuoha DC, Maxwell JA, Thomson LE, Cadet JL, Rothman RB: Effect of dopamine receptor antagonists on cocaine subjective effects: a naturalistic case study. Journal of Substance Abuse Treatment: 14(3); 249–258, 1997.

Ouimette PC, Ahrens C, Moos RH, Finney JW: Enduring treatment changes in substance abuse patients with posttraumatic stress disorder. The influence of specific interventions and program environments. Journal of Substance Abuse Treatment: 15(6); 555–564, 1998.

Pecina S, Berridge KC: Brainstem mediates diazepam enhancement of palatability and feeding: microinjections into fourth ventricle versus lateral ventricle. Brain Research: 727(1–2); 22–30, 1996.

Pedersen W, Skrondal A: Alcohol and sexual victimization: a longitudinal study of Norwegian girls. Addiction: 91(4); 565–581, 1996.

Phillips GD, Robbins TW, Everitt BJ: Bilateral intra-accumbens self-administration of d-amphetamine: antagonism with intra-accumbens SCH-23390 and sulpiride. Psychopharmacology: 114(3); 477–485, 1994.

Piazza PV, Deminiere JM, Le Moal M, Simon H: Factors that predict individual vulnerability to amphetamine self-administration. Science: 245(4925); 1511–1514, 1989.

Piazza PV, Deroche V, Deminiere JM, Le Moal M, Simon H: Corticosterone in the range of stress-induced levels possesses reinforcing properties: implications for sensation-seeking behaviors. Neurobiology: 90(24); 11738–11742, 1993.

Piazza PV, Le Moal ML: Pathophysiological basis of vulnerability to drug abuse: role of an interaction between stress, glucocorticoids, and dopaminergic neurons. Annual Review of Pharmacology and Toxicology: 36; 359–378, 1996.

Piazza PV, Maccari S, Deminiere JM, LeMoal M, Mormede P, Simon H: Corticosterone levels determine individual vulnerability to amphetamine self-administration. Neurobiology: 88(6); 2088–2092, 1991.

Pich EM, Lorang M, Yeganeth M, de Fonseca FR, Raber J, Koob GF, Weiss F: Increase of extracellular corticotropin-releasing factor-like immunoreactivity levels in the amygdala of awake rats during restraint stress and ethanol withdrawal as measured by microdialysis. Journal of Neuroscience: 15(8); 5439–5447, 1995.

Pickens RW, Svikis DS, McGue M, Lykken DT, Heston LL, Clayton PJ: Heterogeneity in the inheritance of alcoholism. A study of male and female twins. Archives of General Psychiatry: 48(1); 19–28, 1991.

Rasmussen DD: Effects of chronic nicotine treatment and withdrawal on hypothalamic proopiomelanocortin gene expression and neuroendocrine regulation. Psychoneuroendocrinology: 23(3); 245–259, 1998.

Reiman EM, Fusselman MJ, Fox PT, Raichle ME: Neuroanatomical correlates of anticipatory anxiety. Science: 243(4894 Pt 1); 1071–1074, 1989.

Richter RM, Pich EM, Koob GF, Weiss F: Sensitization of cocaine-stimulated increase in extracellular levels of corticotropin-releasing factor from the rat amygdala after repeated administration as determined by intracranial microdialysis. Neuroscience Letters: 187(3); 169–172, 1995.

Richter RM, Weiss F: In vivo CRF release in rat amygdala is increased during cocaine withdrawal in self-administering rats. Synapse: 32(4); 254–261, 1999.

Robbins TW, Cador M, Taylor JR, Everitt BJ: Limbic-striatal interactions in reward-related processes. Neuroscience and Biobehavioral Reviews: 13(2–3); 155–162, 1989.

Robbins TW, Everitt BJ: Interaction of the dopaminergic system with mechanisms of associative learning and cognition: implications for drug abuse. Psychological Science: 10; 199–202, 1999.

Robinson TE, Kolb B: Persistent structural modifications in nucleus accumbens and prefrontal cortex neurons produced by previous experience with amphetamine. Journal of Neuroscience: 17(21); 8491–8497, 1997.

Rocha BA, Scearce-Levie K, Lucas JJ, Hiroi N, Castanon N, Crabbe JC, Nestler EJ, Hen R: Increased vulnerability to cocaine in mice lacking the serotonin-1B receptor. Nature: 393(6681); 175–178, 1998.

Rodriguez de Fonseca F, Carrera MRA, Navarro M, Koob GF, Weiss F: Activation of corticotropin-releasing factor in the limbic system during cannabinoid withdrawal. Science: 276(5321); 2050–2054, 1997.

Rohsenow DJ, Corbett R, Devine D: Molested as children: a hidden contribution to substance abuse? Journal of Substance Abuse Treatment: 5(1); 13–18, 1988.

Rosen JB, Schulkin J: From normal fear to pathological anxiety. Psychological Review: 105(2); 325–350, 1998.

Rourke SB, Grant I: The interactive effects of age and length of abstinence on the recovery of neuropsychological functioning in chronic male alcoholics: a 2-year follow-up study. Journal of the International Neuropsychological Society: 5(3); 234–246, 1999.

Sarnyai Z, Dhabhar FS, McEwen BS, Kreek MJ: Neuroendocrine-related effects of long-term, 'binge' cocaine administration: diminished individual differences in stress-induced corticosterone response. Neuroendocrinology: 68(5); 334–344, 1998.

Sawchenko PE: Evidence for a local site of action for glucocorticoids in inhibiting CRF and vasopressin expression in the paraventricular nucleus. Brain Research: 403(2); 213–223, 1987.

Sax KW, Strakowski SM: Enhanced behavioral response to repeated d-amphetamine and personality traits in humans. Biological Psychiatry: 44(11); 1192–1195, 1998.

Scheier LM, Botvin GJ: Effects of early adolescent drug use on cognitive efficacy in early-late adolescence: a developmental structural model. Journal of Substance Abuse: 7(4); 379–404, 1995.

Schneider ML, Coe CL, Lubach GR: Endocrine activation mimics the adverse effects of prenatal stress on the neuromotor development of the infant primate. Developmental Psychobiology: 25(6); 427–439, 1992.

Schnierla TC: An evolutionary and biphasic process underlying approach and withdrawal. In Aronson LR et al. (Eds), Selected Writings of T.C. Schnierla. San Francisco: Freeman, 1959.

Schulkin J: The Neuroendocrine Regulation of Behavior. Cambridge: Cambridge University Press, 1999.

Schulkin J: Rethinking Homeostasis. Boston: MIT Press, 2003.

Schulkin J, Gold P, McEwen B: Induction of corticotropin-releasing hormone gene expression by glucocorticoids: implications for understanding the states of fear and anxiety and allostatic load. Psychoneuroendocrinology: 23(3); 219–243, 1998.

Schwartz RH, Gruenewald PJ, Klitzner M, Fedio P: Short-term memory impairment in cannabis-dependent adolescents. American Journal of the Disabled Child: 143(10); 1214–1219, 1989.

Selby MJ, Azrin RL: Neuropsychological functioning in drug abusers. Drug Alcohol and Dependence: 50(1); 39–45, 1998.

Shannon C, Champoux M, Suomi SJ: Rearing condition and plasma cortisol in rhesus monkey infants. American Journal of Primatology: 46(4); 311–321, 1998.

Sigvardsson S, Bohman M, Cloninger CR: Replication of the Stockholm Adoption Study of alcoholism. Confirmatory cross-fostering analysis. Archives of General Psychiatry: 53(8); 681–687, 1996.

Single E, Robson L, Rehm J, Xie X: Morbidity and mortality attributable to alcohol, tobacco and illicit drug use in Canada. American Journal of Public Health: 89(3); 385–390, 1999.

Smith MA, Davidson J, Ritchie JC, Kudler H, Lipper S, Chappell P, Nemeroff CB: The corticotropin-releasing hormone test in patients with posttraumatic stress disorder. Biological Psychiatry: 26(4); 349–355, 1989.

Smith OA, DeVito JL, Astley CA: Neurons controlling cardiovascular responses to emotion are located in lateral hypothalamus-perifornical region. American Journal of Physiology: 259(5 Pt 2); R943–R954, 1990.

Spak L, Spak F, Allebeck P: Sexual abuse and alcoholism in a female population. Addiction: 93(9); 1365–1373, 1998.

Stein MB, Walker JR, Anderson G, Hazen AL, Ross CA, Eldridge G, Forde DR: Childhood physical and sexual abuse in patients with anxiety disorders and in a community sample. American Journal of Psychiatry: 153(2); 275–277, 1996.

Stein MB, Yehuda R, Koverola C, Hanna C: Enhanced dexamethasone suppression of plasma cortisol in adult women traumatized by childhood sexual abuse. Biological Psychiatry: 42(8); 680–686, 1997.

Stellar E: The physiology of motivation. Psychological Review: 61; 5–22, 1954.

Stellar JR, Stellar E: The Neurobiology of Reward. Berlin: Springer-Verlag, 1985.

Sterling P, Eyer J: Allostasis: a new paradigm to explain arousal pathology. In: Fisher S, Reason HS (Eds), Handbook of Life Stress, Cognition and Health. New York: John Wiley, 1981.

Swanson LW, Simmon DM: Differential steroid hormone and neural influences on peptide mRNA levels in CRH cells of the paraventricular nucleus: a hybridization histochemical study in the rat. Journal of Comparative Neurology: 285(4); 413–435, 1989.

Tapert SF, Baratta MV, Abrantes AM, Brown SA: Attention dysfunction predicts substance involvement in community youths. Journal of the American Academy of Child and Adolescent Psychiatry: 41(6); 680–686, 2002.

Tapert SF, Brown SA: Neuropsychological correlates of adolescent substance abuse: four-year outcomes. Journal of the International Neuropsychological Society: 5(6); 481–493, 1999.

Thorpe SJ, Rolls ET, Maddison S: The orbitofrontal cortex: neuronal activity in the behaving monkey. Experimental Brain Research: 49(1); 93–115, 1983.

Triffleman EG, Marmar CR, Delucchi KL, Ronfeldt H: Childhood trauma and posttraumatic stress disorder in substance abuse inpatients. Journal of Nervous and Mental Disorders: 183(3); 172–176, 1995.

Turnbull JE: Early background variables as predictors of adult alcohol problems in women. International Journal of Addiction: 29(6); 707–728, 1994.

Van den Bree MB, Johnson EO, Neale MC, Pickens RW: Genetic and environmental influences on drug use and abuse/dependence in male and female twins. Drug and Alcohol Dependence: 52(3); 231–241, 1998.

Van den Buuse M: Pressor responses to brain dopaminergic stimulation. Clinical and Experimental Pharmacology and Physiology: 24(9–10); 764–769, 1997.

Van Gorp WG, Wilkins JN, Hinkin CH, Moore LH, Hull J, Horner MD, Plotkin D: Declarative and procedural memory functioning in abstinent cocaine abusers. Archives of General Psychiatry: 56(1); 85–89, 1999.

Volkow ND, Fowler JS, Wolf AP, Hitzemann R, Dewey S, Bendriem B, Alpert R, Hoff A: Changes in brain glucose metabolism in cocaine dependence and withdrawal. American Journal of Psychiatry: 148(5); 621–626, 1991.

Volkow ND, Hitzemann R, Wang GJ, Fowler JS, Burr G, Pascani K, Dewey SL, Wolf AP: Decreased brain metabolism in neurologically intact healthy alcoholics. American Journal of Psychiatry: 149(8); 1016–1022, 1992.

Wang W: Illegal drug abuse and the community camp strategy in China. Journal of Drug Education: 29(2); 97–114, 1999.

Watts AG, Sanchez-Watts G: Region-specific regulation of neuropeptide mRNAs in rat limbic forebrain neurones by aldosterone and corticosterone. Journal of Physiology (London): 484(Pt 3); 721–736, 1995.

Wert RC, Raulin ML: The chronic cerebral effects of cannabis use. II. Psychological findings and conclusions. International Journal of Addiction: 21(6); 629–642, 1986.

Wiers RW, Sergeant JA, Gunning WB: Psychological mechanisms of enhanced risk of addiction in children of alcoholics: a duel pathway? Acta Paediatrica, Nov: 404; 9–13, 1994.

Williams J, Haut JS: Differential performance on the WRAML in children and adolescents diagnosed with epilepsy, head-injury, and substance-abuse. Developmental Neuropsychology: 11(2); 201–213, 1995.

Wills TA, Windle M, Cleary SD: Temperament and novelty seeking in adolescent substance use: convergence of dimensions of temperament with constructs from Cloninger's theory. Journal of Personality and Social Psychology: 74(2); 387–406, 1998.

Wilsnack SC, Vogeltanz ND, Klassen AD, Harris TR: Childhood sexual abuse and women's substance abuse: national survey findings. Journal of Studies on Alcoholism: 58(3); 264–271, 1997.

Wise RA: Neuroleptics and operant behavior: the anhedonia hypothesis. Behavioral and Brain Sciences: 5; 39–87, 1982.

Wise RA, Spindler J, deWit H, Gerberg GJ: Neuroleptic-induced 'anhedonia' in rats: pimozide blocks reward quality of food. Science: 201(4325); 262–264, 1978.

Yama MF, Tovey SL, Fogas BS, Teegarden LA: Joint consequences of parental alcoholism and childhood sexual abuse, and their partial mediation by family environment. Violence and Victims: 7(4); 313–325, 1992.

Yehuda R: Current status of cortisol findings in post-traumatic stress disorder. Psychiatric Clinics of North America: 25(2); 341–368, 2002.

Yehuda R, Resnick HS, Schmeidler J, Yang RK, Pitman RK: Predictors of cortisol and 3-methoxy-4-hydroxyphenylglycol responses in the acute aftermath of rape. Biological Psychiatry: 43(11); 855–859, 1998.

Handbook of Neuropsychology, 2nd Edition, Vol. 8, Part II
S.J. Segalowitz and I. Rapin (Eds)

CHAPTER 32

Eating disorders

Audrey Walker [*]

Department of Psychiatry, Division of Child and Adolescent Psychiatry, Albert Einstein College of Medicine/Montefiore Medical Center, 3317 Rochambeau Avenue, Bronx, NY 10467, USA

Introduction

As societies become wealthier and food relatively available, clinical obesity becomes more prevalent in the population. It is a fascinating paradox that, as societies become more prosperous, the prevalence of serious eating disorders, those which lead to a misuse of the eating function and emaciation in the case of anorexia nervosa (AN), or death in the case of end-stage AN and bulimia nervosa (BN), increase dramatically. In the past, periods of starvation were endemic to human civilizations. In these same civilizations, the artistic convention and ideal of beauty was the obese, heavy-hipped woman, often with a large, pregnant-appearing abdomen. It was as if, to paraphrase Hilda Bruch (Bruch, 1973), obesity was conceived as a defense against the dreaded fate of starvation, as well as a symbol of hope for fertility and fecundity. The earliest female representations currently known date back to 20,000 B.C. They are the products of an ancient hunter–gatherer culture and are known as the Venuses of Willendorf and Lespugne (Fig. 1). Fashioned of mammoth ivory and standing 6 inches high, they characteristically had no feet and small featureless heads. It is the center of the body, with its large, pendulous breasts, wide waists and hips, and pronounced genitals and buttocks, which are the focus of the objects. Understood by anthropologists as sacred relics, these Venuses were almost certainly goddesses of childbirth and seem to bear the symbolic ideas of physical abundance and reproductive fertility. In the Greek and Roman art which remains for us to examine, the female form is typically depicted as fleshy and pear-shaped, as in the Crouching Venus attributed to Doedulus in the early 4th century B.C. (Fig. 2). There are countless examples throughout the Renaissance and into the nineteenth century, well represented by the work of Renoir (Fig. 3). And even as recently as the mid-twentieth century, female symbols of desirability followed the same model (Fig. 4).

Epidemiology

Over the past forty years, something has changed dramatically in the conception of the ideal female form and it is happening alongside a significant change in the epidemiology of the eating disorders in Western societies. Eating disorders are currently among the most common psychiatric disorders in young women and the prevalence of eating disorders has increased steadily over the past fifty years. All studies using rigorous methodology regarding diagnosis and utilizing interview formats with established reliability have reported this recent increase. Two-stage studies refer to studies in which a first stage of a screening questionnaire to identify the at-risk population is followed by a second stage consisting of extensive personal interviews of this at-risk population, as well as of a randomly selected sample of the population not identified as being at risk. These studies have consistently found the prevalence

* Corresponding author. Tel.: +1-718-920-6562; Fax: +1-718-798-3810; E-mail: coventry8@aol.com

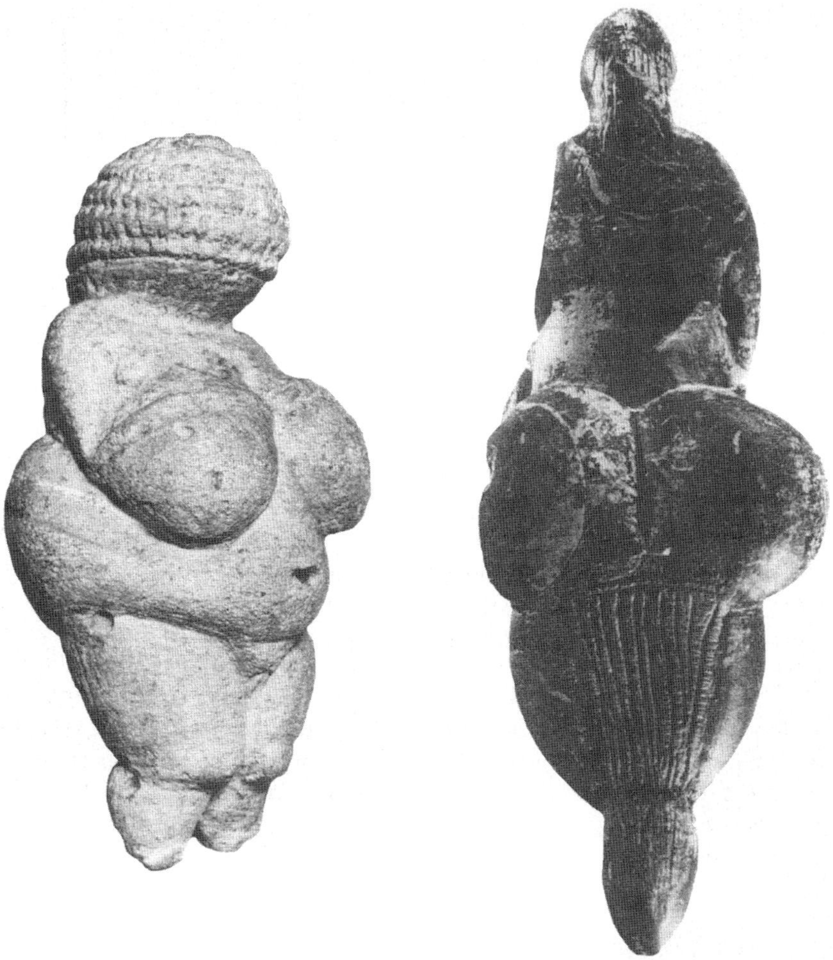

Fig. 1. Venuses of Willendorf and Lespugne.

of AN in young women to be 0.5% and of BN to be 2–3% (Hsu, 1996).

Prevalence of eating disorders among men appears to be much lower than in women, with a male-to-female ratio consistently found across studies to be 1 : 10. According to a recent study published by a research group at New York Hospital-Cornell Medical Center (Braun, Sunday, Huang et al., 1999), an increase in the prevalence of eating disorder admissions in males during the period from 1984–1987 was clearly demonstrated. In a study of all males with eating disorders treated in a general hospital setting over a 14-year period, Carlat, Camargo and Herzog (1997) identified 135 males with eating disorders. Of this group, 46% were found to be bulimic while 22% were anorexic and 32% met criterion for an eating disorder not otherwise specified. The most striking finding in this study was the marked differences in sexual orientation found by diagnostic group. The authors found that 27% of the study group reported being primarily homosexual or bisexual and 32% were asexual, defined as a lack of all sexual interest for one year prior to assessment. This contrasts with recent data on sexual preference in the general population, in which the prevalence of homosexuality in males is reported to be 1–6% (Seidman and Reider, 1994). This is also in marked contrast to the reported 2% prevalence of homosexuality in females with eating disorders (Woodside, Garner, Rockert et al., 1990). Though the clinical picture in males with eating disorders is otherwise remarkably similar to females,

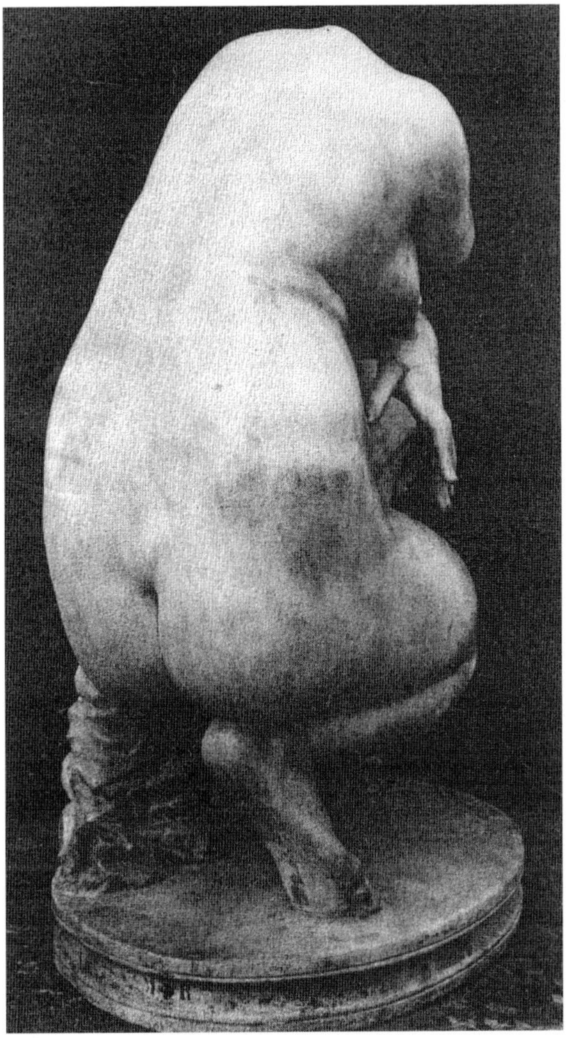

Fig. 2. Crouching Venus, Doedulus.

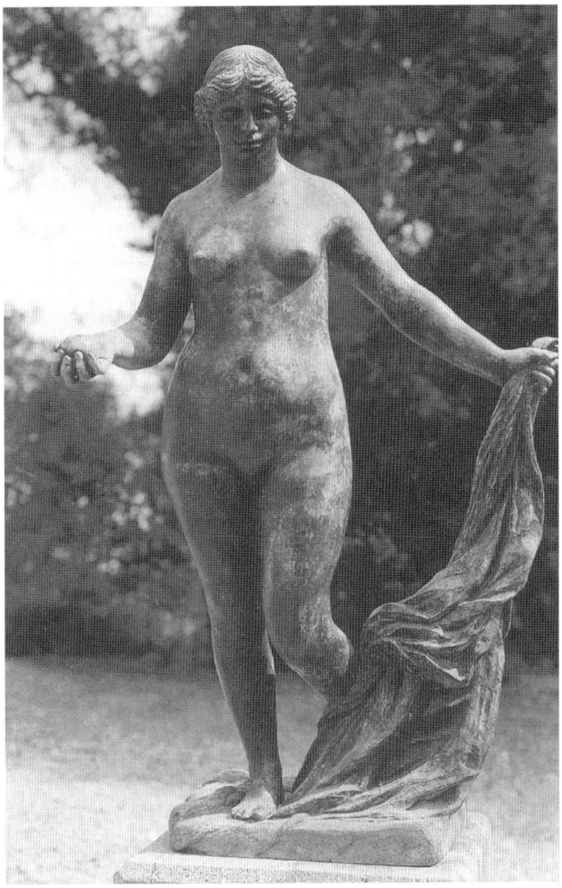

Fig. 3. Nude, Renoir.

homosexuality and bisexuality are clearly significant risk factors in males. This was found in the Carlat study to be particularly true in BN, where the prevalence of homosexuality/bisexuality was 42%. Whether this striking difference is mediated by cultural or biological factors is unknown, and future research on the link between sexual preference and the expression of eating disorders is needed. One additional finding across studies is an older age of onset for males compared with females. The physiological significance of this finding with regard to the onset of puberty in males compared with females will be discussed later in the chapter.

Prevalence data derive from the most rigorous studies and thus exclude borderline and subclinical cases of eating disorders, which are far more common. These subclinical and borderline cases share many of the core features of the true cases and many will later go on to meet full criteria for an eating disorder. Because of the high mortality and morbidity of the eating disorders as well as the discouraging chronicity of their courses, even subclinical cases should be identified and treated. There is much evidence to suggest that the cultural expectations of extreme thinness in women is continuing unabated in western societies (Field, Camargo, Taylor et al., 2001), and thus we can expect to see the incidence and prevalence of eating disorders increase in the coming years.

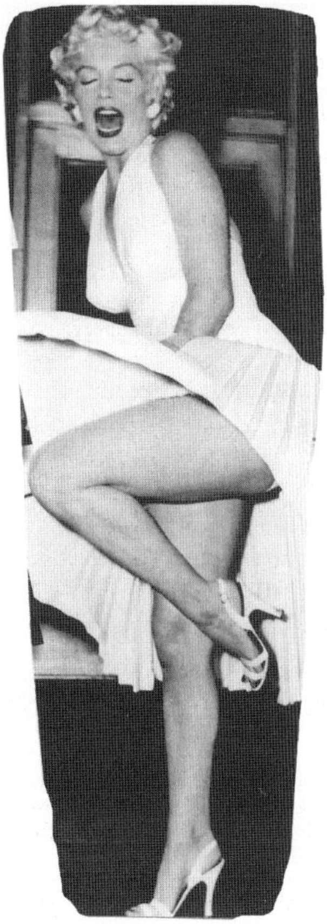

Fig. 4. Marilyn Monroe.

Diagnostic issues

As clinicians, before we can detect and treat a case, we must be able to rigorously define what a case is. The earliest published account of a substantial pressure on women for an ideal of thinness can be found in Terence's Eunuchus. Terence was a Roman comic poet who wrote in the second century B.C. This was a time of rapid expansionism and prosperity in Roman society. A character, speaking of a young women whom he admires, states "She is a girl who doesn't look like the girls of our day whose mothers strive to make them have sloping shoulders, a squeezed chest so that they look thin. If one is a little plumper, they say she is a boxer and reduce her diet. Though she is well endowed by nature, this treatment makes her as thin as a bulrush" (Chabrol, Callahan and O'Halloran, 2000). AN became a clinical entity with the independent reports by Gull (1888) in England and Lasegue in France in the early 1870s (Bruch, 1973) though reports of self-inflicted starvation can be found in earlier literature. According to Gull, the outstanding symptoms were emaciation associated with amenorrhea, constipation, loss of appetite, slow pulse and respiration in the absence of somatic pathology. With the advent of the Diagnostic and Statistical Manual of Mental Disorders, eating disorders have been rigorously defined. AN and BN are understood as psychiatric disorders which are characterized by abnormal eating behaviors and obsessive ideation about body size and weight. Adult patients with AN are defined by DSMIV (American Psychiatric Association, 1994) as having a body weight which is less than 85% of that expected or, in the case of children and adolescents, to evidence of failure to make expected weight gains during a period of growth, leading to a body weight which is less than 85% of that expected. By contrast, patients with BN tend to maintain a near to normal body weight.

The current DSMIV (American Psychiatric Association, 1994) departed from DSM III-R significantly in its organization of the eating disorders. AN and BN were moved out of the section for childhood-onset disorders and a new "Eating Disorders" section was established in the adult section of the manual. This restructuring occurred in response to the growing body of research that supports the fact that eating disorders can develop in adulthood as well as in childhood and adolescence and should therefore be distinguished from the eating disorders which typically present in childhood such as Rumination Disorder and PICA (Pryor, 1995). The signs and symptoms necessary to diagnose the eating disorders currently fall into three broad categories: (1) pathological thoughts and emotions; (2) deviant eating behaviors and (3) alterations in body composition in the case of AN. Full criteria for AN and BN are shown in Tables 1 and 2. DSM IV also introduced two types of AN: the restricting type during which the patient restricts food intake but does not regularly engage in binge eating followed by purging, and the binge eating, purging type during which the patient regularly engages in binge eating or purging through self-induced vomiting or the use of laxatives or diuretics. It is important to understand that "anorexia" is a misnomer for this disorder as anorexia connotes

TABLE 1

DSM IV diagnostic criteria, anorexia nervosa

Diagnostic criteria for 307.1 anorexia nervosa
A. Refusal to maintain body weight at or above a minimally normal weight for age and height (e.g., weight loss leading to maintenance of body weight less than 85% of that expected, or failure to make expected weight gain during period of growth, leading to body weight less than 85% of that expected).
B. Intense fear of gaining weight or becoming fat, even though underweight.
C. Disturbance in the way in which one's body weight or shape is experienced, undue influence of body weight or shape on self-evaluation, or denial of the seriousness of the current low body weight.
D. In postmenarcheal females, amenorrhea, i.e., the absence of at least three consecutive menstrual cycles. (A woman is considered to have amenorrhea if her periods occur only following hormone, e.g., estrogen, administration.)
Specify type:
Restricting type: during the current episode of anorexia nervosa, the person has not regularly engaged in binge-eating or purging behavior (i.e., self-induced vomiting or the misuse of laxatives, diuretics, or enemas)
Binge-eating/purging type: during the current episode of anorexia nervosa, the person has regularly engaged in binge-eating or purging behavior (i.e., self-induced vomiting or the misuse of laxatives, diuretics, or enemas)

TABLE 2

DSM IV diagnostic criteria, bulimia nervosa

Diagnostic criteria for 307.51 bulimia nervosa
A. Recurrent episodes of binge eating. An episode of binge eating is characterized by both of the following: (1) eating, in a discrete period of time (e.g., within any 2-hour period), an amount of food that is definitely larger than most people would eat during a similar period of time and under similar circumstances (2) a sense of lack of control over eating during the episode (e.g., a feeling that one cannot stop eating or control what or how much one is eating)
B. Recurrent inappropriate compensatory behavior in order to prevent weight gain, such as self-induced vomiting; misuse of laxatives, diuretics, enemas, or other medications; fasting; or excessive exercise.
C. The binge eating and inappropriate compensatory behaviors both occur, on average, at least twice a week for 3 months.
D. Self-evaluation is unduly influenced by body shape and weight.
E. The disturbance does not occur exclusively during episodes of anorexia nervosa.
Specify type:
Purging type: during the current episode of bulimia nervosa, the person has regularly engaged in self-induced vomiting or the misuse of laxatives, diuretics, or enemas
Nonpurging type: during the current episode of bulimia nervosa, the person has used other inappropriate compensatory behaviors, such as fasting or excessive exercise, but has not regularly engaged in self-induced vomiting or the misuse of laxatives, diuretics, or enemas

a lack of appetite, a symptom that is rarely present in these patients, who typically describe themselves as experiencing normal sensations of hunger until a very late stage in the disorder.

The clinical picture of the anorectic patient is a striking and unmistakable one. The anorectic adolescent enters the consulting room with the familiar appearance of the wan, thin girl with markedly protruding clavicles and scapulae. Often the patient appears prepubertal, with little or no breast tissue. The patients will attempt to conceal their appearance with baggy clothing, which is often much warmer than the weather calls for, not only to conceal the condition but also to combat the heightened cold sensitivity they experience due to decreased fat stores. The anorectic patient is very restricted in her thinking: usually the timing and calorie content of her next meal vies with her current weight as the most important of her concerns. She is constricted, sad appearing and lethargic, due to inadequate calorie consumption. Anorectic patients often look and feel depressed, even if they do not meet full criteria for a Major Depressive Episode, and accurate evaluation of depression must often be deferred until refeeding and significant weight gain is successfully accomplished. The anorectic patient is withdrawn from her peer group. This social isolation allows for better control of eating as well as the avoidance of the worried, intrusive glances of friends and family members. The daily life of the anorectic patient is full of real misery and plagued by constant anxiety and obsessive concern about food and the body.

Patients with BN who purge are more difficult to identify by clinical observation and physical findings. Dental enamel erosions and abrasions on the dorsum of the hands from repeated contact with the teeth while inducing vomiting may be seen, as well as parotid gland hypertrophy, which can sometimes be identified by inspection. In the diagnosis of BN, episodes of the disorder are accompanied by a feeling of being out of control. Binge eating episodes are terminated by social interruption or feelings of extreme physical discomfort and followed by extreme feeling of guilt which precipitate compensatory purging behaviors. Binges and purges are specifically operationalized in DSM IV by duration and specific behavioral features as described in Table 2. An important change in the diagnostic criteria for BN in DSM-IV is the specific distinction between bulimics whose purging behavior involves self-induced vomiting, laxative or diuretic abuse, in contrast to those who use behaviors such as compulsive exercise or fasting to counterbalance binges.

In summary, several important clinical features distinguish AN from BN. Unlike patients with AN, whose appearance makes the disorder obvious, those with BN are usually able to maintain a normal weight and thus are better able to conceal the disorder. The sense of total control that the anorectic patient feels over her food intake is in marked contrast to the sense of total loss of control over the binge and purges episodes experienced by the bulimic patient. In BN, binge episodes usually precede purging behaviors by one year. DSM IV also allows for a non-purging type of BN in which the patient uses fasting or excessive exercising to control weight rather than purges.

Medical complications of anorexia nervosa and bulimia nervosa

Many patients who are diagnosed with AN will later meet criteria for BN. Thirty to fifty percent of patients with onset of AN will go on to have symptoms of BN within eighteen months (Kaplan and Sadock, 1998). Morbidity in these disorders is myriad and seen in virtually every organ system. Table 3 lists medical complications related to (1) weight loss and (2) purging in order to cover the spectrum of clinical problems a practitioner is likely to encounter when treating a patient with eating disorder over several years.

TABLE 3

Medical complications of eating disorders

Medical consequences of eating disorders
Related to weight loss:
Endocrine: changes in growth hormone; reduced thyroid metabolism; hypothalamic hypogonadism; pubertal delay; hypoglycemia
Skeletal: osteoporosis; peak bone mass reduction (Castro, Lazaro, Pons et al., 2000)
Cardiovascular: loss of cardiac muscle; cardiac arrhythmias including atrial and ventricular premature contractions, prolonged QT interval; bradycardia; ventricular tachycardia; sudden death
Gastrointestinal: delayed gastric emptying; bloating; constipation
Reproductive: Amenorrhea; low levels of FSH and LH
Dermatologic: Lanugo
Hematologic: Leukopenia
Neurologic: Attentional and memory impairment
Related to purging:
Cardiovascular: Dehydration; orthostatic blood pressure changes; myocardial damage with excessive IPECAC abuse
Gastrointestinal: Salivary gland and pancreatic inflammation with corresponding increase in serum amylase; esophageal and gastric erosions; dysfunctional bowel with haustral dilation
Neurologic: Seizures; mild peripheral neuropathies
Dental: erosion of dental enamel
Metabolic: hypochloremic alkalosis (vomiting); hypokalemia (laxative abuse)

Etiology and pathophysiology

Psychiatric disorders are complex disorders, which probably have polygenic inheritance patterns, which are significantly modulated by environmental factors. In addition, little is currently known about the neuroanatomic substrate of these disorders. The current consensus regarding the etiology of eating disorders is that these disorders have a multifactorial origin with reciprocal interactions amongst a number of factors that will be discussed.

Genetics

Genetic factors have been implicated in the genesis of AN. Some twin studies indicate that the concordance rate for anorexia is higher among monozygotic than dizygotic twins. In one study (Holland, Hall, Murray et al., 1984), the concordance rate was 55% for monozygotic twins but only 7% for dizygotic pairs. Sisters of patients with AN are more likely to be afflicted than the general population (Holland, Sicotte and Treasure, 1988), but this association may reflect social influences rather than genetic factors. Holland did a combined twin and family study of patients with AN and found that 56% of the 25 female monozygotic twin pairs and 5% of the 20 female dizygotic twin pairs were concordant for AN. In addition, 5% of other female first degree relatives also had a history of AN, supporting the hypothesis that genetic factors are very significant in the etiology of AN. Genetic effects are less convincingly demonstrated amongst patients with BN. To date, there are no adequate longitudinal studies controlling shared and non-shared environmental factors that would aid in the clarification of the role of heritability in BN.

Puberty

The onset of puberty, in both the physiological and psychological sense, is clearly related to the expression of the eating disorders. Puberty heralds the beginning of the highest risk period for the onset of AN in females and males. The fact that puberty typically begins 1–2 years later in boys than in girls may partially account for the difference in age of onset of the eating disorders in males compared with females. To test the hypothesis that the development of eating disorders represented an accommodation to puberty, a short-term prospective study was conducted. The subjects were 193 girls from 7th through 10th grade who were followed for two years (Fairburn, Cooper, Doll et al., 1999). The authors found that girls who developed the most negative attitudes about their changing bodies were at highest risk for developing an eating disorder, after initial eating problem scores were taken into account. The precise physiological mechanism by which the onset of puberty leads to the development of eating disorders is as yet unknown.

Dieting behavior

The sociocultural emphasis on thinness, both as an ideal of beauty as well as a marker for self-control, has accelerated in the last several decades in western societies. The practices of excessive dieting and exercise which eating disorder patients engage in finds much support in the larger society. In a recent population-based cohort study (Patton, Selzer, Coffey et al., 1999) students age 14 were followed for three years to determine predictors of new eating disorders. The authors found that adolescent girls who dieted were 18 times more likely to develop eating disorder than those who did not diet. This severe dieting may have been an early clinical phase of the disorder rather than a risk factor, as the authors acknowledge in their discussion.

Special populations

Certain special populations have been identified as being at high risk for developing eating disorders. Most studies of athletes who compete in sports that emphasize leanness to enhance performance or appearance show that these individuals are clearly at increased risk. This group includes dancers, gymnasts, distance runners, and wrestlers. Clearly, the pressure to diet and become thin may trigger eating disorders in people with specific vulnerabilities. Alternatively, certain sports may attract athletes with pre-existing eating disorders.

An interesting theory has emerged from the study of physical activity and eating disorders. The 'activity-induced anorexia hypothesis' posits that a program of strenuous physical activity may play a pathogenic role in the development and maintenance of eating disorders by disrupting the normal mechanisms of energy balance. Animal research (Epling and Pierce, 1984, 1988) has shown that food intake is reduced following exercise and that in the face of food restriction, physical activity increases, creating a weight-loss cycle. These studies have shown that 90% of adolescent rats and 70% of mature rats whose access to food was restricted to 60–90 minutes a day and who were given free access to a running wheel progressively increased the amount of running and decreased food intake, sometimes literally running themselves to death. One of the physiological mediators may be the release of endogenous opioid peptides in the brain. In addition the serotonin system is involved in this phenomenon, which will be discussed in the following section. The relationship of compulsive exercise in humans to this animal model of activity-based AN has recently come under investigation. Brewerton (1995) studied a large series of eating disorder patients to determine the frequency of compulsive exercising (CE), defined as daily exercise to control weight for at least 60 minutes a day. One fourth of this sample were defined as CE and AN was much more common in the CE subgroup than BN. Patients who engaged in CE scored much higher on a measure of body dissatisfaction than non-CEs. In addition, CEs were much less likely than non-CEs to vomit or to use laxatives. These results may have important implications for research on the psychobiology of the eating disorders, possibly heralding potential differences in the neurochemical function of individuals with CE versus non-CE.

Neurophysiology and neuroendocrinology

Amongst the major psychiatric disorders, the eating disorders have been the most difficult on which to obtain sound evidence for biological etiologies. There are several reasons for this. As noted previously, the disorders are rare and it has been difficult to establish a good animal model for study. In spite of the primitive stage of research in this field, the study of two substances, the hormone leptin and the neurotransmitter serotonin has begun to shed some light on the neurophysiologic basis of eating behaviors and the possible pathophysiologic alterations which take place in these disorders. The question of whether these substances are causative, an associated pathological finding or one of the many physiological consequences of the malnutrition, starvation or metabolic derangements which accompanies them has not yet been established.

In 1994, a research team from Rockefeller University reported that mutations in the leptin gene caused hereditary obesity in a mutant strain of mice (Gura, 2000). Leptin is a hormone that is encoded by the adipocyte-specific gene *ob*, and under normal physiologic conditions it plays a central role in the regulation of body weight, appetite and energy expenditure. Leptin is secreted by the adipocyte and has receptors in the brain, muscle and fat tissues. In human models, serum leptin levels are proportional to the size of the fat deposits. With elevation in serum leptin levels, either due to overfeeding or with increased fat stores, leptin enters the brain and seems to interact with a number of neuropeptides in the hypothalamus including alpha-MSH (melanocyte-stimulating hormone) to signal appetite suppression. A second class of neuropeptides which act as appetite-stimulants, the SOCS3 (suppressor of cytokine signaling-3) are shut down when leptin levels are high. In patients with clinical obesity, resistance to the appetite-suppressant effects of leptin seems to occur since the presence of elevated leptin in these obese subjects is not accompanied by the usual appetite-suppression seen in normal subjects.

In the eating disorders AN and BN, there is some evidence that the normal physiologic effect of leptin is deranged. Ferron, Considine, Peino et al. (1997) looked at serum leptin levels in three groups of patients affected by severe eating disorders: AN, BN and non-specific eating disorder, and found that serum leptin levels were not correlated to the specific psychiatric pathology but were correlated to the individual body mass index (BMI). Patients with AN with the accompanying severe decrease in BMI had, as expected from studies of normal weight controls, a reduction in serum leptin levels which correlated with BMI reduction as the disorder progressed. In the bulimic subjects in this study, most of whom maintained normal bmi in spite of the binge and purge behaviors seen in this disorder, mean serum leptin levels did not significantly differ from controls. Nakai, Hamagaki, Kato et al. (1999), in a related study, measured the serum leptin levels and BMIs in 152 eating-disordered subjects. In addition the authors also assessed eating behavior by obtaining a detailed history of eating behavior within 48 hours before blood sampling using recall methods. The authors found that plasma leptin levels were significantly correlated with the BMI in the eating-disordered patients. Plasma leptin levels were also correlated with eating behavior scores: higher leptin levels were seen in patients who reported extremely high caloric intakes from binging, while very low leptin levels were found in patients who reported fasting behavior or extremely low caloric intakes. In spite of this, the normal process of increased appetite and feeding with resulting increase in body fat expected with decreased leptin levels is not seen in patients with anorexia. Though clinically, anorectic patients often describe themselves as hungry, this increased appetite does not lead to increase in feeding behavior.

Bulimic patients have the clinical symptom of excessive feeding behavior in the form of binging in spite of normal or elevated serum leptin levels. Once again, as in the case of clinically obese patients, a resistance of appetite, metabolism and feeding behavior to the normal physiologic response to leptin seems to be occurring in patients with both AN and BN. The mediator that produces these effects is not yet known, though several neuropeptides have been found to play a central role in feeding behavior and to interact with leptin. Neuropeptide Y (NPY) and Peptide YY (PYY), predominantly found in the hypothalamus, are two of the most potent endogenous stimulants to feeding behavior thus far identified in the CNS. In animal models, hypothalamic administration of these substances results in rapid and voracious feeding with a preference for carbohydrate-rich foods (Cord, Melville, Gibbs et al., 1990). Kaye, Berrettini and Gwirtsman (1990) assessed CNS NPY and PYY levels in patients with eating disorders when they were symptomatic with their eating disorders and again after nutritional stabilization. The authors found that anorectic patients and normal-weight bulimics had distinct differences in CSF NPY and PYY concentrations compared with healthy volunteers. The CSF NPY level was elevated only in underweight anorectic patients, short-term weight-restored anorectic patients and long-term weight restored anorectic patients with amenorrhea or oligomenorrhea. The CSF PYY level was elevated only in normal-weight bulimic patients after abstinence. The authors comment that these results suggest that although anorectic patients and normal-weight bulimic patients have many behavioral similarities, the finding that they have distinct differences in NPY and PYY function may be a reflection of pathophysiological distinctions between these two disorders.

Recent biological studies indicate that disturbances in the serotonin (5-HT) neurotransmitter system have been implicated in the genesis of a variety of forms of psychopathology that are most frequently found to be comorbid with the eating disorders. These include obsessive–compulsive disorder (Brewerton, 1995), depressive disorders (Jimerson, Lesem, Kaye et al., 1990), substance abuse (Ballenger, Goodwin, Major et al., 1979), and aggressive behavior (Brown, Ebert, Goyer et al., 1982). Recently, attention has been focused on the role of the serotonin system in the genesis and maintenance of the eating disorders. Brain serotonin activity contributes to satiety. It is well known that increase in serotonin function can lead to reduction in food consumption. Kaye, Gwirtsman, George et al. (1991) found that in a group of long-term, weight-restored anorectics in remission, 15 of 17 had elevated CSF 5-hydroxyindoleacetic acid, the major serotonin metabolite. This indicated an increase in serotonin activity, which may contribute to the pathological feeding behavior as well as the inhibited and obsessional trait seen in these patients. Jimerson, Wolfe, Metzger et al. (1997) demonstrated impaired CNS serotonergic responsiveness in patients with BN and hypothesized that this contributes to the onset or maintenance of the binge eating seen in this disorder. The binge eating behaviors seen in patients with BN have been shown to be decreased by treatment with fluoxetine (Fluoxetine Bulimia Nervosa Collaborative Study Group, 1992) and the serotonin reuptake inhibitor fluvoxamine has been shown to significantly reduce the frequency of binges in patients with the DSMIV diagnosis of binge-eating disorder, which is characterized by recurrent binge-eating episodes without the purging behaviors seen in BN (Hudson, McElroy, Raymond et al., 1998). Pharmacologically PYY-induced food intake has been shown to be reduced by the selective serotonin reuptake inhibitor fluoxetine. In addition, Halmi, Eckert, LaDu et al. (1986) reported a decrease in satiety and an increase in food consumption in patients with AN treated with the 5-HT antagonist cyproheptadine. In a follow-up study of the activity based anorexia hypothesis discussed previously, Altemus, Glowa and Murphy (1993) pretreated rats prior to providing them with the food restriction and free access to a running wheel, which was previously described. Rats were treated with fluoxetine, imipramine or placebo. The rats treated with fluoxetine showed significant attenuation of wheel running, anorexia and weight loss compared with the other two groups. This study suggests that food-restriction-induced compulsive running and the associated anorexia are prevented by serotonin reuptake blockade.

Neuropsychology of eating disorders

Neuropsychological assessment

(a) Neuroimaging
In patients with AN, several recent studies using neuroimaging have identified abnormal structural findings which include enlarged CSF spaces and reductions in white and gray matter which are correlated with the degree of malnutrition (Golden, Ashtari, Kohn et al., 1996) and are not fully reversed when weight recovery occurs (Katzman, Zipursky, Lambe et al., 1997; Lambe, Katzman, Mikulis et al., 1997). Kingston, Szmukler, Tress et al. (1996) studied the neuropsychological performance and MRI brain appearance of patients with AN and found that the AN group performed significantly worse than controls on tasks measuring attention, visuospatial ability and memory. In this study, comparison of MRI measures showed a significant proportion of anorexics had enlarged lateral ventricles and dilated sulci on both cortical and cerebellar surfaces. There was only modest improvement in the AN group following treatment both in morphological appearance and cognitive performance. Palazidou, Robinson and Lishman (1990) examined 17 inpatients with AN by computed tomography and also performed neuropsychological assessments utilizing the Bexley Maudsley Automated Psychological Screening and Sorting Test. The patients were found to have enlarged external cerebrospinal fluid spaces compared to controls. The patients also performed abnormally on the Digit Symbol Test and this finding correlated negatively with the cortical score, raising the possibility that enlarged external CSF spaces which occur together with impaired digit symbol performance is an indicator of brain damage. In this study, patients were not retested after weight recovery, so it was not possible to assess whether weight recovery was associated with improvement in test performance or brain morphology.

(b) Neuropsychological function
Neuropsychological factors have not been adequately elucidated in the study of the eating disorders, although a number of studies of neuropsychological function have been carried out. Studies of the cognitive abilities of eating disordered patients compared with normals assessed with standard IQ and achievement measures have yielded confusing and at times contradictory results. Bruch (1962) was the first to identify cognitive deficits in the patients she treated, though she did not study this finding systematically. She observed these patients to have advanced scholastic achievement combined with a dearth of abstracting ability, which she understood to be a failure in the development of formal operational thinking. Fox (1982) compared fifteen individuals with AN with fifteen randomly selected psychiatric patients utilizing the Wechsler Adult Intelligence Scale (WAIS) or the Wechsler Intelligence Scale for Children (WISC), the Mattis Organic Mental Syndrome Screening Examination (Mattis, 1978), the Trail Marking Test (Reitan, 1958), and the Benton Visual Retention Test (Benton, 1974). A significant deviation in cognitive performance was found in the patients with AN, consisting of impaired performance on tasks which assess attention and concentration, poor performance on items requiring detailed factual information about society and the environment, excessive psychomotor activity, and impaired arithmetic skills compared with language skills. Kowalski (1986), utilizing The Proverbs Test developed by Gorham and two tasks assessing the individual's ability to isolate variables in natural experimental contexts, found no differences in cognitive abilities between female adolescents with anorexia and age-matched normal control group. Gillberg, Gillberg, Rastam et al. (1996), using the Wechsler Adult Intelligence Scale-Revised (WAIS-R), contrasted a community-based sample of adolescent-onset anorectics with a school-matched comparison group and similarly found few differences in cognitive abilities. Of note, the comparison group did significantly better on the Object Assembly subtest than the anorectic group, leading the authors to speculate that the ability to disregard concrete details in the construction of a coherent 'whole' is relatively lacking in these anorectic patients, an observation that is compatible with Bruch's original observations. Horne, Van Vactor and Emerson (1991) reported on a group of hospitalized patients with AN. Using the Wechsler Intelligence Scale for Children-Revised (WISC-R) or the WAIS-R, they found that the majority of anorectics had higher

Verbal IQs than Performance IQs. Dura and Bornstein (1989) measured school achievement with the WRAT and general intelligence with the WISC-R or the WAIS-R for older subjects and found that school achievement was advanced in comparison with intellectual abilities in anorectic patients. No comparison group was included in this study. Finally, Mathias and Kent (1988) examined the cognitive performance of 34 female patients with AN and compared them to a community control group with no history of eating disorder or other psychiatric disorders. A variety of measures were used including the WAIS-R for general intelligence, the revised Wechsler Memory Scale (WMS-R), the Austin Maze to assess complex visuospatial learning and the Trail Making Test to assess attention and mental tracking. The study found very few differences between the cognitive performance of the group with AN and controls.

Some investigators have focused on specific subtests to determine whether circumscribed neuropsychological functions are impaired in eating disordered patients and whether this impairment has an impact on outcome. Hamsher, Halmi and Benton (1981) used a neuropsychological assessment battery that included either the WAIS or the WISC on 20 female inpatients with AN. The patients were contacted one year after discharge to assess outcome. Patients with favorable outcomes did not differ from those with unfavorable outcomes with regard to pretreatment IQ. However, at post treatment examination, a significant association between the number of cognitive deficits and outcome was found. Attention–concentration deficits, most notably slow complex reaction times, appeared to be a reliable sign of a poor prognosis for weight maintenance 1 year after treatment. The authors emphasized that this pattern of impaired performance did not suggest a focal or diffuse cerebral disease, though the profile was most characteristic of persons with attentional deficits. The study did not answer the question of whether the attention–concentration deficits identified in the poorer-prognosis anorectics occurred on the basis of a primary organic disturbance in arousal mechanisms or as a secondary consequence of disturbances in motivation and endogenous distractions such as weight and eating preoccupations.

Personality assessment

The assessment of personality and the evaluation of comorbid personality disorders have the potential to enhance the clinical understanding of the risk factors, dynamics, prognosis, and treatment outcome of the patient with an eating disorder. Premorbid personality characteristics and pathology are generally believed to play an important role in the genesis of eating disorders and their specific expression. A number of attempts have been made to group eating disorder patients according to their accompanying personality features. According to Kaplan and Sadock (1998), personality can be understood as "a person's characteristic totality of emotional and behavioral traits apparent in ordinary life, a totality that is usually stable and predictable." Personality disorders refer to "enduring subjective experiences that deviate from cultural standards, are rigidly pervasive, have an onset in adolescence or early adulthood, are stable through time and lead to unhappiness or impairment." Research has focused not only on the question of whether concurrent personality characteristics have an effect on treatment outcome, but also on whether personality features, including personality disorder, precede the development of eating disorders or are a result of the psychiatric distress which occurs as a result of having an eating disorder.

An extensive literature exists on the comorbidity of eating disorders and personality disorder symptoms. A growing literature suggests that the presence of personality disorder is associated with a more negative clinical eating disorder outcome (Wonderlich, Fullerton, Swift et al., 1994). The personality disorders are organized into three clusters in DSM IV, based on descriptive similarities (DSM IV 1994). Cluster A includes the Paranoid, Schizoid and Schizotypal Personality Disorders. Individuals with these disorders appear odd or eccentric. Cluster B includes the Antisocial, Borderline, Histrionic and Narcissistic Personality Disorders. Individuals with these disorders behave in an erratic and overly emotional manner. Cluster C includes the Avoidant, Dependent and Obsessive–Compulsive Personality Disorders. These individuals often appear fearful and anxious. Some research has suggested that the types of personality pathology which are seen in AN and BN differ. Cluster B Personality Disorders, especially those with borderline and narcissistic traits, have been reported to be more prevalent in patients with BN (Johnson and Wonderlich, 1992). In contrast, patients with AN-Restricting Type have been found to have the Cluster C personality disorders characterized by excessive anxiety and drive for perfection, such as Obsessive–Compulsive Personality Disorder (Herzog, Keller, LaVori et al., 1992). A widely used and well-validated instrument for the assessment of personality is the Minnesota Multiphasic Personality Inventory (MMPI-2; Butcher, Dahlstrom, Graham et al., 1989) but many studies which have used it to attempt to identify personality features in AN and BN have yielded disappointing results (Pryor and Weiderman, 1996). In response to the inadequacy of the MMPI identified in previous studies for the delineation of personality disorder differences in AN and BN, Weiderman and Pryor (1997) studied 165 eating disorder patients utilizing the Millon Clinical Multiaxial Inventory-II (MCMI-II, 1987). The authors found that, compared to patients with BN, those with AN restricting type had higher scores on the Dependent scale and lower scores on the Narcissistic, Passive–Aggressive, and Borderline scales. Restricting anorexics scored significantly lower on the Antisocial and Aggressive–Sadistic scales. Patients in the anorexic group also scored significantly higher on the Compulsive scale relative to patients with BN. The results of this study are consistent with previous work with regard to higher scores in patients with BN on the Histrionic and Borderline scales and higher scores on the Dependent and Compulsive scales in patients with AN-Restricting type. A very interesting additional finding in this study concerned the patients with AN-binge-purge type. On the Histrionic, Narcissistic, Antisocial, and Borderline personality scales, these patients occupied a middle position between patients with BN and patients with AN-restricting type. The authors concluded that personality features, or personality psychopathology, may lie along a continuum among patients with disordered eating. Cluster C personality disorder features may correspond to anorexia, restricting type and Cluster B personality features to BN. Anorexic patients with bulimic symptoms may represent a midpoint on the continuum. The authors concluded that patients with pathological eating and weight concerns may seek alleviation of these feeling by behaviors such as binging, purging or restricting, depending on their particular personality features.

As previously discussed, recent biological studies have indicated that disturbances in the serotonin (5-HT) neurotransmitter system are associated with a variety of forms of psychopathology, including aggressive behavior, obsessive compulsive disorder, and eating disorders (Brewerton, 1995; Brown et al., 1982). The clinical symptoms of poor impulse control and aggressive behavior in eating disorder patients has been examined recently by Thompson, Wonderlich, Crosby et al. (1999). In this study, data were gathered from a community-based sample of 3630 girls in grades 6 through 12. The subjects responded to a survey comprised of questions about binges, purging behavior, dietary restrictions, drug use, aggressive behavior, and suicide attempts. The authors found that eating disturbances were significantly associated with aggressive behavior and that subjects who endorsed binge eating, purging or dietary restriction had the highest incidence of aggressive behavior. These results support the findings frequently reported in the clinical literature that BN is associated with behavioral impulsivity and low impulse control (Casper, Hedeker and McClough, 1992). They were surprising, however, in revealing that patients who report dietary restriction also have elevated incidence of aggressivity, a finding which runs counter to the predominant portrait of the restricting anorexic in the clinical literature as a compliant and non-aggressive individual. The authors speculate that these findings may reflect a previously undetected tendency for subjects with eating disturbance, or a subset of such individuals, to exhibit aggression, perhaps due to some trait-based abnormality such as disturbed 5-HT functioning. They further suggest that this subset of patients is unlikely to seek treatment and thus fails to contribute to the prevailing clinical profile of AN, which is derived principally from studies in clinical populations or in individual case reports. This association has important clinical implications for the diagnosis of co-occurring eating disorders and aggressive disorders. It also highlights the problems in the treatment and compliance of eating disorder patients for whom aggression is a prominent clinical feature.

Treatment

Several different categories of treatment have been studied to determine the most effective clinical strategies in the eating disorders. Family therapy has emerged as the most effective. Adolescent bulimic patients and early onset, short history anorectic patients have been shown to have the best outcome with family therapies (Agras, 1991; Russell, Szmukler, Dare et al., 1987). In older patients with eating disorders, superiority of individual therapy has been convincingly demonstrated (Agras, 1991). In successful family and individual treatment of eating disorders, a cognitive/behavioral approach is taken. In cognitive-behavioral therapy, explicit cognitive focus on the identification and modification of attitudes toward body shape and weight is combined with behavioral techniques. These techniques include behavioral contracts, relaxation techniques, graded exposure and response prevention, as well as positive reinforcements using daily logs which include information on feeling states, stressful life events and their relationship to episodes of disturbed eating. Treatment must continue for a sufficient time, not only to restore the weight and eradicate the abnormal eating behaviors, but also to address eating attitudes, depressive affect and family relationships. In one study (Strober, Morrell, Burroughs et al., 1985), significant improvements were observed in weight gain and eating attitudes, as well as in resumption of menses, in patients with AN with the use of both behavioral family therapy and cognitive/behavioral individual treatment.

Psychopharmacologic agents in AN have yielded few promising results in adults. Antidepressants and low dose antipsychotic medications are of little benefit in patients with AN (Becker, Hamburg and Herzog, 1998). There is some recent data (Kaye, Nagata, Weltzin et al., 1998), which suggest that selective serotonin reuptake inhibitors, specifically fluoxetine, may be useful in preventing relapse in weight-restored anorectic patients in remission.

In BN, the news is more hopeful. Antidepressant drugs have consistently proved themselves to be superior to placebo in reducing the binge eating and purging behaviors seen in this disorder (Devlin and Walsh, 1995). Different classes of antidepressants appear to be equally effective (Becker et al., 1998). Recent reports suggest that the combination of antidepressant medication and cognitive behavioral therapy may have a synergistic effect in the treatment of binge/purge cycles, as well as of the depressive symptoms associated with BN (Wilson, Loeb, Walsh et al., 1999).

Recovery and relapse

AN and BN are frequently associated with chronicity and relapse. Fig. 5 presents data from a recent study (Herzog, Dorer, Keel et al., 1999) looking at the full recovery rates over a 7 year period for three types of eating disorders: anorexia nervosa-restricting type (AN-R), anorexia nervosa binge purge type (AN-BP) and bulimia nervosa (BN). As is clear from this graph, the strongest predictor for full recovery was intake diagnosis, with the bulimic patients much more likely to achieve a full recovery than either subtype of AN. At 7 years follow-up, 34% of the ANR subjects, 32% of the AN-BP subjects and 73% of the BN subjects had achieved full recovery. The criteria for full recovery in AN was more stringent in this study than in past studies and was defined as 95% proportion of average body weight (pABW).

A significant majority of the subjects from each of the 3 diagnostic groups, however, attained a partial recovery by a median of 90 months, as Fig. 6 illustrates. Partial recovery was defined in this study as a reduction of symptoms to less than full criteria for at least eight consecutive weeks. 91% of the full sample, 83.7% of the AN subjects and 99% of the BN subjects achieved partial recovery at some time during a median of 90 months of follow-up. In the AN group, longer duration of intake episode, lower pABW and a history of hospitalization predicted delayed onset of partial recovery, while a history of major depressive disorder predicted shorter time to partial recovery. No predictors of recovery emerged for the subjects with BN in this study.

Fig. 7, also from the Herzog study, gives relapse rates for subjects with AN and BN. 40% of AN subjects relapsed after full recovery compared with 35% of BN subjects. No predictors for relapse emerged for either group.

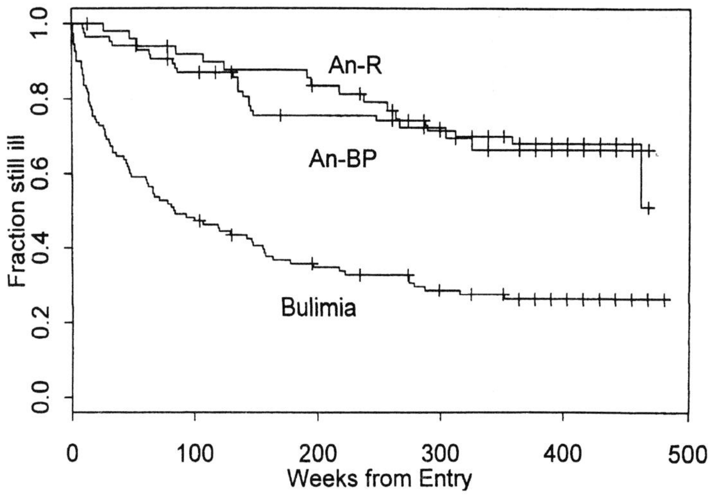

Fig. 5. Full recovery rates.

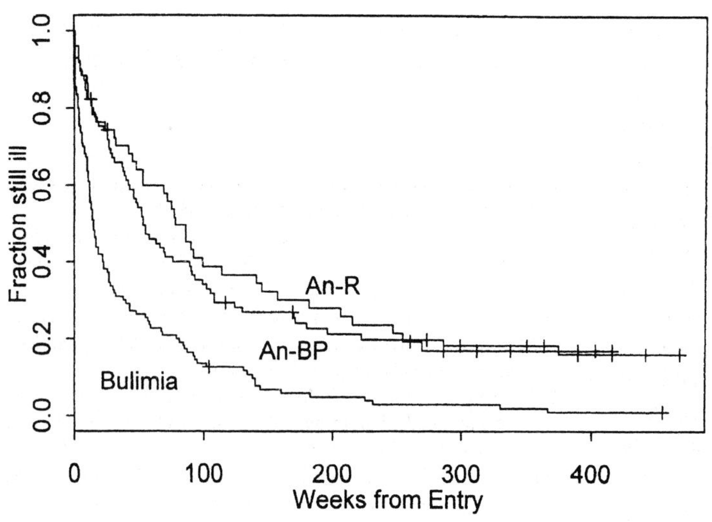

Fig. 6. Partial recovery rates.

Conclusion

Eating disorders occur overwhelmingly in young women and are associated with significant morbidity and mortality. The disorders emerge in mid-adolescence and thus have profound implications for future health as bone mineralization, pubertal development, cardiac health, and cognitive function are major processes which are potentially irreversibly affected by these disorders. Development of an eating disorder during the adolescent years may therefore result in morbidity and mortality many years after the adolescent has recovered from the acute phase of the disorder. The etiology of the eating disorders is still unclear, but a set of factors, including biological, psychological and social, is probably at work in the expression and course of the disorders. Neuropsychological research, including neuroimaging studies, have begun to shed some light on the impact on neuropsychological function of having an eating disorder. In AN, these findings include abnormal structural findings such as enlarged

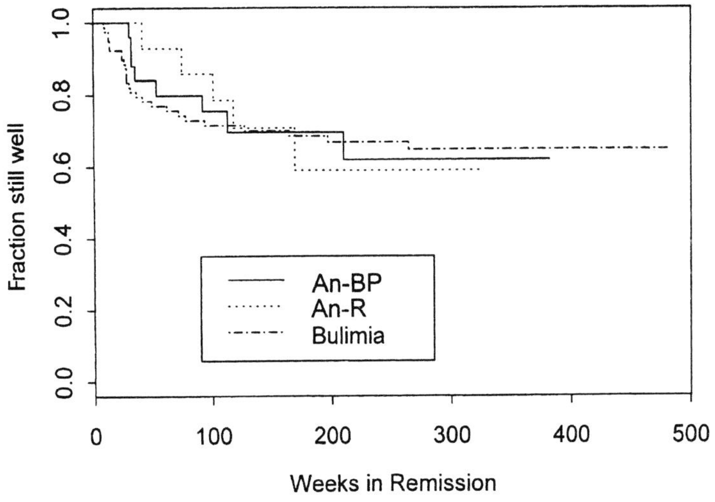

Fig. 7. Relapse rates.

CSF spaces and reduction in white and gray matter. These imaging findings are correlated with the degree of malnutrition, and are not fully reversed with weight restoration. Associated neuropsychological abnormalities in AN include impairment in attention and memory function as well as abnormalities in visuospatial domains. Further investigation will be necessary to fully understand the neuropsychological effects of AN and to discover if BN also affects neuropsychological functioning. In recent, well-designed studies, psychological treatment, both family and individual with a cognitive/behavioral approach, have been shown to be helpful in improving the symptoms of both AN and BN. Studies of antidepressant treatments alone, as well as in combination with psychological treatments, especially family therapy and individual cognitive/behavioral therapy, have been effective in the treatment of BN. Psychopharmacologic agents have not been useful in the treatment of AN, though they may have a role in preventing relapse. The course and outcome of AN and BN are substantially different. In AN, the course is more chronic, with a much lower full recovery rate and a somewhat higher relapse rate than BN.

The chronic course of the eating disorders in many patients suggests the need to identify these problems early and to intervene before the disorders become full-blown and intractable. The association between longer duration of episode and worse outcome may represent greater efficacy of treatment if it is initiated early in the course of these disorders.

References

Agras WS: Nonpharmacologic treatments of bulimia nervosa. Journal of Clinical Psychiatry: 52; 233, 1991.

Altemus M, Glowa JR, Murphy DL: Attenuation of food-restiction-induced running by chronic fluoxetine treatment. Psychopharmacology Bulletin: 29; 397–400, 1993.

American Psychiatric Association: Diagnostic and Statistical Manual of Mental Disorders, Fourth Edition. Washington, DC: American Psychiatric Association, 1994.

Ballenger JC, Goodwin FG, Major LF et al.: Alcohol and central serotonin metabolism in man. Archives of General Psychiatry: 36; 224–227, 1979.

Becker AE, Grinspoon SY, Klibanski A et al.: Eating disorders. New England Journal of Medicine: 340; 1092–1098, 1999.

Becker AE, Hamburg P, Herzog DB: The role of psychopharmacologic management in the treatment of eating disorders. In Dunner DL, Rosenbaum JF (Eds), Annual of Drug Therapy. Philadelphia: W.B. Saunders, pp. 17–51, 1998.

Benton AL: Revised Visual Retention Test: Clinical and Experimental Applications. New York: The Psychological Corporation, 1974.

Braun DL, Sunday SR, Huang A et al.: More males seek treatment for eating disorders. International Journal of Eating Disorders: 25; 415–425, 1999.

Brewerton T: Toward a unified theory of serotonin dysregulation in eating and related disorders. Psychoneuroendocrinology: 20; 561–590, 1995.

Brewerton TD, Stellefson EJ, Hibbs N et al.: Comparison of eating disorder patients with and without compulsive exercising. International Journal of Eating Disorders: 17; 413–416, 1995.

Brown GL, Ebert MH, Goyer PF et al.: Aggression, suicide and serotonin: relationships to CSF amine metabolites. American Journal of Psychiatry: 139; 741–746, 1982.

Bruch H: Perceptual and cognitive disturbances in anorexia nervosa. Psychosomatic Medicine: 24; 187–194, 1962.

Bruch H: Eating Disorders. New York: Basic Books Inc., 1973.

Butcher JN, Dahlstrom WG, Graham JR et al.: Minnesota Multiphasic Personality Inventory (MMPI-2): Manual for Administration and Scoring. Minneapolis: University of Minnesota Press, 1989.

Carlat DJ, Camargo CA, Herzog DDB: Eating disorders in males: A report on 135 patients. American Journal of Psychiatry: 154; 1127–1132, 1997.

Casper RC, Hedeker D, McClough JF: Personality dimensions in eating disorders and their relevance for subtypes. Journal of the American Academy of Child and Adolescent Psychiatry: 31; 830–840, 1992.

Castro J, Lazaro L, Pons F et al.: Predictors of bone mineral density reduction in adolescents with anorexia nervosa. Journal of the American Academy of Child and Adolescent Psychiatry: 39; 1365–1370, 2000.

Chabrol H, Callahan S, O'Halloran S: The pressure to be thin on adolescent girls in ancient Rome. Journal of the American Academy of Child and Adolescent Psychiatry: 39; 1345–1346, 2000.

Charney DS, Goodman WK, Price LH et al.: Serotonin function in obsessive–compulsive disorder: a comparison of the effects of tryptophan and m-chlorophenylperazine in patients and healthy subjects. Archives of General Psychiatry: 45; 177–185, 1988.

Cord FS, Melville D, Gibbs J et al.: Effect of fourth ventricular neuropeptide Y and peptide YY on ingestive and other behaviors. American Journal of Physiology: 259; 1013–1023, 1990.

Devlin M, Walsh T: Medication treatment for eating disorders. Journal of Mental Health: 4; 459–469, 1995.

Dura J, Bornstein R: Differences between IQ and school achievement in anorexia nervosa. Journal of Clinical Psychology: 45; 433–435, 1989.

Epling WF, Pierce WD: Activity-based anorexia in rats as a function of opportunity run on an activity wheel. Nutrition and Behavior: 2; 37–49, 1984.

Epling WF, Pierce WD: Activity-based anorexia: A biobehavioral perspective. International Journal of Eating Disorders: 7; 475–485, 1988.

Fairburn C, Cooper Z, Doll H et al.: Risk factors for anorexia nervosa. Archives of General Psychiatry: 56; 468–476, 1999.

Ferguson C, LaVia M, Crossan P et al.: Are serotonin selective reuptake inhibitors effective in underweight anorexia nervosa? International Journal of Eating Disorders: 25; 11–17, 1999.

Ferron F, Considine R, Peino R et al.: Serum leptin concentrations in patients with anorexia nervosa, bulimia nervosa and non-specific eating disorders correlate with the body mass index but are independent of the respective disease. Clinical Endocrinology: 46; 289–293, 1997.

Field A, Camargo C, Taylor C et al.: Peer, parent and media influences on the development of weight concerns and frequent dieting among preadolescent and adolescent girls and boys. Pediatrics: 107; 54–60, 2001.

Fluoxetine Bulimia Nervosa Collaborative Study Group: Fluoxetine in the treatment of bulimia nervosa. Archives of General Psychiatry: 49; 139–147, 1992.

Fox C: Neuropsychological correlates of anorexia nervosa. International Journal of Psychiatry in Medicine: 11; 285–290, 1982.

Gillberg I, Gillberg C, Rastam M et al.: The cognitive profile of anorexia nervosa: A comparative study including a community-based sample. Comprehensive Psychiatry: 37; 23–30, 1996.

Golden N, Ashtari M, Kohn M et al.: Reversibility of cerebral ventricular enlargement in anorexia nervosa, demonstrated by quantitative magnetic resonance imaging. Journal of Pediatrics: 128; 296–301, 1996.

Grinspoon S, Gulick T, Askari H et al.: Serum leptin levels in women with anorexia nervosa. Journal of Clinical Endocrinology and Metabolism: 81; 3861–3863, 1996.

Gull W: anorexia nervosa. Lancet: 1; 516–517, 1888.

Gura T: Tracing leptons partners in regulating body weight. Science: 287; 1738–1741, 2000.

Hagen M, Castaneda E, Sumaya I et al.: The effect of hypothalamic peptide YY on hippocampal acetylcholine release in vivo: Implications for limbic function in binge-eating behavior. Brain Research: 805; 20–28, 1998.

Halmi K, Eckert E, LaDu T et al.: Anorexia nervosa: Treatment efficacy of Cyproheptidine and Amitriptyline. Archives of General Psychiatry: 43; 177–181, 1986.

Hamsher K, Halmi K, Benton A: Prediction of outcome in anorexia nervosa from neuropsychological status. Psychiatry Research: 4; 79–88, 1981.

Herzog DB, Dorer DJ, Keel PK et al.: Recovery and relapse in anorexia nervosa and bulimia nervosa: A 7.5 year follow-up study. Journal of the American Academy of Child and Adolescent Psychiatry: 38(7); 829–837, 1999.

Herzog DB, Keller MB, LaVori P et al.: The prevalence of personality disorders in 210 women with eating disorders. Journal of Clinical Psychiatry: 53; 147–152, 1992.

Holland AJ, Hall A, Murray R et al.: Anorexia nervosa: A study of 34 pairs of twins and one set of triplets. British Journal of Psychiatry: 145; 414–419, 1984.

Holland AJ, Sicotte N, Treasure J: Anorexia nervosa: Evidence for a genetic basis. Journal of Psychosomatic Research: 32; 561–571, 1988.

Horne RL, Van Vactor JC, Emerson S: Disturbed body image in patients with eating disorders. American Journal of Psychiatry: 148; 211–215, 1991.

Hsu LK: Epidemiology of the eating disorders. Psychiatric Clinics of North America: 19; 681–700, 1996.

Hudson J, McElroy S, Raymond N et al.: Fluvoxamine in the treatment of Binge-eating Disorder: A multicenter placebo-controlled, double-blind trial. American Journal of Psychiatry: 155; 1756–1762, 1998.

Jimerson D, Lesem M, Kaye W et al.: Eating disorders and depression: Is there a serotonin connection? Biological Psychiatry: 26; 443–454, 1990.

Jimerson D, Wolfe B, Metzger E et al.: Decreased serotonin function in bulimia nervosa. Archives of General Psychiatry: 54; 529–534, 1997.

Johnson C, Wonderlich S: Personality characteristics as a risk factor in the development of eating disorders. In Crowther JH, Tennenbaum DL, Hobfoll SE et al. (Eds), The Etiology of Bulimia Nervosa. Philadelphia: Hemisphere, pp. 179–196, 1992.

Kaplan HI, Sadock BJ: Synopsis of Psychiatry. Philadelphia: Williams and Wilkins, 1998.

Katzman D, Lambe E, Mikulis D et al.: Cerebral gray matter and white matter volume deficits in adolescent girls with anorexia nervosa. Journal of Pediatrics: 129; 794–803, 1996.

Katzman D, Zipursky R, Lambe E et al.: A longitudinal magnetic resonance imaging study of brain changes in adolescents with anorexia nervosa. Archives of Pediatric and Adolescent Medicine: 151; 793–797, 1997.

Kaye WH: Paper presented at the 150th meeting of the American Psychiatric Association, San Diego, Ca, 17 to 22 May, 1997.

Kaye W, Berrettini W, Gwirtsman H et al.: Altered cerebrospinal fluid neuropeptide Y and peptide YY immunoreactivity in anorexia and bulimia nervosa. Archives of General Psychiatry: 47; 548–556, 1990.

Kaye W, Gwirtsman H, George D et al.: Altered serotonin activity in anorexia nervosa after long-term weight restoration. Archives of General Psychiatry: 48; 556–562, 1991.

Kaye WH, Nagata T, Weltzin TE et al.: Successful outcome of restricting type anorexia nervosa after the double-blind placebo-controlled administration of Fluoxetine. Manuscript submitted for publication, 1998.

Kaye W, Weltzin T: Serotonin activity in anorexia and bulimia nervosa: Relationship to the modulation of feeding and mood. Journal of Clinical Psychiatry: 52; 41–48, 1991.

Kingston K, Szmukler G, Tress A et al.: Neuropsychological and structural brain changes in anorexia nervosa before and after refeeding. Psychological Medicine: 26; 15–28, 1996.

Kowalski P: Cognitive abilities of female adolescents with anorexia nervosa. International Journal of Eating Disorders: 5; 983–997, 1986.

Lambe E, Katzman D, Mikulis D et al.: Cerebral gray matter volume deficits after weight recovery from anorexia nervosa. Archives of General Psychiatry: 54; 537–542, 1997.

Mathias J, Kent P: Neuropsychological consequences of extreme weight loss and dietary restriction in patients with anorexia nervosa. Journal of Clinical and Experimental Neuropsychology: 20; 548–564, 1988.

Mattis S: Mattis Organic Mental Syndromes Screening Examination. Unpublished, 1978.

Nakai Y, Hamagaki S, Kato S et al.: Leptin in women with eating disorders. Metabolism: 8; 217–220, 1999.

Palazidou E, Robinson P, Lishman WA: Neuroradiological and neuropsychological assessment in anorexia nervosa. Psychological Medicine: 20; 521–527, 1990.

Patton GC, Selzer R, Coffey C et al.: Onset of adolescent eating disorders: population based cohort study over 3 years. British Medical Journal: 318; 765–768, 1999.

Pryor T: Diagnostic Criteria for eating disorders: DSM-IV revisions. Psychiatric Annals: 25; 40–45, 1995.

Pryor T, Weiderman M: Use of the MMPI-2 in the outpatient assessment of women with anorexia nervosa or bulimia nervosa. Journal of Personality Assessment: 66; 363–373, 1996.

Reitan RM: Validity of the Trail Making Test as an Indicator of Organic Brain Damage. Perceptual and Motor Skills: 8; 271–276, 1958.

Russell GF, Szmukler GI, Dare C et al.: An evaluation of family therapy in anorexia nervosa and bulimia nervosa. Archives of General Psychiatry: 44; 1047–1056, 1987.

Seidman SN, Reider RD: A review of sexual behavior in the US. American Journal of Psychiatry: 151; 330–341, 1994.

Strober M, Morrell W, Burroughs J et al.: A controlled family study of anorexia nervosa. Journal of Psychiatric Research: 19; 239–246, 1985.

Szmukler G, Andrewes D, Kingston K et al.: Neuropsychological impairment in anorexia nervosa: before and after refeeding. Journal of Clinical and Experimental Neuropsychology: 14; 347–352, 1992.

Thompson KM, Wonderlich SA, Crosby RD et al.: The neglected link between eating disturbances and aggressive behavior in girls. Journal of the American Academy of Child and Adolescent Psychiatry: 38; 1277–1284, 1999.

Wade T, Martin M, Neale MC et al.: The structure of genetic and environmental risk factors for three measures of disordered eating. Psychological Medicine: 29; 925–934, 1999.

Walsh BT, Devlin MJ: Eating disorders: progress and problems. Science: 280; 1387–1390, 1998.

Warren M, Voussoughian F, Geer E et al.: Functional hypothalamic amenorrhea: hypoleptinemia and disordered eating. Journal of Clinical Endocrinology and Metabolism: 84; 873–877, 1999.

Weiderman M, Pryor T: MCMI-II personality scale scores among women with anorexia nervosa or bulimia nervosa. Journal of Personality Assessment: 69; 508–516, 1997.

Wilson G, Loeb K, Walsh B et al.: Psychological versus pharmacological treatments of bulimia nervosa: Predictors and processes of change. Journal of Consulting and Clinical Psychology: 69; 451–459, 1999.

Wonderlich S, Fullerton D, Swift W et al.: Five-year outcome from eating disorders: relevance of personality disorders. International Journal of Eating Disorders: 15; 233–243, 1994.

Woodside DB, Garner DM, Rockert W et al.: Males with eating disorders. New York: Brunner/Mazel, 1990.

Handbook of Neuropsychology, 2nd Edition, Vol. 8, Part II
S.J. Segalowitz and I. Rapin (Eds)

CHAPTER 33

Autism spectrum disorders

Nancy J. Minshew [a,*], Jessica A. Meyer [b] and Michelle Dunn [c]

[a] *Departments of Psychiatry and Neurology, University of Pittsburgh School of Medicine, 3811 O'Hara Street, Pittsburgh, PA 15213, USA*
[b] *Department of Psychology, Lousiana State University, 2356 Drusilla Lane, Baton Rouge, LA 70809, USA*
[c] *Albert Einstein College of Medicine, 1300 Morris Park Avenue, Bronx, NY 10461, USA*

Introduction

Autism [1] is a behaviorally defined developmental syndrome characterized by distinctive abnormalities in social behavior, verbal and nonverbal language and its use for communication, imaginative play, and a restricted range of interests and activities. It is the prototype for a cluster of disorders formally referred to as pervasive developmental disorders (PDDs) but more popularly as autism spectrum disorders (ASDs). The disorders in this category share the same 'autistic-like' behavior, meaning that the quality of the symptoms are the same (Lord and Risi, 1998). They are differentiated by variations in their severity relative to age and general level of function or, in the case of Asperger's disorder, by an absence of abnormalities in language development. Currently, the ASDs include autistic disorder, Asperger's disorder, pervasive developmental disorder not otherwise specified, childhood disintegrative disorder, Rett's disorder, and, in ICD-10, atypical autism. Rett's disorder was included in this category because of the regression at presentation that also characterizes 25% of cases of autism, but it is otherwise a very different disorder clinically, neurologically, and neuropathologically from the other ASDs. Childhood disintegrative disorder refers to children experiencing neurologic deterioration or regression between 2 and 12 years of age, after the establishment of extensive language. Given the broad age range and differing stages of brain development, this category is likely to represent a diverse group etiologically. Those children regressing at 2–3 years of age after developing extensive sentence language are properly diagnosed as having childhood disintegrative disorder rather than autism; they often have prominent problems with seizures and have been the target of treatment with steroids, if the EEG indicates active temporal lobe epileptogenic activity and therefore unresponsive to conventional antiepileptic medications.

Recent scientific advances

Remarkable progress has occurred in the field of autism in the past 10 years. Estimates of the prevalence of autism have increased 12-fold world-wide from the pre-1980 estimates of 4–5/10,000 for infantile autism to 60/10,000 for autistic disorder, Asperger's disorder, and pervasive developmental disorder not otherwise specified (Chakrabarti and Fombonne, 2001). Some of this increase is thought to represent improved recognition at the two ends of the spectrum, but the actual number of cases has risen significantly due to unknown causes. Diagnostic criteria are now consistent across the two

* Corresponding author. Tel.: +1-412-624-0818; Fax: +1-412-624-0930; E-mail: minshewnj@msx.upmc.edu

[1] The term 'autism' is used instead of 'autistic disorder' or 'classic autism' or 'Kannerian autism'.

classification systems (DSM and ICD), and considerable progress has been made in defining the cognitive and neurologic basis of the odd behavior that is the hallmark of autism. Autism is also now widely viewed as a familial genetic disorder, with family members expressing the broader autism phenotype (BAP), obsessive compulsive disorder, affective disorder, anxiety disorder, developmental language disorder, and possibly attention deficit disorder and macrocephaly. Genetic evidence suggests that it is a polygenetic disorder resulting from at least 4–6 interacting genes, but not the same 4–6 in all cases, and chromosomes 7 and 15 have been the first identified as containing autism-related genes. Candidate genes on chromosome 7 are under active study, including the reelin gene which is adjacent to the selective language impairment gene and a break point identified in an autism case (Persico, D'Agruma, Maiorano et al., 2001). Teratologic studies of thalidomide and valproic acid have suggested that *HOXA1* and *HOXB1* genes may play a role in autism in cases with congenital abnormalities of the facial nerve nuclei (Ingram, Croog, Tisdale and Rodier, 1996; Rodier, Ingram, Tisdale and Croog, 1997) and possibly in other cases of autism (Ingram, Stodgell, Hyman et al., 2000). All such studies require replication before results can be considered to be valid and applicable to autism. Nelson, Grether, Croen et al. (2001) have reported abnormalities in neurotrophin levels in the newborn blood spots of children later diagnosed with autism or mental retardation but not typically developing children or those with cerebral palsy.

The brain localization for the behavioral syndrome is now thought to be at the neural systems level involving the underdevelopment of the connections within and between neural systems (Minshew, Luna and Sweeney, 1999). The sparse data on the histologic and gross anatomy of the brain suggest abnormalities in developmental events, such as the elaboration and pruning of the dendritic tree and synaptogenesis. Clinical studies have reported an increase in mean head circumference with a significant subset having megalencephaly, consistent with reports of increased brain weight and volume. These findings further support abnormalities in brain developmental events. Reports of improvement in outcome with early behavioral intervention have changed the approach to treatment and increased the urgency of early diagnosis. The introduction of the potent serotonin transporter inhibitors has provided an important pharmacological adjunct to environmental modification and behavioral intervention.

Historical background

The clinical syndrome of autism was initially described in elegant detail in a series of papers by Leo Kanner (1943, 1971; Kanner, Rodrigues and Ashenden, 1972) as a developmental disorder of 'affective contact' with an onset in the first 2–3 years of life and a marked tendency towards improvement after the preschool years in the majority of cases. Kanner identified two cardinal symptoms: the inability to relate to people and situations in the ordinary way and an anxiously obsessive desire to maintain sameness, the latter symptom evolving with age into obsessive preoccupations in the speaking children. After a similar early 'autistic-like' presentation (Kanner, 1943), Kanner reported significant gains in function in 60% of the children and a wide divergence in outcome in later childhood and adulthood, leading him to conclude that autism, like most disorders, occurred across a wide range of severity (Kanner, 1971). However, even those non-mentally retarded autistic individuals from Kanner's clinic who were independent and self-sufficient as adults, retained the basic features or qualities of their early deficits, which had a major adverse impact on their job status and personal life (Kanner et al., 1972).

In ensuing decades, two distortions altered 'Kannerian autism'. The first was its categorization as a psychotic disorder. When autism was first added to the diagnostic classification system in DSM-II, it was classified as a form of childhood schizophrenia because of the overlap in negative symptoms that had led to the borrowing of the term 'autism' from the schizophrenia literature. Kanner had attempted to prevent this by emphasizing the absence in autism of the positive symptoms of schizophrenia and the discontinuity in age of onset. Although removed from the psychotic disorders category in DSM-III, this overlap in negative symptoms, together with the general lack of awareness of high-functioning autism among adult psychiatrists and psychologists, remains responsible for the frequent misdiagnosis of verbal autistic adults as having schizophrenia or schizotypal personality disorder.

The second distortion of Kanner's autism was the loss of appreciation of verbal individuals as part of the autism spectrum to the point that 'classic autism' or 'Kannerian autism' came to be equated with those individuals with echolalia or limited stereotyped language and IQ scores between 50 and 70. This stereotype of autism resulted in the hypothesis that low- and high-functioning autism represented different disorders, which was reflected in DSM-III in the distinction made between infantile autism and childhood onset pervasive developmental disorder. Improvement in symptoms with age resulted in the addition of 'residual state' as a modifier. Another notable change apparent in DSM-III was the introduction of the term 'pervasive developmental disorder', which was coined for autism and autistic-like disorders to emphasize the pervasive impact on real life function of the selective deficits in social, communication, and abstract reasoning abilities. This new term created its own problems, though, because it did not connote autism and was therefore meaningless to professionals and families alike.

When field trials failed to support a clinical distinction between low-and high-functioning autism, childhood onset pervasive developmental disorder was eliminated from the classification system and the spectrum of severity originally described by Kanner was once again united as autistic disorder in DSM-III-R. The natural history of improvement was also recognized and the residual state modifier eliminated. The 'disorder' modifier added to autism was a generalized policy of DSM-III-R and did not signify a different clinical syndrome than that previously referred to as infantile autism or autism. The focus of diagnostic research then shifted to defining the boundaries of autism at the two extremes of function and differentiating autism from other disorders within the PDD category. The definition and validity of such distinctions was made possible by the development of structured diagnostic research instruments, the Autism Diagnostic Interview (ADI-R, Lord, Rutter and Le Couteur, 1994) and Autism Diagnostic Observation Schedule (ADOS-G; Le Couteur, Rutter and Lord, 1989), and their uniform and reliable use based on shared training and maintenance of reliability across research centers internationally. The understanding of the diagnostic distinctions arrived at through the use of these instruments did not extend outside of research centers. Such distinctions were based on severity of symptoms relative to age and IQ of the individual and thus were dependent on the evaluator having experience with hundreds of cases of autism spectrum disorder and access to research diagnostic instruments too time consuming and narrowly focused for clinical practice. Such distinctions were also not amenable to the brief checklist format of the classification systems and, thus, the clinical community was left to contend with the resulting diagnostic subgroups without the requisite background or instruments. Distinctions within the pervasive developmental disorder, such as between high functioning autism and Asperger's disorder or autistic disorder and PDDNOS, are not reliably made in clinical practice. In actuality, such distinctions are clinically unimportant as the treatment for all PDDs is the same and the primary factor is the functional level of the individual.

In DSM-IV (American Psychiatric Association, 1994) and ICD-10 (World Health Organization, 1992), the diagnostic criteria for autism achieved uniformity internationally. In addition, Asperger's disorder was added as a formal diagnosis. The introduction of the Asperger's disorder diagnosis some 50 years after its description was largely motivated by the resistance of families and pediatricians to the use of the term autism in verbal children. It was also based on the hypothesis that absence of early developmental language abnormalities would predict a less severe outcome than in high-functioning autism. Research thus far has not supported this hypothesis, in that normal early language development does not portend the absence of later semantic pragmatic language impairments. Differences in various other deficits have also generally been shown to be related to IQ, rather than distinguishing between autism and Asperger's disorder. Additional subdivisions within the PDD category are not likely to be pursued until there is biologic evidence to guide their validity.

The challenge for the future will be to integrate into the classification system the behavioral syndromes associated with fragile-X syndrome, tuberous sclerosis, the nonverbal learning disability syndrome, social phobia, and schizoid personality disorder. Progress is also needed in defining the cognitive basis of the restricted range of interests and repetitive behavior, and there is a great need for new assessment tools that capture the social, communication, and problem-solving deficits found in the ASDs.

Demographics

Prevalence

Epidemiological studies prior to 1985 reported prevalence estimates of 4–5/10,000 for *autism* (for a comprehensive review, see Wing, 1993). Estimates of prevalence have been increasing since then. Most non-U.S. studies since 1985 have yielded prevalence rates of 10/10,000 or 1/1000 for *autism* (for reviews see: Bryson and Smith, 1998; Gillberg and Wing, 1999; see also: Deb and Prasad, 1994; Gillberg, Steffenburg and Schaumann, 1991; Nordin and Gillberg, 1996; Webb, Lobo, Hervas and Scourfield, 1996; Wignyosumatro, Mukhlas and Hirataki, 1992), but not always (for review see: Fombonne, 1998). Even higher prevalence rates of 13–21/10,000 were reported in five of six studies from Japan (Honda, Shimizu, Misumi and Niimi, 1996; Ishii and Takahashi, 1983; Matsuishi, Shiotsuki, Yoshimura et al., 1987; Sugiyama and Abe, 1989; Tanoue, Oda, Asano and Kawashima, 1988). These studies directly evaluated all young children with any developmental or behavioral abnormality, thus avoiding the major limitations imposed on ascertainment in other epidemiologic studies. The most recent study from Sweden reported an even higher prevalence for autism of 31/10,000 (Arvidsson, Danielsson, Forsberg et al., 1997) as has a study from Great Britain (Baird, Charman, Baron-Cohen et al., 2000). The rise in prevalence rates in the past 10 years has been attributed to improving recognition, especially at IQs below 50 and above 70 (Bryson, 1996; Gillberg et al., 1991; Wing, 1993), but there also appears to be an actual increase in prevalence.

The prevalence of *pervasive developmental disorders other than autism* has not been well studied but available evidence suggests that collectively these other disorders are more common than autism. In a review of 19 epidemiological studies, the ratio of the other pervasive developmental disorders to autism ranged from 1.44 to 4.33 to 1 with a mean of 2.6 (Fombonne, 1998). Wing and Gould (1979) examined a broader range of pervasive developmental disorders and reported a total prevalence rate of 21/10,000 for autistic disorder, atypical autism, and pervasive developmental disorder not otherwise specified. This led to the commonly cited prevalence of 1/500 for autism. Gillberg and colleagues have proposed a rate of 40–50 per 10,000 children for autistic disorder, Asperger's disorder, atypical autism, and disintegrative disorder (Gillberg and Wing, 1999), based in part on their prevalence estimates for Asperger's disorder of 26–36/10,000 (Ehlers and Gillberg, 1993; Kadesjoe, Gillberg and Hagberg, 1999). A recent study from England has reported provisional rates of 31/10,000 for autism and 27/10,000 for other PDDs, for a total of 58/10,000 or 1 : 170 for autistic disorder, Asperger's disorder, and PDDNOS (Baird et al., 2000). A recent study of the New Jersey Bricks Township cluster by the United States Center for Disease Control and Prevention reported rates of 40/10,000 for autism, 27/10,000 for other PDDs and 67/10,000 for all PDDs or 1 : 150 for autism spectrum disorders. The Brick township figures are proposed to be higher than earlier estimates as a result of more intense case finding, and thus are a more accurate estimate of true prevalence in the United States. The latest study (Chakrabarti and Fombonne, 2001) reports 17/10,000 for autistic disorder, 46/10,000 for other PDDs, for a total of 63/10,000 or 1 : 160 for autistic disorder, Asperger's disorder and PDDNOS.

Gender

Autism is more common in males with a 3–4 : 1 male to female ratio (Gillberg and Wing, 1999). The proportion of males to females varies with IQ, approaching 1.7 : 1 or less in severe and profoundly mentally retarded individuals and as high as 15 : 1 in those without mental retardation (Bryson, 1997; Ehlers and Gillberg, 1993; Fombonne, 1998; Wing and Gould, 1979). Females with autism are therefore typically more severely affected than males. The lower frequency and greater severity of autism in females has been cited as evidence for a multifactorial polygenic mode of inheritance with differential loading by sex, which predicts greater severity in the less frequently affected sex (Lord, Schopler and Revicki, 1982; Tsai, Stewart and August, 1981). Others have proposed that higher-ability females are underrepresented because they are less socially impaired than their male counterparts and thus escape recognition (McLennan, Lord and Schopler, 1993; Volkmar, Szatmari and Sparrow, 1993).

Socioeconomic status

Epidemiological studies since 1980 have shown no relationship between socioeconomic status and the prevalence of autism (Fombonne, 1998; Gillberg, Schaumann and Gillberg, 1995). There is no documented predisposition on the basis of race, ethnic or geographic origin, but data on these factors are limited to absent.

Severity

Autism occurs across a broad range of severity of which Verbal IQ scores and level of functional language are the best available indices of *relative* severity *within* the autism population. The normal IQ scores of non-mentally retarded autistic individuals do not mean that they are minimally impaired, only that they have a higher level of general ability than mentally retarded individuals with autism and that IQ scores no longer reflect their social, language, and problem-solving deficits. When non-retarded autistic individuals are compared to IQ-matched non-autistic peers, the severity of their disability is as great as for mentally retarded autistic individuals (McLennan et al., 1993; Volkmar et al., 1993). This is reflected in a study of Vineland Adaptive Behavior Scores (VABS) reporting that the discrepancy between IQ scores and VABS scores was small in mentally retarded autistic and non-autistic individuals but was larger in normal-IQ autistic individuals (Schatz and Hamdan-Allen, 1995). That is, the gap between IQ and adaptive function is wider in autism at higher IQs than at lower IQs. The implication of this dissociation is that IQ scores are not predictive of function in real life in verbal individuals with autism and assessment of adaptive function is essential.

IQ distribution

Autism occurs across the entire range of IQ scores. There is no IQ score too high or too low that excludes a diagnosis of autism. However, the majority of individuals with *autism* have been thought to have IQ scores in the mentally retarded range. An analysis of 19 studies conducted over the past 30 years found that approximately 24% of autistic individuals are within the normal range of intellectual functioning, 22% in the mild to moderate range of mental retardation, and 55% in the severe to profound range of mental retardation (Fombonne, 1998). Other studies have reported that about 50% have IQ scores below 50 and are considered to be in the severe range of autism (Gillberg et al., 1991; Tsai and Beisler, 1983).

The proportion of individuals who are mentally retarded is considerably lower for the other pervasive developmental disorders. Individuals with Asperger's disorder are by definition verbal and have IQ scores in the normal or mildly mentally retarded range. In addition, the diagnoses of atypical autism and pervasive developmental disorder not otherwise specified are often used instead of autism for higher-ability individuals. If Asperger's disorder is as prevalent as recent studies suggest, then the proportion of individuals with PDD that are non-retarded could approach 70% as was found in the recent British study (Baird et al., 2000). This shift is supported by the rising proportion of preschoolers who have normal IQ scores at diagnosis. Clinicians should therefore expect that a substantial proportion of individuals identified as having pervasive developmental disorder will be verbal and have IQ scores in the normal range.

Clinical syndrome

Clinical features

Autism is defined by specific qualitative abnormalities in social behavior, language and communication, pretend play, and a restricted range of interests and activities. It occurs across a broad range of severity, which is further modified by developmental changes.

The essential quality of the social behavior in autism is impaired reciprocity, i.e., loss of the coordinated and flexible quality of verbal and nonverbal social interchanges. Reciprocity is independent of the amount of interaction, as it can be equally impaired in those who interact too much and those who interact too little; both are missing the social cues as to what is appropriate. The most severe expression of this impairment is seen in the total detachment of the most severely autistic individuals who fail to respond to or initiate social approaches. The intermediate expression is the individual who approaches others only for wants and needs using functional echolalia, phrases, or stereotyped sentences (simple scripts). Less severely impaired individuals with autism participate in conversational interchanges, but these typically take the form of endless questions or monologues and typically focus on the individual's obsessive interests; the epitome of social reciprocity, chit chat, is beyond them. In the least impaired individuals, the scripted nature of their interchanges is often not appreciated unless: they are seen multiple times allowing an opportunity for chit chat, a topic comes up they have not thought about and created a script for, or an observer is present during their interactions with different conversational partners who can attest to the word for word repetition of their 'conversation'. The deterioration in the content and quality of their conversation on unfamiliar topics and the scripted nature of their conversations on familiar topics is often striking but also often unappreciated.

The cognitive basis of the impairment in social reciprocity involves deficits in multiple abilities, but the defining deficit is in the automatic, non-conscious capacity for making inferences about the knowledge, thoughts, feelings, and intentions of others known as theory of mind abilities. Testable individuals with autism have deficits in theory of mind or perspective-taking abilities. Their understanding of others' minds is further limited by deficits in the comprehension of verbal language, prosody, facial expression, eye contact, and body language. The collective impact of these deficits is that interactions do not have that coordinated and moment-to-moment flexibility inherent to true conversation. Instead, social interchanges become 'collisions' or 'fly-bys'.

The language and communication impairments are characterized by deficits in the comprehension and *use of* language for communication. The inclusion of both language and communication in the characterization reflects the dissociation that occurs when language is present but not used for communication or used inappropriately. In *autism*, but not Asperger's disorder, language development is delayed and displays odd features such as echolalia, pronoun reversals, and stereotyped language. At outcome, language ranges from none (muteness), to echolalia, to the functional use of echolalia, to single words or phrases used spontaneously and appropriately, to a limited number of stereotyped sentences, to simple poorly articulated sentences with grammatical errors and incorrect word order, to sentences with correct grammar but residual deficits in the comprehension of idioms, metaphors, verbal inferences, paragraphs, and themes of stories. Nonverbal language, e.g., eye contact, prosody, facial expression and body language, is also impaired. They do not understand messages communicated nonverbally, nor do they use those modes of communication. Eye contact is absent in the most impaired individuals, glancing or brief at intermediate levels of function, and sustained but lacking in modulation at high levels of function. Facial expression is typically masked, though some have only one expression or have stilted practiced facial expressions. It is therefore difficult to determine how the child feels or is reacting by his or her expressions. Prosody or tone of voice is typically a monotone, too loud and occasionally too soft, or erratic. Gestures are similarly affected, being absent, occasional or limited to a few taught commonly used ones. Impaired body language is often reflected in their lack of appreciation of social space or their stiffness or lack of molding when held.

Impairments in pretend play are also an integral part of autism spectrum disorders. Initially, this is expressed as a lack of interest in toys that require understanding of their symbolic meaning for appropriate use as opposed to infant toys, which do not. With developmental progress, the functional use of such toys develops followed by the emergence of play sequences. Play is typically stereotyped with little variability or creativity, though the verbatim re-enactment of movies or videos or use of television game show or news reporting scripts can often deceive adults into thinking these children are imaginative. In addition to impaired creativity, their play often lacks the social content of typical children's play, focusing instead on the objects. Observation of spontaneous play with figures and responses to play overtures, as is done in the Autism Diagnostic Observation Schedule, gives a remarkably accurate view of social function and the capacity for creating logical and imaginative sequences of events. High-functioning children with autism quickly shift from toy play to video and computer games at which they excel because of their superb rote memory. Preoccupation with game shows, such as Wheel of Fortune and Jeopardy, is also typical.

The restricted range of activities and repetitive behavior category encompasses a range of superficially unrelated behavior. The cognitive basis of this behavior has not been demonstrated but the cognitive constellation of enhanced awareness and focus on details with impaired abstraction is the likely common denominator. The stereotypic behavior (repetitive hand movements, flapping, rocking, vocalizations) is nonspecific to autism but disproportionate to IQ level, reflecting the disproportionate loss of adaptive behavior as a result of the social, language, and reasoning deficits. The preoccupation with object parts and with the elementary sensory aspects of the environment likely reflects the lack of comprehension of the meaning of the whole and a more elementary level of analysis. Difficulties with change are expressed as a range of behaviors from tantrums in response to change, attempts to control change through rituals and directing others' behavior, to difficulty with unusual changes only. The most impaired individuals have little awareness of the external world and appear unaware of change. Personality style also modifies these symptoms with children born to calm parents typically less bothered by change than children born to 'type A' parents. Problems coping with change likely reflect difficulty in predicting the outcome of change (seeing details rather than the whole) and cognitive inflexibility which may reflect limited encoding of concepts at learning. The final behavior listed in this category is a narrow range of interests, which have the quality of obsessions or preoccupations. These interests are furthermore characterized by a focus on facts or details, which can be encyclopedic. For example, one of Kanner's patients had memorized the ball gown that every first lady had worn to the inaugural ball. Individuals with autism typically do not have opinions about the information, but are limited to reciting the facts. Because neither the topics nor the facts are judged through a conceptual lens, their choice of topic may be unusual and irrelevant or trivial details are given equal weight to relevant details.

Autism is also commonly accompanied by a number of other features. About one-third of individuals have sensory sensitivities to sound, taste, texture, or light, or sensory preoccupations. They also may have a low or a high pain tolerance. Motor apraxia is also a consistent element of this syndrome. Gait is also frequently characterized as odd and they typically are poorly coordinated. Hyperactivity is common, especially in young children or in the more impaired; 70% of children diagnosed with autism receive a diagnosis of attention deficit disorder with hyperactivity before the ultimate diagnosis of autism (Lord, 1999). Head circumference tends to be average or above average with about 10–15% being macrocephalic (Fombonne, Roge, Claverie et al., 1999). Tone is reduced and reflexes are variable.

Presentation

About 25–30% of children with autism spectrum disorder present with a period of apparently normal development followed by a clear loss of skills and appearance of the behavior that defines autism; this subgroup is commonly referred to as regressive autism. The presenting problem is usually that of language loss typically of a few words; further questioning elicits evidence of loss of social, play and nonverbal language abilities also. Other children present with acquisition of a few words followed by a long plateau before language acquisition resumes. The remaining 70–75% present with developmental delays recognized in the second year of life. The majority of these children have subtle or nonspecific signs of abnormality in the first year of life with more obvious and specific signs of language, social, and play abnormalities emerging between 14 and 18 months. Retrospective examination of first birthday videotapes in these children typically reveals evidence of deficits in joint attention, social, and motor behavior (Werner, Dawson, Osterling and Dinno, 2000). Other children, though, appear to be entirely normal in the first year of life.

Natural history

The natural history of autism is one of developmental delays in the first several years of life followed by minimal to very large developmental gains between

3 and 8 years of age. Thereafter gains occur, but even in the highest-functioning children there is a growing gap between them and their peers in the areas of social function and abstraction in adolescence.

Temporary or permanent deterioration in behavior and cognition during adolescence was reported in the earliest studies of autism and is a significant concern of parents. Permanent deterioration in cognitive and behavioral function was observed during adolescence in 10% of individuals in one early longitudinal study and typically occurred in association with the onset of seizures (Lockyer and Rutter, 1970). Most but not all of these cases had IQ scores below 50 prior to deterioration. Deterioration during adolescence occurred in 12–22% of children in other studies (Nordin and Gillberg, 1998). Epilepsy has been suggested as a cause of the regression in adolescence and also the regression in early childhood; however, it seems more likely that the epilepsy is a consequence of the same underlying process. In other adolescents, cyclical but temporary exacerbation of behavior problems has been associated with a family history of affective disorder. The hormonal changes of adolescence may also be the basis of behavior problems. A study from Japan of 200 autistic children reported that 43% improved in adolescence, 25% were unchanged, and 32% deteriorated (Kobayashi, Murata and Yoshinaga, 1992). The percentage of the children with permanent deterioration was not specified.

Outcome

Studies prior to 1990 reported that outcome was generally poor in autism with only 10–15% attaining gainful employment, most requiring some degree of ongoing care or supervision, and as many as 50% requiring a large degree of assistance (Bryson, 1997; Gillberg, 1991; Lotter, 1978; Venter, Lord and Schopler, 1992). Outcome appears to have improved over the past decade, although little documentation is available. This improvement has been attributed to better and earlier treatment and better services throughout life. Outcome is likely to improve further as children who have undergone intensive early intervention reach adulthood and the growing proportion of individuals with IQ scores in the normal range at diagnosis impact these figures.

IQ scores and the status of functional language at age 5 years are the best early predictors of later outcome in autism (Stevens, Fein, Dunn et al., 2000; Venter et al., 1992), although other factors such as the degree of behavioral rigidity and co-morbid conditions also modify outcome. IQs of 50 or below are associated with a poor outcome in terms of independent living and self-sufficiency, which is also true of non-autistic mentally retarded individuals. High-functioning autistic individuals are reported to have a better outcome than mentally retarded individuals with autism but their lives are still severely restricted compared to adults without autism.

Outcome in terms of job status in autism is often better for those with mild mental retardation than those with normal IQs. For those with mild mental retardation, their capacity for consistent performance of repetitive tasks, careful adherence to rules, and limited interest in social interactions result in good work performance in sheltered settings. They are also not expected to solve problems or comprehend much beyond that involved in their immediate jobs, and thus their deficits do not interfere with job performance. Their disability is readily apparent to observers, which results in social protection and a willingness of co-workers to adapt to them and help. In contrast, autistic individuals with normal IQ scores have difficulty finding jobs that are consistent with their general ability level but also their limitations in social, communication and problem-solving abilities. Most jobs expect and require adaptive skills that are compatible with job difficulty. Few competitive jobs exist that capitalize on these individuals' enhanced awareness of details, rote memory, deductive logic and capacity for consistent performance on repetitive tasks while avoiding limitations imposed by their deficits in social, communication, and problem-solving abilities. In addition, these individuals are subject to tremendous scape-goating by peers, who perceive them as odd or strange rather than as having a disability. Thus, job status for people with autism also reflects the degree to which vocational programs and society are able to accommodate individuals with ASD. A great deal remains to be done before society achieves the degree of tolerance and job accommodation for autistic individuals that it has for individuals with dyslexia and physical disabilities.

Many high-functioning individuals with autism never do as well in adult life as they did while in school and living at home. School and families provide a highly structured and restricted life experience that compensates for their deficits to a considerable degree. The emphasis on least restrictive living environments often places these individuals in settings that lack sufficient structure for them to function. Neuroleptics and a variety of other medications are commonly used to address the behavior problems that result, without recognition that an even better outcome can be achieved by increasing structure and reducing social, communication and adaptive demands of their environment. This is the reason that many individuals taken to hospital for aggression calm immediately upon entering the doors of the hospital and have exemplary behavior while in the hospital.

Complications

The rate of epilepsy in the autism population is substantial and is cumulative with age. The life-time risk is unknown but cumulative risk of epilepsy by age 18 years is reported to be 20–30% (Deykin and McMahon, 1979; Gillberg and Steffenburg, 1987; Goode, Rutter and Howlin, 1994; Tuchman and Rapin, 1997; Tuchman, Rapin and Shinnar, 1991; Volkmar and Nelson, 1990). There are two peaks of onset: one in the preschool years and a larger one in adolescence. Although it was previously thought that epilepsy in autism was more common in those with mental retardation, the rate is now reported to be the same in those with IQ scores above and below 70 (Goode et al., 1994). Both generalized and partial seizures have been reported, with the latter being particularly difficult to recognize in the presence of the already detached behavior of children with autism (Gillberg and Schaumann, 1983). Seizures may also become apparent or worsen in association with medications, especially tricyclic antidepressants and traditional neuroleptics but also the sustained serotonin reuptake inhibitors.

Depression and mania also occur in autism. Although it may simply represent ease of diagnosis, depression is thought to be most common in high-functioning adolescents and young adults when they develop an awareness for the first time that they are different and are unable to be like others. Depression can occur in verbal children at any age, frequently in response to the social pressures of school. Nonverbal children and adults with ASD also develop depression, but as with partial seizures, it is more difficult to recognize. As a result, any sustained deterioration in function and behavior in a child or adult with ASD not explainable by change should prompt consideration of seizures and affective disorder.

Anxiety is a nearly constant accompaniment of autism and its treatment is thought to account for the frequent improvement in function associated with the administration of the sustained serotonin reuptake inhibitors or SSRIs. As even verbal individuals with autism spectrum disorder lack insight into their feelings and have never felt differently, they do not complain of being anxious or worried nor do they show the typical physical signs that would suggest anxiety to others. A small percentage also has superimposed obsessive compulsive disorder (OCD). This is distinct from the ritualistic behavior that characterizes autism, which is for them the logical way of doing things in contrast to OCD in which the act or thought is viewed as illogical and one the individual would like to resist. Individuals with autism and OCD will repeat the same behavior over and over, for example stepping over and back across a threshold, innumerable times. These individuals are the most likely to respond to SSRIs. Difficulty with change and rigidity are also often considered indications for SSRIs, but success is thought to be the result of reduced anxiety.

Diagnosis

Practice parameters for the screening, diagnosis and assessment of children and adolescents with ASD have been published and provide an excellent resource for instruments that can be used (Filipek, Accardo, Ashwal et al., 2000; Volkmar, Cook, Pomeroy et al., 1999a,b). Diagnosis is primarily clinical, but questionnaires and instruments are available. The Childhood Autism Rating Scale is in common use with mentally retarded individuals with autism, but loses validity when IQ reaches the normal range. The Autism Diagnostic Observation Schedule, a structured instrument designed for research, is now clinically available and has four age- and ability-appropriate versions. It requires a multiple day training course and demonstration of reliability in its use. It is a very helpful diagnostic tool in the hands of clinicians experienced with autism.

Routine screening of all toddlers for autism is now recommended. The Checklist for Autism in Toddlers (CHAT) was the first instrument introduced for this purpose (Baron-Cohen, Cox, Baird et al., 1996). It was designed for use at 18 months; it has proven to be very accurate but has low sensitivity (Baird et al., 2000). A modification of the CHAT can be completed by the parent (Robins, Fein, Barton and Liss, 1999). Another tool for children 4 years and older is the Autism Screening Questionnaire (Berument, Rutter, Lord et al., 1999). Efforts are also being made to develop methods of diagnosing autism in infants. Another screening tool is the Pervasive Developmental Disorders Screening Test (PDDST), which has several versions to be used from screening to diagnosis (Siegel, unpublished) [2]. The Australian Questionaire (Atwood, 1998) is currently in widespread use as an aide to diagnosis in verbal children and adults with ASD.

Differential diagnosis

In the mentally retarded subgroup, the primary differential diagnostic issues are differentiating ASD from non-ASD mental retardation and identifying cases secondary to other disorders, such as tuberous sclerosis and fragile-X syndrome. In the high-functioning subgroup, differential diagnosis is age-dependent. Young children with ASD are commonly misdiagnosed as having receptive–expressive language disorder, attention deficit disorder, oppositional defiant disorder, and sometimes even conduct disorder. Older children and adolescents with ASD are frequently misdiagnosed as having obsessive compulsive disorder or conduct disorder. Adults with ASD, particularly those in the lower end of the normal IQ range, are frequently misdiagnosed as having schizophrenia. Higher-functioning individuals may also be diagnosed as having affective disorder, because of their affective lability or discouragement and sadness over failure in their lives. The erroneous diagnoses reflect the near total lack of familiarity with verbal individuals with ASD. Verbal individuals with ASD are so distinctive as a result of their social oddness, obsessions, and their remarkable memory for odd details that diagnosis would be relatively easy if clinicians had familiarity with ASDs. The misdiagnosis of individuals with ASD as having schizophrenia is of particular concern because of the automatic use of neuroleptics for schizophrenia and the lack of the needed structure in living arrangements and various other programs for individuals with schizophrenia. The basis for this confusion is the overlap in negative symptoms, which is striking; however, hallucinations and delusions are absent in ASD. Because of their cognitive impairments, they are not 'well-organized' to begin with and stress can result in significant deterioration. Again the symptoms are in the negative category rather than the positive. Occasionally, the vivid recall of a past event, which is related out of context, is interpreted as hallucinatory, so caution must be used in questioning.

Etiology and pathophysiology

Etiology

A diverse group of genetic, metabolic, and infectious diseases have been viewed as etiologic of 5–10% of cases of autism. To understand how such diverse causes can produce the same syndrome, etiology must be distinguished from pathophysiology. Different etiologies may trigger or recreate the same pathophysiology and thus the same or nearly the same clinical syndrome. Recent studies have found that medical etiologies are responsible for 10% or fewer cases of autism (Fombonne, 1998; Rutter, Bailey, Bolton and Le Couteur, 1994). The disorders most commonly associated with autism are tuberous sclerosis and fragile-X syndrome (Fombonne, 1998). Rates for neurofibromatosis, Down syndrome, phenylketonuria, fetal rubella, and cerebral palsy do not exceed rates expected by chance co-occurrence in the mentally retarded population. Fetal rubella and phenylketonuria were two of the original etiologies reported for autism, but public health policies have virtually eliminated their occurrence and thus the evidence of their association with autism. In earlier

[2] For a copy, contact Dr. Bryna Siegel at bryna@itsa.ucsf.edu

Abnormalities in Genetic Code for Brain Development

↓

Abnormal Mechanisms of Brain Development

↓

Structural and Functional Abnormalities of Brain

↓

Cognitive & Neurologic Abnormalities

↓

Behavioral Syndrome

Fig. 1. Autism: components of cause.

decades, the presence of underlying medical etiologies for some cases of autism was interpreted to mean that underlying diseases would ultimately be identified for all cases of autism. However, the past decade has seen the emergence of the understanding of autism as a familial genetic disorder, and that the myriad of other diseases associated with a few cases duplicate the syndrome of autism but by a different mechanism. The cause of autism is therefore conceptualized as occurring at multiple levels between gene and behavior (see Fig. 1).

Genetics[3]

Autism not associated with known medical conditions is now thought to be a polygenetic disorder resulting from interacting liability genes. How many genes contribute to liability is unknown, but estimates range from a few to perhaps a score (Risch, Spiker, Lotspeich et al., 1999). The evidence for a genetic basis for autism arose from family and twin studies. The concordance rate for autism in monozygotic twins is 69% for MZ twins and 0% for DZ twins (Bailey, Le Couteur, Gottesman et al., 1995). Estimated heritability is 91–93% (Bailey, Phillips and Rutter, 1996). The recurrence risk for autism is 2.2% (Szatmari, Jones, Zwaigenbaum and MacLean, 1998), which represents a 50- to 100-fold increase in risk over population prevalence. All of these evidences suggest a strong genetic liability for autism. The rapid fall-off in affected individuals from first- to third-degree relatives is taken as evidence for interaction of genes as a critical component of liability.

A common means of discovering genes affecting liability to complex disease is to perform genome-wide linkage analysis using affected sibling pairs (ASP). This approach uses highly variable markers distributed throughout the genome, usually at roughly 10-centimorgan intervals, and seeks to find genomic regions exhibiting co-inheritance of alleles at much greater than chance proportions. ASP are expected to share 0, 1 and 2 alleles identical-by-descent (IBD) from their parents with probabilities 1/4, 1/2 and 1/4. Regions showing substantial excess IBD-sharing potentially harbor liability genes.

Several studies have applied this logic to discovery liability genes for autism (Barrett, Beck, Bernier et al., 1999; Buxbaum, Silverman, Smith et al., 2001; International Molecular Genetic Study of Autism Consortium, 1998 [IMGSAC]; Philippe, Martinez, Guilloud-Bataille et al., 1999; Risch et al., 1999). Unfortunately, no especially noteworthy linkage signals have been produced by these studies, and there is minimal correspondence between the best peaks from the different studies. Arguably the best signal appears to emanate from chromosome 7 (Folstein and Mankoski, 2000; International Molecular Genetic Study of Autism Consortium, 1998). This region is the focus of intense investigation (Bradford, Haines, Hutcheson et al., 2001; Lamb, Moore, Bailey and Monaco, 2000; Wassink, Piven, Vieland et al., 2001), but has so far not yielded any genes.

Other weaker signals occur on chromosome 16p (International Molecular Genetic Study of Autism Consortium, 1998), 13 (Barrett et al., 1999), 2q, 7q, 16p, and 19p (Philippe et al., 1999), and 1p (Risch et al., 1999). Recently, using phrase-speech-delay as a means of partitioning their sample, Buxbaum and colleagues have produced a reasonably strong signal for linkage on chromosome 2q. This new result may turn out to be the best lead yet, but must be replicated by other studies.

Broader autism phenotype

An even larger group of individuals has ‘traits’ of autism, which do not prevent them from functioning in society but are noticeable to others and an obstacle to their function. Recognition of these in-

[3] This section courtesy of Dr. B. Devlin, computational geneticist, Department of Psychiatry, University of Pittsburgh, Pittsburgh, PA, USA.

dividuals came about as a result of family studies, which identified traits or fragments of autism in first- and second-degree relatives of autistic children. These manifestations are called the 'broader autism phenotype'. In autism, the broader autism phenotype is thought to reflect the presence of an autism susceptibility gene. This phenotype clearly occurs in individuals without a family member with autism and so it is not clear how much of a risk factor this phenotype is for having a child with autism. Classification systems do not accommodate individuals with the broader autism phenotype who essentially have an isolated 'developmental specific learning disability' in social, communication, or reasoning abilities of the type seen in autism. They nonetheless experience difficulty as a result of this limitation and would likely benefit from intervention.

Pathophysiology

Regardless of etiology, the syndrome is presumed to be the result of a common pathophysiology, i.e., common structural and functional brain abnormalities and common cognitive deficits. It would be difficult to have multiple different structural and functional abnormalities that faithfully produce this syndrome, given the specific nature of the impairments defining autism and the complexity of the constellation. In profoundly mentally retarded individuals, there may be insufficient behavior to verify the quality of the deficits and the potential for phenocopies resulting from other pathophysiologies is increased.

Neuropathologic data are surprisingly limited given the interest in this syndrome. Less than two dozen brains have been examined by two different groups with half of these only at a preliminary stage of examination (Bailey, Luther, Dean et al., 1998; Kemper and Bauman, 1998). Common findings across studies have been an increase in brain weight in some but not all cases, and a reduction in Purkinje cells in the cerebellar hemispheres. The most thoroughly studied case series reported consistent findings of increased cell packing of immature neurons with truncated dendritic tree development in the hippocampus and amygdala, reflecting a reduction in the neural connections of these structures (Kemper and Bauman, 1998). The other more preliminary results included the cerebellar abnormality, neurons in white matter in some cases, and various abnormalities in the cerebral cortex; abnormalities were not found in the limbic system but the method was less rigorous than in the prior study (Bailey et al., 1998).

Structural imaging data are also limited in autism. One of the most interesting findings that has been replicated across multiple studies is an increase in total brain volume in children with autism but not adults (Aylward, Minshew, Field et al., 2002; Courchesne, Karns, Davis et al., 2001; Piven et al., 1995; Piven, Arndt, Bailey and Andreasen, 1996; Sparks, Friedman, Shaw et al., 2002). The first two of these studies involved a total of 127 autistic individuals between 3 and 46 years and reported an abnormal pattern of brain growth with a premature acceleration in brain growth in the first 3 years of life followed by a very modest reduction in volume in late childhood and then a decrease in adulthood. In contrast, normal controls exhibited a brain growth spurt in late childhood resulting in increased brain volume in adolescence followed by a decrease in adulthood. The 'normalization' of brain volume in the autism group in adolescence was therefore the result of brain growth in the normal controls and not normal developmental processes in the autism group. The early increase in brain volume in autism could reflect increased numbers of neurons and glia, and or premature and accelerated proliferation of synapses, axonal and dendritic arbors, axons and increased myelination. One recent study reporting an increase in brain volume in autistic children also found increased volumes of cerebral cortical gray matter (12%), cerebral white matter (18%), and cerebellar white matter (39%) (Courchesne et al., 2001). These findings suggest that all of the above developmental neurobiologic processes are up-regulated and contribute to the increase in total brain volume in autistic children. One study has reported an increase in four neurotrophins and neuropeptides in blood from newborns later diagnosed with autism (Nelson et al., 2001). These elevations or others could be the molecular basis for the early and accelerated brain growth in autism. Neurotropins typically stimulate the growth of both neuronal and glial elements as well as endothelium. The increased levels of neurotropins suggest that there is early over-expression of genes that lead to the production of neurotropins and neuropeptides. The potential relationship between brain growth in autism and neurotropins has not yet been documented, but the evidence is beginning to outline a sequence of events from gene to brain structure in a previously very poorly understood disorder.

Data on other brain structures are limited and inconsistent. A number of studies have reported a decrease in the size of the corpus callosum but in different regions. Two found a reduction in the body (Manes, Piven, Vrancic et al., 1999; Piven, Bailey, Ranson and Arndt, 1997) and the posterior subregions (Egaas, Courchesne and Saitoh, 1995; Piven et al., 1997). One study reported a decrease in the anterior segments of the corpus callosum (Hardan, Minshew and Keshavan, 2000) and another reported no change in the MR signal intensity, suggesting that there is no change in myelination (Belmonte, Egaas, Townsend and Courchesne, 1995).

Three studies of hippocampal volume have reported no abnormalities (Haznedar, Buchsbaum, Wei et al., 2000; Piven, Bailey, Ranson and Arndt, 1998; Saitoh, Courchesne, Egaas et al., 1995), but two studies have found a reduction in the volume of the hippocampus from early childhood to adulthood (Aylward, Minshew, Goldstein et al., 1999; Saitoh, Karns and Courchesne, 2001). The latter study was limited to the dentate gyrus and CA4 rather than the entire hippocampus. The volume of the amygdala has been reported to be reduced (Aylward et al., 1999) and increased (Howard, Cowell, Boucher et al., 2000). A third study reported reduced volume of the anterior amygdala and increased volume of the posterior amygdala (Abell, Krams, Ashburner et al., 1999). The anterior cingulate has been reported to be reduced in size (Haznedar et al., 2000).

Abnormalities in the size of the cerebellar vermis have been reported but have generally not been replicated by independent laboratories (Courchesne, Townsend, Akshoomoff et al., 1994; Hashimoto, Murakawa, Miyazaki et al., 1992; Holttum et al., 1992; Kleiman, Neff and Rosman, 1992). This group has also reported an inverse correlation between frontal lobe volume (increased) and superior cerebellar vermal volume (Carper and Courchesne, 2000) and a correlation between orienting time on a spatial attention paradigm and cerebellar volume (Harris, Courchesne, Townsend et al., 1999). Two studies have reported an increase in the volume of the cerebellar hemispheres (Hardan, Minshew, Harenski and Keshvan, 2001; Piven et al., 1995). Several studies of the brainstem have not found any abnormalities (Garber and Ritvo, 1992; Hardan et al., 2001; Hashimoto et al., 1992; Hsu, Yeung-Courchesne, Courchesne and Press, 1991; Piven, Nehme, Simon et al., 1992) but two studies have reported parts of the brainstem to be smaller (Hashimoto, Tayama, Miyazaki et al., 1993; Hashimoto, Tayama, Murakawa et al., 1995).

Functional imaging studies are few. One early 2,3-deoxyglucose PET study reported a decrease in the intracortical, intercortical and subcortical functional correlations of frontal and parietal cortices at rest, suggesting reduced cortical connectivity (Horwitz and Rumsey, 1994). A recent 18F-deoxyglucose study has reported decreased metabolic activity in anterior and posterior cingulate (Haznedar et al., 2000). A serotonin PET study reported decreased synthesis in frontal cortex and thalamus and increased synthesis in contralateral dentate nucleus, suggesting abnormalities in the dentatothalamocortical pathway (Chugani, Muzik, Rothermel et al., 1997). A subsequent study of age-related changes in serotonin synthesis found that the very high levels of serotonin synthesis present until 5 years of age and declining thereafter in non-autistic children contrasted with the gradual increase in levels between 2 and 15 years in the autistic children (Chugani, Muzik, Behen et al., 1999). Serotonin levels play an important role in brain development and altered levels in rats reproduce some elements of the neuropathology of autism. Thus, these data suggested that this developmental process might be disrupted in autism but subject number was very small because of the radioactivity involved in PET scanning and findings remain tentative.

An fMRI study of a theory of mind social cognition task (inferring mental states from the eye expression) found that normal individuals activated superior temporal gyrus, amygdala and prefrontal cortex, whereas individuals with autism activated frontotemporal regions (Baron-Cohen, Ring, Wheelwright et al., 1999). It was proposed that the neural network involved in social intelligence did not incorporate input from amygdala in autism. An fMRI study of theory of mind cartoons and stories in normal individuals has reported activation in medial prefrontal and temporo-parietal regions, but only the activation in the paracingulate region of prefrontal cortex was unique to tasks requiring mental state attribution. Thus, there appears to be a neural network for social cognition but its precise composition and abnormalities in autism are not yet clearly defined. An fMRI study comparing face and object recognition demonstrated that normal individuals activated superior temporal gyrus for faces and inferior temporal gyrus for objects, whereas individuals with autism activated inferior temporal gyrus for both faces and objects (Schultz, Gauthier, Klin et al., 2000). A recent study has similarly reported that face processing is accomplished outside the face area in autistic individuals (Courchesne et al., 2001). During an Embedded Figures test which assesses part–whole processing, autistic individuals did not show activation of prefrontal regions and relied on ventral occipitotemporal areas (Ring, Baron-Cohen, Wheelwright et al., 1999). All of these fMRI studies have shown a failure of neural systems to develop, with autistic individuals not activating higher brain or more specialized brain regions, and instead relying on less specialized regions for task performance.

Neurophysiologic studies have reported a pattern of normal early and middle latency auditory evoked potentials with abnormalities in cognitive potentials. Analogous abnormalities of visual evoked potentials have been observed but appear to be less severe, but tasks have not been matched for difficulty. Audiometry and evoked potentials in children reported to be sound sensitive or to have hyperacusis have failed to detect any abnormalities (Gravel, 1994). A recent study of N1b and N1c components reported abnormalities of the latter but not the former, providing support for dysfunction of auditory association cortex but not primary auditory cortex (Dunn, Vaughan, Kreuzer and Kurtzberg, 1999). Investigation of oculomotor physiology has found abnormalities in volitional saccades dependent on frontal systems and no abnormalities in reflexive saccades related to brainstem and cerebellar function (Minshew et al., 1999). These functional studies support impairments in higher-order cognitive abilities and information processing secondary to neocortical systems dysfunction.

Electroencephalographic (EEG) abnormalities are common in autism and are present in approximately 80% of children with autism after three high quality EEGs that include all stages of sleep. This is in contrast to the 20–30% of individuals with autism with clinical seizures by early adulthood (Fombonne, 1998; Olsson, Steffenburg and Gillberg, 1988; Volkmar and Nelson, 1990).

Neuropsychology

IQ scores

The Wechsler Intelligence Scales have commonly been used to assess intelligence in verbal individuals with autism and IQ scores obtained have been demonstrated to be stable over time (Venter et al., 1992). Early studies reported a prototypic pattern of lower Verbal than Performance IQ score. On the Verbal scale, lowest subtest scaled scores were typically found on Comprehension and highest on Digit Span; on the Performance scale, lowest scores were on Picture Arrangement or Coding/Digit Symbol and highest scores on Block Design. These features were sufficiently common that diagnostic significance came to be attached to this pattern. However, these findings were based on studies of mentally retarded individuals with autism. This pattern has not been present in studies of non-mentally retarded individuals with autism (Verbal and Full Scale IQ scores above 70), the majority of whom had no significant disparity. In one such study, 80% of the children with autism had no significant VIQ–PIQ disparity and the remainder were equally divided between VIQ > PIQ and VIQ < PIQ (Siegel, Minshew and Goldstein, 1996; Szatmari, Tuff, Finlayson and Bartolucci, 1990). Consistent with studies in mentally retarded individuals with autism, the subtest pattern for the group revealed Comprehension to be the lowest score and Block Design the highest. Subtest variability was small, though, and the pattern was not universal among the subjects. In addition, factors other than ASD can impact on this profile. Thus, the Wechler profile commonly associated with autism is severity-dependent and such differences are not present when Verbal and Full Scale IQ scores are both above 70. Furthermore the results indicate that disparities can be present in both directions in non-mentally retarded individuals with autism and so such differences cannot be used as the basis for differentiating between autism, Asperger's disorder, and the nonverbal learning disability syndrome. IQ prototypes have been proposed for the latter two disorders too. In Asperger's disorder, the proposed prototype is that of a VIQ higher than PIQ, presumably reflecting their superior verbal skills and poor motor skills. In NLD, VIQ is also higher than PIQ but as a result of poor scores on the arithmetic and visuospatial subtests. However, the validity of the proposed profile prototypes for these two disorders has not been examined and they should not be used in diagnosis.

The assessment of IQ in nonverbal children with autism is more problematic. Choice of instruments depends on age and ability level and can range from the Bailey Scales of Infant Development, to the Leiter, the Raven's Colored Progressive Matrices, and the Performance Scale of the Wechler Intelligence Scales to name a few. Changes from one test to another over the course of development can result in large changes in IQ scores.

The conditions of testing are as important or more so than the choice of instrument. The performance of children with autism is frequently adversely affected by the usual circumstances of testing, i.e., the interruption of the child's regular routine, an unfamiliar setting, a stranger administering the testing, the social intensity of the experience, and the novelty of the activities. Performance is also adversely affected by the social, motor, and time demands of tests. Language comprehension limitations may mean that the child knows the answer to a question when it is phrased in one way but not another. Reliable testing requires familiarization with the tester and testing situation and may require more than one session especially in young children.

Mental retardation

Mental retardation is part and parcel of autism and not the result of the chance co-occurrence of two low-frequency disorders, which could not, in any case, explain the high frequency of this association. The mental retardation in autism is the more severe expression of the pattern of cognitive deficits and intact abilities seen in non-mentally retarded individuals with autism. As a result, the mental retardation retains the peculiarities typical of cognition in autism, which distinguish it from mental retardation resulting from other conditions.

Mentally retarded individuals with autism can be distinguished from non-autistic mentally retarded individuals with comparable IQ scores by their much poorer social, verbal and nonverbal language, and reasoning abilities, the inability to use the skills they do have in these areas in a functional manner, and their greater facility with trivial details. In essence, mentally retarded autistic individuals are functionally much more retarded than their non-autistic mentally retarded peers. This distinction between autistic and non-autistic individuals with comparable IQ scores holds true across the IQ spectrum.

Profile of neuropsychologic functioning

Although most neuropsychologic studies in autism have focused on a single domain, the profile of neuropsychologic functioning has been examined in a few studies. The examination of cognitive function across domains in the same subjects provides an opportunity for assessing the predominance of any single deficit based on disproportionate severity. More importantly, though, such studies provide an opportunity for identifying a common feature or pattern to the deficits across domains that would provide an important clue to the fundamental nature of the underlying brain abnormality.

One of the earliest studies to do this was that of Rumsey and Hamburger (1988) who tested 10 non-mentally retarded men with autism compared to matched normal controls. The resulting profile was characterized by dramatic impairments in verbal and nonverbal reasoning, relatively preserved memory, language, and motor skills, and intact sensory perceptual and visuospatial abilities. However, test selection in the memory, language, and motor areas was limited and performance was mixed. A subsequent study addressed this with a more comprehensive battery (Table 1; Minshew, Goldstein and Siegel, 1997; Minshew, Johnson and Luna, 2000). The results defined a distinctive profile in non-mentally retarded adolescents and adults with autism. Deficits were not found in attention, sensory perception, simple motor skills, simple language skills (fluency,

TABLE 1

Psychometric data used for discriminant analysis

Tests entered into prediction equations	Autistic group		Control group		*P* [a]
	M	SD	M	SD	
Attention domain					
WAIS-R Digit Span	9.88	3.81	10.52	2.46	0.424
Serial Digit Learning, correct responses	16.52	8.17	17.42	7.91	0.648
Continuous Performance Test [b]	0.34	0.62	0.23	0.66	0.487
Letter Cancellation, omissions	1.09	1.63	0.45	1.00	0.061
Number Cancellation, omissions	3.27	4.03	4.39	5.38	0.342
Sensory perception domain					
Luria–Nebraska Tactile Scale:					
Simple touch errors	0.29	0.55	0.17	0.48	0.407
Stereognosis errors	0.46	0.59	0.21	0.42	0.096
Sharp–dull discrimination errors	0.88	0.80	0.58	0.72	0.189
Position sense errors	0.00	0.00	0.08	0.41	0.328
Finger position errors	0.67	1.27	0.46	1.02	0.535
Halstead–Reitan: Fingertip Number Writing, errors	5.38	4.30	2.79	2.84	0.019 *
Motor domain					
Finger tapping, dominant hand	44.27	13.78	45.19	16.24	0.805
DVMI, total points [c]	15.42	32.43	22.18	31.69	0.465
Grooved pegboard, dominant hand, in seconds	86.73	18.30	70.67	16.03	0.000 *
Trail making A, time in seconds	31.52	15.81	20.45	7.99	0.001 *
Simple language domain					
WAIS-R Vocabulary	9.45	3.02	9.70	2.26	0.713
K-TEA Reading Decoding	97.48	13.60	102.79	10.19	0.078
Controlled Oral Word Association (FAS) [d]	36.00	13.31	34.00	16.18	0.586
K-TEA Spelling	102.58	16.93	100.91	11.50	0.642
Woodcock Reading Mastery, word attack	107.24	11.55	103.52	15.53	0.273
Woodcock Reading Mastery, passage comprehension	92.27	15.04	104.27	14.34	0.002 *
K-TEA Reading Comprehension	91.36	14.43	103.06	12.45	0.001 *
Test of Language Competence Metaphoric Expression	6.85	3.25	9.42	3.70	0.004 *
Binet Verbal Absurdities, raw score	9.30	3.64	12.48	3.97	0.001 *
Token Test, number correct	18.03	2.19	18.42	5.19	0.690
Simple memory domain					
Paired Associate Learning, number correct	42.55	23.13	48.76	24.21	0.690
3 Word Short Term Memory [e]	3.24	3.04	2.91	3.15	0.663
Maze Recall, correct/incorrect	0.42	0.61	0.52	0.57	0.534
CVLT A List, Trial 1 number correct	4.50	3.90	6.30	3.90	0.072
Complex memory domain					
Paired Associates, delayed recall	16.00	7.46	17.45	6.13	0.390
CVLT A List, long delay	7.00	5.49	9.00	5.55	0.146
Nonverbal Selective Reminding, CLTR	19.94	15.09	37.39	16.09	0.000 *
WMS-R Logical Memory, delayed recall	5.58	5.79	8.45	6.02	0.052 *
Rey–Osterrieth Figure, delayed recall	16.83	8.58	21.94	7.49	0.012 *
Reasoning domain					
Trail Making B, time in seconds	65.48	37.19	52.42	23.31	0.093
Halstead Category Test, errors	46.24	28.71	40.73	22.46	0.388
Wisconsin Card Sorting Test, perseverative errors	16.45	15.48	13.27	11.13	0.342
Binet Picture Absurdities, raw score	20.00	11.46	27.52	6.12	0.002 *

[a] *t*-test results are provided to identify domains not entered into the equations but still demonstrating a significantly different performance between groups.

[b] Mean reaction time correct responses.

[c] Developmental test of visual–motor integration.

[d] Number of words.

[e] Number of correct sequences.

[f] Tests with statistically significant results.

reading decoding, spelling, vocabulary), memory for simple information, the rule-learning aspects of abstraction, or visuospatial abilities. These intact abilities indicated the integrity of information acquisition abilities and of visuospatial processing but also of the simpler abilities within the motor, language, memory and reasoning domains. Deficits were found in motor praxis, higher-order interpretive language (reading comprehension, complex sentence comprehension, understanding of inferences and metaphors), memory for information that was inherently complex or involved a large number of simple units, and in the concept formation aspects of abstract reasoning. With the exception of visuospatial abilities, the common denominator of the strengths or intact abilities was that they involved simple information processing. The common denominator of the deficits was that they selectively involved the most demanding abilities in domains with the highest information processing demands. Thus, it was proposed that autism is a disorder of information processing that disproportionately impacts complex information processing abilities. The presence of deficits in the motor and memory domains analogous to those in other domains suggested that the localization of the brain abnormality was not defined by involvement of the three neural systems involved in social, language, and reasoning abilities. Rather, the more widespread involvement of domains suggests that the brain abnormality is more likely to involve specialized connections or dendritic architecture used throughout the brain to deal with higher-order cognitive and neurologic abilities.

The complex information processing construct is important to understand for a number of reasons. First, it allows all of the clinical deficits to be embraced under a single category, making it possible to move to the next level of the pathophysiology and think about neurologic localization and developmental neurobiologic processes. Second, this construct also provides an explanation for why the deficits in autism travel together. Third, it focuses attention on the information processing demands of tasks and this perspective can help in identifying the differences between tasks an individual with autism can do and those he or she cannot do. This profile also defines a new type of learning disability.

There are several important constraints that define this complex information processing construct. The first is that deficits in complex abilities are defined domain by domain not independent of domains. Otherwise, any language task could be viewed as more complex than any motor task. Second, visuospatial processing is complex but is spared and so the model stipulates that this neural system is spared. The third important constraint of this model is that complex information processing is disproportionately impacted, i.e., this is not a general processing deficit.

The generalization of this construct to more severely impaired individuals with autism requires that test selection include a range of abilities within each domain; for subjects with minimal ability, the profile within domains may have to be defined by testing individuals at several levels of severity. In fact, Fein, Dunn, Allen et al. (1996) have completed a large-scale study of neuropsychologic functioning in children with a broad range of IQ scores and found a similar pattern with ability-appropriate tests.

Attention

Although a subset of individuals with autism have attention deficit disorder responsive to medications for this condition, abnormalities of attention have not proven to be a core component of the cognitive profile in autism unless the tasks involved executive function or motor demands. Deficits in all aspects of attention have been proposed at one time or another as the underlying cause of the social and behavioral abnormalities in autism, but research has ultimately demonstrated their absence despite the clinical appeal of the hypothesized relationship to behavior. The history of attention research in autism has therefore been one of theories being advanced based on limited data and compelling logic, but then disproven when investigated more critically.

Failure to modulate attention and arousal was proposed as the basis for the propensity to repetitive stereotyped behavior, atypical responses to the environment, and the aversion to social contact (Dawson and Levy, 1989). However, studies assessing arousal failed to confirm these hypothesized relationships (Hutt, Forrest and Richer, 1975; Lake, Ziegler and Murphy, 1977; Van Engeland, 1984; Zahn, Rumsey and Van Kammen, 1987). Overselective attention was proposed to explain the intense focus on detail and failure to interpret multiple cues in the environment (Pierce, Glad and Schreibman, 1997), but the evidence cited for this deficit was later found to be related to developmental level and was not replicated with higher-functioning and older individuals with autism (Burack, Enns and Johannes, 1997). Deficits in reflexive orienting were proposed to explain perseveration on irrelevant environmental stimuli (Casey, Gordon, Mannheim and Rumsey, 1993). However, a number of studies have demonstrated that reflexive orienting is intact and that apparent deficits in orienting are a function of the information processing demands of the directional cues (Burack et al., 1997; Wainwright and Bryson, 1996). The possibility of deficits in sustained attention or vigilance has also been proposed (Casey et al., 1993) but not supported by continuous performance test results (Goldstein, Johnson and Minshew, 2001; Ozonoff, Strayer, McMahon and Filloux, 1994; Pascualvaca, Fantie, Papageorgiou and Mirsky, 1998). An impairment in shifting attention has been the most recent focus of attention theories. An early version of this theory proposed a deficit in the capacity to shift between intrapersonal and extrapersonal space, i.e., bilateral neglect (Ornitz, 1988), as the cause of autism but cancellation and sensoriperceptual tasks have demonstrated the absence of neglect (Minshew et al., 1997). Deficits in the capacity for intra- and inter-modal shifts of attention and in disengagement from stimuli in preparation for a shift have been proposed as a result of several studies (Courchesne et al., 1994; Wainwright and Bryson, 1996). A number of studies examining the component cognitive processes involved in shifting attention behavior have demonstrated that the behavioral difficulties are the consequence of the executive function demands of the task and not the attentional demands (Ozonoff et al., 1994; Pascualvaca et al., 1998). In addition, a study of saccadic eye movements using methods similar to those employed by Goldman-Rakic and others demonstrated the absence of deficits in reflexive shifts of attention subserved by the cerebellum and the presence of deficits in volitional shifts subserved by executive abilities and frontal systems (Minshew et al., 1999).

A recent comprehensive study of attention using the Mirsky four-factor model for test selection (focus, encode, sustain, and shift-execute) addressed many aspects of attention and the findings indicated that purported attention deficits in autism are actually primary deficits in complex decision-making or psychomotor abilities (Goldstein et al., 2001). The attention research in autism is therefore consistent in demonstrating that abnormal attentional behavior is the result of deficits in executive abilities, the processing of directional cues, or the psychomotor demands of tests.

Sensory perception

Behavior involving reactions to sensory stimuli is commonly associated with autism and descriptions of the syndrome often include under- and overreactivity to sensory stimuli. Thus, behavior attributed to abnormalities in 'sensory processing' range from children's lack of response to their names being called to a terrified response to vacuum cleaners. Although the provoking stimulus has a sensory component, in these two cases auditory, the cognitive or neurologic basis of the behavior is likely related to the social impairment in the first case and any of a number of deficits in the second (sound sensitivity, lack of understanding of what will happen, or persistent memory of fear from an initial unexpected exposure).

The behavior most likely to be related to sensory processing abnormalities in the brain are the sensory preoccupations, sensory sensitivities, high or low pain tolerance, and inability to filter extraneous sounds (dichotic listening deficit). Despite the presence of these symptoms in approximately one-third of verbal individuals with autism, there is no objective evidence of alteration in sensory perception using the sensory perceptual scales of the Luria Nebraska Neuropsychological Battery or the Halstead Reitan Battery. The presence or absence of sensory sensitivities and preoccupations does not predict performance on these scales and vice versa (Minshew, unpublished data). Conversely, occasional individuals will perform poorly on these scales and this is not associated with sensory symptoms. Auditory and visual evoked potentials have found intact latencies and accurate perception of stimuli, also demonstrating intact perception.

Motor

Although not part of the diagnostic criteria, motor problems are an integral component of the autism spectrum disorders. The motor deficit has multiple components described clinically as awkwardness, clumsiness, uncoordinated gait, postural instability, and difficulty with complex motor tasks. One prominent element is apraxia, which extends to both fine and gross motor abilities. The simplest tests used to demonstrate this deficit are finger tapping and the Grooved Pegboard Test. Although some individuals with autism also have reduced coordination and poor performance on finger tapping, it is not uncommon for performance to be selectively impaired on the Grooved Pegboard Test. The expression of the praxis problem in school-age children is often in handwriting, which is either sloppy or very slow and neat, and in noticeable clumsiness when running. In preschool, the praxis difficulty is apparent in difficulty holding a pencil, using scissors, tying shoes, and bike riding. The capacity for and quality of sign language has also been correlated with motor apraxia. Gait may also be visibly odd. Adaptive strategies can be used for the fine motor problems and ultimately a computer can be used to circumvent the handwriting problem. Adaptive physical education is important, as performance is impaired by the motor, social, and comprehension deficits relevant to group sports.

Language and communication

As described above, delayed and disordered language development is an integral part of the course of autism and is the primary feature, in addition to the requirement of an IQ in the normal range, that distinguishes high-functioning autism and Asperger's disorder in DSM-IV. The disordered features include immediate and delayed echolalia, functional use of echolalia, pronoun reversals, idiosyncratic words or phrases, sentences with missing articles and adjectives or words out of order, delayed echoing of television or video segments, and stereotyped or scripted sentences. As language emerges, children with autism typically pass through a stage in which they refuse to use the language they have to communicate even needs, preferring to get what they want themselves or go without. Eventually, they go to adults more spontaneously for needs and then to impart information on their topics or to ask questions. Thus, there are two parts to the language problem, the first is the delay and disorder in language development and the second is in the social use of language; these appear to be two separate impairments. The dissociation between the presence of language and failure to use it socially suggests that neural connections must develop between the brain's neural system for language and that for social function in order for language to be used for communication.

Nonverbal language (eye contact, facial expression for social communication, and prosody) is also delayed in developing but abnormalities appear to be more closely linked to the social impairment than to verbal language, since nonverbal language is impaired even in the absence of developmental delay in verbal language. This association between social and nonverbal language impairments may reflect the right frontal localization of theory of mind ability and nonverbal language. The social use of eye contact is delayed in developing. Skill levels range from total absence of eye contact to watching others at a distance to glances during social encounters to longer but not sustained eye contact, and finally more sustained eye contact. Children with autism are delayed in developing the capacity to point to indicate needs, use head nods for yes and no, and use gestures with symbolic meaning. Facial expression is absent or limited to a few often-stilted expressions during social interactions, even though laughter, smiling, or an angry look may accompany their own internal emotional experiences at other times. Use of body language for communication is also impaired with failure to orient themselves in a socially appropriate manner during interactions. Prosody is subtly to dramatically abnormal in terms of loudness (too soft or too loud), tone fluctuation (monotone or sing-song), and rate (too fast without pauses between words), which may be sufficiently severe to interfere with intelligibility, the latter occurring more often in mildly mentally retarded individuals with autism. The expressive deficits in nonverbal language are also accompanied by equally severe comprehension deficits for nonverbal language, which often go unappreciated. The expressive deficits in nonverbal language are also accompanied by equally severe comprehension deficits for nonverbal language, which often go unappreciated.

Unfortunately, there are no clinically available instruments for quantitatively measuring nonverbal language impairments and assessment is therefore dependent on clinical observation. The Autism Diagnostic Observation Schedule (ADOS) may partially address this problem.

A variety of language outcomes occur in autism, depending on the severity of the disorder. A significant subgroup develops little to no verbal or nonverbal language expression or comprehension. Others make some progress but remain in one of the disordered stages of development described above. Non-mentally retarded verbal children with autism spectrum disorder including Asperger's disorder have grammatically correct sentence language by age 5 years but have life-long residual semantic–pragmatic deficits (Boucher, 1988). Comprehension of idioms, metaphors, verbal inferences, complex sentences, stories and books is impaired. They may finish reading a story or book and be unable to answer questions not because of memory problems but because of comprehension problems. Their expressive language reflects these same language limitations. Thus, what they mean by what they say may be different than what others would mean if they said the same thing. They also have difficulty writing essays that may be expressed as difficulty choosing a topic (no plan for narrowing the options or forming a concept), to developing a logical sequence and theme, to differentiating between relevant and irrelevant details. Some adults are prolific writers, but it is often in a stream of consciousness style. Reading and writing are often easier than auditory comprehension and speaking because of the elimination of the social element, the increased time for re-reading, planing and revising, and the restriction of information sources to the printed word. A variety of standardized tests are available that assess these skills; some are listed in the table of instruments used to define the profile of neuropsychologic functioning in autism.

Memory and learning

For several decades, research on memory in autism focused on an analogy to Korsakoff's syndrome based on a shared pattern of impaired recall and recognition memory and improvement of recall with cuing (Boucher and Warrington, 1976). A critical difference overlooked in this analogy was that the memory impairments in autism were mild and did not result in the severe inability to form new memories that typifies amnesia. Ultimately, the amnesia theory was disproven (Bennetto, Pennington and Rogers, 1996; Minshew and Goldstein, 1993; Rumsey and Hamburger, 1988). Memory studies have otherwise consistently demonstrated that individuals with autism recall digits and nonsense words as well as matched controls but that their memory fails to improve with the addition of semantic meaning or patterns. Studies of recall of related word lists such as the California Verbal Learning Test in non-retarded individuals with autism demonstrate a general inefficiency of memory with slightly less learning than matched controls (Bennetto et al., 1996; Minshew and Goldstein, 1993). Other studies have shown that even when autistic children categorized words at encoding, they fail to use these categories to support memory (Tager-Flusberg, 1989). One comprehensive study examined memory as a function of information complexity, since increasingly complex material requires increasing use of strategies for optimal performance (Minshew and Goldstein, 2002). This relationship was confirmed in both the auditory and visual modalities, for immediate and delayed recall, and for span tasks. Thus, digit span was normal but word span and sentence span were progressively more impaired and recall of related word lists was subtly impaired and better than complex sentence and story recall. The clinical impact of this memory impairment was demonstrated by Boucher (1981), who reported that high-ability autistic children recalled significantly less about recently experienced activities than language- and IQ-matched controls. The practical implications of this relationship are that learning can be improved by simplifying the material, reducing the amount of the material, and increasing processing time.

A few studies of working memory have been reported. Although the initial study reported deficits in verbal working memory (Bennetto et al., 1996; Russell, Jarrold and Henry, 1996), subsequent studies have not.

Reasoning

Impaired abstract reasoning has long been viewed as an integral part of autism. Kanner described children with autism as being extremely literal in their thinking and having difficulty with generalization. Rutter observed that abstract reasoning fell disproportionately with declining IQ scores. Clinically, individuals with autism are concrete in their thinking, focus on details, have difficulty grasping concepts, and have little insight or judgement beyond that provided to them by others or by rules. Their behavior is often described as rule-bound with difficulty in novel situations.

Using a test battery to examine all the major domains, Rumsey and Hamburger (1988) reported marked impairments in verbal and nonverbal reasoning abilities not explained by impairments in any other domain. Thereafter, Ozonoff, Pennington and Rogers (1991) reported deficits in executive function (EF), which became a research focus for nearly a decade. The Wisconsin Card Sorting Test and the Tower of Hanoi were commonly used to document EF deficits in autism. Decomposition of the Wisconsin Card Sorting Test into its cognitive components resulted in the identification of cognitive inflexibility as the basis for impaired performance. Ultimately, executive dysfunction as defined by cognitive inflexibility and difficulty shifting cognitive set proved not to be universal in autism and impaired performance on the WCST was ultimately found to be ability-dependent. An earlier study had reported the absence of deficits on the Wisconsin Card Sorting Test in non-mentally retarded individuals with autism and a dissociation between the intact performance on rule-learning and rule-identification tests and impaired performance on concept formation tests such as the Twenty Questions procedure and Picture Absurdities (Minshew, Goldstein, Muenz and Payton, 1992). This absence of impairments on rule-learning tests may result in failure to recognize reasoning deficits if concept formation tests are not also administered. This characterization of abstraction in autism is consistent with behavior in that the lowest-ability children with autism have no rule-learning or concept-formation abilities, the moderately impaired have rule-learning abilities but are inflexible in their application and so they rotely apply rules without the capacity to alter them to the situation, and the highest-functioning individuals can flexibly apply rules to situations based on past experience but continue to have difficulty with concept formation as well as with judgement and insight, which are dependent on concept formation.

Executive dysfunction

As described above, executive function deficits are frequently present in all but the most able individuals with autism or in children who have had intervention focusing on flexibility and concept training. A minority of individuals have problems with organization, which will become apparent on plan of search tests. The Behavioral Assessment of the Dysexecutive Syndrome (BADS) is useful for assessing executive function with real-life tests, except in non-mentally retarded individuals who only have trouble with the cork and water test which requires concept formation. Executive dysfunction is one of the reasons that some academically able children with ASD require an aide in order to function; in these cases the BADS may be very helpful in documenting the need for externally imposed structure.

Visuospatial, arithmetic, facial recognition and savant abilities

One stereotype of autism is superior visuospatial abilities as reflected in high Block Design subtest scores and facility with puzzles, a remarkable capacity for mental calculations, and the ability to recognize and remember every person's name. This stereotype applies to group comparisons but each of these skills is subject to large individual variations. Although a subgroup of individuals with autism have poor visuospatial, arithmetic, or facial recognition skills, these skill deficits do not co-occur. Together they define the nonverbal learning disability (NLD) syndrome; the social and reasoning impairments in these individuals are less severe than those of individuals with autism and they lack the restricted range of interests and activities. Because of their social and nonverbal language impairments, individuals with NLD may be diagnosed as having Asperger's disorder or PDDNOS (Klin, Volkmar, Sparrow et al., 1995).

Academic achievement

Children with autism spectrum disorder capable of functioning in a regular classroom often enter kindergarten with the 'self-taught' capacity to read, frequently with poor comprehension. They often read at very advanced grade levels but with comprehension skills at a much lower level (hyperlexia). Math facts are also often acquired quickly and spelling and grammar are excellent in this type of child. As with visuospatial skills, this is not typical of all children with autism; some have average abilities and a few have difficulties with reading and calculations. Report or essay writing is often difficult because of difficulty with making logical sequences of events and differentiating between relevant and irrelevant details, but is aided by story webs or the graphic organizers described below. Towards the end of elementary school or beginning of middle school, the demands for comprehension and use of abstract reasoning begin to escalate, and the basic skills become a means to acquire and process large amounts of information and form concepts and insights. The transition to middle school and then high school are also associated with increasing demands on these higher-order skills. It is at these transitions that the previously excellent academic performance (except in the area of handwriting and sports) begins to deteriorate. Social demands also increase and create another set of severe problems that may cause a child with autism to leave the regular education system in order to survive emotionally. At this point, classes that are factually and memory-based, such as science, mainstream history classes, and rule-based math classes, may remain areas of achievement. However, English literature classes are typically their most difficult academic subjects because they require strong skills in the areas of greatest weakness for individuals with ASD. Understanding literature and writing essays require the capacity for knowing peoples' thoughts, feelings, intentions and motives, intact comprehension of idioms and metaphors, and the capacity for identifying themes and cause-and-effect relationships between people's actions.

A major limitation of the educational curriculum at all levels is the lack of textbooks adapted to the cognitive strengths and limitations of children with autism of varying levels of severity. Adaptation of materials by dedicated personnel is feasible in the elementary-school years but becomes impossible at higher-grade levels. Planning for post-highschool education is subject to these same basic limitations. Success in the work place, which unfortunately remains uncommon, depends on the identification of a job that taps their strengths and does not require social, problem-solving or communication skills beyond the elementary. Kanner commented long ago on the marked contrast between academic achievement and job status (Kanner et al., 1972).

Educational intervention

Fifty to seventy per cent of the children now being diagnosed with autism are non-mentally retarded. It will therefore be increasingly important to have an understanding of educational intervention for these more able children. Most verbal children on the autistic spectrum have impaired ability to organize concepts in their expression and comprehension of verbal material. This deficit is evident from early in development and tends to persist even when other language-related deficits abate. Visual perception, concrete visually based problem-solving, and simple visual memory are frequently strengths. In addition, children on the autistic spectrum benefit from memorizing a plan or set of rules for how to do something. Direct teaching of scripts can be very effective. An intervention approach that is particularly well suited to the remedial needs, learning style, and neuropsychological profile of these individuals is graphic organizers (Parks and Black, 1990, 1992; Pehrsson and Robinson, 1985, 1988). Instead of scripting a series of individual utterances, this concrete visual approach to language organization scripts a finite set of plans for organizing expression and for identifying the organization of concepts in oral and written language. The child is taught to identify main topic, subtopics and details and to give more importance to main topic than subtopics and to subtopics than lower-level details.

There exist a wide variety of graphic organizers in the literature. This is confusing for children and teachers especially when different visual formats represent the same hierarchic semantic structure.

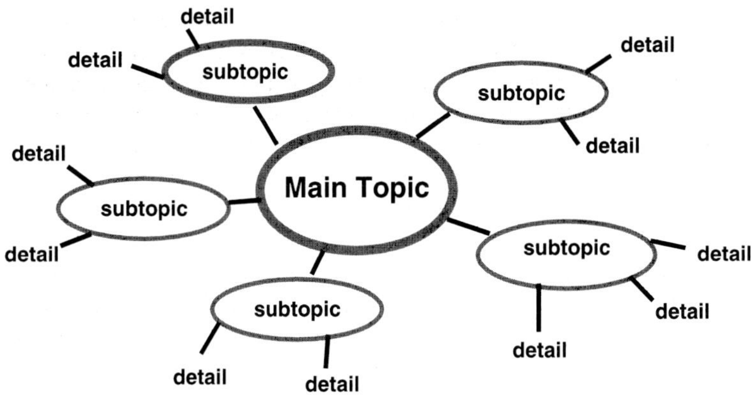

Fig. 2. Description organizer: model.

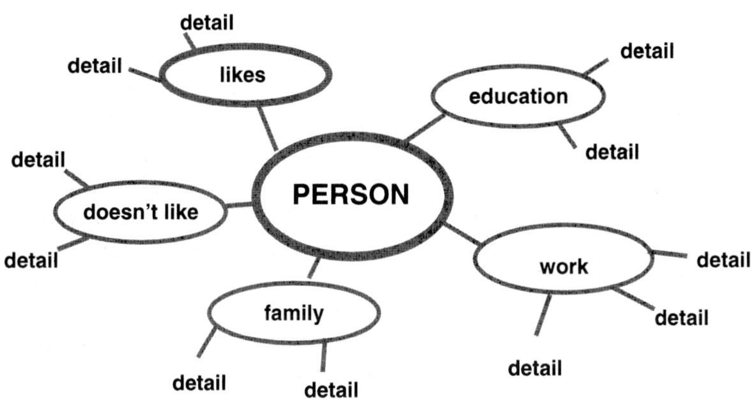

Fig. 3. Description organizer: example 1.

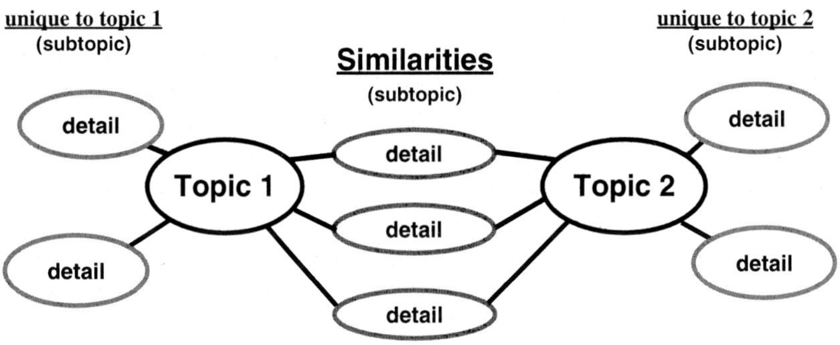

Fig. 4. Comparison organizer: model 1.

The recommended approach (Dunn and Sebastian, 2000) utilizes the following four formats: (1) the description organizer, (2) the comparison organizer, (3) the sequential organizer, and (4) the cause and effect organizer (Figs. 2–5).

Initially the description organizers are used to help the child structure expression. Children who are initially able to generate single sentences are taught to use the visual cues to generate 'paragraphs' and conversations. For more verbal children, the organiz-

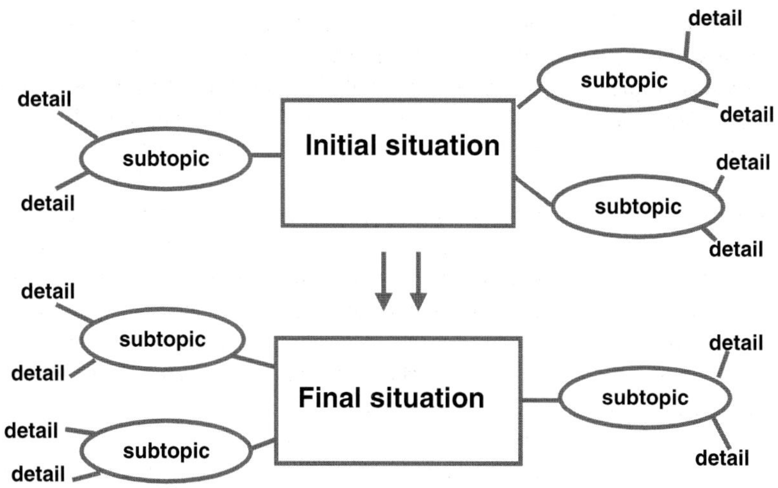

Fig. 5. Cause and effect organizer: model.

ers focus the child on a main topic as being more important than subtopics which should have more importance than lower-level details. With the benefit of concrete visual cues, the child is taught to generate topic sentences prior to providing details and to maintain topic. Once the child has some facility with the use of the description organizer for expression, the focus shifts to the use of organizers for comprehension as well. First the child is given practice identifying the categories to which words belong, the topic of pictures, and the topic of connected speech or written language. The most difficult activity for communication-impaired children is typically identification of subtopics and shifts in subtopic. To teach subtopic identification, it is often necessary to help the child to list details from the material and then sort them and give the categories of information labels. Once the child can do these tasks, description organizers are used to map main topic, subtopics and details. The other organizers are then taught in turn.

The graphic organizer approach teaches children on the autistic spectrum to identify the overall concept prior to attending to individual details (see the forest before the individual trees). It teaches an alternative to the natural tendency to rote memorization. It helps the child to emphasize what is important and to de-emphasize what is less important. Finally, improved organization of verbal material supports ability to make inferences and to integrate current learning with information to be acquired in the future or that which was learned in the past.

The description organizer is used for descriptions or explanations of people, places, objects, events or ideas. This organizer can be used for definitions of words that include specification of category membership. It is used to improve comprehension of factual and fictional material. A special use of the description organizer is to work on topic maintenance in conversation. The organizers may be generated by a group of children employing the same main topic and perhaps the same subtopics. Children in the group are asked to speak using the graphic organizer. The other children in the group are required to comment, ask questions and add information to the topic under discussion. Children are taught to explicitly mark shifts in topic.

Comparison organizers are used for comparison of people, places, things, events and ideas. Sequential organizers are used for sequential narrative or expository expression. Cause-and-effect organizers are used to outline initial and resulting situations to aid understanding of causes and consequences (specifically, what in the initial situation produced the final situation?).

The use of graphic organizers with each individual child must be tailored to the child's neuropsychological profile of strengths and weaknesses. Graphic organizers can, for example, be color-coded in order to focus the child's attention. If the child is having difficulty with topic maintenance, coloring each subtopic along with its corresponding details a different color can help the child stick to each subtopic. If a child is having difficulty with the hierarchic structure of language, specifically, having a tendency to emphasize a single detail over central ideas, the main topic can be one color, subtopics another color, and details a third color. If the child is distracted by color, the organizers can be presented in black and white. The number of subtopics or details may have to be limited in children who are hyper-verbal and perseverative. If a child has problems with visual sequencing the sequential organizer would simply not be used.

Treatment

Behavioral intervention

Behavior modification programs are used in autism at all ages. The principles are simple (operant conditioning, positive reinforcement, token or reward systems, ignoring negative behavior, use of activities that reduce the opportunity for engaging in negative behavior), but they must be applied within the framework of autism. Because of the particular constellation of cognitive deficits and abilities, autistic individuals 'see' the world far differently than other people. Their behavior and reactions to the world are logical if one sees the world through their minds' eye. Individuals with most other developmental disabilities have the same basic constellation of cognitive abilities or frame of reference as non-disabled individuals. This is because their brains are still wired in the normal pattern, perhaps with less wiring or with focal glitches, but the computations of the brain produce the same type of answer as in non-disabled people. However, in autism these relationships are not present; they have selective problems with higher-order skills and intact or enhanced simpler skills that result in an entirely different interpretation of the world. A typical example from the *Rain Man* of these differences was when Raymond began to tantrum because there were only four fish sticks instead of eight; the solution that satisfied him was for his brother to cut them in half. To other people, the details or precise number of pieces would not have been the issue; the quantity of fish would have been. They would also be likely to know that they could ask for more or would get more when they ate what they had. Raymond's tantrum could have led to considerable effort with traditional behavior modification techniques to try to achieve 'normal' behavior or to the prescribing of medications. Ultimately, though, an understanding of how the person with autism sees the world and a simple modification of the environment (and of the mindset of those who insist the person with autism act 'normal') solves the problem. As this example demonstrates, the world (inanimate and human) will always have to be adapted to these individuals because their deficits severely compromise their capacity to be flexible, to cope, and to adapt. Determining the purpose or function an undesirable behavior serves for the person with autism is key to addressing it. The same problem behavior, for example, aggression, may reflect frustration from inability to communicate needs, interruption of rituals, or violation of social space. The solution obviously differs greatly for each of these possibilities. In the absence of the capacity to identify needs, which requires concept formation, the individual with ASD is dependent on the problem-solving abilities of those around him to determine what is upsetting them.

Early childhood intervention programs are a current major focus of treatment in autism. A number of university-based model programs have reported substantial improvement in children with autism participating in programs that involve 15–40 h per week of school-based intervention (reviewed in: Dawson and Osterling, 1997; Howlin, 1998; Rogers, 1998). These programs report better than expected gains in IQ scores, language level, autism severity, class placement, and sometimes also social and adaptive behavior. The gains are greatest in children with less severe symptoms at entry and with evidence of the emergence of social and communication skills. Programs that take more severely impaired children report less dramatic improvements. It is also clear that the response to treatment is variable, with some children making little progress in programs that produce remarkable gains in other children. The National Academy of Sciences Committee on 'Educating Children with Autism' has released a report on non-pharmacologic treatment for autism, which reviews supporting data for each intervention and makes recommendations regarding treatment programs. This report can be found at the National Academy Press Web site.[5]

Each of the early intervention programs in autism has a different approach, but all focus on training five basic skills: (1) the ability to attend to people and to cooperate with teaching exercises; (2) the ability to imitate others both verbally and motorically; (3) the ability to comprehend and use language, which begins with providing immediate positive reward to the child's smallest attempt to communicate, such as a glance or the slightest body movement; (4) the ability to play appropriately with toys; and (5) the ability to socially interact with others. There are eight common elements to these programs: (1) a specific established curriculum delivered by highly trained and educated professional staff with ongoing monitoring of program fidelity and child response; (2) intervention beginning early, continuing year-round for 1–2 or more years, and involving 25 or more hours per week of intervention; (3) highly structured teaching environments with a high staff to student ratio, often 1 : 1 or 1 : 2, followed by systematic procedures for generalization of skills to more complex natural environments; (4) recognition of the importance of predictable routines with support through transitions; (5) use of functional analysis of problem behaviors; (6) a focus on the transfer of skills acquired in intervention programs to school classrooms; (7) training and active participation of family in the intervention process, and (8) individualization of the treatment program to consider the abilities of each child.

Intervention programs are multifaceted and comprehensive and have evolved largely through the use of applied behavior analysis (ABA). ABA is not, however, an intervention program or a specific method, but applies to any method that changes behavior in a systematic way to produce objective improvement. Using an ABA perspective, intervention research led to many procedures or methods such as discrete trial training, massed trials, discrimination training, pivotal response training, incidental teaching, and peer-mediated treatment. An ABA approach to problem behavior similarly led to the use of functional analysis of problem behaviors, reinforcement of competing behavior, identification and elimination of provocations of the behavior or prompting of alternative desired behavior, ignoring the behavior until it is extinguished, and rarely aversive or negative responses.

There are some notable limitations to these studies and thus to their conclusions. Outcome data are remarkably limited for all of the model programs, often reflecting a small number of subjects. There are no comparison studies of these programs and so no data to demonstrate the superiority of one program over another. Also, to date, there have been no true replication studies that have required random assignment to treatment groups and outcome assessment by individuals blind to treatment status. Some programs have also used entry criteria that select children with evidence of communicative intent, the absence of dysmorphic features, and low rates of stereotypic behavior, which are early signs of less severe autism. It is not clear whether such programs would be equally effective in an unselected population or in more severely impaired children with autism. One additional significant limitation of early intervention research is the failure to consider the natural history of improvement that has characterized a substantial subgroup of children with autism since Kanner's original reports (Kanner, 1943, 1971; Kanner et al., 1972). This being said, no one is contesting the importance of early intervention.

The major unresolved problems with regard to early intervention include: the successful translation of model programs into local public intervention programs, their availability, the identification of all children at the earliest age possible, and the identification of child indicators of the timing, intensity, and type of intervention that will result in maximal success. A variety of approaches including training and monitoring programs, routine screening of toddlers and young children, and research will be needed to address these issues.

Pharmacologic intervention

Medications are an adjunct only and their use should be preceded and accompanied by an intense effort to modify the environment and the use of behavioral techniques. Medication is typically prescribed either to address specific complications, such as attention

[5] URL: http://www.nationalacademies.org

deficit disorder, seizures, or affective disorder, or more commonly to reduce problem behavior such as aggression, verbal outbursts, non-compliance, or ritualistic behavior. There can be many underlying reasons for the latter nonspecific behavioral responses and success in treatment depends to a great extent on identifying and specifically addressing these problems, i.e., use of functional analysis of behavior. Excellent reviews of pharmacologic treatment in ASD are provided by Cook and Leventhal, 1995, McDougle, 1997, and Posey and McDougle, 2000.

Pharmacologic treatment in ASD is severely hampered by the paucity of controlled trial data on efficacy and side effects for most of the medications in common use. There is considerable variability in response, and what may be very helpful in some individuals may make others worse. Data are not yet available to make individual predictions about response. In the interim, clinical practice awaits the availability of controlled trial data and relies on experienced clinicians.

A few caveats have emerged that may represent idiosyncrasies in drug response specific to ASD. The two best known are the near universal tolerance that develops to clonidine (Catapres) after several weeks or months of treatment and the response to very low or 'subtherapeutic' doses of the potent serotonin transporter inhibitors. Perhaps a third caveat is that anxiety is the largest unrecognized contributor to behavior problems in ASD and can be responsible for aggression, increased ritualistic behavior, and social withdrawal. Its relief is thought to be the basis for the success associated with the use of serotonin transporter inhibitors in ASD. Perhaps a fourth is that complex partial seizures are far more prevalent than appreciated in ASD, and may account for the not uncommon positive response of aggression, irritability, and sleep disturbances in young children to Depakote (valproic acid) and Tegretol (carbamazapine).

Sertonin transporter inhibitors

These agents were the first to make a major difference in ASD and their use has become widespread. These agents include Prozac (fluoxetine), Zoloft (sertraline), Paxil (paroxetine), and Luvox (fluvoxamine), Celexa (citralopram), and the less selective tricyclic Anafranil (clomipramine). All but the last are categorized as selective serotonin reuptake inhibitors and are commonly referred to as SSRIs. These agents are most likely to be effective when individuals appear constantly and highly anxious, manifested by worrying or anger when encountering change or by aggression when routines are disrupted. It is also indicated for obsessive–compulsive symptoms and for ritualistic behavior that is interfering significantly with function. The most data are available for the first two agents released, Prozac and Anafranil. However, the side effect profile and long half-life make them less desirable than the newer agents. In addition, both lower the seizure threshold. Although the newer SSRIs are thought to be associated with a lower or no risk for seizures, all may reduce the seizure threshold, but not nearly to the extent that tricyclic antidepressants do. Zoloft and Paxil have shorter half-lives and have the advantage of not altering the metabolism of Tegretol and Risperdal (Risperidone). The side effects include restlessness, insomnia, irritability and loss of appetite. Occasional children become hypo-manic on SSRIs.

Tricyclic antidepressants other than Anafranil

Little data exist for efficacy in autism, but what has been published suggests that tricyclic antidepressants other than Anafranil worsen symptoms in the majority of individuals with autism even at very low doses. Worsening comes in the form of worsening hyperactivity, irritability and insomnia and, in some, signs of psychosis. The tricyclics also lower the seizure threshold. Wellbutrin (bupropion) is commonly effective in children with ADHD as a second-line treatment but its efficacy in ASD is not known. Generally these medications are also avoided in favor of the SSRIs because of their cardiac and strong anticholinergic effects.

Stimulants

Stimulants such as Ritalin (methylphenidate) and Adderall (dextroamphetamine and amphetamine) are effective in the treatment of ADHD symptoms in some children with ASD. The important distinction is between the random inattention seen in ADHD and the inattention in autism that is the result of the social impairment, deficits in comprehension, or internal preoccupations especially of children with strong visual memory abilities. Other children are worsened by stimulants becoming either more irritable or dazed. Patients should be closely monitored for tics, and parents instructed to call at the first evidence of tics so that medication can be discontinued before a permanent movement disorder occurs. Also, if there is a family history of tics or movement disorder, stimulants should be avoided.

Sympatholytic agents

Tenex (guanfacine) and Catapres (clonidine) have been used in the treatment of hyperactivity, impulsivity, and inattention in ASD. What little evidence exists, especially for Tenex, suggests that they are not effective. The development of tolerance after a few weeks or months of improvement is very common with Catapres. Catapres and perhaps Tenex are best used for sleep only (given once at night), after non-medication interventions have been tried.

In contrast, the beta blockers, Inderal (propanolol) and Corgard (naldolol), have shown efficacy in treating aggression and impulsivity related to interruption of routines in some individuals. Individuals who become aggressive when an anticipated event does not occur are the most likely candidates to respond. Propanolol has been the only agent to work in some cases of this type. Antihypertensive doses are required. Appropriate use of these agents may reduce the dose or use of neuroleptics.

Anxiolytics

Ativan (lorazepam) and Klonopin (clonazepam) are sometimes effective in reducing anxiety. Most experience is with adults, and efficacy in children is unknown. Buspar (buspirone) is infrequently helpful but when effective can help avoid or reduce the dose of neuroleptic.

Traditional neuroleptics

Because of the risk of permanent tardive dyskinesia and the life-long nature of the symptoms in autism, the traditional neuroleptics are usually avoided. All other possibilities should be exhausted before considering these agents. If individuals are on them, attempts should be made to substitute another agent or at least reduce the dose.

Atypical neuroleptics

The atypical neuroleptics are considered to have a reduced but not absent risk of tardive dyskinesia. Risperdal is the current favorite and efficacy in both children and adults with ASD has been demonstrated in initial trials. It has been used effectively for the treatment of aggression, agitation, hyperactivity not responsive to other agents, self-mutilation, and severe ritualistic or stereotypic behavior. Again, the lowest dose for the shortest time possible should be used after trials of other medications that reduce anxiety, impulsivity and aggression have failed. Agents associated with obesity are to be avoided as this readily becomes a chronic intractable medical problem.

Anticonvulsants

Seizures are treated in the same way as in other individuals. In ASD, though, unrecognized partial complex seizures appear to be relatively common in the presence of behavior problems and may underlie cyclical irritability and aggression, sleep disturbances particularly insomnia, and deteriorations in behavior. Treatment of seizures in such cases is typically associated with a generalized improvement in the autistic symptoms; conversely, loss of seizure control is associated with increasing severity of the autism. Thus, any sustained worsening in function not explained by change or environmental overload requires consideration of partial complex seizures as well as depression and rarely mania. Depakote in particular, but also Tegretol, used for 'mood lability' have been reported anecdotally to produce significant improvements in ASD children, most likely in relation to unrecognized seizures. However, it is important to be aware that Depakote commonly results in obesity, which itself can become a significant health problem. It goes without saying that phenobarbital is to be avoided in this population because of the high rate of adverse behavioral side effects.

Naltrexone and lithium

These medications are generally ineffective. Lithium of course is effective in the treatment of mania but use as a mood stabilizer in the absence of bipolar disorder is usually of no benefit.

Conclusion

Considerable progress has been made in the understanding of autism and the pervasive developmental disorders in the past 5–10 years. Prevalence estimates for autism and autism spectrum disorders (autism, Asperger's disorder, and pervasive developmental disorder not otherwise specified) have risen dramatically to 60/10,000 and 50% of the children being diagnosed today are non-mentally retarded. Cognitive and neurologic impairments have been identified to account for nearly every feature of the disorder. This has demystified autism and brought it clearly into the realm of neurologic disorders. The majority of cases (90%) are now thought to be the result of multiple interacting genes but not the same genes in each case. Family members have been found to have a high rate of social and communication impairments and preoccupations with particular interests. These symptoms are milder than those in autism but of the same type. The rates of affective disorder, anxiety disorder and possibly attention deficit disorder are also increased in family members. An increase in brain weight in autistic children under 12 years of age, an accelerated growth of the head in the early years of life, and an increase in imaging brain volume in children under 12 have strongly implicated disturbances in developmental neurobiologic processes, particularly those involved in the elaboration and pruning of neuronal processes. Treatment remains primarily behavioral. Early intervention programs report an improvement in outcome with intensive behavior training in very early life. Behavioral intervention and environmental modification remain the mainstays of treatment in autism throughout life. Such interventions must be applied within the framework of autism. Identifying the specific trigger for an undesirable behavior is important to effectively addressing it. Pharmacologic treatment is an adjunct and has been improved with the introduction of the selective serotonin reuptake inhibitors, which reduce anxiety, aggression, and obsessive–compulsive behavior. The future holds great promise for progress in the treatment of these disorders. The decoding of the human genome has provided the foundation for a medical revolution and for radically improved biologically based treatments in the future.

Acknowledgements

I would like to thank Evelyn Herbert for her devoted and excellent work and her patience. I would also like to thank Dr. Bernie Devlin for his contribution of the genetics section. Finally, I would like to thank Dr. Isabelle Rapin for considerable patience. This chapter was supported by HD35469 grant and by the NICHD Neurobiology and Genetics of Autism Network, Collaborative Program of Excellence in Autism.

References

Abell F, Krams M, Ashburner J, Passingham R, Friston K, Frackowiak R, Happe F, Frith C, Frith U: The neuroanatomy of autism: a voxel-based whole brain analysis of structural scans. Neuroreport: 10(8); 1647–1651, 1999.

American Psychiatric Association: Diagnostic and Statistical Manual of Mental Disorders, 4th ed. Washington, DC: APA, 1994.

Arvidsson T, Danielsson B, Forsberg P, Gillberg C, Johansson M, Kallgren G: Autism in 3 to 6-year-old children in a suburb of Goteborg, Sweden. Autism: 1; 163–173, 1997.

Atwood AJ: Asperger's Syndrome: A Guide for Parents and Professionals. London: Kingsley, 1998.

Aylward EH, Minshew NJ, Field K, Sparks BF, Singh N: Effects of age on brain volume and head circumference in autism. Neurology: 59(2); 175–183, 2002

Aylward EH, Minshew NJ, Goldstein G, Honeycutt NA, Augustine AM, Yates KO, Barta PE, Pearlson GD: MRI volumes of amygdala and hippocampus in non-mentally retarded autistic adolescents and adults. Neurology: 53(9); 2145–2150, 1999.

Bailey A, Le Couteur A, Gottesman I, Bolton P, Simonoff E, Yuzda E, Rutter M: Autism as a strongly genetic disorder: evidence from a British twin study. Psychology Medicine: 25(1); 63–77, 1995.

Bailey A, Luthert P, Dean A, Harding B, Janota I, Montgomery M, Rutter M, Lantos P: A clinicopathological study of autism. Brain: 121(Pt 5); 889–905, 1998.

Bailey A, Phillips W, Rutter M: Autism: towards an integration of clinical, genetic, neuropsychological, and neurobiological perspectives. Journal of Child Psychology and Psychiatry and Allied Disciplines: 37(1); 89–126, 1996.

Baird G, Charman T, Baron-Cohen S, Cox A, Swettenham J, Wheelwright S, Drew A: A screening instrument for autism at 18 months of age: A 6-year follow-up study. Journal of the American Academy of Child and Adolescent Psychiatry: 39(6); 694–702, 2000.

Baron-Cohen S, Cox A, Baird G et al.: Psychological markers of autism at 18 months of age in a large population. British Journal of Psychiatry: 168; 158–163, 1996.

Baron-Cohen S, Ring HA, Wheelwright S, Bullmore ET, Brammer MJ, Simmons A, Williams SC: Social intelligence in the normal and autistic brain: an fMRI study. European Journal of Neuroscience: 11(6); 1891–1898, 1999.

Barrett S, Beck JC, Bernier R, Bisson E, Braun TA, Casavant TL, Childress D et al.: An autosomal genomic screen for autism: collaborative linkage study of autism. American Journal of Medical Genetics: 88; 609–615, 1999.

Belmonte M, Egaas B, Townsend J, Courchesne E: NMR intensity of corpus callosum differs with age but not with diagnosis of autism. Neuroreport: 6(9); 1253–1256, 1995.

Bennetto L, Pennington BF, Rogers SJ: Intact and impaired memory functions in autism. Child Development: 67(4); 1816–1835, 1996.

Berument SK, Rutter M, Lord C et al.: Autism screening questionnaire: Diagnostic validity. British Journal of Psychiatry: 175; 444–451, 1999.

Boucher J: Immediate free recall in early childhood autism: another point of behavioural similarity with the amnesic syndrome. British Journal of Psychology: 72(Pt 2); 211–215, 1981.

Boucher J: Word fluency in high-functioning autistic children. Journal of Autism and Developmental Disorders: 18(4); 637–645, 1988.

Boucher J, Warrington EK: Memory deficits in early infantile autism: some similarities to the amnesic syndrome. British Journal of Psychology: 67(1); 73–87, 1976.

Bradford Y, Haines J, Hutcheson et al.: Incorporating language phenotypes strengthens evidence of linkage to autism. American Journal of Medical Genetics: 105; 539–547, 2001.

Bryson SE: Epidemiology of autism. Journal of Autism and Developmental Disorders: 26; 165–167, 1996.

Bryson SE: Epidemiology of autism: Overview and issues outstanding. In Cohen DJ, Volkmar FR (Eds), Handbook of Autism and Pervasive Developmental Disorders. New York: Wiley, pp. 41–46, 1997.

Bryson SE, Smith IM: Epidemiology of autism: Prevalence, associated characteristics, and implications for research and service delivery. Mental Retardation and Developmental Disabilities Research Reviews: 4; 97–103, 1998.

Burack JA, Enns JT, Johannes EA: Attention and autism: behavioral and electrophysiological evidence. In Cohen DJ, Volkmar FR (Eds), Handbook of Autism and Pervasive Developmental Disorders. New York: Wiley, pp. 226–247, 1997.

Buxbaum JD, Silverman JM, Smith CJ, Kilifarski M, Reichert J, Hollander E et al.: Linkage and heterogeneity in autism. American Journal of Human Genetics: 68; 1514–1520, 2001.

Carper RA, Courchesne E: Inverse correlation between frontal lobe and cerebellum sizes in children with autism. Brain: 123(Pt 4); 836–844, 2000.

Casey BJ, Gordon CT, Mannheim GB, Rumsey JM: Dysfunctional attention in autistic savants. Journal of Clinical and Experimental Neuropsychology: 15(6); 933–46, 1993.

Chakrabarti S, Fombonne E: Pervasive developmental disorders in preschool children. Journal of the American Medical Association: 285; 3093–3099, 2001.

Chugani DC, Muzik O, Behen M, Rothermel R, Janisse JJ, Lee J, Chugani HT: Developmental changes in brain serotonin synthesis capacity in autistic and nonautistic children. Annals of Neurology: 45(3); 287–295, 1999.

Chugani DC, Muzik O, Rothermel R, Behen M, Chakraborty P, Mangner T, da Silva EA, Chugani HT: Altered serotonin synthesis in the dentatothalamocortical pathway in autistic boys. Annals of Neurology: 42(4); 666–669, 1997.

Cook EH, Leventhal BL: Autistic disorder and other pervasive developmental disorders. Pediatric Psychopharmacology: 4(2); 381–399, 1995.

Courchesne E, Karns CM, Davis HR, Ziccardi R, Carper RA, Tigue ZD, Chisum HJ, Moses P, Pierce K, Lord C, Lincoln AJ, Pizzo S, Schreibman L, Haas RH, Akshoomoff NA, Courchesne RY: Unusual brain growth patterns in early life in patients with autistic disorder: An MRI study. Neurology: 57(2); 245–254, 2001.

Courchesne E, Townsend J, Akshoomoff NA, Saitoh O, Yeung-Courchesne R, Lincoln AJ, James HE, Haas RH, Schreibman L, Lau L: Impairment in shifting attention in autistic and cerebellar patients. Behavioral Neuroscience: 108(5); 848–865, 1994.

Dawson G, Levy A: Arousal, attention, and the socioemotional impairments of individuals with autism. In Dawson G (Ed), Autism: Nature, Diagnosis, and Treatment. New York: Guilford Press, pp. 49–74, 1989.

Dawson G, Osterling J: Early intervention in autism: Effectiveness and common elements of current approaches. In Guralnick MJ (Ed), The Effectiveness of Early Intervention: Second Generation Research. Baltimore, MD: Paul H. Brookes, pp. 307–326, 1997.

Deb S, Prasad KBG: The prevalence of autistic disorder among children with a learning disability. British Journal of Psychiatry: 165(3); 395–399, 1994.

Deykin EY, McMahon B: The incidence of seizures among children with autistic symptoms. American Journal of Psychiatry: 136; 1310–1312, 1979.

Dunn M, Sebastian M: A neuropsychological approach to language intervention in autistic children. In Accardo PJ, Magnusen C, Capute AJ (Eds), Autism: Clinical and Research Issues. York Press: Iimonium, pp. 57–75, 2000.

Dunn M, Vaughan H, Kreuzer J, Kurtzberg D: Electrophysiologic correlates of semantic classification in autistic and normal children. Developmental Neuropsychology: 16(1); 79–99, 1999.

Egaas B, Courchesne E, Saitoh O: Reduced size of the corpus callosum in autism. Archives of Neurology: 52; 794–801, 1995.

Ehlers S, Gillberg C: The epidemiology of Asperger's syndrome. A total population study. Journal of Child Psychology and Psychiatry: 34; 1327–1350, 1993.

Fein D, Dunn M, Allen DA, Aram DM, Hall N, Morris R, Wilson BC: Language and neuropsychological findings. In Rapin I (Ed), Preschool Children with Inadequate Communication: Developmental Language Disorder, Autism, Low IQ. London: Mac Keith Press, pp. 123–154, 1996.

Filipek PA, Accardo PJ, Ashwal S, Baranek GT, Cook EH Jr, Dawson G, Gordon B, Gravel JS, Johnson CP, Kallen RJ, Levy SE, Minshew NJ, Ozonoff S, Prizant BM, Rapin I, Rogers SJ, Stone WL, Teplin SW, Tuchman RF, Volkmar FR: Practice parameter: Screening and diagnosis of autism: Report of the Quality Standards Subcommittee of the American Academy of Neurology and the Child Neurology Society. Neurology: 55(4); 468–479, 2000.

Folstein SE, Mankoski RE: Chromosome 7q: where autism meets language disorder? American Journal of Human Genetics: 67; 278–281, 2000.

Fombonne E: Epidemiology of autism in France. Psychologie Française: 43(2); 119–125, 1998.

Fombonne E, Roge B, Claverie J, Courty S, Fremolle: Microcephaly and macrocephaly in autism. Journal of Autism and Developmental Disorders: 29(2); 113–119, 1999.

Garber HJ, Ritvo ER: Magnetic resonance imaging of the posterior fossa in autistic adults. American Journal of Psychiatry: 149(2); 245–247, 1992.

Gillberg C: Outcome in autism and autistic-like conditions. Journal of the American Academy of Child and Adolescent Psychiatry: 3; 375–382, 1991.

Gillberg C, Schaumann H: Epilepsy presenting as infantile autism? Two case studies. Neuropediatrics: 14; 206–212, 1983.

Gillberg C, Schaumann H, Gillberg IC: Autism in immigrants: children born in Sweden to mothers born in Uganda. Journal of Intellectual Disability Research: 39; 141–144, 1995.

Gillberg C, Steffenburg S: Outcome and prognostic factors in Infantile Autism and similar conditions: A population-based study of 46 cases followed through puberty. Journal of Autism and Developmental Disorders: 17; 273–287, 1987.

Gillberg C, Steffenburg S, Schaumann H: Is autism more common now than ten years ago? British Journal of Psychiatry: 158; 403–409, 1991.

Gillberg C, Wing L: Autism: not an extremely rare disorder. Acta Psychiatrica Scandinavica: 99(6); 399–406, 1999.

Goldstein G, Johnson CR, Minshew NJ: Attentional processes in autism. Journal of Autism and Developmental Disorders: 31(4); 433–440, 2001.

Goode S, Rutter M, Howlin P: A twenty-year follow-up of children with autism. Paper presented at the 13th biennial meeting of ISSBD, Amsterdam, 1994.

Gravel JS: Auditory integration training: Placing the burden of proof. American Journal of Speech–Language Pathology: 3(2); 25–29, 1994.

Hardan AY, Minshew NJ, Harenski K, Keshvan M: Posterior fossa structure in autism. Journal of the American Academy of Child and Adolescent Psychiatry: 40(6); 666–672, 2001.

Hardan AY, Minshew NJ, Keshavan MS: Corpus callosum size in autism. Neurology: 55; 1033–1036, 2000.

Harris NS, Courchesne E, Townsend J, Carper RA, Lord C: Neuroanatomic contributions to slowed orienting of attention in children with autism. Cognitive Brain Research: 8(1); 61–71, 1999.

Hashimoto T, Murakawa K, Miyazaki M, Tayama M, Kuroda Y: Magnetic resonance imaging of the brain structures in the posterior fossa in retarded autistic children. Acta Paediatrica: 81(12); 1030–1034, 1992.

Hashimoto T, Tayama M, Miyazaki M, Murakawa K, Shimakawa S, Yoneda Y, Kuroda Y: Brainstem involvement in high functioning autistic children. Acta Neurologica Scandinavica: 88(2); 123–128, 1993.

Hashimoto T, Tayama M, Murakawa K, Yoshimoto T, Miyazaki M, Harada M, Kuroda Y: Development of the brainstem and cerebellum in autistic patients. Journal of Autism and Developmental Disorders: 25(1); 1–18, 1995.

Haznedar MM, Buchsbaum MS, Wei TC, Hof PR, Cartwright C, Bienstock CA, Hollander E: Limbic circuitry in patients with autism spectrum disorders studied with positron emission tomography and magnetic resonance imaging. American Journal of Psychiatry: 157(12); 1994–2001, 2000.

Holttum JR, Minshew NJ, Sanders RS, Phillips NE: Magnetic resonance imaging of the posterior fossa in autism. Biological Psychiatry: 32(12); 1091–1101, 1992.

Honda H, Shimizu Y, Misumi K, Niimi M: Cumulative incidence and prevalence of childhood autism in children in Japan. British Journal of Psychiatry: 169(2); 228–235, 1996.

Horwitz B, Rumsey JM: Positron emission tomography: Implications for cerebral dysfunction in autism. In Bauman ML, Kemper TL (Eds), The Neurobiology of Autism. Baltimore, MD: The Johns Hopkins University Press, pp. 102–118, 1994.

Howard MA, Cowell PE, Boucher J, Broks P, Mayes A, Farrant A, Roberts N: convergent neuroanatomical and behavioural evidence of an amygdala hypothesis of autism. Neuroreport: 11(13); 2931–2935, 2000.

Howlin P: Practitioner review: psychological and educational treatments for autism. Journal of Child Psychology and Psychiatry and Allied Disciplines: 39(3); 307–322, 1998.

Hsu M, Yeung-Courchesne R, Courchesne E, Press GA: Absence of magnetic resonance imaging evidence of pontine abnormality in infantile autism. Archives of Neurology: 48(11); 1160–1163, 1991.

Hutt C, Forrest SJ, Richer J: Cardiac arrhythmia and behaviour in autistic children. Acta Psychiatrica Scandinavica: 51; 361–372, 1975.

International Molecular Genetic Study of Autism Consortium: A full genome screen for autism with evidence for linkage to a region on chromosome 7q: International Molecular Genetic Study of Autism Consortium. Human Molecular Genetics: 7; 571–578, 1998.

Ingram JL, Croog VJ, Tisdale B, Rodier PM: Valproic acid treatment in rats reproduces the cerebellar anomalies associated with autism. Teratology: 53; 86, 1996.

Ingram JL, Stodgell CJ, Hyman SL, Figlewicz DA, Weitkamp LR, Rodier PM: Discovery of allelic variants of HOXA1 and HOXB1: genetic susceptibility to autism spectrum disorders. Teratology: 62; 393–405, 2000.

Ishii T, Takahashi O: The epidemiology of autistic children

in Toyota, Japan: Prevalence. Japanese Journal of Child and Adolescent Psychiatry: 24(5); 311–312, 1983.

Kadesjoe B, Gillberg C, Hagberg B: Autism and Asperger syndrome in seven-year-old children: A total population study. Journal of Autism and Developmental Disorders: 29(4); 327–331, 1999.

Kanner L: Autistic disturbances of affective contact. Nervous Child: 2; 217–250, 1943.

Kanner L: Follow-up study of eleven autistic children originally reported in 1943. Journal of Autism and Child Schizophrenia: 1(2); 119–145, 1971.

Kanner L, Rodriguez A, Ashenden B: How far can autistic children go in matters of social adaptations? Journal of Autism and Developmental Disorders: 2; 9–33, 1972.

Kemper TL, Bauman M: Neuropathology of infantile autism. Journal of Neuropathology and Experimental Neurology: 57(7); 645–652, 1998.

Kleiman MD, Neff S, Rosman NP: The brain in infantile autism: are posterior fossa structures abnormal? Neurology: 42(4); 753–760, 1992.

Klin A, Volkmar FR, Sparrow SS, Cicchetti DV, Rourke BP: Validity and neuropsychological characterization of Asperger syndrome: convergence with nonverbal learning disabilities syndrome. Journal of Child Psychology and Psychiatry and Allied Disciplines: 36(7); 1127–1140, 1995.

Kobayashi R, Murata T, Yoshinaga K: A follow-up study of 201 children with autism in Kyushu and Yamaguchi areas, Japan. Journal of Autism and Developmental Disorders: 22; 395–411, 1992.

Lake CR, Ziegler MG, Murphy DL: Increased norepinephrine levels and decreased dopamine-β-hydroxylase activity in primary autism. Archives of General Psychiatry: 34; 553–556, 1977.

Lamb JA, Moore J, Bailey A, Monaco AP: Autism: recent molecular genetic advances. Human Molecular Genetics: 9; 861–868, 2000.

Le Couteur A, Rutter M, Lord C: Autism diagnostic observation schedule: A standardized observation of communicative and social behavior. Journal of Autism and Developmental Disorders: 19; 363–387, 1989.

Lockyer L, Rutter M: A five to fifteen year follow-up study of infantile psychosis: IV. Patterns of cognitive ability. British Journal of Social and Clinical Psychology: 9: 152–163, 1970.

Lord C: Autism spectrum disorders and ADHD: In Accardo P, Blondis TA, Shitman BY, Stein M (Eds), Attention Deficit Disorders and Hyperactivity in Children and Adults. New York, NY: Marcel Dekker, pp. 401–417, 1999.

Lord C, Risi S: Frameworks and methods in diagnosing autism spectrum disorders. Mental Retardation and Developmental Disabilities Research Reviews: 4; 90–96, 1998.

Lord C, Rutter M, Le Couteur AL: Autism diagnostic interview revised: A revised version of a diagnostic interview for caregivers of individuals with possible pervasive developmental disorders. Journal of Autism and Developmental Disorders: 24; 659–685, 1994.

Lord C, Schopler E, Revicki D: Sex differences in autism. Journal of Autism and Developmental Disorders: 12; 317–330, 1982.

Lotter V: Follow-up studies. In: Rutter M, Schopler E (Eds), Autism. A Reappraisal of Concepts and Treatment. New York: Plenum Press, pp. 475–495, 1978.

Manes F, Piven J, Vrancic D, Nanclares V, Plebst C, Starkstein SE: An MRI study of the corpus callosum and cerebellum in mentally retarded autistic individuals. Journal of Neuropsychiatry and Clinical Neuroscience: 11(4); 470–474, 1999.

Matsuishi T, Shiotsuki Y, Yoshimura K, Shoji H, Yamashita Y: High prevalence of infantile autism in Kurume City, Japan. Journal of Child Neurology: 2(4); 268–271, 1987.

McDougle CJ: Psychopharmacology. In Cohen DJ, Volkmar FR (Eds), Handbook of Autism and Pervasive Developmental Disorders, 2nd ed. New York: Wiley, pp. 707–729, 1997.

McLennan JD, Lord C, Schopler E: Sex differences in higher functioning people with autism. Journal of Autism and Developmental Disorders: 23(2); 217–227, 1993.

Minshew NJ, Goldstein G: Is autism an amnesic disorder?: Evidence from the California Verbal Learning Test. Neuropsychology: 792; 209–216, 1993.

Minshew NJ, Goldstein G: The pattern of intact and impaired memory functions in autism. Journal of Child Psychology and Psychiatry and Allied Disciplines: in press, 2002.

Minshew NJ, Goldstein G, Muenz LR, Payton JB: Neuropsychological functioning in non-mentally retarded autistic individuals. Journal of Clinical and Experimental Neuropsychology: 14(5); 749–761, 1992.

Minshew NJ, Goldstein G, Siegel DJ: Neuropsychologic functioning in autism: profile of a complex information processing disorder. Journal of International Neuropsychology Society: 3(4); 303–316, 1997.

Minshew N, Johnson C, Luna B: The cognitive and neural basis of autism: A disorder of complex information processing and dysfunction of neocortical systems. In Glidden LM (Ed), International Review of Research in Mental Retardation. New York: Academic Press, pp. 111–138, 2000.

Minshew NJ, Luna B, Sweeney JA: Oculomotor evidence for neocortical systems but not cerebellar dysfunction in autism. Neurology: 52; 917–922, 1999.

Nelson KB, Grether JK, Croen LA, Dambrosia JM, Dickens BF, Jelliffe LL, Hansen RL, Phillips TM: Neuropeptides and neurotrophins in neonatal blood of children with autism or mental retardation. Annals of Neurology: 49(5); 597–606, 2001.

Nordin V, Gillberg C: Autism spectrum disorders in children with physical or mental disability or both: II. Screening aspects. Developmental Medicine and Child Neurology: 38(4); 314–324, 1996.

Nordin V, Gillberg C: The long-term course of autistic disorders: update on follow-up studies. Acta Psychiatrica Scandinavica: 97; 99–108, 1998.

Olsson I, Steffenburg S, Gillberg C: Epilepsy in autism and autistic-like conditions: a population-based study. Archives of Neurology: 45; 666–668, 1988.

Ornitz EM: Autism: A disorder of directed attention. Brain Dysfunction: 1(5–6); 309–322, 1988.

Ozonoff S, Pennington BF, Rogers SJ: Executive function deficits in high-functioning autistic individuals: relationship to theory of mind. Journal of Child Psychology and Psychiatry and Allied Disciplines: 32(7); 1081–1105, 1991.

Ozonoff S, Strayer DL, McMahon WM, Filloux F: Executive function abilities in autism and Tourette syndrome: an information processing approach. Journal of Child Psychology and Psychiatry and Allied Disciplines: 35(6); 1015–1032, 1994.

Parks S, Black H: Organizing Thinking (Book 2). Pacific Grove, CA: Critical Thinking Press and Software, 1990.

Parks S, Black H: Organizing Thinking (Book 1). Pacific Grove, CA: Critical Thinking Press and Software, 1992.

Pascualvaca DM, Fantie BD, Papageorgiou M, Mirsky AF: Attentional capacities in children with autism: is there a general deficit in shifting focus? Journal of Autism and Developmental Disorders: 28(6); 467–478, 1998.

Pehrsson RS, Robinson HA: The Semantic Organizer Approach to Reading and Writing Instruction. Rockville, MD: Aspen, 1985.

Pehrsson RS, Robinson HA: Semantic organizers. Topics in Language Disorders: 8(3); 24–37, 1988.

Persico AM, D'Agruma L, Maiorano N et al.: Reeling gene alleles and haplotypes as a factor predisposing to autistic disorder. Molecular Psychiatry: 6; 150–159, 2001.

Philippe A, Martinez M, Guilloud-Bataille M, Gillberg C, Rastam M, Sponheim E, Coleman M, Zappella M, Aschauer H, Van Maldergem L, Penet C, Feingold J, Brice A, Leboyer M, van Malldergerme L: Genome-wide scan for autism susceptibility genes: Paris Autism Research International Sibpair Study. Human Molecular Genetics: 8; 805–812, 1999.

Pierce K, Glad KS, Schreibman L: Social perception in children with autism: an attentional deficit? Journal of Autism and Developmental Disorders: 27(3); 265–82, 1997.

Piven J, Arndt S, Bailey J, Andreasen N: Regional brain enlargement in autism: a magnetic resonance imaging study. Journal of the American Academy of Child and Adolescent Psychiatry: 35(4); 530–536, 1996.

Piven J, Arndt S, Bailey J, Havercamp S, Andreasen N, Palmer P: An MRI study of brain size in autism. American Journal of Psychiatry: 152; 1145–1149, 1995.

Piven J, Bailey J, Ranson BJ, Arndt S: An MRI study of corpus callosum in autism. American Journal of Psychiatry: 154; 1051–1056, 1997.

Piven J, Bailey J, Ranson BJ, Arndt S: No difference in hippocampus volume detected on magnetic resonance imaging in autistic individuals. Journal of Autism and Developmental Disorders: 28(2); 105–110, 1998.

Piven J, Nehme E, Simon J, Barta P, Pearlson G, Folstein SE: Magnetic resonance imaging in autism: measurement of the cerebellum, pons, and fourth ventricle. Biological Psychiatry: 31(5); 491–504, 1992.

Posey DJ, McDougle CJ: The pharmacotherapy of target symptoms associated with autistic disorder and other pervasive developmental disorders. Harvard Review of Psychiatry: 8(2); 45–63, 2000.

Ring HA, Baron-Cohen S, Wheelwright S, Williams SC, Brammer M, Andrew C, Bullmore ET: Cerebral correlates of preserved cognitive skills in autism: a functional MRI study of embedded figures task performance. Brain: 122(Pt 7); 1305–1315, 1999.

Risch N, Spiker D, Lotspeich L, Nouri N, Hinds D, Hallmayer J et al.: A genomic screen in autism. American Journal of Human Genetics: 65; 493–507, 1999.

Robins D, Fein D, Barton M, Liss M: The Autism Screening Project: How early can autism be detected? Paper presented at the American Psychological Association Meeting, Boston, 1999.

Rodier PM, Ingram JL, Tisdale B, Croog VJ: Linking etiologies in humans and animal models: Studies of autism. Reproductive Toxicology: 11(2/3); 417–422, 1997.

Rogers SJ: Empirically supported comprehensive treatments for young children with autism. Journal of Clinical Child Psychology: 27(2); 168–179, 1998.

Rumsey JM, Hamburger SD: Neuropsychological findings in high-functioning men with infantile autism, residual state. Journal of Clinical and Experimental Neuropsychology: 10(2); 201–221, 1988.

Russell J, Jarrold C, Henry L: Working memory in children with autism and with moderate learning difficulties. Journal of Child Psychology and Psychiatry and Allied Disciplines: 37(6); 673–686, 1996.

Rutter M, Bailey A, Bolton P, Le Couteur A: Autism and known medical conditions: myth and substance. Journal of Child Psychology and Psychiatry and Allied Disciplines: 35(2); 311–322, 1994.

Saitoh O, Courchesne E, Egaas B, Lincoln AJ, Schreibman L: Cross-sectional area of the posterior hippocampus in autistic patients with cerebellar and corpus callosum abnormalities. Neurology: 45(f2); 317–324, 1995.

Saitoh O, Karns CM, Courchesne E: Development of the hippocampal formation from 2 to 42 years: MRI evidence of smaller area dentata in autism. Brain: 124(Pt 7); 1317–1324, 2001.

Schatz J, Hamdan-Allen G: Effects of age and IQ on adaptive behavior domains for children with autism. Journal of Autism and Developmental Disorders: 25(1); 51–60, 1995.

Schultz RT, Gauthier I, Klin A, Fulbright RK, Anderson AW, Volkmar F, Skudlarski P, Lacadie C, Cohen DJ, Gore JC: Abnormal ventral temporal cortical activity during face discrimination among individuals with autism and Asperger syndrome. Archives of General Psychiatry: 57(4); 331–340, 2000.

Siegel DJ, Minshew NJ, Goldstein G: Wechsler IQ profiles in diagnosis of high-functioning autism. Journal of Autism and Developmental Disorders: 26(4); 389–406, 1996.

Sparks BF, Friedman SD, Shaw DW, Aylward EH, Echelard D, Artru AA, Maravilla KR, Giedd JN, Munson J, Dawson G, Dager SR: Brain structural abnormalities in young children with autism spectrum disorder. Neurology: 59(2); 184–192, 2002.

Stevens MC, Fein DA, Dunn M, Allen D, Waterhouse LH, Feinstein C, Rapin I: Subgroups of children with autism by cluster analysis: A longitudinal examination. Journal of the American Academy of Child and Adolescent Psychiatry: 39(3); 346–352, 2000.

Sugiyama T, Abe T: The prevalence of autism in Nagoya, Japan: A total population study. Journal of Autism and Developmental Disorders: 19(1); 87–96, 1989.

Szatmari P, Jones MB, Zwaigenbaum L, MacLean JE: Genetics of autism: overview and new directions. Journal of Autism and Developmental Disorders: 28; 351–368, 1998.

Szatmari P, Tuff L, Finlayson MA, Bartolucci G: Asperger's syndrome and autism: Neurocognitive aspects. Journal of Autism and Developmental Disorders: 29; 130–136, 1990.

Tager-Flusberg H: Semantic processing in the free recall of autistic children: Further evidence of a cognitive deficit. In Dawson G (Ed), Autism: Nature, Diagnosis and Treatment. New York: Guilford Press, pp. 92–109, 1989.

Tanoue Y, Oda S, Asano F, Kawashima K: Epidemiology of infantile autism in southern Ibaraki, Japan: Differences in prevalence in birth cohorts: Journal of Autism and Developmental Disorders: 18(2); 155–166, 1988.

Tsai LY, Beisler JM: The development of sex differences in infantile autism. British Journal of Psychiatry: 142; 373–378, 1983.

Tsai L, Stewart MA, August G: Implication of sex differences in the familial transmission of infantile autism. Journal of Autism and Developmental Disorders: 11(2); 165–173, 1981.

Tuchman RF, Rapin I: Regression in pervasive developmental disorders: seizures and epileptiform electroencephalogram correlates. Pediatrics: 99(4); 560–566, 1997.

Tuchman RF, Rapin I, Shinnar S: Autistic and dysphasic children. II: Epilepsy. Pediatrics: 88(6); 1219–1225, 1991.

Van Engeland H: The electrodermal orienting response to auditive stimuli in autistic children, mentally retarded children, and child psychiatric patients. Journal of Autism and Developmental Disorders: 14; 261–279, 1984.

Venter A, Lord C, Schopler E: A follow-up study of high-functioning autistic children. Journal of Child Psychology and Psychiatry: 33: 489–507, 1992.

Volkmar F, Cook EH Jr, Pomeroy J, Realmuto G, Tanguay P: Practice parameters for the assessment and treatment of children, adolescents, and adults with autism and other pervasive developmental disorders. American Academy of Child and Adolescent Psychiatry Working Group on Quality Issues. Journal of the American Academy of Child and Adolescent Psychiatry: 38(12 Suppl); 32S–54S, 1999a.

Volkmar F, Cook E Jr, Pomeroy J, Realmuto G, Tanguay P: Summary of the practice parameters for the assessment and treatment of children, adolescents, and adults with autism and other pervasive developmental disorders. Journal of the American Academy of Child and Adolescent Psychiatry: 38(12); 1611–1616, 1999b.

Volkmar F, Nelson D: Seizure disorders in autism. Journal of the American Academy of Child and Adolescent Psychiatry: 29; 127–129, 1990.

Volkmar FR, Szatmari P, Sparrow SS: Sex differences in pervasive developmental disorders. Journal of Autism and Developmental Disorders: 23(4); 579–591, 1993.

Wainwright JA, Bryson SE: Visual–spatial orienting in autism. Journal of Autism and Developmental Disorders: 26(4); 423–38, 1996.

Wassink TH, Piven J, Vieland VJ et al.: Evidence supporting WNT2 as an Autism Susceptibility Gene. American Journal of Medical Genetics: 105; 406–413, 2001.

Webb EVJ, Lobo S, Hervas A, Scourfield J et al.: The changing prevalence of autistic disorder in a Welsh health district. Developmental Medicine and Child Neurology: 39(3); 150–157, 1996.

Werner E, Dawson G, Osterling J, Dinno N: Brief report: Recognition of autism spectrum disorder before one year of age: A retrospective study based on home videotapes. Journal of Autism and Developmental Disorders: 30(2); 157–167, 2000.

Wignyosumatro S, Mukhlas M, Hirataki S: Epidemiological and clinical study of autistic children in Yogyakarta, Indonesia. Kobe Journal of Medical Sciences: 38; 1–19, 1992.

Wing L: The definition and prevalence of autism: A review: European Child and Adolescent Psychiatry: 2(2); 61–74, 1993.

Wing L, Gould J: Severe impairments of social interaction and associated abnormalities in children: Epidemiology and classification. Journal of Autism and Developmental Disorders: 9(1); 11–29, 1979.

World Health Organization: The International Classification of Diseases, Mental and Behavioural Disorders — Clinical Descriptions and Diagnostic Guidelines. Geneva: WHO, 1992.

Zahn TP, Rumsey JM, Van Kammen DP: Autonomic nervous system activity in autistic, schizophrenic, and normal men: effects of stimulus significance. Journal of Abnormal Psychology: 96; 135–144, 1987.

Subject Index *

* Underlined page numbers indicate in-depth treatment.